Y0-CXJ-306

Understanding Abnormal Behavior

Understanding Abnormal Behavior

L. E. COLE

EMERITUS, OBERLIN COLLEGE

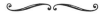 **CHANDLER PUBLISHING COMPANY**
An Intext Publisher • Scranton, Pennsylvania 18515

COPYRIGHT © 1970 BY CHANDLER PUBLISHING COMPANY
ALL RIGHTS RESERVED
STANDARD BOOK NO. 8102-0005-8
LIBRARY OF CONGRESS CATALOG CARD NO. 68-12429
PRINTED IN THE UNITED STATES OF AMERICA

Book designed by Joseph M. Roter

To James and Marie

CONTENTS

PREFACE

It was more than ten years ago that I set myself the task of translating Pierre Janet's *De l'angoisse à l'extase*. The task led to my discovery of how great a gap existed in the English-language accounts of abnormality and to my ambition to present some of Janet's views to American students. The rise of psychoanalysis and of behavioristic theories had eclipsed the work of this successor of Charcot as the dean of French psychiatrists.

The effort to place Janet's views in a modern setting has led me to an eclectic approach to the study of abnormal behavior and to a review of the major influences in the psychiatry and psychology of the past eighty years. I have tried to be critical without being dogmatic and to search for whatever would help in shaping a more adequate psychology for our time. Advances in genetics, in social psychology and anthropology, in neurology and physiology have forced me to broaden my studies almost beyond the scope of those limits which had to be observed if a useful text was to emerge.

In recent decades awareness of the light thrown on the human condition by abnormal forms of behavior make this type of study imperative for everyone whose ambition is to deal with other human beings, whether as administrator, therapist, or theorist. The pitfalls that lie in wait for those who have not appreciated the complexity of psychological problems, and who have too-ready answers, call for a disciplined study—a process that is bound to teach us humility and to motivate further inquiry.

In addition to saluting Pierre Janet, whose writings gave me the initial inspiration for this book, I should like to make special acknowledgement of the encouragement given by Theodore Sarbin and Leslie Rabkin in the days when the manuscript was taking shape.

Chapel Hill
November 1, 1968

L. E. C.

Understanding Abnormal Behavior

Chapter 1 • Concepts of Abnormality

Four main issues are raised in this introductory chapter. The first one, "Who are the abnormal?" has one easy answer and several difficult or partial ones. The head count of the census taker is the simplest of all: these persons either are under custodial care or are now seeking treatment for their symptoms. We do not have to raise any questions about the precise nature of abnormality: the courts and the experts have decided. We are certain, however, that there are others among us, outside of institutions and all outpatient rolls, who have similar symptoms, and some of whom are equally ill, but for one reason or another are getting no treatment. Attempts to project estimates of abnormality within the general population have been made, and they have raised questions about the precise meaning of the term. Samples of "abnormally normal" populations have been studied; spot surveys have covered representative urban and rural populations. These surveys have called for methods of testing, examining, and evaluating data that are still much in need of improvement, and have also shown that normal-abnormal discrimination is not an all-or-none affair. Even the normal have symptoms similar to those found among the hospitalized. When abnormality is viewed as a social question, we are forced to seek a sociological definition of it as well as individual biological and psychological ones: a medical certificate is not a completely satisfactory label.

Another approach to our first issue proposes a culture-relative definition. The work of clinic and court is already hampered by confusions in this area. Even the church leaders, as perplexed arbiters of values, have felt called upon to make some discriminations in borderline areas. One mass delusion that brought tragedy to thousands of persons will illustrate the tragic consequences that follow a false cultural consensus. And, as a corollary to the generalizations that arise from the facts about witchcraft, we are forced to confront the possibility that even the normal may have delusions.

The second issue arises as soon as we attempt to identify and classify the abnormal ones by some criterion for each category that we make tends to imply a theory of causation and to define the types of effort that we must make if we

1

are to cope with the problem. We need to be alerted to the implications of our categories: seven views of abnormality are examined.

The third issue is prompted by our ambivalence about the term *freedom.* We like to be free agents; we relish liberty and we are inclined to treat our fellow citizens as responsible agents, blaming them for their errors. Yet at the same time we accept the notion that all behavior is caused. Our dilemma is sharpened as we consider the varieties of determination and attempt to assess our degrees of freedom, which seem to vary from one individual to another. And we have to face the practical question about when it is useful to assume that the person with symptoms (or behavioral deviations) should be encouraged to accept full responsibility for them and when we should accept him as the helpless product of forces and agencies over which he has no control.

Finally, our introductory survey leads us to examine the "metapsychology" that forms the assumed basis of our own beliefs and practices. Doing so will force us to clarify the foundations of that psychology which underlies our concept of the normal and our procedures for dealing with the abnormal. The study of the abnormal can thus provide a pathway to self-knowledge, and even to a clarification of the nature of the scientific quest itself.

WHO ARE THE ABNORMAL?

A preliminary answer to our first question can be found in the reports of the National Institute of Mental Health. Excluding the mentally retarded, there are approximately 800,000 persons now in mental hospitals or under treatment in psychiatric outpatient clinics in the United States. These are minimal figures: those who are hospitalized are so ill that they are regarded as (1) a threat to those around them, (2) in danger of harming themselves seriously, e.g., by committing suicide, (3) incapable of managing their own affairs, as in senile dementia, (4) too great a burden for the family, or (5) in need of special kinds of professional care that the family cannot provide. For the most part the outpatients who visit psychiatric clinics (and some 200,000 of these are reported in addition to those who visit clinics managed by the Veterans Administration) do so under their own power, either because they are unable to work at an effective level, or are disturbed by their symptoms, or are unable to manage their habits (e.g., alcoholism).[1] In spite of their impairment, this second group is able to carry on outside of the hospital. In recent decades, as clinical facilities have developed and a public awareness of the nature of mental illness has spread, the size of this outpatient group has increased.

These minimal figures give a kind of public audit of our mental health. Other methods of assessment show that they must be expanded to cover borderland

---

[1]In addition, there are many among the patients who visit the general practitioner for what they believe to be bodily illnesses. Underlying these complaints, and intermingled with their physical symptoms as causes or sequelae, are psychological components. Some students of psychosomatic medicine estimate that this admixture occurs in half or two-thirds of the cases visiting the general practitioner (see Chapter 7).

cases that are not now identified on this public roll. The study of the army draft population in World Wars I and II suggest that at least an equal number should be added to our totals, and that illnesses as grave as those now hospitalized have escaped identification and treatment (Landis and Page 1938, p. 25).[2] During World War II, when the psychiatric examinations, though improved, were still minimal, the figures show that one in six of this youthful age group were either rejected at their induction examination or subsequently discharged from the service for neuropsychiatric reasons.[3] It should be emphasized that the "unfit for military service" criterion was not severe, the psychiatric and psychological assessment not searching.

An additional expansion of our figures will be required if we are interested in the "lifetime incidence" of serious abnormalities in addition to the incidence found in a single age group sampled at one limited period. When New York and Massachusetts were reporting that between one and two in every 100 persons over age 20 were incapacitated by mental illness *at any one time,* their lifetime rates showed that at least one person out of every 20 would become a mental-hospital patient at some time during his life (Landis and Page 1938, p. 24). Combining these figures with their educated guess that less than half of the mentally ill are hospitalized, Landis and Page offered one in ten as being the most likely probability that a person would have a serious and incapacitating mental illness *at some time in his life.*

Still one more expansion of the figures would have to be made if, instead of waiting for a major mental problem to develop to the point where it would warrant hospitalization or professional attention, a medical team could interview and examine a reasonably large and representative sample of our population. We might then discover the extent of all degrees of abnormality that exist *as of now.* Such a thorough survey has so far not proved practicable, although several rough approximations have been made. One of these, called the Midtown Manhattan Study (Srole *et al.* 1962), reported figures based upon extensive interviews of some 1,700 respondents, chosen so that the sample was as representative as possible, but only for ages 20 to 59. Interview data contained answers to questions that probed for symptoms that had been found to occur frequently among the mentally ill, both in the hospital and during outpatient treatment. Although these interviews were rather intensive and ran to more than an hour's length, they did have to depend upon the memory of the respondent,[4] his willingness or capacity to furnish accurate answers, the skill (and possibly the bias) of the investigator, and the as yet uncertain validity

---

[2]For full citations, see the Bibliography at the end of this book.

[3]The one-in-six ratio is the more striking when we discover that as older age groups are examined, a sharp rise in the rates of mental illness begins in the period between 40 and 50.

[4]For example, the memory of patients for recent symptoms or past illnesses is notoriously faulty. Their description of their performance fluctuates with their mood. And there are many symptoms which they cannot report, such as an abnormal electroencephalogram, or ulceration of the intestinal wall, or high blood pressure, or their physiological reactions to effort.

of the method. The results cannot be considered equivalent to the data that would have emerged from an equal number of complete clinical (and experimental) examinations of the patients. Nonetheless, the expert clinicians among the investigators were willing to estimate that abnormal symptoms were reported by at least one-fourth of the respondents in such saturation as to indicate impairment that would warrant professional assistance. Their reported symptoms would have placed them among the groups now treated by hospitals or outpatient services. And of the total group examined, less than a fifth were estimated as free from any degree of impairment.

Thus, beginning with the kind of symptoms which are being treated in our mental hospitals and outpatient clinics, we have had to expand the group who are abnormal by our public-accounting criterion until we have found one in four seriously impaired and a total of 80 per cent with some degree of impairment of the same type. Thus, if we define the abnormal personality as "the person with symptoms," we have caught four out of five of us in our conceptual net.

Perhaps less than 3 per cent of our population is at this moment so ill as to seriously need professional care. The one-in-four figure that emerges from the Midtown Manhattan Study may represent professional enthusiasm; yet if one holds a high ideal for mental health and is very optimistic about our ability to make it available (and attainable) for all, the figure is probably too low. From the seriously ill core group to a fringe where the symptoms are only mildly or occasionally incapacitating, and of the type that a confident and independent person would want to handle himself, any "abnormality scale" that we might construct would show such steadily varying saturations of disabilities, from category to category, that the borderlines would have to be arbitrary points, like those we use in separating intelligence quotients.

We would find not only many shades of gray, instead of clearly defined black and white areas, but also, when we turn to an intensive study of individuals, that the man whom an interviewer might describe as symptom-free today will turn up among those hospitalized tomorrow. Or, today a patient may strike his family as merely lazy or apathetic, and lacking in motivation, as he complains of emptiness, boredom, or a mild chronic anxiety. At worst his family might see him as hypochondriacal, or neurotic, or a weak character. Two years later, when a schizophrenic process has developed unmistakable symptoms, he will have to be hospitalized for psychosis. Or again, a teenager who is a dropout, who seems to be full of inner conflicts and involved in an identity crisis, will tomorrow begin a course in rehabilitation, and shortly thereafter appear to be well-launched upon a professional career. Thus we need to note that the label "abnormal personality" should not be applied as though the person were a fixed and self-consistent thing. An individual can move into and out of disease categories, up and down the scale of abnormality.

And while we have been seeking our easiest answer to the question "Who is abnormal?" we have raised no questions about our criterion. We have assumed the existence of an expert body of evaluators, whose business it is to know which symptoms are danger signs and which fall within the range we would want to call normal.[5]

THE ABNORMALLY "NORMAL"

When we shift our attention to that symptom-free fifth who are found to be most normal according to interviewing methods of the type just referred to or by self-ratings on questionnaires designed to reveal those abnormal traits that are counted as liabilities, we find them to be stable, responsible, and contented individuals. In addition to being symptom-free, they are so well-adjusted and so blandly contented that their interviewers judged them to be "uninteresting." Golden, Glueck, and Feder (1962) describe one such group of "normals" as not only well-adjusted but lacking in aspiration:

"The major focus of interest of the subjects appears to be in the home. Those who were married expressed a high order of contentment with their wives and children. There were no separations or broken marriages; with one outstanding exception, the men tended to idealize their wives and the wives were, again with one exception, content with their husbands as stable, responsible, dependable, supportive individuals. . . . These men were found to have little imagination, and generally limited interests and social activities. They indicate limited educational and vocational aspirations for themselves, and also for their children."

A comparable group of male undergraduates was studied by Grinker and Grinker. They were found in a college that trains potential YMCA secretaries. Using a variety of screening devices (a series of tests and extended clinical interviews), these investigators also eliminated all subjects with symptoms, ending up with a "mentally healthy" group. A few in this residual group, when studied intensively, proved to have minor conflicts, slightly exaggerated suspicions, occasional compulsive actions, but there were no crippling disabilities and no handicapping traits. Instead, one of the authors noted (p. 445) that:

". . . the average subject can work well on his job, and with the usual American student's procrastination and rapid cramming, passes his school examination and graduates with a C average. He plays well and with satisfactions. He copes adequately with stimuli that arouse emotional reactions. There is adequate adjustment to reality. The subject has a firm sense of identity; he feels good and has hope for the future. Also, he has had warm human relationships with parents, teachers, friends, and girls.

"Within the general population of the United States, this group is relatively silent. Its members are goal-directed, anxious only in striving to do their jobs well,

---

[5]Such a clinician would have to be clear about the difference between neurotic guilt and real guilt, between an exaggerated reaction to interpersonal pressures and a "normal" one, between a reasonable shyness and a schizoid withdrawal, between a healthy jubilation and a manic excitement, and so on. And we might want to press him, one day, to give us a more than negative answer to the question of normality. Is the goal of his therapy merely to rid the person of incapacitating symptoms and to strengthen his integrative forces so that these negative signs do not reappear? Is the "normal" man merely one who has no more than the statistically common load of anxiety and quiet desperation? Or is the clinician's work carried on with one eye upon some ideal of health and full productivity that he is almost embarrassed to state? (See the discussion of this ideal of mental health in Grinker and Grinker 1962.)

in which they will have moved up from their fathers' positions, but with little ambition for upward social or economic mobility. By the nature of their aspirations to do well, to do good, and to be liked, they plan to carry on their lives quietly, in simple comfort, marry and raise their families, and retire on small pensions plus social security. The psychiatrist does not often see this population of *homoclites*, and, should he chance to come in contact with them, he will be as surprised as I was."

These recent studies are interesting for several reasons. For one thing, they reveal the startling impact that interviews with this type of subject made upon the psychiatrists, who had developed a kind of inner standard, or set of expectations, from interviews with clients who have had difficulties in their marriages, who cause difficulties for the school authorities, whose alcoholism and absenteeism make them poor employees, who have fallen afoul of the law because of sexual deviations that violate public decency or threaten the immature, or who bring crippling disabilities to a specialist for help because they feel helpless, overwhelmed by something they cannot deal with. They had developed a "science of the abnormal" suitable for the maladjusted, the self-destructive, the incapacitated, who had somehow failed to measure up to the social tasks and opportunities confronting them. It was a shock to meet those who had no need for their services. "Here was a type that I had not met before in my role as a psychiatrist and rarely in my personal life," the senior author of the second study confessed as he reported his results to a professional group; and one of his fellow practitioners was moved by his summary to observe, "These boys are really sick; they have no ambition."[6]

Both of these studies point to a mixture of contentment and very modest ambitions. These "normals" are not infected with that peculiar American virus called "status seeking." They are not torn by inner torment nor filled with messianic dreams, nor does their imagination generate discontent with their life. If one considers the men who have made the deepest impact upon our culture in science, the fine arts, politics, their journals and biographies reveal them to be full of symptoms, discontent, self-doubt, pathological anxieties, periods of depression, genuine "deviations." Van Gogh, André Gide, Cardinal Newman,

---

⁶The avant-garde groups would call them "squares," without imagination. Social reformers and protesters would count them criminally complacent. The soul-searching devout person would find them as complacent as Kierkegaard found the Copenhagen bishops. And all of the discontented would see them as horribly content with a life that is indescribably dull. The professional who is prepared to deal with "persons with problems" finds the simply uninteresting. These possibilities warn us that when various groups serve on a panel to discuss the objectives of psychotherapy, along with the meaning of that kind of normality which one would count the best of all possible adjustments, we should be prepared for expressions of divergent values. Freud felt that when he had freed the individual of his symptoms, given him some notion of their origin and some way of warding off their return, he could terminate the therapeutic relationship: the patient could be released when he had no more severe anxieties, or symptoms, than the average man carries. Even so, his conception of "insight" required a self-knowledge that was both complex and highly specialized. To deal with all that hampers the best which is within us is something that, in all modesty, the working counselor would have to decline to undertake. This does not mean that none of his clients will ask him to do just this.

Willard Gibbs, to pick a random handful, offer much more to interest a clinician; and if we could add Strindberg, Mary Baker Eddy, Joseph Smith, Henry James, Virginia Woolf, and one or two others, we could find representatives of all the major forms of mental illness within this group of talented artists, scientists, and religious leaders.[7]

Placed at a moment in history when men are caught up in great conflicts, possessing unusual susceptibilities, developing a life plan that carries them into stress, these men of "genius with symptoms" were made strong and creative. As a childhood disease can leave antibodies that provide greater resistance to disease, the very causes that create symptoms can also make adults tolerant of stresses, creative in the midst of conflict, interesting and self-actualizing in spite of the overhead of symptoms.

The creative labors of these men of genius are to be contrasted with the simple recipes used by the normals studied by the Grinkers. When these students felt depressed or in conflict with their surroundings or themselves, they took a nap, had a good workout in the gym, went out for the evening. They threw off their difficulties with such ease that the professionals who interviewed them must have found them "disgustingly healthy." And sometimes such a professional will suspect that these adjusted ones have deeper problems, problems that would require a great deal of probing, since they have repressed them so well.[8]

Perhaps, too, we should remind ourselves of the tenuous nature of our normal "future-making" actions. We need constantly to correct our orientations and revise our plans. The delicacy of this process is revealed in the experiments on sensory deprivation reported in Chapter 8. In these it has been discovered that a mere separation from the orienting cues of our environment (through severe reduction of sensory input) produces confusion about the boundary that separates dream from reality; hynagogic images form and take on a "too real" quality. Behavioral fields, which are in essence organized postures of expectancy, are never absolutely accurate. At their fringes there is always a "beyond" which is not well-structured but which seems to penetrate the "real." Our well-structured consciousness seems to float on a billowy deep; in the depths are the cellular and biochemical processes beneath our ken, old and forgotten (or

---

[7]Some of the symptoms appearing in these lives were a kind of psychological overhead. The great achievements were made in spite of their disabilities, not because of them. Often the pressures that they suffered from were created by these men of genius themselves, as when they reacted against what they felt to be injustice, oppression, or corruption (consider Zola's *J'accuse*). Sometimes their "problems" arose from an unusual susceptibility and intelligence and from that lack of fit so often noted between the genius and his times. Occasionally, as with Nietzsche and Strindberg, their illnesses brought their productive period to a close so gradually that one is at a loss to point out the moment when their creative imagination ceased and illness began, so inextricably intertwined were the two.

[8]Like Kierkegaard's bishops of Copenhagen who *know* that they are Christians and whom he therefore viewed as being in the gravest danger, the normals of these psychiatric investigations are suspected of having repressed the awareness of things they need to face. Their "unawareness of problems" is abnormal.

repressed) action sequences, infantile imaginings, and, a Jungian would add, archetypes from a racial unconscious. It was Freud's view of dreams as the key to the unconscious that led him, at the end of his life, to judge his *Interpretation of Dreams* as his most substantial claim to fame as a scientist. The point which James, Janet, Freud, Jung, and a host of others wanted to emphasize is a simple one: these subconscious or extraconscious processes affect our action-structuring, our central behavioral field that we call conscious.

A Sociological Definition

In an effort to be as matter of fact as possible and to suggest definitions that would be useful in research, Eaton once identified five concepts of abnormality. "This action is abnormal" might refer to (1) a clinical judgment by the experts, (2) a self-judgment by an individual who believes that he is different from his fellows, (3) a group judgment, such as that of the judge who acts as an agent for society and its laws when he has to pronounce upon homosexuality, obscenity, or some violation of what is counted common sense or decency, (4) any action that lies outside an operationally defined and objectively measurable zone that a society agrees upon as the average, or (5) a measurable departure from a typological ideal that best represents the aspirations of some culture or subculture (Eaton and Weil 1955, pp. 17-26; see also Hollingshead and Redlich 1952, and Grinker and Grinker 1962).

It is clear that different research tools would be needed to deal with each of these varieties of "abnormal," that both the amount and the distribution of abnormalities would vary, and that some identifying subscript will have to be used whenever the term is employed. Each definition has its shortcomings and raises special problems for the research worker, and in spite of all the effort to make the definitions objective, each will be found to conceal value judgments. This is also true of the definition used by the clinician who tries to state his task in terms of relationships that center in the individual he is treating. For example, we could describe the abnormal person as one who (1) does not produce harmonious relationships with others, (2) cannot achieve a satisfactory synthesis of his conflicting drives, (3) cannot perceive himself and the surrounding world correctly, or (4) is unable to work toward and adjust to constructive changes in the physical and social environment. So many disturbing questions are prompted the moment one announces that this quartet of goals is precisely what our society expects of a man that, like the golden apple, it becomes a source of contention. (Harmonize with John Birchers? Synthesize slavery and gracious living? Accept whose definition of reality? Admit that *their* reforms are constructive?)

Any method of classifying abnormalities according to the current working model of the science is also a social product that will have to be changed as the categories of science change. Once we grouped our abnormalities according to the major faculties affected, and we could speak of affective disorders, intellectual disorders, or defects in willing (e.g., see Ribot 1914). As our notions of behavior change, we can expect each new system maker to produce a new classification of abnormalities that will emphasize his new insight. In a science like psychology, which is not only a recent arrival on the field but still badly split into "schools," the classifications (and consequent clinical and experimental studies) of one group will seem wholly inadequate to rival theorists. While the Pavlovian is highlighting the differences between men that alter the course of conditioning and extinction, a psychoanalyst will want to focus upon the process of repression and upon that splitting of the mind into conscious and unconscious portions, or will direct his questions toward revealing the relationships between ego, superego, and id (entities which the behaviorist might disregard altogether). In short, the classifications of mental illnesses will reveal a theorist's predilection and the state of his science.

Pierre Janet once told the story of a letter he had received from the physiologist and physician, Grasset of Montpelier. The latter announced his intention of reforming the classification of nervous and mental illnesses. The new classification needed to be based upon psychology, of that he was certain. But, lacking a first-hand knowledge of the latest clinical and experimental work, he felt that Janet might supply him with a simple statement that would enumerate the psychological functions. It would not take more than a page or two. "Give me a list of these functions and my work will be simplified. I can then take up each function, and describe the various ways in which it is disturbed (through hypertrophy or deficiency), and the work will soon be accomplished" (Janet 1932, p. 301).

We know, now, that there is no such list, certainly not one that can be regarded as basic, or final, in a science that is developing and changing its categories as it develops. The functional disorders that Grasset wanted to classify do not walk into the clinic, with one patient suffering from a memory defect and another person with sensory disturbances (anesthesias) and a third person with a defect in willing. Instead of such distinct and easy-to-identify disorders, patients bring clusters of symptoms. Even when we call them syndromes, or clinical pictures, we imply a greater constancy than actually exists, for the contents of these clusters are varied enough to give rise to disputes among clinicians: a psychopath may have schizophrenic features, schizophrenics may have manic-depressive features, and manics may have schizophrenic features. In short, the illnesses which exist often show a lack of respect for our categories. And there is often some friction between the clinician, who is interested in the person bearing the symptoms, and that statistician at the state office of mental hygiene who must keep an orderly account of the numbers of patients treated in each disease category.

The Clinic, the Courts, and the Church

Without belaboring each of the points we have raised in opening the discussion of a sociological approach to the problem, we can illustrate by an example one of the difficulties that have to be faced. Whether it is a question of the opinions of the experts, or of the categories and data of the science of our times, or of that central social consensus that produces a statistical norm, it soon becomes apparent that we are dealing with a changing scene, with shifting norms, and with conflicting opinions, not with a single and self-consistent harmonious whole. Consider the current discussions of homosexuality.

Statistically the homosexuals are deviates, a minority of "different" ones, and as long as new generations are born out of heterosexual unions, they will continue to make up a fringe group, whose members will necessarily be children of heterosexuals. Beyond this inevitable fact, the majority in our society look upon the homosexual with a certain revulsion, and see his attachments as a kind of unpleasant caricature of love. We have even constructed out of the voice and gestures of the male stereotype (which is not an accurate image of the male homosexual) a figure of fun, suitable for broad farce.[9]

The courts have taken the matter seriously: the homosexual's acts are viewed as criminal, and as against nature. Convicted, he is severely punished. In England and in various states of the union, commissions have been appointed to study both the offenses and the laws, and from these studies proposals for new and more temperate legislation have emerged. Although the "principle of unripe time" has operated to reject most of these proposals, the adoption of the central recommendation of the Wolfenden Committee into British law suggests that it may not be very long before there is public recognition of our changed attitudes.[10]

While the legal battle was shaping up and before any changes in legislation had been made, an international conference of writers was held in Edinburgh (1962). In the course of one of the meetings, a participant introduced his remarks with the blunt statement, "I am a homosexual." And he proceeded not only to defend his right to be one but to speak for his special capacity to write of love. He was immediately challenged; and the discussions which followed in the succeeding hours of the conference became so heated that it seemed at

---

[9]The committee that prepared a report on homosexual offenses for the British Parliament (known as the Wolfenden Report) censured these attitudes. Admitting the prevalence of the problem, the committee added that many believe "conduct of this kind is a cause of the demoralisation and decay of civilisations, and that therefore, unless we wish to see our nation degenerate and decay, such conduct must be stopped, by every possible means. We have found no evidence to support this view, and we cannot feel it right to frame the laws which should govern this country in the present age by reference to hypothetical explanations of the history of other peoples in ages distant in time and different in circumstances from our own. Insofar as the basis of this argument can be precisely formulated, it is often no more than the expression of revulsion against what is regarded as unnatural, sinful, or disgusting. Many people feel this revulsion, for one or more of these reasons. But moral conviction or instinctive feeling, however strong, is not a valid basis for overriding the individual's privacy and for bringing within the ambit of the criminal law private sexual behavior of this kind (Wolfenden Report, p. 22).

[10]The committee recommended, among other things, that actions between consenting adults in private should no longer be subject to criminal prosecution, that *adult* be defined as "aged 21 years," and that the words "consent" and "in private" be interpreted by the courts according to the same criteria governing heterosexual acts between adults. Recognizing the winds of change and the need for expert knowledge, the Wolfenden Committee urged that "research be instituted into the etiology of homosexuality and the effects of various forms of treatment" (*ibid.*, para. 355).

one point that the conference was going to have to go on record as supporting or condemning homosexuality by vote. (For an account of the meeting, see Condee 1962, or *Times Lit. Supp.,* Aug. 31, 1962.)

And while these discussions were going on in Edinburgh, whose Presbyterian editors studiously avoided such subject matter, a committee of Quakers was preparing a report dealing with the church's responsibility in shaping the sexual attitudes of its members, and in particular of its youth. This report urged, among other things, that "it is the nature and quality of a relationship that matters: one must not judge it by its outward appearance but by its inner worth. Homosexual affection can be as selfless as heterosexual affection, and therefore we cannot see that it is in some way morally worse" (Heron 1963).

The secular experts, the courts, the elected representatives of the voters, the ecclesiastical authorities, the playwrights and the novelists who give us emotionally charged images of reality, and, finally, the general public—all become involved in establishing the criteria that determine what is abnormal. Arriving at their convictions at different rates and for most divergent reasons, this confusing array of persons with opinions forms the milieu in which the odd one must develop. Such a deviant as the homosexual, who in the nature of things must internalize and suffer from some of the heated confusion in our society, might read an account of the *berdache* with a certain wistfulness. Described by Ruth Benedict in her *Patterns of Culture* (pp. 243 ff), this role devised by the Plains Indians for the deviant males spares the odd one from inner conflict and stress and from the blackmailer, the gossips, and the officers of the court that trouble him in our society.

Thus, our illustration shows us that a sociological view of the abnormal personality leads directly to these critical evaluations of our criteria:

1. A deviant is not a simple entity, an isolated monad determined by inner mechanisms, a biological sport, or a disease.

2. As a member of society he gains from internalizing his portion of the social surplus and at the same time suffers from the social values which mark him as a guilty deviant.

3. Living within a changing matrix, he internalizes his society's conflicts and confusions, and some of his symptoms may be traceable to the relationship between his own deviating life style and the mores which punish what, in some measure, they produce.

4. A scientist, who, by training and preference, would study individual life-histories, genetic endowments, and personal experiences, neglects at his peril the matrix within which human development must take place.[11]

---

[11]As Benedict points out (p. 245), "When the homosexual response is regarded as a perversion . . . the invert is immediately exposed to all the conflicts to which aberrants are always exposed. His guilt, his sense of inadequacy, his failures, are consequences of the disrepute which social tradition visits upon him; and few people can achieve a satisfactory life unsupported by the standards of the society. The adjustments that society demands of them would strain any man's vitality, and the consequences of this conflict we identify with their homosexuality."

The Belief in Witchcraft

There was a time, in our own past, when witches existed. Not only in the popular imagination, but in the statutes which defined the witch's crimes for judges and prosecutors who sentenced these poor creatures to torture, burning, hanging, the witch belief became a substantial thing. And the public spectacles afforded by the trials and the tortures burned the witch concept into the popular memory, validating the belief by the horrible sanctions. As though to clinch the issue and remove all doubt, some of the witches confessed to abominable crimes: they had made pacts with demons, flown through the air to conclaves, devoured human flesh, drunk the blood of infants, made men impotent and wives barren, caused cattle to die and crops to fail.

Freely circulating as believed-in realities, the tortures, the confessions, as well as strange happenings, made the witch concept a potent force that produced new victims. Men and women could feel themselves bewitched. In turn the belief furnished the form in which all manner of vaguely apprehended anxieties could find a clearly channeled expression: a wide variety of misfortunes as well as free-floating anxieties were laid at the doors of these agents of the Evil One. The highest ecclesiastical authorities felt that their powers were being threatened; and inquisitors and witch-finders were dispatched to seek out these offenders and to hear the complaints of those who suffered from their work. The manuals which the authorities designed as guides for the witch-finders can now be looked upon as curious precursors of our manuals of psychiatry that guide the young intern in his practice today, for they were full of specific advice on how to identify the witch; the diagnostic signs were so accurately described that some modern clinicians believe they can identify the illness from which these odd ones suffered.[12]

Zilboorg, as a medical historian, and Parrinder, as an anthropologist reporting on contemporary witchcraft in Africa, describe the victims of this massive social fantasy; and there is a strange contrast between the helplessness of most of these unhappy persons and the supposed evil powers they were supposed to possess. Most of them were defenseless women, old, odd, ill. For the most part they were poor, and sometimes their reported behavior, seen today, would be counted as evidence of hysteria, schizophrenia, depression, obsession. That their accusers were frequently relatives may indicate they were also a burden to their families.

Accusations of witchcraft were also leveled against troublesome heretics, such as the Cathars ("the pure ones"), who were a threat to the ecclesiastical and

---

[12]The presence of anesthetic areas on the skin was one of these signs, a fact which has persuaded some medical historians to look upon these victims as hystericals. The older women who freely confessed to all manner of evil doings were also full of guilt, much as in the cases of depression seen in the modern clinics, for the latter also feel to blame for all manner of misfortunes that had befallen their family. The witch category was a broad one, and it undoubtedly covered a wide range of types that would be allocated to many different categories in the modern clinician's classification system. And there may have also been many that would today be counted normal: occasionally the property they possessed motivated the judge, for the witch's belongings were confiscated. In a few instances there were undoubtedly political reasons behind the accusation.

civil authorities. The witch concept thus managed to fuse concerns about evil influences, subversion, heresy, and all manner of disasters; and the sanctions imposed by the highest authorities were so severe that some may have confessed in the hope of escaping the tortures.[13]

The social historian is tempted to see such a witch concept, embedded as it is in the network of practices and beliefs of a people, as actually *pathogenic,* that is, as *producing* the very abnormalities that the witch-doctor or the ecclesiastical courts investigate and exterminate. And the social psychologist, viewing the spectacles in which torture and confession give public proof of the guilt of the witch, is apt to underscore the way in which a belief that is transformed into such practices can serve to validate error. Succeeding generations transmit the pattern; it becomes codified; a permanent body of "truth" is established.

In the contexts in which this strange body of truth operated, there were undoubtedly many factors at work outside of the conscious formulations which men made of these events. Even the historian and anthropologist who select what they believe to be the significant and relevant facts to record have their peculiar preoccupations. Evans-Pritchard, for example, is moved to emphasize that witchcraft is an *imaginary offense,* that it does not exist now, and never did. If one adds that "the fear of witchcraft and the measures taken to counteract its powers must be symbolic," then the door is opened to all manner of sociological analogies. It is a symbol of the position of women in primitive society. It is one more bit of evidence of the male's fear of the female. It is a symbol of the fact that the healer's power is based upon the collective. It symbolizes something that still exists, even when we believe that we have banished it by the disciplines and the knowledge that have been ushered in with modern science and technology.

Using moderate restraint, therefore, can we be reasonably certain that witchcraft's history warrants a few generalizations? For example:

1. The content of abnormal preoccupations, delusions, may be drawn from a body of ideas that circulates among the normal without creating marked disturbance in them. It seems reasonable to hesitate to call these ideas pathogenic when the stolid citizens do not use them in a pathological way. Other more susceptible ones become overwrought, possessed; in these the idea is "made flesh" and carried to a pathological extreme.

2. It is clear that concepts such as the witch belief can and do interfere with proper diagnosis and treatment of the abnormal. Nonetheless, by their use, cures have also been produced, and these too can validate error. An easygoing pragmatism is a poor test for the validity of a theory. In our own society we have been slow in applying adequate measures to our efforts at therapy; and

---

[13]Zilboorg's account (1941) of the church's role in prosecuting witches discusses the history of this mass delusion from 1500 to 1800. Parrinder (1963, p. 21) notes that the Cathars were accused of flying to their meetings on broomsticks anointed with oil, and of drinking potions made from the bodies of captured children. With such a belief to justify it, "scapegoating" could find its easy targets in any hated or feared person. For discussions of what may be parallel phenomena in African cultures, see Parrinder 1963, Evans-Pritchard 1937, and Field 1937, 1955, and 1958.

as a result rival and contradictory views claim equal authority. Unable to discriminate in some of our internal quarrels, we obviously cannot compare modern methods with the ones used by the witch-doctor of Ghana. From our present knowledge one might guess that the hystericals among those who seek the help of the witch-doctor would show the highest percentages of cures, that the psychotics would be less susceptible to their rituals. But although this would hold true for our own cases, we do not possess the proper diagnosis of the bewitched of Ghana to make the required projection. What happens when the peculiar behavior of the senile dement carries him to the witch-doctor we do not know, though we can make an educated guess.

3. The specialist (whether he is psychiatrist, witch-finder, or member of the ecclesiastical court) can serve a wide variety of aims other than those which he avows: ecclesiastical, moral, political, personal. Taking the Hippocratic oath, reading the reports of the ethical-standards committee of the American Psychological Association, undergoing the discipline that makes a young man of Ghana into a witch-doctor, do not guarantee that agreed-upon aims will be pursued in practice. Even the concept of mental illness which we have developed in Western nations can be used to absolve an individual from social responsibility, to break a marriage, to imprison a man guilty of subversive activities, and for many other extraneous purposes.[14]

4. As we follow the history of our notions of the abnormal, we can see that the delusions of the patient have sometimes been matched by the delusions of his judges and of the experts. They are often shared by the entire society whom these "professionals" serve. The case of witchcraft warns us that, even while we are examining the empirical data, we also need to be sharply critical of the categories that have guided the collection of facts, categories which rest upon mass beliefs often uncritically held. And we have to entertain the possibility that some of the data may have been produced by the theories developed to explain deviant behavior.

Delusions of the Normal

There is an additional aspect to the discussion of the witch concept worth a moment of reflection. If we use the term *delusion* to designate a well-organized belief in something that *objectively* may not exist, we might conclude that the jurists and theologians, as well as the rank and file of European society in the years between 1250 and 1800, were deluded. For every witch who confessed, and for every one who anxiously sought help from some witch-doctor, there were thousands in the surrounding society, including even the best-informed

---

[14]Consider, for example the case made by Valeriy Tarsis (1965), who describes a special ward that is set aside in a mental hospital to imprison those suspected by Moscow of subversion.

An American psychiatrist, Thomas Szasz, has made a valiant effort to correct what he believes are abuses of psychiatric authority. He sees that what are basically "problems in living" are often converted into "mental disorders"; and he charges that patients are often confined to mental hospital on a trumped-up diagnosis for reasons entirely unrelated to their mental health. The vigor of his attack has been matched by that of the profession's counterattack; and the controversy aroused underscores the fact that a passionate personal involvement can overwhelm and distort what the clinic requires, namely, patient, critical, and experimental work required to validate our theories and procedures. See Szasz 1961 and 1964, and Davidson 1964.

minds, ready to nod in understanding, adding their consensual validation to the beliefs of these sensitives even as they were drawing from the latter's existence, and confessions, the facts to validate their own delusions.[15]

Witch and witch-finder, populace and its victims, formed an interlocking system. At this comfortable and secure distance we are inclined to call the witch hysterical (or obsessed, or schizophrenic). We might also consider the diagnosis for the witch-finder, so obsessed with ferreting out the evidence of an old crone's witchery, searching for anesthetic areas in her private parts. Taken together, these doctors and their patients enacted a weird and ghastly scene, a kind of absurd black comedy. We might venture further and ask, "Who is the more hysterical, the Mohammed who accepted his visions as proof of a visit from the messenger of Allah, or the 360 million who now support that delusion by their belief, adding the weight of numbers until the sheer mass of believers makes absurdity seem true?"

Potentially, at least, the study of the abnormal can test and improve our own concept of normality. It is a study that deserves a dual approach: the empirical testing of hypotheses needs to be accompanied by a constant and lively examination of the categories that underlie the work of the data collectors, for even the specialist who represents the most highly differentiated thinking in a culture can also share some of the delusions of that culture, even though his procedures, at their best, serve to correct them.

Today we no longer use such concepts as "pacts with the devil." We prefer to speak of uncontrolled impulses, or of forces in the unconscious mind, or of death instincts and libido, or of constitutional psychopathic inferiority, or of a schizophrenic process. We entertain speculations about sex chromosomes that have "gone wrong," or about inhibitory substances that spread over the cortex; and while, here and there, the speculations pay off in improved understanding and control of behavior, a few may very well serve—as delusions have in the past—to mask and conceal reality.

IDENTIFYING AND CLASSIFYING THE ABNORMAL

In the United States, the standard diagnostic system for mental disorders is that appearing in the *Diagnostic and Statistical Manual of Mental Disorders* of the American Psychiatric Association. The following are the major categories in the 1968 edition of this classification system:

    I. Mental Retardation
   II. Organic Brain Syndromes
      II-A. Psychoses Associated With Organic Brain Syndromes
      II-B. Non-Psychotic Organic Brain Syndromes

---

[15]Still, the exceptional wisdom and expertise of a few kept them from rash conclusions, and allowed them to resist the tide and speak out. Montaigne (1580) observed, "it is setting a high value on one's conjectures, if for their sake one is willing to burn a human being alive.... The lives of witches in my neighborhood are in danger whenever a new writer appears who takes their dreams for fact.... One should not always respect the confessions of persons involved in a crime, for there have been too many cases in which people accused themselves of having killed others who were afterward found alive and in good health. Those extravagant accusations!"

   III. Psychoses Not Attributed to Physical Conditions Listed Previously
   IV. Neuroses
    V. Psychotic Disorders and Certain Other Non-Psychotic Disorders
   VI. Psychophysiologic Disorders
  VII. Special Symptoms
 VIII. Transient Situational Disturbances
   IX. Behavior Disorders of Childhood and Adolescence
    X. Conditions Without Manifest Psychiatric Disorder and Non-Specific
       Conditions

A few words should be said about mental retardation, which is largely beyond
the purview of this book. Aiken (1968) defines this category as "a general
term for disorders in which there is some degree of impairment in the ability
to learn and to solve problems of the type found on intelligence tests." Aiken
goes on to say that 2.2 per cent of the population would have IQ (intelligence
quotient) scores below 70 on a standard test such as the Wechsler Adult Intelligence Scale, "and these individuals are usually classified as mentally retarded."
The alert reader will note that most of the venerable, and still widely used,
terms of psychopathology—hysteria, paranoia, schizophrenia, manic-depressive,
psychopath—are omitted altogether from this classification system.

   A name is more than a label. Even as we identify the abnormal ones, we establish a class that relates them to conditions and causes.

THE ETHICAL-DAEMONIC VIEW

   As we have noted, we once called the abnormal one a sinner, a witch, a person possessed or pursued by the devil, and blamed him for having invited the
latter to take charge of his actions. For 500 years the witch-hunters and the
courts treated these odd ones as though they had freely chosen their course. If
now we should regard them as having been punished in the first place by a
chain of causal circumstances that made them so peculiar, we would see the
tortures and prosecution as a second punishment that adds insult to injury.

   Now that we have moved away from this daemonic view, its injustice inclines
us to look upon our alcoholics, psychopaths, homosexuals, drug addicts, psychotics, and neurotics as mentally ill, as the product of circumstances or heredity. But we are not quite sure. We are repeatedly forced to assess a deviant's
degree of responsibility in the present, and to maintain the distinction between
the cause that has determined his actions in the past and his present responsibility for their consequences. Both our legislation and our therapies betray an
interesting and uneasy mixture of moral evaluations and scientific analysis. Is an
alcoholic helped by being told: "You are a sick man. Your alcoholism is a
disease. You have no way of controlling this illness until you admit your helplessness and place yourself completely in the hands of a therapist who will
direct your efforts. This is not a moral question. You have no cause for guilt"?

THE GENETIC VIEW

   We sometimes look upon the abnormal person as a twisted product that has
developed from bad seed. We have discovered the very chromosomes that are

abnormal in a few cases: the mongolian idiot with an extra twenty-third chromosome, the sterile male with underdeveloped genitals and an extra sex chromosome (Klinefelter's syndrome). Can we also extend our genetic studies to other abnormalities, to depressions, schizophrenias, and other constitutional inferiorities susceptible to fixations or special motivations? Where we can do so, we shall have to take a sharp turn away from that all-too-human tendency to blame and exorcise, and look in the long run toward a program of eugenics or toward that most remote possibility, finding a way of altering the DNA itself.

THE ENVIRONMENTALIST POSITION

Given a society that is in flux, in which social mobility is visible, and which is aware that differences in environment produce differences in ability, even public policies are framed in America with this belief in the potency of environment in mind. We look on some of the abnormal as *sociopaths,* using this name to put the finger upon the cause, and to blame the disorganizing forces in our social structure for his existence. This view attributes the fact that so many of his kind are found in the city slums, where crime and disease also flourish, to our lack of social responsibility in cleaning up this "illth."

The geneticists among us, who concentrate their attention upon the bad seed, will, of course, see the slums as traps into which the disorganized, the social misfits, and the biologically weak will inevitably drift. The slum is a trap or catch-basin for, not the producer of, its inhabitants. True or false, each of these theories is related to our own feelings of guilt and responsibility, feelings which may enter into our choice of a theory. Does not the discovery that mongolian idiocy is due to a defect in one of the chromosomes, not to that often-invoked "lack of maternal love," bring great relief to the mother of such a child? And so the search for adequate concepts to deal with the abnormal ones is heavily charged with emotions.

THE HABIT VIEW

There is a view of the personality that looks upon it as a bundle of habits. The conditioned responses of the deviant, it suggests, are established by the working of the same laws that produce good habits. Habits are simply a serial unfolding, a coupling and uncoupling of reflexes under patterned sequences of stimulation. If the experimenter can make his laboratory animal into a maze-runner, a paper-tearer, a bar-presser, a dominant fighter, or a submissive follower by appropriately designed schedules of reinforcement, should the clinician not ask, "What were the peculiar patterns of stimulation which shaped the patient?" For behavior is caused. Given a set of reflexes, an assortment of drives needing release, is it not the arrangement of the stimuli that orders the flow of behavior? And does it not follow that to redesign the patterns will require us to arrange reconditioning situations, even if doing so requires special rehabilitation centers where the laws of operant conditioning can produce healthy actions instead of abnormal ones?

Those who hold this view are apt to stress the importance of the earliest years, even the earliest months. Realizing that the tree tends to grow as the twig is bent, both psychoanalysts and behaviorists have been focusing upon this most vulnerable period, where fixations, breakdowns, separation anxieties, and exaggerated needs are most easily produced. And since, in our society, it is the mother who is primarily responsible for the first conditionings, this view would open the discussion of abnormality by a description of abnormal mothering.[16] As we shall discover in Chapter 4, this view arouses sharp controversy. When the World Health Organization drafted Dr. John Bowlby to study the relationship between maternal care and mental health, it seemed that medical opinion, the world over, had turned in this direction. But it was not long before the storm of criticism aroused by the Geneva report proved so great that, just four years after his publication appeared, the author publicly warned against those who were using his evidence to overstate the case for this particular brand of environmentalism. In addition he warned against blaming hospitalization or other forms of institutional life for the development of psychopathic or "affectionless" characters. It is only a small minority, he insisted, who show these institution-based "disabilities in personality." (See Bowlby 1952 and 1953a, Bowlby et al. 1961, Ainsworth et al. 1962, Yudkin and Holme 1963, and Rimland 1964.)

Behavioristic psychotherapists are chiefly influenced by the work of laboratory scientists, whereas psychoanalytic therapists derive their ideas primarily from clinicians. The psychoanalytic tradition has evolved from the experience of clinicians like Janet and Freud in treating patients. The behavioristic tradition has been more strongly affected by laboratory experiments, often on animals. The spiritual father of behaviorism was the Russian physiologist Pavlov (Nobel laureate in 1903), whose experiments established the principle of classical conditioning. Techniques of classical conditioning—as well as other principles of learning (or losing) habits—have been applied to the correction of abnormal behavior. A degree of rivalry always has existed between therapists of psychoanalytic and behavioristic inclinations, as will be seen at the end of Chapter 6. Many behaviorists charge the psychoanalysts with being metaphysical and unscientific, while the latter group often dismiss behavioristic therapies as superficial and unconcerned with the psychodynamics of the whole person.

INTRAPSYCHIC CONFLICT: REPRESSION AND SOCIETY

Another view of the abnormal personality attributes it to a greater than normal amount of intrapsychic conflict which implies that the half of the personality that would go forward toward creative and productive living is neutralized and sometimes overwhelmed by another half that is self-destructive, fearful, as though it were bound for death. When Freud postulated a death instinct—which seemed at first to be a self-contradictory notion, since instinctive patterns were believed to have been selected in the course of a struggle for survival and therefore to be of biological value—and placed it on equal footing with all of the

---

[16]In Chapter 4 we shall discover, for example, the concept of the "schizophrenogenic mother," who is responsible for the pathogenic interchanges that initiated and reinforced a process that culminated in a particular form of mental illness.

life-saving and life-producing forces, he made intrapsychic conflict into an inevitable and universal thing. The existence of a special abnormal group naturally raises the questions:

1. Are these odd ones simply endowed with a stronger dosage of this death instinct?

2. Has their conditioning, more frustrating and self-defeating than that of others, forced the energies that might have flowed out to master their world to turn back upon the self?

3. Have these odd ones had to repress so much that was a part of them and which would otherwise have led to gratification that, in retaliation, these instinctual demands strike at the very ego that repressed them?

4. Does intrapsychic conflict represent conflicts between a pair of parents that have been internalized in such a way that the child is divided within?

5. Has a mother's hatred of her spouse been internalized by a son who now fears maleness lest he, too, be deprived of her love?

What Freud's theory implied, finally, was that the mind of the individual can be divided into conscious and unconscious halves by this process of intrapsychic conflict, so that an instinct-charged stream of intentionally suppressed forces produces what the conscious ego never understands or intends.

In any case, this view of the abnormal person emphasizes the inner structure of the self-system that has been divided by repression. It calls for a therapy that will redistribute the self's energies, make the repressed conscious, redeploy the forces locked in conflict. The social reformers who accepted Freud's basic premises insisted that this therapy and redeployment of energies required the patient to discover the real enemy in those social institutions which must be changed.[17]

ABNORMALITY AS DISEASE

The abnormal one can be viewed as sick, with a special kind of sickness. Following the program first outlined by Hippocrates, the clinician will want to order the phenomena so as to be able to trace the typical course of the illness from onset to final outcome, establishing the conditions which modify its course and seeking the drugs or regimen suitable for each disease. The painstaking work of Kraepelin, aimed at assembling all of the facts about dementia praecox, sought this type of cause-course-outcome sequence. He centered his attention upon the regularities, beneath which he hoped to discover some organic disease process: in the brain, in metabolism gone wrong, in the ductless glands, within

---

[17]That such definitions of the abnormal are embedded within social contexts and serve social values is demonstrated by the official Communist view of psychoanalysis, which is that Freud's doctrines are the natural outgrowth of capitalist individualism, are a tool to be used by the haves against the have-nots. The revisions of Fromm, on the other hand, are considered by conservatives to be a sophisticated version of socialism. One critic of Fromm asks, "Which should a man do first of all, join the party or clear up his own inner conflicts?" "Only the sciences can generate a fruitful axiology," writes Kimmelman (1948), seeming to agree with Fromm's naturalistic ethics expounded in *Man for Himself*; but then adding, "man to me seems doomed to eternal frustration" and "it is this very immanence of human suffering which has made and always will make morality possible."

the cells. The great advance in nineteenth-century psychiatry would come, he believed, with the full realization that mental processes are the functioning of organic structures and that for every mental illness there is an underlying derangement in the functioning "down among the cells."

Some of the odd ones, like those suffering from senile dementia, may be suffering from as yet irreversible intracellular degenerative changes. Their memory losses will be traced to such cellular decay, and, in turn, this decay will have to be followed to its causes: atheromatous plaques of fatty substances, reduced bore of cerebral blood vessels, dietary deficiencies that reduce cortical functioning. Still other degenerative changes will be traced to the destruction of nerve cells by such invading microorganisms as the spirochetes of syphilis. Where such relations hold, the psychology of the abnormal will become a joint concern for psychologist and physician, a type of collaboration still hindered by an overspecialization in our disciplines that robs each of these workers of a full understanding of the views of the other.

Most mental disorders, including those that are specifically designated as organic, show symptoms that arise from a multiplicity of causes. Genetic, biochemical, physiological, environmental (physical), and intrapersonal factors have been at work; as the person who bears the illness develops, he also develops an identity, a set of goals, a power of integrating his actions toward aims that the cultural matrix will reward or punish. He is surrounded by those who support him, make demands, and occasionally contribute to his delinquency. Since diverse causal factors are at work, these "diseases" will require all manner of strategies of the therapist. The cardiac patient will not be simply a man with a defective heart: person, symptoms, milieu are interrelated. And so it will be with family, schizophrenic process, and developing personality even when Kraepelin's hypothetical underlying organic process is discovered.

As a result of these complex interrelationships, the classifications of abnormal personalities now in use may create false simplifications that hinder therapy. No one of our languages satisfies all of the experts or fits all of the data. Experimenters and clinicians lack any kind of scientific Esperanto based on a grand consensus. The stable structure of laws that the organicist aimed at is not only something for the future, but possibly a chimera. Sometimes the psychopathologist grows envious of his fellow workers in such fields as astronomy and physics, imagining that things are simpler there. He may sigh, in his discouragement, and say, "I am tired of 'dynamics,' of holism, of all this controversy about interrelatedness. I would like to get back to the organic simplicities of Kraepelin, Watson, Pavlov, where things had a way of staying put." And a literature that contains such harsh evaluations as the following helps to explain his conflict:

"Mental illness is a myth, whose function it is to disguise and thus render palatable the bitter pill of moral conflicts in human relations" (Szasz 1961).
"Psychiatrists menace a free society" (Szasz 1960).
"Mental health cannot be defined scientifically" (Hoffman 1960).
"A psychiatrist, by profession, is called upon to treat 'mental illness' without a

definitive outline of what it is... [and] he cannot define that 'health' to which he hopes to return his patients" (Grinker and Grinker 1962).

"Most psychoanalysts, and this holds true even for Freud, are not less blind to realities of human existence and to unconscious social phenomena than are the other members of their own social class" (Fromm 1959).

A statement such as the first one, made by Dr. Szasz in a meeting of his fellow psychiatrists, can convert a forum for the dispassionate evaluation of ideas into a gathering of angry men who sometimes forget the rules of order and professional courtesy and counterattack with charges of carelessness, irresponsibility, and misguided enthusiasm. Some of the other discouraging words quoted do not prevent clinicians and therapists from working toward improved definitions of mental health and those rigorous methods that will satisfy the criteria of science, nor from continuing to treat the abnormal. A few carry on their work, with schizophrenics for example, insisting all the while that they are dealing with a "psychosis of unknown origin." Classifications endorsed by professional associations are constantly changing. Goals for therapy that are more relevant to culture than health are being recognized as such. Unstable mixtures of scientific testing and moral evaluation are being analyzed and clarified. And new generations of clinicians are being disciplined for a task that still requires a combination of the skills of the artist, the spiritual guide, and the scientist; yet they are still biased by their training to believe that it is a finished science they are entering.

Before concluding the discussion of this concept of diseases of organic origin, it might be well to remind ourselves that there are deteriorative changes, also organic, of functional origin. For example, the pitting of the stomach wall produced by a chronic hyperacidity may be related in turn to chronic emotional stress created by interpersonal difficulties. A season of stress can be written into the bone structure of a developing child just as a dry season can affect the amount of growth in a tree (Sontag and Comstock 1939). But it also important to realize that changes of a more positive character can also be built in, even to the point of changing an organism's capacities for stress tolerance, for decision and for effective work, for managing one's tendencies so as to control disorganizing emotions, for remembering, perceiving, and expressing, and so on.[18]

The changes in this positive direction, and the procedures which produce them, have long been the stock in trade of our spiritual guides and religious healers, although some who promise these positive gains have been charlatans who prey upon those patients rejected by the experts. We sometimes tolerate them, observing that after all these patients have no others to turn to. And among these healers there are some who generalize so enthusiastically that they seem to believe that they can summon forces that will invade and dominate our

---

[18]Consider the example of the humble laboratory rat whose thoracic capacity is altered, along with its intercostal muscles, as it is reared in a special environment with a low concentration of oxygen in the air it breathes. On this area, see Cole 1953, Chapters 2-6.

material being at any moment, neutralizing every contrary law.[19] Such a "spiritual view" of mental illness arouses suspicion in the minds of those trained in objective and experimental science, for it seems to invite us to return to an earlier daemonic world where, as in the case of witchcraft, spirits could be summoned or exorcised, and to abandon all of our hard-won scientific discriminations. Having barely emerged from these superstitions, we are somewhat in the frame of mind of the adolescent who, having just learned the shape of a tough social reality, has no notion of letting himself be taken in.

That there is a sthenic force in a new enthusiasm, or in a new insight, or in a new organization of one's efforts; that there are changes which can be brought about by the effort of a therapist (or a spiritual guide); that some of these changes can penetrate to the very tissues—these are also facts we cannot afford to lose sight of in our eagerness to avoid the pitfalls of an earlier enthusiasm for miraculous types of healing.

THE EXISTENTIALIST APPROACH

A seventh approach to abnormal personalities would describe them as "lost souls" who for one reason or another have not found their way to a meaningful role in our society. Freudianism caught on, Fromm believes, because it found groups of urban intellectuals who had lost their religious beliefs and who were floundering about without any ideals or profound convictions to give shape to their disordered lives. Viktor Frankl and Rollo May, to name but two who call themselves existentialists, agree with the diagnosis and dislike the Freudian answer. They would provide other touchstones of meaning. Frankl's logotherapy, he writes, "focuses on the meaning of human existence as well as on man's search for such meaning . . . the primary motivational force in man." Basing his views upon his own experience in a Nazi death camp, where he concluded that only the prisoners who could find and keep alive this spark of meaning could continue to exist, he offers a mixture of logic and inspiration for those who suffer from what he calls a *noogenic neurosis* (see Frankl 1959, 1960, and 1956; see also Maslow 1962).

Like the theologian Paul Tillich, who also imagined that modern man is suffering from a kind of meaningless drift, these existentialists carry their death-camp analyses into society as a whole. And some very ancient ethical principles that have long characterized our Judaeo-Christian tradition are used to explain that loss of vital relationship to reality which they advance as the underlying cause of the abnormal person's behavior. Thus there is a brand of existentialism that seeks to reinstate an essentially moral and religious evaluation of the abnormal, once so distorted in theory and practice by the witch-hunters, and we are brought full circle back to some very old traditions. St. Theresa of Avila also

---

[19]One definition of miraculous healing might run: "an event with an extremely low probability of occurring." The Theological Council of the American Lutheran Church is bolder in its statement: "God has power to heal in whatever way and whatever time he wills to do so" (reported in the *New York Times*, Oct. 23, 1966). Warning against false expectancies, the Council lays down the guidelines for correct healing procedures, but at no place suggests consulting those most expert in diagnosis.

had some very positive notions about the moral roots of that *acedia,* or spiritual dryness, that sometimes appeared among her Carmelites, and she was ready to encourage, chide, punish (and to recommend to the Mothers Superior that the defectors be put on bread and water, solitary confinement, or hard labor) in order to restore to them that moral force that comes with the right relationship with God. Though they resembled women who were ill, their illness was a sickness of the spirit. They had lost their way. Existentialism in counseling practice becomes a new effort along ancient and honorable lines: a form of spiritual (and inspirational) guidance that would restore to the abnormal the lost core of meaning. Pierre Janet described the *aboulia* (loss of will) in his psychasthenics, and Ribot published a treatise on *Les maladies de la volunté.* Both were eclectics who viewed this loss of the power to decide and to center one's life upon significant central tasks as the product of a multitude of factors, some of them physiological, some of them attributable to poor habits; Janet discussed more than a dozen causes of psychasthenia. The existentialists seem to want to restore mind (or consciousness, or spirit) to its dominant position, and to center upon the life-style of the whole man rather than upon the pieces of which he is composed. Their program could be described as a reaction against mechanism, materialism, and all of those types of analysis which reduce man to a bundle of bits, a helpless bundle that includes one highly verbal strand called the persona or ego. The existentialists might argue: this bundle hypothesis represents the way the abnormal person feels, whereas in the normal healthy self, the spirit infuses and dominates the whole, charging the parts with deeply felt meanings and keeping them in line with a central goal that is beyond a mere self-actualization (see Janet 1926, pp. 227, 276-77, and 1928, pp. 216 ff; May, Angel, and Ellenberger 1959).

SUMMARY OF CONCEPTS

The seven approaches we have sketched do not do justice to the diversity that exists in our time. Each of them will have to be developed as we take up the disorders described in the chapters which follow. Each will have to be examined critically, for each involves assumptions that organize the clinical data, and each can exaggerate special facts and conceal others. No view is adequate to include all of the facts, and our science is an unfinished one, full of unknowns, requiring compromises and balanced assessments that are never wholly satisfactory or convincing. Even the wholly discarded "witch concept" was able to put us on our guard against too great certitude in our own times.

THE PROBLEM OF FREEDOM

We like to think of man as a free agent, capable of making promises and of assuming responsibility. Slavery is abhorrent to us. And there is a residue, in many of us, of that adolescent revolt against authority that we passed through when, in haste to outgrow all dependence, we fought against every imposed restriction. Perhaps because of this residue we are quick to resent any restrictions upon our freedom, even those assumptions of determinism that underlie the scientific view of man. The innocent phrase, "behavior is caused," has to be converted to "the understanding of the causes makes us free to create our own destiny."[20] Our political and religious ideals announce this love of freedom. And yet we know that this freedom is limited, that the power to make promises and to assume responsibility varies widely from man to man. We have set up court procedures so that, where it is necessary for the protection of an individual or those around him, a man may be declared incompetent and of unsound mind, "unable to appreciate the wrongfulness of his conduct or to conform his conduct to the requirements of law."[21] And we are prepared to take away his freedom, confining him to the locked wards of a hospital for the insane, certain that free and rational choices are no longer possible *for him*.

THE BELIEF THAT ALL BEHAVIOR IS CAUSED

Even in thus policing our own society we discover that absence of freedom is not an all-or-none thing: there are all degrees of this power to integrate a good life, to behave in rational and responsible fashion, to make a future that is desirable for oneself and tolerable for one's neighbors. This kind of freedom varies even within the groups that we call abnormal and to which we attach the label "mentally ill." We believe that we are being both compassionate and sensible when we say to our neighbor the alcoholic, "You are sick. You need help. Until you realize this and place yourself in the hands of a competent therapist, you are not going to improve." And should he, in his pride, invite us to mind our own business, or insist "There is nothing the matter with me that I can't take care of," his counselor sometimes concludes that this insensibility to his true predicament (and his lack of integrative power) is also a part of his illness. A man, we conclude, may not realize how very unfree he is, even when in fact his habits possess him. For such a man the first step in therapy would be the discovery that he is *not* free, that his mechanisms *are* running him. ("Oh, I could stop smoking any time, *if it were important!*" said the man who was secretly worried about lung cancer.)

There are other times when we are not so sure. We argue that treating a youth as an adult, throwing him upon his own responsibility, is the kind of challenge which will make him mature into that responsible freedom which is his birthright. Keeping him dependent, supervising his going and coming, looking out for him, is a kind of prolonged "swaddling" care, and we can cite instances where dependency and immaturity are the outcomes of maternal overprotection. Yet we also know that there must be rules, even for men and women of college age. We even invite them to make their own.

---

[20]Vance Packard's *Hidden Persuaders* is charged with this resentment against being used by others. There is even an anti-science, anti-intellectual hatred of knowledge that colors the public's attitude toward the psychologist: he aims to predict and control *others*. This view has its classic expression in Dostoevsky's *Notes from the Underground*.

[21]The uneasy vacillation from the McNaughten Rule to the Durham Rule and back again may indicate uncertainty on the part of the court, and the difficulty in making the criterion work properly.

In short, we are ambivalent. We are keenly aware that the medieval witch-hunters went too far when they insisted that the witch's misfortunes had been brought on her by her own pact with the devil, that she was in fact wholly responsible and therefore guilty. We are doubly certain when we discover that the witch-finders went still further in their generalizations, and insisted that all physical diseases were of this same type, that the sick were in need of prayer rather than a purge or a bloodletting by some barber-surgeon, much as we doubt the efficacy of the treatments by those healers. When St. Theresa punished her depressed nuns, certain that they had sinned against the Holy Ghost and that their souls were in danger, we are disturbed, certain that in a modern convent there would be psychiatric help available for similar cases.[22] Mothers Superior are required to be sensitive to that difference between those who should be subjected to discipline and those who should be given special psychological therapy (even as the courts must assess a defendant's degree of responsibility).

On college campuses the student health service has to make similar discriminations within that tenth of the student body who consult them with their problems. When should a student be protected, excused from exams, sent home, advised to undergo psychotherapy? And when should he be exposed to the full scholastic discipline, encouraged to "stick it out," forced to meet his responsibilities, encouraged to act like a grownup? Governing boards are sometimes reluctant to assign funds to such a health service, on the grounds that these counselors, in defending their clients and sheltering them from the full impact of academic discipline, are making mollycoddles instead of helping youth to mature. The same conflict about social policies arises in Newburgh, New York, and in Washington, D.C., where legislators are concerned about contributing to the delinquency of relief clients and to the flabbiness of our culture. An impartial observer of trends would see in the extension of student health services, in the expanding costs of social legislation, clear evidence that—whether we are aware of it or not—we act as though we believe that man is less free than he once assumed he was in a pioneer society.

From the days of witchcraft to the modern college campus, this question of the freedom of the individual has been debated. With the slow emergence of a medical psychology with its concept of mental illness, we have moved away from an older, more absolute position. A man is as free as he is. And he may be less free than he imagines himself to be. Some of us are even ready to assume that such a predicament is universal. Psychoanalysis, on its part, with a doctrine of unconscious determination of behavior, offers a pointed warning to those who are sure of themselves at the top of their voices. And behaviorism, ready to demonstrate to any willing subject that his reflexes will obey the laws of conditioning, leaves little room for an ego to decide *on its own* to take a course of action. Even the ego's sense of its own freedom, of being in charge of its destiny, becomes a determined thing, an attitude with causes.

---

[22]And in studies of recent war casualties, now called "combat fatigue," we have found that a hard-boiled commander who is determined that his men shall not escape duty by reporting sick can actually increase the rate of severe mental illness in his brigade by his methods (even though, in one sense, he flatters the men by assuming that they are both free and courageous).

Varieties of Determinism

Organic Changes

The changes in the physiological and anatomical substrate that supports our actions offer the most obvious form of determinism. In the third stage of syphilis, as the spirochetes are gnawing their way into the cerebral tissues and disrupting that network so vitally important for our powers of integration, the self can remain blandly unaware of the changes. In the aging person, troubled with cerebral atherosclerosis, the fatty deposits that form the fatal plaques on the inner surface of the artery walls do not announce their presence in any clear-cut conscious change. Only as immediate memory begins to fail is there any visible sign of those changes that give the cerebral surface its moth-eaten appearance when viewed at post-mortem. Like a Dutch windmill that swings slowly with the changes in air currents, these selves show altered dynamic properties that are not of their choosing and not within their ken. It is a determinism of which the self is ignorant and over which it has little control.

Fluctuations in Physiological States and in Integrative Powers

There are changes in attitude, such as those that accompany a depression, which sometimes can be traced to biochemical changes, down among the cells. In the depression of the hangover we can see that chemical factors have affected a whole outlook on life; and in the exhilaration of the mountaintop experience we can identify the lowered oxygen pressure in the inhaled air as the cause of the behavorial changes. The individual may know nothing of the chemical changes. The young male, whose drinking companions expect him to tolerate alcohol and to be happy-go-lucky, may be so convinced by their attitudes that he will turn against his own weakness or project his mood changes upon the surrounding world. And the man on the mountaintop may accept his vision as proof of the supernatural. A neuritis, anoxia, or aftermath of hepatitis may be at work beneath the level of his awareness, and without his decisions ever taking these causes into account; and while he makes his decisions as though he were a free agent, these biochemical changes are developing according to the impersonal laws governing chemical changes, and can sweep him into such an irreversible act as suicide, or initiate some withdrawal from responsibility that will alter his destiny. In his ignorance he is determined.

There are surges and troughs in our integrative powers, as though there were some tide of life that rises and falls for reasons we know nothing of. We feel them as mood changes, as altered powers to act, produce, create. Sometimes, as in the LSD experience (on which see Chap. 8), we know the cause; a few, even so, accept the experiences as a genuine expansion of consciousness, even as a kind of mystic communion. At other times we are swept downward, so that the world appears as a wasteland, dull, uninviting, immovable. And these transformations of outlook can be quite unwarranted, in one respect: we are neither as good as we feel we are when in ecstasy; and the world is not, in fact, as impossible as it seems in depression. And the moods, the shifts in integrative power, need not announce their causes. Determined, we are unaware of the determining factors, are falsely aware of ourselves and the world, and are something less than free agents because of this.

The Automatic Coupling and Uncoupling of Reflexes

There is a third group of effects, which emerge from the unceasing coupling and uncoupling of reflexes that the world imposes upon us. Some of these associative processes occur insidiously, beneath our imaginative and insightful structuring of our actions, even beneath consciousness. We neither attend to the items which cumulatively change our attitude nor sense the drift in our outlook. The changes follow intensity-contingency laws, until their effects can choke the very sources of invention or shunt our creative powers into some self-destructive channel; the "aha-moment" of insight may occur long after we have consolidated our new position. The teacher of creative writing often complains of the sodden clichés that his students scatter through their themes, as though their ability to see and communicate what lies before them had been overlaid by an inhibiting screen. Such a teacher would understand the editor who wrote:

"The writing of almost any child has freshness and energy. Then, usually in late adolescence, the serpent enters the garden. Clichés start to rustle through the undergrowth. Tired phrases press forward. Such a decline cannot be attributed entirely to bad teaching. It is as though experience and evocation have, save in the exercise of a few talents, begun to pull apart; as though, in response to new experience, there is nothing good in the word-hoard" (*Times Lit. Supp.,* Dec. 24, 1964, p. 1163).

The slow and silent attrition and combination of attitudes, by processes that work below the level where conscious intentions operate, can produce even more serious and pervasive effects. Ernest Renan, who left the priesthood and his church, admitted to a Breton friend that his faith had been undermined by a force independent of his will. The change had not been of his seeking. New truths had forced themselves upon him. Accumulating from small events, a conviction had grown until an "identity crisis was upon him. Surprised, he wakened outside the church" (Wardman 1964).

In his subjective account of the matter, an individual may discover that he has fallen into (or out of) love, or that he is suddenly in the opposition party politically, or that he no longer has confidence in his ability to fulfill promises, or that his vocation is no longer of any interest to him. However we describe the processes of attrition or recombination of reflexes that alter attitudes in this silent fashion, their results surprise the unsuspecting subject as though they had been secretly formed, down among the cells, in response to stimulations that had gone unnoticed. Unintended, these fateful changes reveal that the very groundwork for action has shifted.

The saltatory character of the new insights, and the hidden character of the slowly accumulating base to the new decisions, make us want to speak of an unconscious process. How fateful for a man's sanity it would be if such a cumulative process should lead toward schizophrenia! Then his new insight, "I am being persecuted," or "I am Jesus Christ returned," becomes one of the clinical signs that mark the beginning of true alienation. The bloody truth to the individual becomes a basis for commitment to an institution.

As we become increasingly aware of the causes behind our choices, examining our own lives and expanding our area of responsibility, we find ourselves confronted with new ethical and rational choices; novel and lively options emerge in the midst of determinisms (or automatisms). Our new awareness does not always free us from the compulsion to act as we always have. The old "determinism," which operated while we were ignorant of its existence, is now pitted against our new insights: the man as a whole can be pitted against his part-processes. It seems clear that a knowledge of the existence of atherosclerotic plaques will not promptly brighten the day for the aging patient. Nor will the study of conditioning principles abruptly give the smoker the power to terminate his habit or to extinguish the incentive qualities of the cigarette. Even the widely publicized facts about lung cancer, coronary attacks, and emphysema do not suffice to reduce the consumption of tobacco. Two obvious barriers limit the efficacy of the partial insights we possess: organic processes and the inertia of habits.

Unconscious Processes

There is another type of determinism that also hinges upon relationships between our awareness and those other processes that determine our actions. No student of psychology in the twentieth century can miss what two pioneers made so clear before our era had scarcely opened. Freud, on his part, was inclined to view the failure of consciousness to regulate action effectively as due, basically, to a prior act of repression: we have forgotten things we once knew; we have denied what we felt; we have looked away from what was too horrible or anxiety-laden *within us*. Yet in willfully forgetting these events, we did not eliminate them from our systems: their traces persisted, developed outside of our awareness, and were able to determine our actions. Sometimes they throw up their symbolic products (that half-express and half-conceal their existence) into awareness so that, like foreign invaders whom we sense as enemies, they have to be repelled again, and disowned as no part of us. And it sometimes seems that the more we repress them, the more we deny ownership, the more they are freed to work out consequences that we cannot accept. Uninterrupted, their surreptitious work can be completed without our knowledge. And it was toward the undoing of this split within the mind that the work of Freud and his disciples was directed: the repairman has to assist in derepression, to expand awareness and responsibility, to negotiate new relationships between two alienated parts of a self-system.

Pierre Janet was also concerned with this failure in the power of the conscious self to regulate its automatisms. Looking upon a man's action tendencies as arranged in a hierarchy, with automatisms at the lowest rungs of the ladder and the rational-voluntary-conscious regulations at the top, he studied his patients as an expert accountant might study a business venture, for he believed that failures in the top-level functions could arise out of poor investments, wasteful expenditures of energy, poor plans of action. With the failure of a regulative consciousness, the bare bones of automatisms began to stick out, uncovered by the loss of the normal reactions-to-reactions. And so he worked out his own version of counseling: advising against identified waste, simplifying expenditures, introducing new economies and new learnings, liquidating unfinished business, exhorting and encouraging those who were tired and bored, in-inspiring the patient until his top-level powers began to function (Janet 1889).

Whether by psychoanalysis, as a follower of Freud would urge, or by Janet's type of "cost-accounting," a clinician can present a patient with a fresh understanding of the determinisms, or automatisms, that he has not been able to regulate. Such treatment confronts the individual with new choices, new self-regulative tasks. As we discovered above, this procedure, too, can lay bare the structure of action, reveal causes and consequences, and still find that its work is not carried through to full recovery. We are almost tempted to resurrect that hoary concept of the will, since these self-regulators with all of their new understandings can still fail to make good choices.[23]

How far can a therapy aimed at restoring this regulative power to the conscious individual go? Must it be counted unsuccessful when the symptoms persist, and successful if the abnormality is removed, even temporarily? Or must the therapist continue until his patient's new capacities for self-regulation make any recurrence improbable, until the patient can not only identify a new ideal of mental health but move toward it effectively? These questions will haunt us as we examine specific disabilities in the chapters to come. The analysis of a case in which symptoms recur will sometimes be regarded as "unfinished," with the implication that a thorough job would have led to a longer span of health. What ideal of mental health all therapists should be working for has been a source of discussion, a problem so discouraging to some that the answers have been described as "a clutter of words," the guidelines as "a rope of sand," and the objectives as without any operational definition.[24]

---

[23]The therapist who probes into the unconscious roots underlying the behavior of the alcoholic, or who tries to assist in the reorganization of his life plans, reports that even with his best efforts to bring insight and new integrative powers, two out of three of his clients may have to be judged either partially or wholly unimproved. For example, one follow-up study of 100 alcoholics, treated in a private hospital with excellent facilities and a highly skilled staff, reported that, when they were seen from three to eight years later, 24 were recovered and an additional 19 were managing somewhat better (Wall and Allen 1944). When we add to this the facts that more than two-thirds of American adults drink alcoholic beverages, that among those who drink some 10 per cent experience difficulties as a result of their drinking and do not seem to be able to manage the habit, and that therapy of the quality just reported is available to only a very small percentage of these "problem drinkers," we can see that our therapeutic resources, at present, cannot match the problem.

[24]These epithets were offered by Aubrey Lewis, who then modestly, and disparaging his own efforts, suggested the following alternative ideal of mental health: "(1) active adjustment or attempts at mastery of his environment as distinct both from his inability to adjust and from his indiscriminate adjustment through passive acceptance of environmental conditions; (2) unity of his personality, the maintenance of a stable, internal integration which remains intact notwithstanding the flexibility of behavior which derives from active adjustment; and (3) ability to perceive correctly the world and himself" (A. Lewis 1958, p. 170).

THE PROBLEM OF METAPSYCHOLOGY

The term *metapsychology,* which designates something beyond psychology, is analogous in meaning to its companion, metahistory. History, beginning as a tale told about some campfire, grew critical as rival accounts of the same group of events competed to capture belief. It grew scientific and factual, and it not only organized the facts but developed a grand theory of historical changes that embraced all the little histories. Or should we not admit that the grand philosophies of history are rivals, divergent views that aspire to replace all hitherto existing histories, but never quite make it? In thus going beyond the bare facts so as to look down upon all rival accounts as from some absolute vantage point, metahistory develops into an eschatology, a science of the future, a view of the very last things, toward which the whole march of history should be oriented.

Psychology, too, has a way of going beyond itself into metapsychology; and each system builder is prone to criticize his colleagues and his forebears, as though, by the process of criticism of criticism of criticism, an ultimate and grand view of man had been found, a view that can now put an end to all controversy. Standing above man and his institutions, the metapsychologist seeks to establish what must be, in the nature of things. Not always self-consistent, Freud offered us several metapsychologies. A few of them, we suspect, expressed his mood at the time of writing. When he applied his own discoveries to the views of others, he could describe their views as projections; and the unfriendly critic of Freud has already returned the compliment, suggesting that his writings should be used as documentary evidence in "The Case of Sigmund Freud" (Natenberg 1955; see also Fromm 1959). Consider the following paragraph from Freud's *Future of an Illusion* (1928b, pp. 11-12), on the relationship between man and his culture:

"Every culture must be built up on coercion and instinctual renunciation; it does not even appear certain that without coercion the majority of human individuals would be ready to submit to the labour necessary for acquiring new means of supporting life. One has, I think, to reckon with the fact that there are present in all men destructive, and therefore anti-social and anti-cultural, tendencies, and that with a great number of people these are strong enough to determine their behavior in human society.

"This psychological fact acquires a decisive significance when one is forming an estimate of human culture. One thought at first that the essence of culture lay in the conquest of nature for the means of supporting life, and in eliminating the dangers that threaten culture by the suitable distribution of these among mankind, but now the emphasis seems to have shifted away from the material plane onto the psychical. The critical question is whether and to what extent one can succeed, first, in diminishing the burden of the instinctual sacrifices imposed on men; secondly, in reconciling them to those that must necessarily remain; and thirdly, in compensating them for these. It is just as impossible to do without government of the masses by a minority as it is to dispense with coercion in the work of civilization, for the masses are lazy and unintelligent, they have no love for instinctual renunciation, they are not to be convinced of the inevitability by argument, and the individuals support each other in giving full play to their unruliness. It is only by the influence of individuals who can set an example, whom the masses recognize as their leaders, that they can be induced to submit to the labours and renunciations on which the existence of culture depends. All is well if these leaders are people of superior insight into what constitutes the necessities of life, people who have attained the height of mastering their own instinctual wishes. But the danger exists that in order not to lose their influence they will yield to the masses more than these will yield to them, and therefore it seems necessary that they should be independent of the masses by having at their disposal means of enforcing their authority. To put it briefly, there are two widely diffused human characteristics which are responsible for the fact that the organization of culture can be maintained only by a certain measure of coercion: that is to say, men are not naturally fond of work, and arguments are of no avail against their passions."

Lazy, slothful, pleasure-seeking, hostile to anyone who would control his coming and his going, yet sadly in need of a coercing authority if his life is to be organized above the level of the Do-as-you-likes, deaf to the appeal to reason, this is the creature who becomes abnormal when the coercion is severe, or when it is applied too weakly or too late. This is the creature who, chronically ungratified, sinks into emptiness and indifference or grows violent when his lethal death instinct is aroused. This is the creature who, socialized too well, carries a punishing conscience (or superego) that can turn the bottled-up impulses against his own tissues in some suicidal or self-destructive action. Such a metapsychology provided the framework within which Freud viewed both normal and abnormal, an odd framework for a man who at heart was also one of the great rationalists, reducing to order the world of dreams and of psychotic phenomena so resistant to analysis and experiment.

While Freud was writing his *Interpretation of Dreams,* he observed, in a letter to Wilhelm Fliess, "It seems to me that the theory of wish-fulfillment gives us only a psychological solution, not the biological or, better, the metapsychological one. (I would ask you seriously whether I may use the term metapsychology for my psychology that takes one beyond consciousness.)" His use of the term suggests that although Freud's interests were always ready to carry him beyond medicine, beyond that realm of mental phenomena open to direct observation, down into the unconscious, back into the prehistory of childhood (and even into prenatal development), and down into the biochemistry of the cells where instinctual forces must ultimately dwell, in so indulging this metapsychological interest he also had the sense that he was striking bedrock, getting to understand some of the riddles of the world, arriving at some conception of how man came to be what he is. Yet this bedrock is at the same time poetry, the least substantiated part of his theories, and the most revealing of his projections. It was almost with a sense of guilt that he forced himself to come back to the task of scientific observation, and it was with some difficulty, for his metapsychology kept injecting interpretations (Jones 1953, pp. 27 f, 294, and 357).

It is well for the student of the abnormal to realize that his search for scientific certitudes will be dogged by a similar tendency to project, by his own

unconscious determinisms; he must stand ready to confess that his most profound convictions can reveal something highly personal. Pressed thus to its
limits, the study of the abnormal can become not only one of the many paths
to self-knowledge but also one to a fresh understanding of the shape of things
in the world around us. But it will require constant vigilance and a readiness
to examine not only the categories and the methods we use to collect our
knowledge, but those assumptions upon which these classes and procedures are
based. There is but one metapsychology that should be taboo: it is betrayed by
the man who says, "I am a scientist. I deal only in facts."

Chapter 2 • The Gene Hypothesis

Among the definitions of the abnormal personality we examined in Chapter 1 there was one which pointed to a precise type of causation. Easy to state, it has proved difficult to validate in living human subjects. In a rare instance, here and there, the electron microscope can be turned upon cells scraped from the lining of the mouth to reveal a faulty sex chromosome that produces a defective development of the reproductive organs, or, in mongolian idiocy, to identify the presence of an extra chromosome responsible for these "unfinished" children. In both of these situations, the basic defect in the building blocks of the body contributes to a series of adjustment failures in the developing person.

Usually the proof of the role of the genes has had to rely on indirect evidence, on family studies and correlations between twins; the data are not easy to collect and, at best, require critical analysis. At times the investigators have not matched the enthusiasm that prompted their studies with an equivalent caution. At times we have had to turn to animal studies for the truly experimental evidence. These have certain special advantages, in that (1) the generations pass swiftly, (2) matings can be controlled, and (3) experimental designs can be used to test a variety of factors that alter the end-results of genetically transmitted differences. Such experiments have the insuperable defect of being limited to problems that are much less complex than those we have to deal with in studying the human being in his society.

A few studies of human patients have provided statistical evidence for a genetic factor in mental illness. Those that have dealt with schizophrenia, although still open to criticism, have produced some of the most impressive evidence; but there are signs which suggest that similar findings will be forthcoming when the neurotic and his relatives are as intensively studied. As we pass from the severe and unmistakable psychoses to the borderline (and milder) forms of neuroses, the convincing demonstrations are more difficult to come by and the role of heredity a more controversial one.

One disorder deserves a special place in the discussion. Epilepsy, which is subject to a wide variety of influences, can be said to have both genetic and exogenous causes. The data accumulated in the study of this disorder point up the need for discriminative diagnoses, for the category contains divergent types of this single disorder. So-called mongolian idiocy is cited as an example of an abnormality that is traceable to genetic defects, yet is not inherited from parents with a similar set of defective genes.

Four studies of individual pairs of twins will direct attention to instances both of correlation and of divergence; the latter will remind us that even in identical twins nongenetic factors can make the difference between normal and abnormal development.

A chemist's view of abnormality makes an appropriate contribution to the chapter, since the gene hypothesis centers attention upon small chemical packets carried in the chromosomes.

A final section warns us that a great many intervening steps have to be covered before the genes can be firmly related to those types of action that are seen by the clinician. The complexity of these intervening stages, at each one of which there are important transactions with the environment, warns us against expecting a simple one-to-one correspondence between genetic endowment and human behavior in society. And we are also warned against those prophets of doom who fear that our humane efforts to rehabilitate the abnormal may actually increase the pool of defective genes. On the one hand, the trends that are now visible do not support their prophecies, and, on the other hand, as we make our studies of the genetic factor more respectable scientifically, we will have a more rational basis for a sound eugenics program than has so far existed.

THE GENE CONCEPT AND MENTAL ILLNESS

The gene concept is today so firmly embedded in biological theory that it seems inappropriate to suggest that there is anything hypothetical about these tiny molecular packets that organize and regulate the growth of the organism. Their relationship with the abnormal personality, however, and with those classifications of mental illness that are used in the clinics, is still a highly controversial question. There are other factors that enter into the functioning of inherited structures so that the tie between chromosomes and conduct is still obscure. Applied to the human personality, the gene concept has the status of a live hypothesis.

To pause for just a moment, and to inject the proper note of doubt, let us look at the reports of Alexander Leighton and his associates (1963). Studying Yoruba witch-doctors, he found them using ways of classifying deviant behavior that were unfamiliar to physicians trained in Western medicine. They gather symptoms into groups in a way that we do not, separate what we unite, and get some rather good results. They are, of course, ignorant of the classification of mental disorders used by the American Psychiatric Association (and changed so many times). It is highly unlikely that specific constellations of genes would obey the categories of a particular culture, or of a particular stage of medical research. If we were to assume, in advance of the facts, that mental illness is basically the outcome of abnormalities in the genes, it might follow that until we know in detail how these abnormalities are transmitted, we cannot make the most useful classification of mental illnesses. As it is, we have tried to fit our genetic research into the presently existing categories. And since, as some clinicians suggest, there may be seven (or more) varieties of schizophrenia, we may discover that the gene hypothesis will fit three of these very well, and the rest poorly. This consideration, alone, is enough to explain why some of these issues are slow to resolve themselves. Because we now use the same name to cover each of the subvarieties of a clinical classification, it does not follow that each is as closely linked with genetic factors. Schizophrenia$_a$ may be closely linked with inherited determiners, schizophrenia$_b$ much less so. Epilepsy$_a$ may be found in a high percentage of cerebral injuries; epilepsy$_b$ may be more closely linked with a genetic factor that can be identified in relatives. The genes do not respect our names.

To choose another example: it is conceivable that the chronic alcoholic, who has both a poor resistance to the poison and at the same time a strong craving for its effects, also has an atypical genetic endowment. We do not know in advance of the studies. If alcoholism runs in families, our suspicions are aroused, although habits acquired during a lifetime can be transmitted too, the family environment accomplishing another type of inheritance. If the children of alcoholic parents, adopted into nonalcoholic families when still very young, are no more prone to alcoholism than samples from the general population, our suspicions would be allayed. If careful studies should show that when one identical twin is alcoholic, the other is also alcoholic in nine cases out of ten, and that among nonidentical twins and among brothers and sisters in general the correlation is much lower, the findings would confirm our suspicion. If we could then carry the problem to the laboratory and find a way of producing addiction in experimental animals, we might find the task easy in a precisely selected and genetically pure strain and very difficult in an equally pure but different strain; thus our hypothesis would have further validation. Finally, if we could identify some structural-molecular anomaly in one of the chromosomes of our experimental animals, and find visual confirmation via the electron microscope, what had begun as a mere hunch would now approach the dignified status of a well-tested theory. We would then know more precisely what to search for in the human organism with its unique genetic structures.

We would still have to face further problems. How can such an anomalous chromosome produce the unusual craving? Does it govern the growth of some atypical "appetite-center" in the visceral brain, where, according to some experimental studies, palatabilities and satiations seem to be regulated?[1] Or does it produce a general instability and weakness so that the normally depressing effects of alcohol offer one way of dulling the pains of existence? Does this

---

[1]Klüver and Bucy (1939) showed that monkeys deprived of both temporal lobes were unable to discriminate visually between objects. The animals also portrayed strong oral tendencies, mouthing and smelling whatever captured their attention. They were also hypersexed, and manifested, in addition to indiscriminate coupling with male or female, excessive masturbation and bizarre forms of oral-sexual behavior rarely shown in normal animals. Experimental studies have also shown that sharp rises in blood pressure, changes in respiration, increases in food intake, and increases in aggressive behavior can be produced by electrical stimulation with electrodes implanted in specific locations in the rhinencephalon (MacLean 1949).

anomalous chromosome control some secretory processes that produce enzymes, so that some deficiency robs the organism of a normal "buffering effect" against the poison's influence? Or do the chromosome-defective animals form neuroses under specific types of stress, and subsequently make food-choices that reveal a change in the palatability of this toxin which also happens to counteract some of the symptoms of stress?

These speculations make it clear that our gene hypothesis, partially confirmed, would then lead to a long series of experimental tests. And as these continued, and both the understanding and the mastery of the problem were completed, the now-missing links between chromosomes and symptoms would be gradually filled in. In the general area of mental illness, we are still at the very beginning, but there is enough evidence to warrant intensive work.

RESULTS OF A FEW ANIMAL STUDIES

In the genetics laboratory, where breeding of pure strains has gone hand-in-hand with behavioral research, the expert management of the chromosomes has produced strains of mice that: (1) show a susceptibility to breast cancer, (2) hoard food and eat to obesity, (3) do not learn mazes with noisy and rickety culs-de-sac, (4) experience seizures under auditory stimulation that resemble an explosive epileptic fit and are followed by coma, (5) show excessive emotion under stress, (6) behave abnormally toward their litters, (7) are sterile, (8) are aggressive, (9) have a visible appearance that betrays hidden susceptibilities and proclivities, and so on.

The traits that can thus be selected by systematic inbreeding for specific purposes include structural traits (such as size, weight, bone growth, fur color), physiological traits (such as resistance to cancer, high or low metabolic rates), and dynamic traits (such as emotionality, sex drive, susceptibility to seizures and experimental neurosis, tendency to seek isolation). The "epileptic" mice, the neurosis-resistant animals, the animals with atypical and sometimes lethal behavior toward their own litters suggest that in the near future, with appropriate selection of genetic types, clear-cut testing of deviations in behavior, and measurement of behavior under specified conditions of stress, the animal studies can provide clues for an experimental analysis of human neurotic and psychotic behavior, clues that could not be found in a hundred generations of clinical observations on human subjects. But they can provide clues *only insofar as the basic psychobiological laws can be formulated in simple stimulus-response terms.*[2] Because breeding can be so controlled as to permit genetic factors to be isolated, because stresses can be applied in ways that would be neither practical nor ethically tolerable for human subjects, and because the generations have

---

[2]Without implying any supernatural factors that would elude such analysis, it may prove, nonetheless, that man, as a complex social creature who "makes his own world as he goes" and who binds together the biologically separate lives of the generations into a human history, operates at a level far above those laboratory animals with their very limited behavioral environments. As suggestive as their concept of subjective environment was, the experiments of Köhler (1917) and Koffka (1921) did not altogether succeed in bridging the gap between a simplistic behaviorism and the more complex social levels where human conduct takes place.

such brief lives that an experimenter can study many successive transmissions of traits during his own limited working time, the animal studies promise a most fruitful testing ground for hypotheses about mental illness.

The final testing of the animal studies, which is their application to human subjects, will prove much more difficult for both scientist and therapist, and it will take much longer. The human being has a way of "fighting back." He too has theories, some of which embrace the experimenter and therapist. Whereas a laboratory clinician could create a kind of Walden II, in which he could train experimental animals to opt for what he is sure they ought to want (even to the point where they die from their choices), human beings would likely want a vote in selecting their goals. The miniature "closed society" that the therapist-reformer imagines will probably become a battleground before the results are all in. The history of the utopian settlements that sprang up in America in the last century reminds us that the therapeutic tests involve a larger society, and that our very culture is itself only one of a series of experiments.

STUDIES OF PATIENTS AND THEIR FAMILIES

FAMILY AND TWIN CORRELATIONS

Many of the family studies to date have had more propaganda value than scientific worth. Carried out by enthusiasts who were certain that "blood will tell," they dealt with royal families and men of genius, as well as with those families that keep social workers and the police busy. Too often the figures, so precise in themselves, have depended on hearsay evidence, curbstone diagnoses, and the reports of relatives and other prejudiced observers. Critics have pointed out that, to judge by the actual number of cases included in the record, often these family histories have obviously lost the argument, for sometimes less than a tenth of the probable progeny have been reported; and in the nature of the data, these studies could not report what control groups would show under similar circumstances. As a result, rival critics evaluating the data have found validation for contradictory interpretations.

A more carefully controlled type of study began to appear at the turn of the century. Darwin, whose *Origin of Species* had directed the attention of his generation to the problem of selecting the fit, had been dead for some twenty-three years when Diem's study of the families of mentally ill patients was published (1905). Beginning with 2,515 patients whose family histories had been recorded, he found that 77 per cent of them had at least one relative with some form of "taint." Matching these patients with 1,193 controls who had been seen in medical practice for reasons unconnected with mental illness (for fractures, infections, childbirth, etc.), he made an equally intensive search for "taint" among their relatives, and found that 66.9 per cent of them had at least one relative who showed one of the abnormalities he had included in his criterion: a psychosis, a nervous disease, alcoholism, apoplexy, senile dementia, abnormal character, suicide.

His criterion for "taint" as well as for some degree of genetic relationship may have been rather crude, yet the study marked a distinct advance. It could not

TABLE 1. *Probability of Schizophrenia in Relatives of Proband Cases.* (According to Kallmann 1946b and Kallmann and Barrera 1942; taken from Fuller and Thompson 1960, p. 274.)

Relationship to Proband	Probability (Per Cent)
Step-siblings	1.8
Half-siblings	7.0 to 7.6
Full siblings	11.5 to 14.3
Children:	
One parent affected	16.4
Both parents affected	68.1
Parents	9.3 to 10.3
Grandparents	3.9
Grandchildren	4.3
Nephews and nieces	3.9

match in precision Morgan's studies of drosophila that were to appear eight years later, but it had introduced the practice of reporting a control series, and it had raised the question, "What is the base rate that expresses the prevalence of disorders in the general population?" If, as Diem found, 77 per cent of the *patients* have relatives with some mental illness, this fact could have been published as exciting evidence of genetic factors in mental illness. But when his controls revealed the base rate of 66.9 per cent, the emphasis had to shift to the identifiable difference in rates, to the precise examination techniques, and to the validity of the evidence upon which the small difference had to rest.

Diem's study also showed the importance of going beyond "taints in general." Selecting patients with the more severe psychoses from his total list, he found that psychoses occurred three times more frequently among their relatives than among the relatives of nonpsychotic controls (45.9 per cent as against 15.1 per cent). Apoplexy, on the contrary, appeared with a greater frequency among the nonpsychotic's relatives than among the relatives of the psychotic (18.4 per cent as against 5.5 per cent). And for this "unwanted" finding he could offer no good explanation. The same contrary trend, weakening the geneticist's expectations, was observed for senile dementia. Diem's study also showed that a direct inheritance of taint (from parent to offspring) occurred more frequently in the psychotic group.

When we turn to the more recent studies of family correlations, two changes emerge: (1) the studies tend to be concerned with specific illnesses, or with bits of behavior that can be operationally defined and measured; and (2) they specify the precise degree of correlation that is found between identical twins, dizygotic twins, siblings, and parents. These refinements have resulted in more precise statements about the inheritance of mental disorder, with high correla-

TABLE 2. *Probability of Schizophrenia in Dizygotic and Monozygotic Twins of Schizophrenics.* (Data taken from Fuller and Thompson 1960, p. 276.)

Author of Study	Dizygotic		Monozygotic	
	No.	Probability (Per Cent)	No.	Probability (Per Cent)
Luxenburger (1928, 1930)	60	3.3	21	66.6
Rosanoff *et al.* (1934)	101	14.9	41	68.3
Essen-Möller (1941)	24	16.7	7	71.4
Slater (1953)	115	14.0	41	76.0
Kallmann (1938 to 1953)	685	14.5	268	86.2

tions revealed for some types of illness, and with mere chance correlations revealed for others.

Kallmann's Study of Schizophrenia[3]

Kallmann's studies began to appear in 1938 and have continued into the present decade. His first studies dealt with patients who had been admitted to hospital between 1893 and 1902. His records of 691 pairs of twins, published in 1945, were drawn from a total resident population of 73,252 cases hospitalized in New York State. Table 1 shows the frequencies of schizophrenia in the relatives of patients (probands). Even the step-siblings show a higher rate of incidence of the disorder (1.8 per cent) than is usually found in the general population (0.5 to 1.4 per cent).

Kallmann's data show that the highest correlation is found between identical twins (86.2 per cent), whereas the figure for dizygotic twins (14.5 per cent) is not greater than for siblings in general. Thus in these "experiments of nature" in which the gene systems are identical, a psychosis in one identical twin is matched by a psychosis in the other twin in almost nine cases out of ten! Four other investigators (see Table 2) have published values for correlations between identical twins that are slightly lower than Kallmann's figures, but in each case they support his insistence on the great difference between the cor-

[3]Schizophrenia, a term introduced by Bleuler, has come to replace dementia praecox, a term in vogue when Kallmann's basic data for his first studies were being collected. The patients placed in this new category were described as lacking in emotional responsiveness, as showing inappropriate mood, as responding with silly and bizarre behavior. A progressive disintegration or regression in behavior that frequently ended in a dementia, or a complete withdrawal into a world of fantasy, may also occur. On the other hand, patients diagnosed as schizophrenic may be discharged from hospital as social recoveries and never suffer further attacks. There are all degrees of arrests and remissions among the total schizophrenic population. The fixed onset-course-outcome that Kraepelin once looked for has not proved to be everywhere present within this broadened category. Indeed, the present category is so inclusive that various investigators have wanted to subdivide it into as many as twenty-two varieties. Thus the very measure of the disorder that obtained when Kallmann's studies began has stretched until today it includes borderline cases that are near-normal. The inclusion of such borderline cases undoubtedly alters whatever correlations an investigator finds.

TABLE 3. *Correlations between Types of Neurotic Disorders in Patients and in Their Relatives.* (According to Brown 1942; taken from Fuller and Thompson 1960, p. 295.)

Type of Disorder of Patients	Per Cent of Affected Relatives					
	Anxiety Neurotics		Hysterics		Obsessionals	
	Parents	Sibs	Parents	Sibs	Parents	Sibs
Anxiety neurotics	21.4	12.3	1.6	2.2	0	0.9
Hysterics	9.5	4.6	19.0	6.2	0	0
Obsessionals	0	5.4	0	0	7.5	7.1

relations for siblings and dizygotic twins and those for identical twins. In one of his reports Kallmann presented figures for identical twins reared together in the same home. He contrasted the correlation for these pairs (which was 91.5 per cent) with that for twins reared apart (which was 77.6 per cent) in homes whose dissimilarity, unfortunately, he could not measure.

Studies of the Neurotic Patient and His Family

The neuroses, which are usually counted less severe than schizophrenia, and which assume such divergent forms that some psychiatrists despair of finding one accurate definition that will cover this group of disorders with any precision,[4] have been studied with a view to finding family correlations similar to those found by Kallmann.

Brown (1942) has studied patients that had been placed into three diagnostic categories. He showed (see Table 3) that the parents and siblings of these patients were more likely to have a history of the same (or a similar) illness than to have either of the other two forms of neurosis. This fact argues that there is something specific in the genetic constitution which breaks down in a particular way. If the members of a family could be characterized as having a certain life style and as training their young to assume a similar outlook on the world and a similar type of action, Brown's figures could point to a kind of

---

[4]Karl Menninger wrote, in a recent popular article, "I hold that the words *neurosis, psychoneurosis, psychopathic personality,* and the like are valueless....I do not use them, and I try to prevent my students from using them, although the latter effort is almost futile once the young psychiatrist discovers how conveniently ambiguous these terms really are" (*National Observer,* Feb. 11, 1963, p. 20). Oskar Diethelm (1950), in a section dealing with the psychotherapy for these disorders, admits that the term *psychoneurosis* is unsatisfactory. When he uses it as a chapter heading, it is to designate anxieties, obsessive-compulsive behavior, hysteria, phobias, and concerns about the body's appearance and its somat'c functions. Gould's pocket medical dictionary defines neurosis tersely as "a nervous affection without lesion." Since there has been no significant observation of the nerves of neurotics, this is defining what we observe in terms of what we have not seen. Blakiston's longer definition emphasizes that they are *functional disorders,* and then adds the gratuitous and confusing information that they have a "nonorganic basis." Although the disorder of functioning might be expected to be reversible, some neurotic conditions are resistant to therapy and persist throughout life. The comment on nonorganic basis merely indicates that no known basis can be identified, rather than that a supra- or infra-organic base is known. In this respect neuroses are like schizophrenia, which is also of unknown origin.

TABLE 4. *Correlations of Neuroticism and Intelligence Scores for Monozygotic and Dizygotic Twins.* (From Eysenck and Prell 1951.)

Scores	Correlations	
	Monozygotic	*Dizygotic*
Intelligence	0.905	0.67
Neuroticism	0.851	0.217

social heredity, a transmission by learning. They do not have the weight, as evidence, that Kallmann's studies of identical twins and siblings do, for example. Brown found a higher correlation between parents and offspring than between siblings, whereas the higher correlations in Kallmann's study of schizophrenia, as Table 1 shows, were between siblings.

A second study (Eysenck and Prell 1951) approached the problem of heredity by means of a statistical correlation technique. In an effort to identify particular traits (since the major categories that divide the neuroses into syndromes are rather vague), Eysenck developed a battery of tests that would identify and measure precise bits of behavior. Those traits which he counted as neurotic signs were revealed by measures of suggestibility, perseveration, static ataxia, judgment discrepancy, rigidity. As these tests were developed and applied to patients, Eysenck found evidence of a correlation with a clinical estimate of the patients' neuroticism (whatever this term may have meant to those making the diagnosis). The correlations of the individual items with the clinical estimate were not high; only three were higher than 0.40, and some were as low as 0.05. Thus the battery of tests which Eysenck chose as a good measure of neuroticism contained some items that were poor measures if the clinical estimate was to be trusted.[5]

Administering these tests to twins, both monozygotic and dizygotic, along with conventional intelligence tests (widely accepted as measures of native capacity), he was able to show that his measures of neurotic traits yielded high correlations between monozygotic pairs (0.85), whereas the comparable value for the dizygotic pairs was 0.22. Placing his values beside the values obtained from the intelligence scores, we can see why Eysenck concluded that the neuroticism he measured behaved as other genetically determined traits do (see Table 4).

A Summary with a Caution

Recent genetic studies have tended to shy away from any attempt to measure the transmission of such vague entities as "neuropathic diathesis," "psychopathic taint," or "neurotic personality." Precision in diagnosis and in measurement

---

[5]In order to duplicate Eysenck's study, one would have to use his precise measures for the traits. Other tests of suggestibility, for example, correlate poorly with his measures; and the same would probably hold for the other traits.

has revealed a few clear relationships that, hopefully, may do something to clear away present confusion. We now ask an investigator to prove that his figures, intended to show that a common genetic factor is at work affecting the relatives and the patients, demonstrate a relationship higher than could be obtained from a sample of random pairs taken from the general population. We now know the base rates for some of these clusters of symptoms. He must also show the precise figures for specific family relationships: parent-child, sibling-sibling, dizygotic twins, and monozygotic twins. And the correlation for the monozygotic twins must be higher than that for the other relationships.

The samples of data which we have presented represent some of the more convincing work. Even these studies have been found to be open to certain reproaches. Pastore (1949a, 1949b) has pointed out that the basic data which Kallmann reworked, as statistician, were obtained between 1893 and 1902, when diagnostic procedures were less than adequate. Records for the probands were sketchy, and the data on the relatives more so. As a result, the records had to be assessed according to the educated guess of a research worker with a hypothesis to prove. Borderline cases could be placed inside or outside the schizophrenic territory according to hunches that other investigators might not have shared; and the borderlines of schizophrenia are notoriously foggy. Pastore also discovered errors in reporting findings, as when a 10.4 per cent correlation is given for parents and patients when the relation was with all ancestors. These and other methodological weaknesses suggest that Kallmann's figures may have to be revised downward, even though his basic conclusion is supported by other workers whose findings are not subject to the same criticisms. New and more critical studies may revise all figures downward (or upward) as the enthusiasm of investigators is corrected by improved methods.

Although loose in diagnosis and with occasional lapses in their mathematical summaries, the reports of Eysenck look like the ultimate in precision: his tests are objective and reproducible, and his statistical reliabilities usually satisfy the mathematician. Yet the meaning of his tests must rest upon their correlation with that familiar old criterion, clinical judgment, which is comfortably loose and vague, and the correlations between the items that he has selected and such clinical judgments are not always impressive, nor are all of his items of acceptable validity; suggestibility $_{Brown}$ is not the same as suggestibility $_{Eysenck}$, and some highly suggestible persons (defined as suggestible because they can be hypnotized with ease) have no more than their share of other neurotic traits. Eysenck's study shows, therefore, that twins are similar in certain precisely measured behavioral traits, but what this resemblance has to do with mental illness is less certain. The individual traits are measured with some precision, but those larger significant shapes we have been calling "the neurotic personality" are most elusive.

EPILEPSY: ILLUSTRATING THE NEED FOR DISCRIMINATING DIAGNOSIS

Epilepsy is a much more clearly defined disorder than either "psychoneurosis" or "neuropathic diathesis." Although some schizophrenics are so severely disorganized that no one can mistake them for normals, schizophrenia has borderline, ambulatory, and pseudoneurotic forms that shade into near-normal forms that are more difficult to identify. Compared to such a disorder, epilepsy seems precisely identifiable; when it takes the explosive form of the *grand mal* attack it is unmistakable. Even the more hidden *petit mal,* which may involve no more than momentary blackouts, yields to modern diagnostic techniques, for it writes its unmistakable signature on the electroencephalogram (see Fig. 11, Chapter 9).

Are these attacks related to some inherited weakness? The somewhat analogous susceptibility to audiogenic seizures that can be segregated and propagated in genetically pure strains of laboratory mice seems to be. Are there some few inherited types of the disorder, and some other forms that are traceable to other causes: metabolic disorders, environmental stress, brain injuries? Must our understanding of this class of disorders differentiate between those types which have endogenous causes that are not related to genetic factors and those that are clearly inherited? What light do the studies of family correlations throw on these questions?

Taking up the last question first, we can answer with precise figures. Relatives of epileptics suffer from seizures in 2.8 per cent of the recorded cases. *This rate is more than five times the frequency with which epilepsy appears in the general population.* Among some 12,119 relatives of the 2,000 patients whose records he examined, Lennox found more than 300 with records of seizures. The data from the 1917 draft population suggest that only one in 200 young males is afflicted. Stating the relationship in another way: less than a fifth of the patients have a family history of epilepsy. Therefore, Lennox concludes, "seizures are not inherited, but only the tendency to seizures" (Lennox, Gibbs, and Gibbs 1940).

Studies of epilepsy in twins have found a correlation of 52 per cent for monozygotic twins, but of only 12 per cent for dizygotic twins. These figures are based upon a study of all types of epilepsy of whatever cause. If the pure form (called idiopathic epilepsy) is isolated, the correlation for identical twins runs up to 86.3 per cent. Where the epileptic attacks in one twin have followed a brain injury, their identical twins, where found, show a correlation of only 15.8 per cent.[6] This last figure is still very high compared with the base rate for epilepsy in the general population, and for this reason some clinicians have argued that when overt attacks of epilepsy follow brain damage, the patient has a genetically determined susceptibility to seizures.[7]

---

[6]Cobb (1943) refers to the electroencephalograms of 77 pairs of twins. In five identical pairs where one twin had epilepsy and the other was judged normal, the epileptic twin had suffered a brain injury in each case. The normal twin, when studied, was found to have abnormal brain waves also, but the condition was subclinical and no attacks had been experienced. Penfield and Jasper (1954, p. 301) report a study of 33 patients from whom cerebral abcesses were removed by surgery, and of whom eight developed seizures. Their search, where carried out, for correlative data in relatives was unsuccessful. (See also Rosanoff, Handy, and Rosanoff 1934.)

[7]This point has been challenged by Penfield and his associates, and will be discussed in Chapter 9.

An additional set of clinical and experimental studies adds further weight to the geneticist's hypothesis. Although the clinically observable forms of epilepsy are found in less than 0.5 per cent of the population, abnormal brain waves (subclinical but similar to both those found during epileptic seizures and those found between seizures) are found in from 10 to 15 per cent of the general population, in 60 per cent of the relatives of patients with overt epilepsy, and in all those identical twins (who themselves have no overt attacks) of epileptic parents. Some clinicians are led to speak, therefore, of a latent form of epilepsy, of an epileptic constitution. Whether this abnormal electroencephalogram can also be related to other behavioral traits that might make up an epileptic personality type is a research problem for which we have no good answers as yet, although many clinicians have gone on record asserting that such a type exists.

STUDIES OF INDIVIDUAL PAIRS OF TWINS

There are a great many studies of individual pairs of twins in the literature. Whether each pair that is called identical is so in fact is not always clearly established, but even where the evidence seems complete and their genetic identity is established, there are three things we have to bear in mind: (1) There are frequently such large gaps in the records that revelant data may not have been considered. Too much has to be left to conjecture. (2) The reports often include so much varied and sometimes irrelevant data that the reader is tempted to advance ad hoc hypotheses. The essential relations are sometimes obscured, and the lack of statistically impressive samples and of controls prevents one from discovering precisely which relationships are essential. Thus the studies are often worth more as an example than as a proof. (3) Clinicians who report these studies frequently have a point of view or a theory to substantiate. Knowing just how exceptional a single case is depends on our obtaining statistically impressive series.

In spite of these limitations, the concrete data in these studies have enriched our understanding, even when they create more questions than they answer. Consider the following case reports.

Schizophrenic Twins: Anna and Emma

This study, reported in Landis and Bolles 1950 (pp. 315-16), is from the series gathered by Kallmann. The twins were born in 1894. What kind of mothering they had prior to separation, we do not know, nor do we know to what degree the two environments into which the separated twins were placed diverged. Born to a mother who had been both psychotic and tubercular, the twins were taken away from her when nine months old. At the end of their second year they were placed in separate foster homes. One completed high school and taught in country schools; the other finished the eighth grade only, and then worked as a domestic servant. At age 24 both showed marked changes in personality. Emma was admitted to hospital when she was 26. Anna was returned to the farm of her father, now remarried. There she grew so irritable, suspicious, sarcastic, and seclusive during the next three years that she finally had to be hospitalized. Both twins were in hospital at the time of the study, and both had progressed to an advanced and chronic state of deterioration.

What causes may have operated in this case (defective mothering prior to separation, a genetic weakness, a combination of events that operated in childhood and adolescence, or some unrecorded illness in early infancy), we cannot know precisely. To Kallmann, and to those who are persuaded on other grounds that the genetic factor is primary, this case offers a striking demonstration of the way in which inherited factors can unfold with the precision of some biological clock, carrying these separated sisters into hospital at the same point in their lives.

Schizophrenia in One Identical Twin

Even where the correlation between identical twins is as high as 85 per cent, as Kallmann found, there are individual pairs who show marked divergence in development, and these too are worth study.

A. and B. were brothers, so identical in appearance that the physician who had attended their birth and had treated them until they were grown had never been able to tell them apart. He had noted that there was a single placenta at their birth. Blue-eyed, weighing 161 and 162 as adults, they had grown up together, followed similar interests, had similar, strong religious convictions. A., who became schizophrenic, had pneumonia when six years old. Both youths developed a hearing loss on the left side. At graduation from high school the twins separated. B. accepted the offer of an uncle and went to Detroit, where he earned good wages as a carpenter, machinist, and cabinetmaker, saved his money, and went into an engineering school. A., the patient, stayed at home, drifted from one odd job to another, suffered an injury to his right eye while sharpening a tool, and developed a cataract that made him partially blind in that eye. He grew deeply religious. He also conceived the notion that he could write, but his manuscripts were returned to him. And he grew suspicious: some person or organization was persecuting him. Believing that he was followed, he fled to Boston. Without funds, he turned to dishwashing and took a series of temporary jobs. Finally he drifted to New York. There he was recognized by a sister who had become a successful department-store manager. She persuaded him to return home. Still haunted by his imaginary persecutors, he complained to the police; and on their advice the family had him committed to hospital, where he was diagnosed as schizophrenic. He remained in hospital for two years, and was discharged when one of the many attempts to reestablish him on the outside finally succeeded.

The healthy twin had always been described as the more active member of the pair. Vigorous, extroverted, he made a successful life (or should we say: "Life smiled upon him"?) His business ventures prospered; he even weathered the onset of the depression of the thirties. [Adapted from Kasanin 1934, p. 27.]

In the one twin a childhood illness, a hearing loss, an injury to an eye that resulted in partial blindness, a drifter's lack of success, and a series of episodes that built and cumulatively validated a false interpretation, all conspired to land him in hospital, where the diagnostic label *schizophrenia* was written into the record. This twin stayed back while his brother made a successful voyage into adulthood, and his clinging to the safety of home makes us wonder about a special dependent relationship to one of the parents which may have existed without being entered into the record. Even if we were to accept a hypothetical "schizophrenic-process-determining" gene in both twins, we would be forced to find the "pathology that made the difference" in those transactions with the environment which built a paranoid weakness in the one twin. His brother had an identical genetic constitution, but other healthful transactions produced an accumulating strength in him.[8]

In addition to the apparent causes of divergent development that this record shows, there may have been unreported events that were crucial. As will be noted below (p. 52), differences in the attitudes of parents toward one of a pair of twins can produce radical differences in development.

Twins and Suicide: Homer and Elmer

The records of 2,500 pairs of twins examined by Kallmann and Anastasia (1946) revealed only 11 suicides. In no pair did both twins commit suicide; three of the pairs containing a suicidal member were judged to be identicals. Just how similar the pair can be in all respects save this one is indicated in the record which follows.

Homer and E'mer came from an old New England family. Reared together, they had the same friends, similar interests, similar musical talents, and similar good performance in school. Trained to be teachers, both ended long careers as high-school principals in the same county. Homer had three children, Elmer three. Homer's wife was a little less thrifty, Elmer's was less selfish and better adjusted to married life. Both wives complained that the twins were closer to each other than to their spouses.

Both twins developed a mild tubercular lesion at 52, and both became restless, anxious, self-absorbed, dissatisfied with teaching and home conditions, forgetful, irritable. Both were hospitalized for a "nervous breakdown" at this period. Both recovered, Elmer more completely. Homer found his wife discontented and quarrelsome; he had to borrow money from his slightly more prosperous brother. Readmitted to a mental hospital with signs of an agitated depression, he was diagnosed "psychosis with arteriosclerosis." Discharged after six months, Homer seemed on the way to recovery, but a short time thereafter he drowned himself in a lake near his twin brother's home. His brother was prostrated with grief, for a while. Recovering, Elmer moved to another community, and, at 70, though depressed, seemed resigned to his melancholy lot.

---

[8]The skeptic may even question the validity of a diagnostic process which sometimes labels "drifters" and other "problem cases" as psychotic as a way of: (1) avoiding our shared responsibility for these cases of atypical development, (2) fooling ourselves into thinking we have provided all of the rehabilitation and therapy needed, or (3) relieving a family of its responsibility. The label helps us forget such cases and soothes our consciences with the illusion that there are adequate human resources in these institutions to accomplish what we have not. In a book which some have found marred by errors and by the author's heated polemic, Thomas Szasz (1965) has emphasized these "institutional errors." Any mislabeling produced by these motives would, if applied to only one of a pair of twins, produce evidence that would not fit in with the geneticist's hypothesis.

The historian of a culture sometimes deals with such varied data as the mean annual rainfall, crop failures, birth rates, ethnic composition, political parties and leaders, cultural goals, the morale of a ruling class, and their response to a challenge from below. The effort to weave a consistent and understandable theory or pattern of relationships is made difficult by the fact that the patterns he finds seldom recur. The "laws of history" have a way of turning out to be ad hoc analyses that do not fit, precisely, other cultures and other periods. His sequences are frequently more dramatic and charged with evaluations, more a matter of myth-making or of the poetry of human existence, than logically tight and convincing "scientific" expositions. He is repeatedly tempted to develop his hypotheses around striking events that stand out clearly. In our present pair of histories, a clinician (particularly one whose own family life contained conflicts) might be moved to say, "Poor fellow, if Homer had only had a wife like his brother's, he would have recovered from his depression, and there would have been no suicide." We recall the nursery rhyme about the battle that was lost, all because of a twopenny nail. Certainly there had to be some twopenny nail in Homer's life, some nongenetic cause, for behavior is caused, is it not?

The case of Homer and Elmer is as exceptional as that of Anna and Emma; it contributes to the environmentalist's rather than to the geneticist's interpretation. Perhaps we should conclude that the cause of a particular mental illness lies in whatever makes a difference, including such states as "a loss of nerve," which can arise from a multiplicity of causes, and that unanalyzed cause we call "spirit" or "will," which rises to meet a challenge, or surrenders, hopeless, or runs away.[9]

MONGOLIAN IDIOCY:
A SPECIAL TYPE OF GENETIC INFLUENCE

Mongolian idiocy is comparatively rare, occurring in one out of 410 births. These children are born "unfinished," and the upper limit of their mental development is between two and five years of age. For several decades clinicians have looked for the causes of this developmental arrest in some prenatal factor, such as glandular deficiency of the mother or uterine conditions which affect foetal development, or in other physiological factors supplied by the maternal environment, for these abnormal births occur more frequently in older mothers, as they near the end of their reproductive period. For example, for mothers between ages 20 and 24 the incidence of mongolian idiocy is eight in 10,000 births. For mothers between 40 and 44, the rate rises to 420 in 10,000; and for mothers over 50, the chances have risen to one in four. (Øster 1953, Benda 1946).[10]

We now know that mongolian children have an extra chromosome that is produced during an imperfect separation of these trait-bearers at gameto-

---

[9]An interesting example of the historian's effort to grapple with this problem is Toynbee's analysis of the problem of "Challenge and Response" (1961, pp. 254-262).

[10]Benda also cites a series of mongolian births in which, out of 255 cases, 59 per cent of the mothers were 35 years or older.

genesis. Although the environment of the foetus, in the older mothers and in those who have frequently aborted, may have something to do with this basic pathology, its role is not yet clear. It does not always act upon both members of a pair of twins if the two are dizygotic; one may be mongolian, the other normal (Morris and MacGillvray 1953). In identicals both are mongolian if one is affected. This chromosomal accident, which blights development, is not a repetition of a similar accident in the parents, nor will it be transmitted. Thus, we have a genetically determined development that is not inherited.

A CHEMIST LOOKS AT GENE THEORY

"I am sure," writes Linus Pauling (1956), "that most mental disease is chemical in origin, and that the chemical abnormalities involved are usually the result of abnormalities in the genetic constitution of the individual." Such assurance gives us pause, when it is voiced by a Nobel Prize winner. Another chemist might urge, "We are what we eat," and he would be interested in the dietary habits of a culture, its consumption of fats, and its blood-cholesterol levels. Such a chemist might envision dietary controls that would affect the rate of incidence of mental illness. We shall later see another chemically minded therapist proposing a treatment for schizophrenia that involves heavy dosage with niacin. Pauling, however, is speaking of the little chemical packets that act as the organizers of growth and development, the genes, and there are facts which support his emphasis on the power of these inner chemical determiners.

Consider phenylpyruvic oligophrenia, a form of mental retardation that arises in the child because of defective genes, so that the child lacks an enzyme that normally catalyzes an oxidation reaction which converts the amino acid phenylalanine into tyrosine. As a consequence, the child develops a defective integrative system: he cannot profit from experience, form conditioned reflexes in normal fashion, reason, speak, or solve the problems created by his needs and by the pressures from his environment as other children do.[11]

Or consider the abnormal molecules in the hemoglobin, found in sickle-cell anemia. This disorder, which occurs almost exclusively in Negroes (10 per cent of whom have these sickle-shaped cells), could also spring from a genetic factor that is responsible for these odd molecular structures. Are not other, macroscopic bodily structures controlled by the genes?

These efforts to link the genes with chemical and structural abnormalities are matched by current efforts to relate psychotic behavior to body chemistry, an effort that has received an enormous boost from the discovery of psychotomimetic drugs, such as psilocybin or lysergic acid diethylamide. In the study of schizophrenia, controversy has centered around some of the products of the adrenal glands (and their derivatives, adrenochrome and adrenolutin). When we remember that the secretions of the adrenal, thyroid, and pituitary bodies

---

[11]The *New York Times* (Jan. 4, 1965) reports a new law that requires a blood test for all babies born in New York State. One out of 12,000 babies is affected by phenylketonuria. A simple blood test reveals the presence of this chemical imbalance, which, untreated, produces permanent brain damage within the first month of life. A simple test, costing less than half a dollar to administer, and a special diet low in phenylalanine can circumvent the deficiency.

are responsible for many of the symptoms of stress, we begin to see how a gene that affects these glands might alter their secretions (or their resynthesis) enough to change the person's capacity to adjust to the pressures of the environment. Such a chain of consequences springing from a gene-produced glandular abnormality might provide some of the missing links between the statistical measures of correlation, such as Kallmann has found, and those behavioral trends we diagnose as psychotic. So long as the latter must be called "diseases of unknown origin" (in our present state of ignorance), we cannot afford to discard these hypotheses without careful study of the possibilities.

It is natural, perhaps, that a chemist should look upon the organism as a complex chemical factory, and use his own language to describe the chemical aspect of all manner of actions. Is there not a chemistry of digestion, of fatigue, of the reproductive hormones? Why not a chemistry of inspiration, of despair, of mental exhaustion and boredom? The linkages between the genes and the final products will, no doubt, prove to be complex, and subject to various environmental effects which distort them. While the chemist is trying to reduce the language of the behaviorist to what he regards as a more basic plane, the psychologist and the existentialist will keep setting new problems for him, until he too can begin to consider the ways his molecules must behave in these larger, macroscopic dimensions. At the moment, we need many languages other than that of the chemist to grapple with the "factors which make a difference."[12]

FROM GENES TO BEHAVIOR

When the French psychiatrists Deschamps (1919), Hartenberg (1921), and Janet (1903) tried to characterize a group of their patients as "sensitives," or as "*timides*," or as lacking in a normal psychological tension, they considered the possibility of inheritance, even at that date when modern gene theory had not been developed. These patients they were called upon to treat seemed to lack some vital force, some integrative power, some willpower (or courage to be) that the normal person possesses. Experiences that might have toughened another person had made them increasingly emotional. Their interests were turned inward; they grew preoccupied with fantasies, engrossed in speculation, while outwardly they settled into a morose inaction. Introspective, often idealistic, they seemed to be a separate breed from their more practical fellows. They blushed, suffered from a social neurosis (abnormal shyness), showed mixtures of envy, hate, contempt, and feelings of both inferiority and superiority toward

---

[12]As he examined the development (and death) of civilizations, Toynbee found that he had to avoid the "apathetic fallacy" as well as anthropomorphism and all mystification. It is as serious an error to restrict oneself to the language of physics and chemistry in describing human behavior, as it is to limit oneself to the shaman's language of "invading spirits." In our effort to avoid all mystification, all psychoanalogy and vague holism, we can commit the opposite error of confining all of our descriptions to physiological, chemical, and physical aspects, as though consciousness and human personality did not exist, or as if existences were *merely* matter in motion. We can squeeze the drama out of existence in our struggle for objectivity, and in our very efforts to help the faltering spirits among us, we can deprive them of decision, choice, awareness, and that vital spark of spirit that remains.

their tougher contemporaries. They saw crudity and vulgarity in power; ideal-
izing their own sensitive egos, they allied themselves with the persecuted, the
exploited, the humiliated, the crucified, or at least some of them did.

When these "sensitives" were evaluated by their families and friends, they
were often described as dull, inhibited, neurotic, withdrawn, or as egocentric,
selfish, complaining, hypochondriacal, childish, or a few, as demanding, tyrannical, paranoid. However they appeared to these outside judges, these "sensitives" would no doubt have written a quite different evaluation of themselves:
some would have outdone their accusers as the guilty and depressed are apt to
do; others would have claimed for themselves the special privilege that "the
elect" have always claimed. In the obsessive, as we shall see, this mixture of
inferiority and superiority is common. Alfred Adler was to emphasize the one
side of this mixture, seeing both the inferiority and the compensation for the
inferiority as springing from a central psychosexual root.

These "sensitives" provide us with three classes of facts:

1. Careful study of their development reveals that they are surrounded by
environing conditions which nurture and shape their particular life styles. Some
have stressed the "tenderizing" influence of maternal overprotection; others
have pointed to a strict Catholic (or mid-Victorian) education. Interacting with
whatever genetic peculiarities may exist, these causal conditions do not fit any
single simple formula. Although today's clinician will certainly look upon such
behavior as caused, he is frequently at odds with his colleagues when he tries to
identify the essential factor or trace development through typical sequences
which produce the individual combinations of traits. From the gene to the outcome there is no simple straight line of relationships.

2. The organism, with its measurable set of capacities, emerges, finally, as
a person with observable ways of interacting with other persons. These persons
with unique histories, subjected to multiple causal factors, are the ones who
enter the clinic to challenge the therapist to make a clear and consistent account
of how they got that way. Like the biographer and historian who have to weave
together a plausible tale out of the scraps of information available, and who
frequently dramatize and emphasize in order to make the account interesting
and credible, the clinician is also an artist, justifying, evaluating, projecting, and
expressing his own values, even when he is also objective and factual.

3. A person's account of his own actions may include his attempt to understand how he came to be, an attempt which is not always accurate and which
can complicate and even worsen his struggle. The self thus not only lives a
history, in the sense of enduring a series of forced responses, it views that history, organizes its own account of it so as to justify and defend its actions, and
may even react *against* the image of the self that forms in awareness. In *The
Hound of Heaven* Francis Thompson put the accusing words in the mouth of
his pursuer:

> "And human love needs human meriting:
> How hast thou merited—
> Of all man's clotted clay the dingiest clot?"

Occasionally, overwhelmed by the judgment of significant others, he accepts their version of his doings, his guilt, his triumphs, his virtues, his defects (even as some of the witches accepted the accusations of their judges as true). More often the self defends itself against these judges, or calls on God to be its witness and to judge its accusers harshly in return, or withdraws in a hurt but lofty isolation, a suffering hero in deep need of both human understanding and professional help.

When, as psychologists, we try to take into account the rich and complex inner life of the person, placing it against the social matrix that has challenged, molded, threatened, and supported him, we begin to see that, important as they are, the raw materials first organized by gene substances are subject to social and interpersonal controls; the emerging self is formed into a many-layered structure with a grand upper story that looks out into a field. It was down in the very foundations of this structure that the tiny chemical packets, the genes, began their work. Their influence will be woven, of course, into the texture of each of the upper stories of controls. In man especially, the social nexus, and that slow maturing process during which the family's shaping influence is at work, give opportunity for a steady dialogue between the developing inner commentator and the objective forces. The gradually forming ego reacts continuously to the gap between what is happening and what it had hoped for; and these charged feelings of hope and disappointment make its reactions anything but simple mathematical functions of the objective conditions at any given moment. The genes undoubtedly play their part in the sensitive's reactions, in his emotionality, but they alone do not set up the distant goals that orient and charge the individual's actions and subsequently give rise to frustrations, nor do they specify in advance the kinds of self-evaluation which must arise in that upper, conscious, vigilant level of the self-structure.

One might speak of first-level responses in referring to reflexes, including those bodily reverberations that penetrate to glands and viscera. Second-level responses would be conditioned reflexes and habits, which emerge as the first-level reflexes are integrated into larger patterns, which in turn regulate and channel these parts. The third level in our structure of behavior arises as soon as the human being begins to look before he leaps, to hold back incipient reactions, to evaluate the more remote consequences with feeling. At this third level the "person in an extended field" will normally dominate his habits, while they in turn regulate his reflexes. It is at this third level that our language begins to describe the personality.

It is the absence of any simple one-to-one relationship between the gene-determined bodily structure and the structure of action of a "person in a field" that we are here emphasizing. The "epileptic gene"—if we can speak of such a thing—that was at work within Dostoevsky did not determine his outlook on Russian society, or provide anything more than grist for his mill when he fashioned his characters, or account for his creativity. As a kind of "thorn in the flesh," his susceptibility may have sharpened his compassion for the perplexed of this world in a peculiar way, but no critic of his art would dream of making this "thorn" the secret of his genius.

In an analogous way the genes might have something to do with a schizophrenic's aloofness, supplying (as some suspect) defective or excessive hormones or enzymes, but they do not provide an adequate account of, say, his delusion of Messiahship. To understand this inner awareness, we must construct a personal history, and employ our understanding of how the great myths of a culture operate. We may have to include disease processes, evaluate the effects of infections, estimate the current pressures at work upon the man. Even his faulty diet may have to be worked into the story. And the end-product may be a patchwork of odds and ends that rivals the sign carried by a beggar: "Crimean war veteran, battles nine, wounds six, children five, total 20." It would be a neat logical device that could project each and every event upon some one-language baseline so that, with appropriate programing, a computer could integrate a patient's formula.

Divergent Development of Twins

Even where the evidence is strongest in support of a genetic factor in mental illness, as in the identical-twin studies, some degree of divergence appears. In schizophrenia in twins, studies have shown that somewhere between 10 and 30 per cent of the samples deal with one identical who has the illness and a twin who failed to develop the disorder. The divergence can begin to appear even in the prenatal period: the blood supplies may differ, for at birth one twin is usually heavier than the other. The disease history of the two is seldom identical: one twin may suffer from measles, typhoid, pneumonia, spasms, while the other twin is spared. Different life experiences may operate, cumulatively, to increase these congenital and disease-produced constitutional factors, until that total power to resist and master environmental pressures is markedly different in the two.

Some pairs of twins are encouraged to dress differently, and to develop different interests and friendships. Knowing that the day of separation must come, and hoping to develop an autonomy in advance, the families may work to assist in this process of ego-differentiation. It has been clear, in some case studies, that the pressure to differentiate may exist before the birth of a child, as when a parent desires a child of a particular sex, and is disappointed, but selects one to fulfill this desire. A recent study of twins (Rainer *et al.* 1960) in which only one member of each pair was homosexual offered an opportunity to test the gene concept and to search for possible parental attitudes which may have influenced these divergent outcomes.

Using a specimen from the mucous lining of the mouth, the chromosomal sex of each patient and twin was studied. All showed a normal genetic makeup. No significant differences in body build, genitals, or endocrine glands were found, so these were eliminated as possible sources of divergent outcome. The interview data obtained from the twins and from their families were suggestive, however. From these findings the research team selected the following items for emphasis:

1. Fantasies and wishes of the parents were found concerning the anticipated sex of the twins. One mother admitted that she had longed for a son

but had been given a pair of daughters. She had allocated to one of these girls the task of fulfilling her wishes. A second mother felt that she had been responsible for distorting the development of one of her twins in this same fashion.

2. Attitudes toward a difficult birth made one mother blame (and reject as a consequence) the second twin, ascribing her invalidism to him. She favored the other twin, who was weaker. This favored twin developed maleness and a stronger ego.

3. In the naming of the child one family betrayed an expectation of maleness. The girl, a disappointment to a mother who had wanted a boy, was called Roberta; and she was trained as though she were the Robert hoped for. A name may help to identify a child with a grandparent or other relative whose sex role influences the sex-typing of the child.

4. Parental efforts to distinguish identical twins may fasten upon very small differences and raise them to a position of importance. When these markings also couple a child with a preferred or nonpreferred parent, making him the object of either unusual affection or rejection, the sex role may be similarly affected.

5. Parental attitudes and practices may include encouragement to play with dolls, to play the piano as mother did, to learn dancing, or discouragement of all participation in rough sports. When these encouragements run counter to the genetic sex, homosexual trends are started. One father recognized the fact that he had a girlish son as early as the latter's sixth year. One girl had been encouraged to find companionship with boys; she participated in their games, became a skillful baseball player, rejected the dress of a girl, scorned feminine interests. At the onset of menstruation she attempted to deny her sex, and developed delusional ideas about being a male. A physically healthy twin was checked from all expressions of anger against his weaker brother, who had suffered from rheumatic heart disease; the healthy twin, rewarded by his mother's affection, shunned all competitive sports, inhibited all occasions for triumph over the brother, and became a homosexual.

One mother warned her preferred male twin against women and against any attachment that would interfere with his career, encouraged him to study ballet, and produced a homosexual.

DIVERGENCE IN IDENTICAL TRIPLETS

Sontag and Nelson at the Fels Institute published a study (1933a, 1933b) of monozygotic triplets which shows how similar genetic endowment can still result in divergent life styles.

From the beginning, when the children were first brought to the clinic for intensive study, Henry was the aggressive one who got into the pocketbook of the psychologist, upset the order of the clinic, barged into the houses of neighbors, acted as leader in the play-group of children. Aggressive, unabashed at reprimands or punishment, he threw off reproof the way water runs off a duck's back, and showed little or no trace of either improved discrimination or harbored resentment. Henry had been the congenitally weak one of the trio, the one of whom the family almost despaired, at first, and he had been reared with an extra dose of tender, loving care. He became so demanding, finally, that the mother consciously diverted her interests to the middle-sized child, who now seemed to need her the most.

John, the middle-sized child, was soon recognized as "momma's boy"; and he rewarded his mother by his affection, his precocious development in language, his gentler nature, but he was also the sensitive one, and could not be punished by those methods the family used on Henry.

Fred, the largest, placidly went his way; he seemed to need his mother less than John, and was little disturbed when she had to be away.

Henry's transformation from the weakling to the most aggressive one emphasizes the manner in which nongenetic factors can operate. In the barnyard, the runt of the litter is often crowded aside, while the others root in the trough and grow fatter and more aggressive. The runt becomes the weakling, the anxious one that the others can chase away with a bluffing gesture. In Henry's case, the intervention of the mother, who gave him extra attention and care, brought the weakling through infancy until, finally, this extra support had to be withdrawn, but by then he had become the confident and aggressive leader of the trio. His strength was the built-in strength of that twosome, mother and son, and it persisted. Fred became "good old reliable Fred," unruffled when others were angry or frightened, the one who was neither a burden to others nor given to introspective analyses. John, who finally became his mother's "special one," also became the tale-bearer, the thoughtful one, the linguist, the one who could get the cooperation of adults when he was in trouble, the one who was apt to show "the right attitude" toward authority. (An analyst would say that he had introjected more of the maternal attitude into his own superego.)

THE HERMAPHRODITE: GENETIC SEX AND "SEX BY ASSIGNMENT"

The anomalies of sexual development remind us that genetic sex, endocrine sex, genital sex, and the psychosexual behavior of the matured adult do not always coincide. Sometimes, through an error in diagnosis at birth, a child may be assigned to a sex other than the one his body was designed for, and later development (plus surgical interference) then belatedly forces a reassignment. In a study by Money and his associates (1957), 14 of 100 hermaphrodites were reassigned, five later than the third year. The investigators found that only one of these five assumed this new role without conflict.

Coupled with the study by Rainer et al., this study brings additional evidence to show that a process of selection, assignment, role-casting, and training is at work at a very early age. This "basic training" affects those inner attitudes that later become important in the selection of a mate, in the assumption of adult roles and interests, and in attitudes toward the self, the body, and the opposite sex. So quickly and so firmly are these attitudes established that reassignment postponed beyond the fifth year seems difficult to achieve, *even though it operates in the direction favored by the person's genetic endowment.* Money and his associates conclude their report with this comment:

"The sex of assignment and rearing is consistently and conspicuously a more reliable prognosticator of a hermaphrodite's gender role and orientation than is the chromosomal sex, the gonadal sex, the hormonal sex, the accessory internal reproductive morphology, or the ambiguous morphology of the external genitals."[13]

In the clinic where older homosexuals are received for treatment, Money's assessment is supported, in two respects. In the first place, the confirmed homosexual has no intention of changing his outlook or his practices; they are not only natural, he insists, but superior. In the second place, the evidence at hand demonstrates that their patterns have not arisen from atypical chromosomal arrangement. A study by Pritchard (1963), utilizing the most recent methods of studying the chromosomes, eliminated this possibility in each of six cases studied. Perhaps we should be content to limit our generalization, and merely insist that *in the cases studied* interpretation had to seek an explanation of the pattern in some factor or factors other than the genes.

When the adult product of this atypical development is studied, we discover that, to him, his object-choices are *natural,* whereas the object-choices of his "normal" contemporaries seem vulgar and disgusting. Between the genetic endowment and that inner evaluator who passes judgment on the world and on his own reactions to it, experience has interposed a screen: the normal perceptual processes are inverted and convictions carry a kind of absolute quality. He is as prepared to rationalize his conduct as his "normal" brother. Nature is obviously capable of playing tricks on what we had assumed to be Nature, producing psychobiological "sports" that are not viable in the long run.

GENETICS AND PSYCHOTHERAPY

Rationally speaking, there is no good basis for a quarrel between geneticist and environmentalist. The question is: "What are the facts?" or "How heavily should the genetic factor be weighted in this particular case?" The facts become loaded, however, with personal and cultural issues, racial animosities, the struggle against being typed in some subordinate role, the grand myths of a culture (and, in particular, of a despised people). One can see, too, how a psychotherapist, committed to trying to change the lives of the mentally ill, might be angered by an enthusiastic geneticist who asserts not only that mental illnesses are the outcome of genetic defects, but that any attempt to tamper with or extend the reproductive periods of these gene-deficient creatures will merely

---

[13]To which we might add "when the sex is assigned at the very beginning of life." The same assignment made at maturity would not have this force. Here we have more evidence to support the theme: "We are what we are because of things done to us, especially things done early, before self-consciousness dawns. The transplanted ego, the infant reared among the aliens, takes on the tribal outlook of his foster-culture, and wakens to make its strongest assertions in the new vernacular." This imprinting in the beginning seems to have a potency whether it is in line with or opposed to the genetic factors, even when the genetic factors are related to the sex role. That is, in the human being, the relationship between the genes and the sex-typing seems relatively loose. This looseness permits some 2 to 15 per cent of adult males to arrive at roles and attitudes contrary to their genetic sex, and at overt behavior that we call homosexual.

intensify the problems we face as a society. However hospitable a Kallmann may be to a wide range of therapeutic efforts, his assertion, that between identical twins, one of whom is schizophrenic, the studies find a correlation as high as 91 per cent when they are reared together, obviously leaves little room for psychotherapy. He urges, for example (1946b), that:

"Psychiatrically it should be evident that the genetic theory of schizophrenia as it may be formulated on the basis of experiment-like observations with the twin family method, does not confute any psychological concepts of a descriptive or analytical nature, if these concepts are adequately defined and applied. There is no genetic reason why the manifestations of a schizophrenic psychosis should not be described in terms of narcissistic regression or of varying biological changes such as defective homeostasis or general immaturity in the metabolic responses to stimuli. Genetically it is also perfectly legitimate to interpret schizophrenic reactions as the expression either of faulty habit formations or of progressive maladaptation to disrupted family relations. The genetic theory explains only why these various phenomena occur in a particular member of a particular family at a particular time."

This statement did not appease everyone, for although, as he suggests, the genetic theory does not "confute any psychological concepts" of causation, it suggests that these concepts provide something less than the basic reason for the illness that strikes a particular patient.

The facts that we have reviewed seem to indicate that Kallmann's figures for correlations are probably high, and that diagnoses such as schizophrenia, epilepsy, manic-depressive psychosis, or neurosis may have to be broken up into subvarieties, some of which will depend less on genetic factors and some of which will depend upon environmental causes that invite both prevention and therapy. Both the genes and the personal history will continue to be invoked as causal factors, when the whole range of abnormalities is considered. The studies of sex-typing suggest that nongenetic factors can turn out to be the crucial ones despite our tendency to look on sexual behavior as instinctive. As large a factor as it is, the genetic basis of mental illness leaves a great deal of room for a preventive mental hygiene, for psychotherapy, and for all other means of reversing the abnormal trends.

PROPHETS OF DOOM: WEIGHING TRENDS AGAINST A QUALITY OF LIFE

A few theorists, impressed by the large genetic component in mental illness, have suggested that all our humanitarian and therapeutic endeavors may create a steadily deteriorating pool of genes unless we also take countermeasures. We assist the hard of hearing with aids that magnify sounds; we rescue the diabetic with insulin injections; we improve the adjustment of schizophrenic children so that they marry and reproduce their kind. Our humane impulses become entangled in that struggle for life, and as we assist the genetically impaired, we are also making the man of the future. We can almost picture him as rising in the morning to take his tranquilizer (or pep pill), adjust his hearing aid, put in his false teeth, put on his glasses, take an injection for his allergy, make an appointment with his counselor because of troublesome insomnia and hallucinations that his barbiturates have not been able to control. More and more children will require protection against phenylpyruvic oligophrenia, receive dilantin to control *petit mal* seizures, receive dietary supplements for metabolic weaknesses. Considering what medical science has done in adding approximately 40 years to the average life expectancy since the days of the Romans, these gloomy geneticists foresee that, with all of the ailments that afflict the aging, our population will have to run faster and faster to stay alive. We shall spend larger and larger portions of the gross national product to prolong lives that, in turn, will contribute to an expanding pool of bad genes.

It is true that with an altered distribution of ages in our society there is more atherosclerosis and more senile dementia. More men and women living into what we euphemistically call the golden years are now subject to coronary attacks, agitated depressions, and neurotic preoccupations that arise from failing energies and invading microorganisms. The surprising fact is that the rates have not risen for hospitalized mental illness in society as a whole, despite an increase per 100,000 in hospitalizations for age-associated disorders, such as atherosclerosis and late-life deterioration in cerebral functioning. We are at least keeping pace with this problem. Medical science and psychological counseling are also improving, so that we are waging a more effective battle even against those disorders that have genetic causes. It is not clear that the quality of human life is deteriorating because of these humane and therapeutic efforts. It is even possible that the program of the eugenicists, which has not yet been seriously applied, may one day be freely adopted by an educated public, and in some humane way. (See Dubos 1959, A. Huxley 1958, Muller 1956, and Glass 1956.)

Chapter 3 • The Social Factor

For many centuries men have cherished a variety of dreams of that perfect society in which men could live in harmony and which, in turn, would foster the optimum growth of every individual. From each according to his abilities, to each according to his needs! Then men could become all that their nature permits. In trying to sketch that better world, every utopian has implied that his present society has stunted, maimed, distorted the growth potentials of its citizens. And when the utopian thinker has a psychiatric turn of mind, he is likely to name mental illness as one of the products of man's inhumanity to man, produced by a faulty organization of our lives, an evil that, hopefully, will be eliminated when the new order comes.

From Sir Thomas More's *Utopia* to Erich Fromm's *The Sane Society,* descriptions of utopias have hinted at what life in a society *properly organized* could be like. Some of these accounts, to use the term of Chad Walsh (1962), strike a modern reader as actually *dystopias;* he shudders at the controls that beneficent dictators imagine will be necessary. A few such accounts (e.g., A. Huxley 1932, 1958) have been satires, a kind of socialized crime-fiction whose horrors are intended to warn us away from types of controls that are even now damaging our lives. But most such accounts have been imaginative attempts to set up guidelines for that human engineering which could produce the man who ought to be, the man his nature would have permitted him to become if other human beings and their social arrangements had not intervened. When cataclysmic social events have interrupted these utopian dreamers, a few have hastily announced to the world, "This is it! The Great Society is here! Now that the revolution" (once it was the American revolution, later the French, still later the Russian, and most recently the Chinese) "has succeeded, a new man will appear! New capacities will be released! The old disabilities will be liquidated along with the old organization" (or class structure, or corrupt nobility, or decadent ruling class) "that was responsible for so much disease, unhappiness, alienation from life," and so on.

In our own time we hear slogans that announce that mental health is purchasable, or that a war against poverty and the elimination of slums can reduce both insanity and delinquency. The conservative wing of our society, and those who count themselves the prudent guardians of the exchequer, argue as conservatives have always argued, that the poor and the mentally ill have been with us for a long time, that these misfortunes are inherent in our very constitutions and in human weaknesses, and that accidents in individual life histories will continue to happen in any society we are likely to construct. While the one group passionately calls for reforms, the other group attacks the optimistic reformers as visionaries (and sometimes as communists, beatniks, pinkos) to be mistrusted. Where in this country conservative broadcasters and newspaper editors may seek to have these advocates of change removed from pulpit or classroom (or barred from the air), in a dictatorship such a visionary's dangerous thoughts can land him in a hospital for the mentally ill—a curious demonstration of society's role in identifying and classifying this type of patient. Occasionally one of the contenders in this arena where public opinion and policy decisions take shape will appeal to statistical studies, some of which we are about to examine. More often than not these passionate convictions arise before statistics, indeed, have shaped some of the facts, have set the very coordinates for the measures, and, needless to say, have also affected the interpretation of the findings.[1]

THE STATISTICS OF MENTAL ILLNESS

We cannot experiment with human societies at will, even though our utopian essayists dream of doing so. And the experiments of nature, which the historians of all societies have attempted to analyze, seldom permit pure or unequivocal answers; otherwise we should not be engaged in rewriting history with each fresh forward surge of civilization (or decline, a Spengler would add). The variables which stand out and catch the eye of the classifier of societies cannot, as in the experimental situation, be changed one at a time, according to good experimental design, and with control societies matching the experimental group. So we try to accomplish by statistical analyses of masses of carefully gathered data what experiment cannot do. We have been asking such questions as:

1. Are there some cultures with high rates of mental illness, and others where mental health is almost universal?

2. Are there spots, or enclaves, within our own society where illness is common, and other spots where the individual seems to be "protected"?

---

[1]One man's design for utopia may strike his neighbor as a fantasy of horrors. Commenting on B. F. Skinner's *Walden Two,* Walsh (1962, p. 26) speaks of the little society there envisioned as "so repulsive to me that I should like to think it was intended as a dystopia. But I know it isn't. Prof. Skinner is plainly out to present an ideal world, from his point of view. I must accept his intention. He intends *Walden Two* as a utopia; a utopia it is."

Negley and Patrick (1962, pp. 589-90) are less charitable, setting down as a "shocking horror" the sterile cubicles and mechanical reinforcement routines which Huxley once satirized, but which Skinner now soberly offers as a way to force the infant to want to become what he must, to want what he ought to want: a design calculated to produce, these authors suggest, "a nadir of ignominy" and a nation of pigeons to be shaped at the will of some Central Committee who needs no guide other than the professor's "principles of human engineering."

3. Are there consistent long-term trends within our own society which support the notion that we are winning (or losing) the war against mental illness?

4. Are there findings which will support the generalization: "Ours is a sick society"? Do the social changes during the time we have been interested in such a question, and for which we have reasonably firm figures, throw any light on the question raised by those "prophets of doom" who insist that the pool of genes contains increasing amounts of "bad" determiners, thanks to our social policies which allow defectives to mate and reproduce their kind?

5. Are there massive and catastrophic events (wars, depressions, concentration camps, battles, mass migrations or displacements of populations) which permit large-scale studies of the concomitant (or resultant) mental changes?

6. Does the nature of mental illness (and both therapy and theory designed for it) change as we cross the boundaries of a culture?

A medical man might set up three indices for each of the diseases he sets out to study: (1) existing cases, (2) cases that are reported on some public record, and (3) cases treated. The first index number would have to be an educated guess, based on an intensive study of a representative sample of the population, and on a carefully controlled extrapolation to society as a whole. There is no complete census, backed by clinical and experimental analysis, of every living member of our society for any single illness *of any type.* The second index figure might be based on such public sources as the draft, or insurance records. For example, incidence of venereal disease can be estimated from the samples of population in those states where blood tests are required of all who obtain marriage licenses. However, the cases "reported," as we shall see, do not include all cases treated by private physicians, and so are not equivalent to all cases *treated.*

Venereal Disease: Illustrating the Difference between Existing, Treated, and Reported Illness

More easily identified and diagnosed than many mental diseases, syphilis would seem to be the kind of disorder that could be submitted to statistical analysis. And, although it is not a mental illness, it is related to one form of dementia. Arriving sometimes twenty years after the first infection, syphilis of the central nervous system and the vascular system of the brain produces a general paralysis which, if not properly treated, ends in death.[2]

When we read about an increase in the incidence of infectious syphilis, we need to ask about the source of the data. In 1964 there were 22,733 cases of infectious syphilis *reported* to the United States Public Health Service from all sources. Private physicians had treated 75 per cent of all cases treated, a pilot study revealed, but they had reported only 11 per cent of the cases they had treated. Estimating the total number of cases treated privately, and adding those

---

[2]When the medical statistician estimates that one case in 200 infected reaches the stage of general paralysis, we are not certain what his figures really refer to. With changing public-health programs and new methods of treatment, and with an unknown ratio between existing cases reported, cases treated, and that group who die in hospitals of syphilis of the central nervous system, the figure of 0.5 per cent given by Grinker (1937, p. 746) is not very firm.

treated in public facilities, we can accept a total of 100,000 cases of *treated* syphilis as an educated guess. There is no firm figure for the number of cases existing, although case-finding techniques that use interviews with cases treated have turned up an average per case of 3.7 sex contacts, many of which were neither reported by any physician or agency nor treated.

With the present large gap between cases treated and cases reported, any comparison of rates between urban and rural areas, between one city and another, between Gold Coast and slum, will have very little significance when it has to rely on the presently published figures. San Francisco reported a rate of 37.7 per 100,000 population in 1964, while rural New Hampshire was reporting 1.1 per 100,000 in the same year. Our uncertainty is increased when we learn that not all states require laboratory directors to report positive indications of the presence of syphilis. Some physicians take the position that such a report, where not specifically required, is a breach of medical ethics, and even where reports are required, some physicians choose to "protect" their patients.

One incidental finding discovered in trying to measure the effectiveness of an educational program is worth mentioning. In the groups involved, the rates of infection have shown no decline as a result of the educational work. There has been some increase in *concern*, and in the number who seek *treatment*, but there has been no measurable change in sex *practices*. Promiscuity and prostitution continue to spread the disease. Counting all forms of infectious venereal disease, the health service estimates that there are 200,000 cases among teenagers every year. With each infectious case interviewed naming three to four sex contacts, it would appear that this disorder has reached epidemic proportions.

The introduction of intensive programs of education into public schools (against the rather strong resistance of parents in some areas) would have an uncertain effect. Some argue that matter-of-fact presentations of existing sex practices, and of the types of treatment for the infections that are anticipated (presentations resembling those informative lectures given to military personnel), might cause a further deterioration in the sex attitudes of children. Some argue that a syphilophobia will arise to add to other sources of anxiety, make the task of maturing more difficult, and possibly hamper a normal sexual development.[3] If such educational programs have no more effect on sex practices than those now measured, they would probably not decrease the number of cases of congenital syphilis, now reported at about 4,000 per year.

THE INCIDENCE OF MENTAL ILLNESS

Many mental illnesses are much more difficult to diagnose and identify than venereal disease. Without clinical and laboratory studies of a rather large sample of the population, we cannot know precisely how prevalent such illnesses are. Such samples as we now have reveal the great gap between the census figures for all mental institutions and the actual prevalence of the illnesses

---

[3]Thomas Parran (1937) observes bluntly: "Syphilophobia never killed anyone; never brought a handicapped child into the world; never infected an innocent person."

in our population. We are again confronted with (1) a mass of abnormalities of unknown size, inferred from limited samples studied intensively, (2) a restricted group known because treated in public institutions and accurately reported, and (3) a larger group treated by private physicians and clinics, and not reported in any census.

When Malzberg (1959, p. 162) reports a steady increase in mental illness from 1880 to 1923, with the rate per 100,000 in the general population rising from 183 to 245, we need not conclude that the strains of modern living and of urban life, or alternatively some hypothetical breakdown in the morale in our society, are creating an increase in mental illness: these increases are merely in the reported cases treated in public institutions. Consider the effects of such variables as the following:

1. Our population is tending to live longer. The rates of hospitalization rise in the older age groups. An increase in total rates of hospitalized illness would be expected along with the increase in the life expectancy of our population (just as one would expect an increase in the rate of coronary attacks).

2. Hospital bed space is expanding, and the quality of treatment is improving. Families are more willing to hospitalize their mentally ill.

3. We have come to be a nation of city-dwellers. More people are near a center where mental illness is treated, and city-dwellers are more likely to be referred to such a center by physicians, social workers, or the courts. (Studies have shown that distance from a hospital affects the rate of hospitalized and reported mental illness.)

4. More than half a century of effort by mental-hygiene associations, physicians, and schools has changed our concept of mental illness. And hospitals are less feared today than they used to be.

5. Rising living standards have been accompanied by higher expectancies for health and well-being. Mental health is now regarded as purchasable, not as a fateful condition that depends on a combination of good fortune and good genes.

6. The proportions of those treated in public hospitals and by private physicians may have changed, just as the proportions educated privately and at public expense have changed. The severity of the illnesses entered in the public records may also have changed. We are not able to evaluate such changes, and since an unrecorded change in the admission standards would influence the census rates, there is a concealed and imponderable factor behind the figures.

7. Urban life, crowded living, in contrast to the life on a farm, may be forcing into institutional treatment or custodial care mentally ill persons who were formerly taken care of in rural homes. A weakening of family ties and of a sense of responsibility for the aging and mentally ill would operate in the same direction.

In addition to these points, Malzberg offers still another hypothesis to account for what he evidently accepts as a real increase in mental illness. He suggests that, "A generation ago, those surviving to middle age probably constituted a better physical selection, on the whole, than those reaching the same age periods today." When one argues that only the fit survive, and adds that advances in medicine have helped the unfit persist into middle age, one makes a case for this interpretation. We might remind ourselves, however, that as recently as 1770 half the children born in London did not live to see their second birthday (Dubos 1961, p. 69). One wonders just how discriminating a selector the death-dealing factors were. (War is another selector; when we excuse the "unfit" from military service, the selection must operate in a negative fashion.) Even though we grant that those who survived were more resistant to specific microorganisms and to whatever "accidents" befall infants, we do not know that they were more resistant to coronary thrombosis, cerebral arteriosclerosis, or marital conflict.

Malzberg's figures, based on *reported* rates, show that, while figures for mental illness as a whole were ascending, the figures for first admissions for general paresis (syphilis of the central nervous system) and for manic-depressive insanity were falling. Dementia praecox, as reported, was on the increase. We wonder whether the conception of the latter disease, more recently coded as schizophrenia, had changed so that it is now a more popular diagnosis, or whether a real change in the character of hospitalized illnesses has, in fact, taken place. We do not know.

TREATED CASES AND SOCIAL CLASSES

Careful studies of hospitalized and privately treated mental illness in metropolitan areas have come from Chicago, New York, New Haven, Bristol (England), Buffalo, St. Louis, Philadelphia. One consistent trend emerges: the rates for existing mental illness are higher in the areas inhabited by the lower socioeconomic groups. Some of the studies have used hospitalized cases, others have studied all patients reported as under treatment (including private clinics and physicians), and one study used an interviewing technique to discover evidence of illness or of symptoms that might be diagnosed as psychoneurotic. Even such widely varying samples and methods have produced figures that agree on this trend. It also appears that, although the rates for mental illness are higher in the lowest stratum, the proportion under treatment is smaller.

The New Haven study has added a new dimension to these class differences. The fifth (lowest) class contains a very low proportion of neuroses among its *treated* cases (see Fig. 1). In all probability this fact means that a neurosis in this class is likely to go untreated; and where it is treated, some social worker or some officer of the court is likely to be the source of referral. Hollingshead and Redlich (1958, p. 240) believe that persons of this class are more likely to be externally maladjusted, whereas in the two upper classes patients come to their physician with internal conflicts. In the authors' words: "The class V neurotic behaves badly, the class IV neurotic aches physically, the class III patients defend fearfully, and the class I-II patient is dissatisfied with himself."

A small proportion of existing neurotics is seen in clinic. Those who enter the clinic because they do not feel well, because they are having difficulties in their love life, because they are not achieving what they had hoped for, and who pay for their own treatment are quite a different sample from the class V

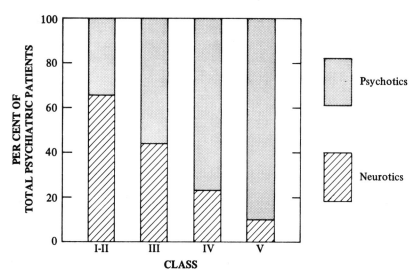

FIGURE 1. PERCENTAGE OF NEUROTICS AND PSYCHOTICS AMONG TOTAL PSYCHI-
ATRIC PATIENTS BY CLASS — AGE AND SEX ADJUSTED. (Reprinted by permission of
John Wiley & Sons, Inc., from August B. Hollingshead and Frederick C. Redlich,
Social Class and Mental Illness [1958], p. 223.)

patients who are referred by public agencies and treated at public expense. If
we add to these facts the screen of prejudice commonly found in the physician's
class position, we can see why we should use these caricatures by a physician
with caution. They may have more to do with attitudes and social practices
than with existing mental illness.

Although the Hollingshead-Redlich study represents an advance over studies
that rely on the census of public institutions, we must remember that, as with
the figures on venereal disease, we are dealing with samples reported as under
treatment. Even the wide sampling of the New Haven area was incomplete.
One of the physicians queried responded with, "I cannot lay my hands on the
records," another with "I have 2,000 patients and I am too busy to search for
the charts from New Haven." And we do not know how many physicians were
treating psychosomatic disorders as though they were in fact organic disorders,
and as a consequence did not report them in the proper category.[4]

SYMPTOM-FINDING IN THE METROPOLITAN AREA

Instead of waiting for "cases" to be diagnosed and reported, some research
teams have interviewed selected samples of the population in the hope of discovering symptoms, assessing degrees of impairment, and so arriving at some
index number that would reveal the existing *potential* case load. Such a case

---

[4]The *Journal of Psychosomatic Medicine* was founded in 1939. The attitude it represents has
penetrated medical circles slowly. Some conservative physicians still regard it as an enthusiasm
that exaggerates the psychological factor. Others insist that as many as two-thirds of the general
practitioner's patients bring symptoms that depend on psychological factors. Under such conditions the gathering of statistics is also a sampling of medical opinion.

load would materialize in a society that could provide free clinical and hospital facilities to all who need it, although even with a maximum effort to educate the public there would be many who would avoid the services. In midtown Manhattan such a survey (Srole *et al.* 1962) revealed that, in the sample interviewed (all between 20 and 59 years of age), four out of five had symptoms that were to some degree impairing their efficiency and peace of mind. All the index numbers obtained by such a method are approximate. Epidemiologists (e.g., Pasamanick 1962) have shown that reliance upon verbal reports and interview techniques, in the absence of clinical and laboratory records, leads to overreporting of some illnesses and underreporting of others. As in the New Haven study, the upper third, which had fewer symptoms of illness and a higher proportion described as mentally sound, had a higher proportion of those who were judged as needing treatment actually under such treatment.

Symptom-Finding in Nova Scotia and Nigeria

A research team (D. Leighton 1956) using still other case-finding methods reported a similarly high incidence of psychological impairment in a small-town sample. Dealing exclusively with adults, they estimated that 370 in every 1,000 were psychiatric cases *in need of help,* suffering from recognizable psychiatric disorders and having more than 10 per cent impairment.[5]

When comparable research methods were applied among the Yoruba people of Nigeria, a corresponding high rate of incidence of symptoms was again found. The close resemblance to the Nova Scotia data, in spite of the marked cultural differences, led these investigators to conclude that, in our theories of personality as well as in our theories of causation of mental illness, the cultural factor may have been overemphasized.[6]

---

[5]The research team secured records from all hospitals serving the area (Stirling County) to find all who had ever been hospitalized and for what reason, and used a follow-up questionnaire interview of each case that had some psychiatric significance to determine health status and possible impairment. They then took a random sample of the population (about 20 per cent), again using questionnaires, to turn up cases who had never been treated. They obtained more data from two general practitioners who were well acquainted with the community and from other sources that included teachers and police, and assessed the degree of impairment for each case. They present their 37 per cent figure as "the firm core of a prevalence figure for our population"; by prevalence they mean lifetime prevalence in the histories of adults (over 18). In contrast to this thorough search for symptoms and lifetime history of illness, it is worth noting that 55 of 1,000 were rejected by Selective Service on neuropsychiatric grounds, that Baltimore found 61 of 1,000 on the active list at various agencies at some time during the year of a survey (1953); and that Williamson County, Tennessee, reported a one-day prevalence for both active and inactive cases of mental disorder of 69.4 per thousand. The Leightons indicate that if their data for Stirling County had included all cases who had significant psychiatric symptoms (regardless of degree of impairment), the figure would rise to 65 per cent.

[6]"By and large . . . the similarity in the two samples is much more impressive than the differences. . . . While the present study does not demand a swing from one extreme to the other or eliminate the view that culture is important in the origin, course, and outcome of psychiatric disorder, it raises some question as to whether the emphasis on cultural difference has been overdone" (A. Leighton *et al.* 1963, p. 274). Both the prevalence rates and the distribution of "pattern quality" (anxiety, depression, etc.) proved to be markedly similar. Other studies, based on hospital statistics alone, have stressed differences, emphasizing the prevalence of excitement and violence, and the absence of depression; these authors believe this result to be a methodological artifact. See also D. Leighton *et al.* 1963.

This conclusion is noteworthy for two reasons:

1. The focus of interest for this research team was upon possible socio-cultural causes of mental disorder; every effort was made to include pertinent social factors in the Nova Scotia study, such as family health, misfortunes, broken home, type of schooling, language and ethnic-group identification, marital status, place in the family, migration history, religious affiliation, occupational history and attitudes, details of housing and possessions, and to explore similar aspects of the tribal life of Yoruba.

2. Their findings do show that, both in Yoruba culture and in Nova Scotia, there are villages with an extremely high rate of disabilities. These high-rate villages also showed marked signs of deterioration in institutional life: poverty, cultural conflicts, weakening of practices and sentiments associated with religion, effects of migrations, epidemics, disasters. One of the indicators of disintegration proved to be less significant than others: there were very poor villages that were well-integrated socially, and in these villages there was a low incidence of personality disorganization.[7]

The findings of the Leightons open up further problems for research; they do not identify the precise causes. It is even possible that some assortment process segregates the less-integrated personalities, so that they collect within these "social traps." It is also possible that the dilapidated milieus *produce* personality disorganization. From the days of Robert Owen, Engels, and Marx, we have not lacked men with a passionate certitude about these matters.[8] Although the data of the Leightons do not contradict the social-causation hypothesis, they do not prove it. While men of Owen's temperament proceed to found their new communities, the social scientists continue to ask: Are the slums of our cities and these broken-down villages havens which attract the apathetic, detached, rebellious? Are the disorganized ones rejected by their communities and unable to find anchorage elsewhere than in these social "traps"? Should we, in recognizing the importance of infancy and those first years of socialization, look upon this period as one in which such "breeders of disorganization" can get in their ill effects and so produce disorganization in the majority of the successive generations that grow up within these traps (or in all who do not, by some unexplained process, escape from the trap)? This last question invites the research worker to examine the patterns of child care in these deteriorated areas in order to discover the precise causes in operation. It becomes clear that a

---

[7]Parrinder's notion (1963, p. 273) that the belief in witchcraft reflects the culture's low opinion of women makes one of the observations of the Yoruba study of special interest. In contrast to Stirling County, where the prevalence of psychiatric symptoms was higher among women than among men, the Yoruba women showed lower rates than the men.

[8]See, for example, Owen 1813. In his introduction (p. x) to the Everyman's edition, G. D. H. Cole identifies the core of Owen's philosophy: "Man's character is made for, and not by, him." And to prove it Owen established a community, paid better wages, worked his employees shorter hours, gave them better conditions, employed no children under ten, and made his factory pay.

mere correlation does not answer the question in the way some massive (but impossible) human experiment might, were some psychological dictator to alter each of the indices of disintegration in some planned fashion.[9] Used instead by reformers and policymakers with passionate convictions, the data take on a bludgeon quality, but the blunt edge of the facts can strike in two quite different directions.

METROPOLITAN CONCENTRATIONS OF MENTAL ILLNESS

One puzzling fact that has been noticed often since Faris and Dunham (1939) first pointed it out is the difference between the distributions of schizophrenia and of manic-depressive psychoses on the city map. While the genetically minded research workers were showing that for *both* these psychoses there is a high correlation between identical twin pairs and a much lower one between siblings, and concluding that a pronounced genetic factor existed in both psychoses (see Rosanoff *et al.* 1934 and 1935, and Kallmann 1938, 1946b, and 1954), the Chicago studies were demonstrating a marked difference in the city-wide distribution of the two psychoses (see Faris 1938 and 1939, Faris and Dunham 1939, and Cavan 1932; these are summarized in Faris 1944). They found, along with vice, disease, and a high suicide rate, high rates of schizophrenia in the poorest residential districts, whereas manic-depressive psychoses were as prevalent in good residential districts as in the poorest, those we euphemistically describe as afflicted with anomie (personal and social disorganization).[10]

Two studies, one in the United States and one in England, have identified a possible factor affecting the distribution of cases of schizophrenia. In Worcester, Mass., Gerard and Houston (1953) reported a city-wide distribution of cases of schizophrenia that showed rates of incidence which were correlated with class position; but when they turned their attention to first admissions who were *living with their families at the time of admission*, they found a random distribution. When we consider that single-person households are concentrated in a central rooming-house district, where so many hospitalized schizophrenics are also spotted on any metropolitan ecological map, a fresh view of the matter becomes possible. If the frequent moves of these patients, beginning with an alienation from their own family, end up in the so-called "schizophrenogenic" zone, we would be witnessing a selection of an environ-

---

[9]Both social scientists and politicians may have the same sorts of reservations about Professor Skinner's fantasies in *Walden Two,* even though the latter envisions a rather specific kind of conditioning procedure.

[10]The youth among the faceless poor do not suffer from the kind of personal "identity crises" that one finds among the middle and upper-middle classes. The lower-lowers do not have much of any identity, in this sense. The poor will remain faceless as long as we do not know them, as long as none of those who have participated in their lives speak for them, as long as students of class attitudes and class-structured experience use little imagination in treating of their plight. Warner and Lunt (1941), Oscar Lewis (1965), Drake and Cayton (1945), and Davis and Dollard (1940), to name but a quartet, have shown what we could expect from a widening stream of such studies.

ment by a disorganized personality. A person who is seeking to avoid close personal relationships might seek the sweet anonymity of the slum, along with hobos, narcotic addicts, and others who for one reason or another are "in flight."

Hare (1956) followed up this lead, analyzing the data for psychotics entering a mental hospital in Bristol, England. The cases that he found entering hospital from some point "out of the family setting" showed a marked concentration in the central wards, and the ward rates for the city as a whole showed a high correlation (.88) with the proportion of single-person households in the wards. The schizophrenics who entered hospitals *from a family setting* were not concentrated in such districts. Pursuing his hunch that alienation from the family may have been the primary factor, Hare discovered that in 30 out of 64 cases the principal cause of the patient's separation from the family lay in his abnormal personality:

"Such patients tended to be selfish, suspicious, and unpredictable. Commonly they had a history of several admissions to mental hospitals. They had often lived with a succession of relatives, quarrelling with each in turn until none of the family wanted anything more to do with them. Quarrels with, or paranoid ideas about, landladies or fellow lodgers, caused them to change their address frequently. Their behavior tended to worsen over the years and in many cases it was hard to say when they crossed the border between abnormal personality and chronic psychosis."

Although this statement applies to less than half the cases, the description of this group implies that a schizophrenic process was at work before their migrations began. Multiplied, and appearing in widely divergent families and localities, such a succession of moves would result in the concentration of cases on the ecological maps which so many research workers have produced and which show high rates of this illness in the slum areas. In an additional 21 cases, Hare found that the separation from the family had been forced upon the patient by conditions over which he had no control, e.g., by the death of a parent. Hare thought that such forced separation may have had some etiological significance in 18 of these cases. He described another 11 cases as schizoid personalities who chose to live alone. Hare did not believe that living alone, per se, was in any way a factor hastening the development of the disorder in these 18 cases, inasmuch as they did not seem to him to be sufficiently deviant to make them difficult to live with.

In Hare's study, as in earlier ones, the raw data suggested that the central wards were either breeders or points of attraction (and possibly both). Close examination of the data suggested that the attraction hypothesis might have merit in a few cases; in a larger group the drift seemed secondary to a personality change that had led to their rejection by family and relatives. The data which Hare reports did not seem to support the "breeder hypothesis."

THE SOCIALLY MOBILE PERSON

The notion that some primary process within a patient's personality creates a gravitation toward a lower class status and a selection of a type of residence has appeared in other studies. Social mobility, especially downward, could result from some primary disability such as the one that emerges in a full-blown psychosis; and the milder neurotic disabilities might produce vocational impairment, unemployment, and the obvious social and economic consequences. Using a cross-section sample of a metropolitan population that included wide ranges in socioeconomic status (rather than a patient sample), Srole and his associates (1962, p. 226) studied occupational levels of patients and their parents. They identified three groups of approximately the same size: upward mobile, stable, and downward mobile (comparing the status of respondents with that of their parents). The sick-well ratios for the three groups were 65,104 and 235 (that is, 13.6% impaired/21% well, 23.6%/22.6%, and 30.1%/12.7%, respectively). When the data for the respondents over 40 years of age were examined separately, the contrasts were even greater. This group had had more time to make the "voyage" to a different class status. But again, the correlations do not identify causes.

The editors of the study cautiously suggest (p. 236) two hypotheses:

"[The postulates which guided this study] hold that toward one pole of the status range, in both preadult and adult life, [sociocultural processes] tend to penetrate the family unit with eugenic or prophylactic effects for personality development, whereas toward the opposite pole they more often work with pathogenic or precipitating effects....

"For targeting of social policy, Midtown zones C and D, and likely their psycho-socioeconomic counterparts elsewhere on the national scene, convey highest priority claims for milieu therapy in its broadest sense. Ultimately indicated here may be interventions into the downward spiral of compounded tragedy, wherein those handicapped in personality or social assets from childhood on are trapped as adults at or near the poverty level, there to find themselves enmeshed in a web of burdens that tend to precipitate (or intensify) mental and somatic morbidity; in turn, such precipitations propel the descent deeper into chronic, personality-crushing indigency. Here, we would suggest, is America's own displaced-persons problem....

"[The] status system [is] an apparatus that differentially sows, reaps, *sifts,* and *redistributes* [my italics] the community's crops of mental morbidity and of sound personalities [from whatever causes they originate]."

Where this type of study collects data that extend over several generations, the selection and redistribution process (that reallocates abilities to the different social strata) and the biological transmission process begin to operate in conjunction. Not only do the lowest class positions entrap the feebler specimens, their dysgenic effects penetrate family life and affect child-rearing practices, levels of aspiration, and physical development. The upper strata, also selective and difficult to penetrate (for climbers), are rewarding, providing the means to achieve desired goals (including mental health). The rival hypotheses become complementary ways of accounting for the facts.

One of our social myths asserts: ability *seeks* its own level. A second social myth is in the process of formation: the levels which exist in our society *produce* characteristic rates of mental health or illness. The transition from a pioneer society to a modern urban and industrial society has brought the second myth to the fore. The Great Society concept of our time (see Toynbee

1939, VI, 6) thus joins with Robert Owen's New View of Society to complete a century and a half of plans for the improvement of the human character.

Psychophysiological and Psychoneurotic Symptoms

In their search for symptoms, the Leightons (both in Nova Scotia and among the Yoruba of Nigeria) questioned those interviewed about every physiological system—skin, sense organs, respiratory, cardiovascular, muscular, genito-urinary, and endocrine—about body weight, bodily sensations, and headaches, and about psychoneurotic symptoms: anxieties, depressions, excitements, suspicions, fatigue (brain-fag), and conversion hysteria. The relationship between these two types of symptoms is worth noting.

In Nova Scotia, *all* respondents who reported six or more psychophysiological symptoms also had psychoneurotic symptoms; 88.9 per cent with five psychophysiological symptoms also had psychoneurotic symptoms; and, similarly, 75.0 for four, 70.4 for three, 54.3 for two, 41.7 for one, and 8.5 for none. Thus a multiple spotting of psychophysiological symptoms is a strong indication that psychoneurotic symptoms will also be present. The entire system, physiological, behavioral, interpersonal, tends to act as a unit and to show "taints" in each of the three aspects. The authors suggest that their findings may be of advantage to those who want to make cross-cultural comparisons, particularly when both the deviant and his cultural pattern are unfamiliar, which make "psychoneurotic" aspects difficult to assess without proper clinical and laboratory procedures, even more difficult to interpret. They note that this same association of psychophysiological and psychoneurotic complaints was found among the drafted soldiers in World War II. Their findings also suggest that any notion of a closer linkage between social factors and the more purely "mental" traits (closer than between social factors and physiological traits) may need reexamination.

Stated in another way, the physiological symptoms do not in any way take the place of or preclude the formation of psychoneurotic symptoms. There are many case reports in the literature which indicate that the onset of a severe and incapacitating illness (of a physical type) which enables a patient to assume the role of an impaired person, with full medical sanction, is also the occasion for the disappearance of mental symptoms that have been under treatment. The Leighton study shows that these are exceptional cases. The main trend of the data suggests:

1. Impairment is commonly a general affair: physical and mental disorganization and disability tend to be associated. (Long ago Terman pointed out that the gifted child was also likely to be well-endowed physically.)

2. Multiple physical impairments make social adjustments difficult and add to stress.

3. A personality structure that is weak, for whatever reason, will also contribute to stress, which in turn affects the major physiological systems. In the resultant somatic disabilities, there are some that can be called psychosomatic,

although the two series of events may not be related in a direct and specific way. (For example, we would scarcely anticipate a specific coronary personality or a gastric-ulcer personality.)

A Summary and a Caution

Two emphases emerge from this brief sampling of the statistical evidence: (1) the index numbers are still poorly related to *existing* mental illness (in contrast with treated mental illness); and (2) a measurable relationship between two variables (such as an index of mental illness treated and class position) does not in itself establish a causal relationship.

In the New Haven area, Hollingshead and Redlich found almost 2,000 patients under treatment in a base population of slightly less than 240,000. Srole and his associates estimated that in their Manhattan sample 25 per cent of those interviewed had symptoms that were sufficiently numerous and serious to merit professional attention. If we assume that there is no essential difference in the two populations as far as true incidence is concerned (and that the professional judges are not overenthusiastic), we would have to conclude that about one-thirtieth of the existing illness is being treated. If mental health is viewed as a purchasable thing, even those who can afford it are not buying it, for one reason or another.[11] In the lower economic brackets, especially among the indigent aged, where the rates of disability are high (and Srole did not interview any respondents over 60), the rates of untreated illness would give any policymaker interested in providing free medical care reason to hesitate.[12]

Our second generalization arises from a contradiction in the data, and in the interpretations that have arisen from a consideration of the fact of social mobility. As we noted above, Srole and his associates found that those who had moved upward from the class position occupied by their fathers were well-integrated, healthy, "tough and capable," whereas those who had dropped to a lower rung on the ladder had multiple physical symptoms and more psychoneurotic symptoms. These authors cite numerous other studies which

---

[11]Among the reasons which come to mind one might mention: the patient may not recognize he has a problem that could be helped in a clinic; he may fear "exposure" if he confesses to a psychiatric problem; he may have friends who have had bad experiences with mental-hygiene clinics; he may doubt the efficacy of such treatment; he may believe that he can be his own "self-regulator"; he may place other values higher and choose to purchase another type of "commodity"; he may value the very pattern the clinician judges abnormal (when, for example, it excuses him from military service); his lack of insight may itself be a part of his illness.

[12]First-admission rates (for all Canadian mental hospitals, 1951) for males aged 20 to 29 are 97/100,000, but for males 70 years and over are 275/100,000 (Gregory 1956, p. 115). Landis and Page (1938) give the figures for similar age groups in the U. S. (1933) as 55.1 and 272.3 per 100,000. Without some improvement in the present public institutions for this large pool of indigent aged with mental symptoms (both in treatment and in the living conditions), it is an open question whether any increase in the proportion hospitalized would mean an improvement in their condition. It would, it is true, "dispose of them," and perhaps relieve their families of responsibility, while giving the general public the illusion that the problem is being cared for.

show that the same differences apply to adolescents (whom Srole did not include in his sample) who have scarcely begun to ascend or descend the social ladder. The premobile personality (like the premorbid schizoid personality) has developed a typical pattern before he has really been tested in social competition. The race is to the swift and the strong. Douvan and Adelson (1958) note:

"The upward aspiring boy is characterized by a high energy level, the presence of autonomy, and a relatively advanced social maturity. These attributes may be viewed as derivatives of a generally effective ego organization....

"The downward mobile boys [show] an apparent blocking or impoverishment of energy which should ideally be available to the ego. There is a relatively poor articulation among the psychic systems; impulses threaten the ego's integrity; the superego seems overly severe and yet incompletely incorporated. These boys seem humorless, gauche, disorganized—relatively so, at least. Perhaps the most telling and poignant datum which the study locates is their response to the possibility of personal change, their tendency to want to change intractable aspects of the self, and the degree of alienation revealed by their desire to modify major and fundamental personal qualities."

Hollingshead and Redlich (1958, pp. 367-70), whose data came from *patients under treatment,* offer radically different interpretations. Using a sample of schizophrenics under treatment, they found no evidence of downward drift toward slum areas within their lifetime. The majority of patients had always lived in the spots from which high commitment rates are found. And, searching the family histories, they report the same absence of downward drift. These findings contrast markedly with those reported by Hare.

Basing their view on neurotic patients under treatment, Hollingshead and Redlich describe the upward-mobile person:

"The 'climber' who appears to move more successfully... [impresses] an observer as pleasant, successful, and very able if he *is* successful; and he appears well integrated. Only on longer acquaintance and after a deeper search does one become aware of the climber's conflicts and defenses. His deeper anxieties become manifest when his mobility drive becomes blocked; then his defenses do not function properly.... [And] when these social climbers were rejected by those who 'are there' socially, their reactions were characterized by severe anxiety, depression, sometimes by anti-social acting out, and in some extreme cases by suicidal attempts which were related, in part, to blocked mobility."

The "strainer," the one who has not moved successfully but who has high aspirations, is an even more unpleasant type:

"The strainers tend to be ambitious dreamers, the type James Thurber so beautifully portrayed in his *The Secret Life of Walter Mitty* and Steig in *Dreams of Glory.* If they do not dream, they constantly plan and scheme, rush from one pursuit to another, or from one 'big deal' to the next, hoping to succeed sufficiently to climb upward in the social system, but always disappointed and frustrated, complaining and rationalizing about what they consider bad luck and failure."

To their impressionistic sketch of the upward-mobile person, these authors add a sketch of the way such patients[13] strike their counselors:

"The upward mobile person, and particularly the strainers, have a certain proneness for neurotic disorder and are apt to cause social troubles. They need not be highly unconventional or flout accepted values—actually, many highly mobile persons are quite conventional—but they are uncertain about their values and some of them can be, at times, obnoxious and hard on others as well as on themselves in their attempt to reach their goals. Psychiatrists encounter many mobile persons with such unpleasant character traits that, behind external conformity, they cannot get along with anybody and do not care for anyone but themselves and their goals.

"The downward mobile persons...are recognized by the community as trouble-makers. As their behavior becomes overtly anti-social they are referred with increasing frequency to psychiatrists when they do not obey the subtle rules of the game expected of them by persons in higher status positions. These patients present the psychiatrist with severe problems, such as alcohol or drug addiction, crime, and most of all with serious character disorders. They are labelled clinically as sadistic-masochistic characters or as destructive and self-destructive personalities. Some of their disorders present the syndrome of a 'fate' neurosis. The spell of gloom, failure, and disaster which these patients exude, even when they are not depressed, makes them rather unapproachable and dreaded by therapists. Treatment of such persons is exceedingly difficult and even more so of families who like that in Faulkner's *Sartoris* march inexorably toward annihilation. Even when insight is reached in downward mobile patients by dynamic psychotherapy, their self-destructive urges in the form of negative therapeutic reactions prevent any real success in treatment."

These authors imply that, in this affluent society, anyone who is born in a family that is not "top flight" is bound to be guilt-ridden, anxious, full of inferiority feelings. Such a person's attempt to move upward, even if successful, will generate and motivate a display of repulsive character traits. Exceptions that should be noted are those who are content with their lot, who know their place, who accept or overlook the claims of those of superior status. Worst of all is the man who tries and fails, weakly complaining and rationalizing the while: the mixture of guilt, resentment, and impotence that he expresses makes him an object of contempt.

We might recall here the "abnormally normal" described in Chapter 1. It seems clear from the choice of adjectives, in both the present and the earlier studies, that those who study the contented ones also find them curiously wanting in those traits which make a person interesting. Such words as uncreative, unimaginative, insensitive to social questions, contented plodders, and happy in their simple home life have distinct overtones. In addition to their descriptive language, Hollingshead and Redlich make explicit statements which illustrate how these mobility orientations affect the patient-physician relationship:

---

[13]The reader should remember that in this free-wheeling interpretation the authors are generalizing from the upward-mobile patient seen in therapy to the whole class of mobile persons, most of whom they did not study.

"In the upward mobile patients the differences in value orientation between the psychiatrist and the patient are overcome by the patient's identification with some of the values of the therapist. Such patients have a desire to sublimate, to achieve, to obey the rules of the game, and yet to enjoy. It is particularly the dynamic psychiatrist who has become the 'sage' for upward mobile persons who have lost their bearings in their exhausting and frantic climb toward the 'top.' *Lower class patients in this study who had a good relationship in dynamic psychotherapy with their psychiatrists were invariably upward mobile* [my italics].

"[In] the downward mobile patient,... the lack of a capacity to sublimate, unwillingness to achieve, often an extraordinary dependency, a tendency to regress and to destroy himself and others, makes insight therapy particularly difficult. Downward mobile patients arouse more antagonism in psychiatrists than any other single group; it is easier to accept a patient with standards different from one's own than someone who, so to speak, has abandoned and betrayed the standards the therapist values as desirable."

We are confronted with several rival hypotheses about these animadversions and the facts which prompted them:

1. "Studies of mental illness have suggested that people moving up in America are more likely to have mental breakdowns than the nonmobile." This quotation from Lipset and Bendix (1959, pp. 65, 251) may have been founded upon the New Haven data, but if so it involves a misinterpretation of the findings. These sociologists have read the prejudices of the authors correctly, but they have not looked too closely at the data.

2. Studies of schizophrenia under treatment give no basis for either the social-mobility hypothesis (of Lipset and Bendix) or the drift hypothesis (of Hollingshead and Redlich).

3. Studies of a representative sample of nonpatient populations show that, on the basis of interview material, the upward mobile have higher morale and better health (Srole).

4. Impressionistic sketches of patients and psychiatrists give the downward mobile a bad name and suggest that these patients both lack insight and resist any that the therapist tries to impart (Hollingshead and Redlich).

These hypotheses, and the contradictions in data and interpretations, suggest the need for further studies of both patient and nonpatient samples (and of both healthy and mentally ill). Perhaps some attention should be paid to the class origins and social mobility of the therapists themselves. The hypotheses also suggest that:

1. Schizophrenia may prove to have different social-mobility characteristics than those found among neurotics, with the schizophrenics showing fewer typical mobility findings and neurotics more.

2. The evaluation and interpretation of the social factor are affected by the prejudices and class attitudes of patient, physician, and research worker. Those who possess highly charged convictions seem to have no difficulty in converting correlations into causes and effects, and, where objective data are lacking, tend to accept impressions as facts.

3. To the healthy and successful, competition can be a stimulus for growth, a morale builder, a source of strength. The struggle keeps them "in training." To those who fail, or who fall afoul of the law and social agencies, or who seek treatment for self-diagnosed disabilities, the social structure is apt to appear responsible for their failure. It is possible that for some of the downward-mobile the social process is indeed responsible for their symptoms, whereas other individuals use the existing opportunities in an abnormal way for personal reasons.

THE SELF AND SOCIETY: MENTAL HEALTH AND OTHER VALUES

Men live by their dreams. Lured by the vision of becoming a perfect knight, or a Jesuit warrior for the Lord, or a business executive, or an Olympic athlete, men have striven to actualize their ego-ideals; passionate pilgrims, severely critical of their own performance, they are bound to become "strivers and strainers" if their goals are high. Charged with such patterned desires, a man can create trouble for himself and for his contemporaries. Given a spark of genius and a deeply rooted personal commitment, a man might become the conscience of an age, a tremendous social force in his own right.

In this relationship between the individual and his society, there is a mutual exchange of influence and power. The society shapes the self. Is it not the repository of tradition, the home of heroes, the educator of the young, the guardian and possessor of all manner of roads to gratification? Did not Sparta make warriors, train her citizens to fight in a phalanx, discipline her boys to endure pain and to despise the Helots? Does not a culture absorb and use the talents of its citizens, and in the process hammer the latter into shape as well as reward them? Is it not true also that the individual fights back, reshapes the culture, acting as a counterforce? Does he not sometimes join with others to form an internal proletariat, and set out to destroy all hithertoexisting values and social arrangements?

The culture can act as a mentor, looking over the shoulder of her pupil, interpreting his tensions for him, shaping his perception of both his world and of himself. Kroeber once made this point by his story of a woman who, having lost her infant son, began to have visions, hear voices, and display other symptoms. Had she lived in an American upper-class family, her relatives would have urged her to seek psychiatric treatment. Her physician would most certainly have described her experiences to her as hallucinations; and he would have evaluated them, privately, as warnings of incipient psychosis. If this physician had also been trained in psychoanalysis (which we might describe as a special subculture), he might entertain the hypothesis, privately, that the voices symbolized something in her unconscious. Noting the mother's depression, and her freely expressed guilt feelings, he might proceed to look for evidence of a death wish toward her child. By the analysis of the mother's dreams and her free associations, he then might lead this mother to reexperience her first ambivalent relationships with her own mother. And all these efforts would be directed toward stopping the voices and restoring the woman to health. Accepting the proffered role of a patient in need of help, the woman would be given in turn a deeper insight into her own personality structure. If she rejected the proffered role, it is possible that her physician would then regard her as lacking in insight. To get well such a woman would have to arrive at a realistic view of all that had occurred to her, that is to say, a view that corresponded to that of her physician and of other sensible people in her culture. For schizophrenia, our culture insists, is a disease in which reality is distorted.

As matters turned out, in Kroeber's account (1952, pp. 310-19), this mother was a Lassik Indian.

"'I bet you are a doctor.' 'Well, I nearly was,' she answered. 'My baby died. I was sitting around the next afternoon. All at once I heard a baby cry overhead, and fell over unconscious. My sister brought me back; but from time to time I heard the crying again, and became more and more sick. I gave an old doctor twenty dollars to cure me, and he said it was my baby's shadow coming to me to tell me to become a doctor. But I did not want to; and when the shadow began to talk, urging me, I told him, "No! I won't," and I urged him to go away. So at last he left off, and I got well, and did not become a doctor.'"

Kroeber urges:

"One may at once suspect the functioning of a cultural pattern, because all through native northern California the onset of shamanistic power is marked by a seizure in which the candidate experiences a hallucination—always auditory and sometimes visual also—in which objectively he is unconscious, or unaware of his surroundings, and acutely ill. To his family and village mates he seems actually stricken with disease. But the older shaman who is consulted promptly diagnoses the disease as the onset of shamanistic power, predicts cure as soon as the patient adjusts himself to his new power, and, with other shamans, helps to 'train' the novice, that is, to find the adjustment. In most cases, apparently, the novice accepts the power which has come upon him: considerable prestige attaches, in a simple society, to one who can cure or exercise other special faculties."

In a similar fashion, Kroeber notes, an effeminate transvestite, who enjoys wearing women's clothes and acting out atypical roles, is sometimes absorbed into shamanism, trained to communicate with spirits, and allowed to enjoy honors, gifts, and the respect of his fellow Yokhuts. How completely inverted these men were and to what degree they found a free erotic expression for their peculiar needs are matters of dispute. One of Kroeber's informants, obviously thoroughly masculine in his outlook, suggested that these nonphysiological "women" took on this institutionalized role "in order to have free association with women and special opportunities for secret heterosexual activity with them."

So we may look upon the society that surrounds the individual as accepting, rejecting, or channeling his unique qualities: it invites, cajoles, arouses, punishes. It provides him with ready-made roles that either fit his special needs or enrage him as it frustrates and punishes him. Since a society is neither unitary nor stationary, since individuals are not struck from the same mold, the tensions which develop between the individual and his milieu involve him in a constantly changing set of dynamic relationships: he is punished and forced to change; or he attacks, pitting his will against those around him. He may strive to achieve a oneness, a feeling of belonging, a *Gemeinschaftsgefühl*; or he may stand, like a proud Jeremiah, to denounce evil in high places, almost inviting personal disaster; or he may suffer, secretly, torn with an inner conflict and filled with guilt, until he learns how to repress a half of what is within him. Such conflicts are social in essence. They could never be predicted on the bases of the individual psychobiological facts. But as we note some of these patterns as they arise in family settings, we can see that it is necessary to include facts of a very personal history; and in each of the three examples we shall examine, there may also have been some very unique genetic factors.

We shall consider, as examples, three persons: a young woman who became a member of the Nazi party, a young journalist who was the upward-mobile son of immigrant parents in America, and a middle-class French girl who rejected the role designed for her by her parents. Each of the three histories rests upon introspective and autobiographic accounts. None of them was a patient under treatment, was given clinical examination, or served as experimental subject. Like the socially mobile who "make the grade" and preserve their health, the personalities we are about to sketch were sound of mind and limb even when unhappy and distressed. The "solutions" which they worked out may not have been the ones the reader would have chosen, or the best possible ones on some hypothetical absolute scale of values. This should remind us that whether an adjustment is ethically valuable or not is not the sole criterion that separates "patients" from "healthy persons." From the standpoint of the clinic, a tough sinner may be "sound as a nut" and sleep well of nights, while his sensitive brother may experience painful and symptom-producing conflict as he strives to stay well within some code of moral perfection. To confuse the issue, the sensitive one often phrases his own illness in terms of personal sin and guilt; his pastor will, on occasion, aid and abet this self-diagnosis when responding to a plea for counseling. To still further confuse the issue, when he accepts spiritual guidance and does the penance recommended, he may achieve a spiritual unity and a sense of wholeness that marks those who are "symptom-free"; here the entire drama of illness and recovery is enacted in spiritual and ethical terms. How easy for us, as observers, to couple the man's self-announced guilt, his disobedience to God's law, with his neurosis, and to accept the pragmatic test of "what produces a cure" as a measure of the correctness of the diagnosis. But it is also possible that such ethical conflicts are a special case of a much more general type of tension between the individual and his society, and that some "resolutions" we would reject as most unethical also "work."[14]

To deviate from the comfortable norm of conformity, where a feeling of belonging is the rule, is to risk isolation, loneliness, inner conflict. A certain kind of personality makeup may find these consequences difficult to endure. Whoever violates the rules and the values of a proximate culture risks experiencing guilt and self-hate. Only the tougher deviant can safely incorporate and

---

[14]For extended expositions of this ethical viewpoint, see Mowrer 1961, Szasz 1961, and May 1959.

at the same time indulge in behavior that lacks respect for these local rules and values. To make judgment more difficult, two forms of guilt have been identified, and both may exist within the same person: a neurotic form that is either exaggerated or displaced (and might conceivably arise from too great dependence) and a legitimate form that is related to a shared ethical code. Either form may exist and produce symptoms, and either may be contained and carried along with other conflicts that are managed without visible impairment by a reasonably well-integrated individual. The *objectively guilty* (as judged by those who have absolute values) may or may not show neurotic signs, may or may not enjoy health and long life, may or may not feel punished.[15]

A JEWISH SCHOOLGIRL IN NAZI GERMANY

How shall we describe the conflict within the self when the forces that are in power within a culture violate the individual's sense of what is decent and right? What kind of an outer mask (or persona) will be shown to her youth group when the person in question is the daughter of a German scientist who also happens to be a Jew? What will happen when the "blood purges" begin? This is the problem proposed by Bruno Bettelheim in his *Informed Heart* (1960, pp. 291 ff). And it is a drama that must plague every Jew who survived the Nazi terror.

Bettelheim writes:

"I once spoke with a young German psychologist who was a child at the beginning of the Hitler regime. Her father was a strong opponent of the Nazi movement and she felt as he did. But life went on and she had to go to school. At school she had to swear allegiance to the Führer, to give the Hitler salute repeatedly. For a long time she mentally crossed her fingers. She told herself that the oath and the salute didn't count because she didn't mean them. But each time it became more difficult to hang on to her self-respect and still keep up the pretense, until finally she gave up her mental reservation and swore allegiance like anybody else."[16]

---

[15]Perhaps if the writers of the Book of Job had not added a Hollywood ending to their story of a good man's "passion," there might be more of us who could identify, even now, persons who are not punished or rewarded according to the moral law. Saying so, I must admit this viewpoint is not easily founded on any statistical summary of clinical evidence. I might say, of course, that it rests on common sense, on a reasonable view of the limited evidence of experience. Since other men, with another variety of common sense and with an equal access to "right reason," seem passionately convinced that all neuroses arise from the breaking of certain basic laws of human decency (God's laws), I should admit that all such views carry us into metapsychology, into pre-science and ambiguity. Such conflicts in viewpoints make clinical psychology, like horse racing, a matter of great interest, but they also suggest that our "science" is shot through with subjectivity.

[16]What Bettelheim suggests here is expressed in Psalms I:1, which describes the transition from "containment of resistance," which the psychoanalyst calls suppression, to the complete form of repression: "Blessed is the man that walketh not in the counsel of the ungodly, nor standeth in the way of sinners, nor sitteth in the seat of the scornful." Here lies a whole implied transformation of the type Bettelheim is talking about. Suppression, once a conscious struggle carried on behind clenched teeth, becomes an automatic process, carried out even before any self-critical thought can occur.

Here the consequences of revealing a loyalty to the family and its values include death itself. The person who wishes to stay alive has to be vigilant, lest in some unguarded moment the deeper layers of the self speak out and betray what is going on behind the facial mask. In the effort not to say the wrong thing, one may even be led to outdo those who seem to have come by their views easily and naturally. Doesn't the new convert or initiate sometimes outdo the faithful (and the secure) in his hatred of the infidels to whom he once belonged?

Bettelheim's informant revealed other changes that were going on within:

> "While this development was still going on, a parallel process was taking place in her inner relation to her father. At first his morality had given the girl strength to go on without wavering in her convictions. But as time went on, she felt herself more and more projected into a most difficult conflict. First she had sided with the father and simply resented the state that forced such a conflict upon her. But eventually there came a time when she blamed her father for being the source of her difficulties."[17]

To use the language of psychoanalysis, one might say "Now the ego is taking up the cudgels against the superego." It is as though the girl had suddenly turned against the father and shouted, "You and your dandipratted morality! You are the one that is causing all of the trouble." Once such a girl has crossed the divide and stands with "the others," she begins to see that the world is not like the one her father has been showing her. She *knows* this. And if we favor the father's view and call her ego treasonable, we have to admit that it is strong enough to destroy the old self, to root out the vestiges of the family religion, to destroy that father-image which had earlier seemed so lovable, so serene, *violently!* And at some cost.[18]

---

[17]The conflicts within the family of a Negro intellectual within our own time are of a similar order: a father who has already made his way some distance into white society can find it almost impossible to communicate with his son who has been caught up into the struggle for Black Power.

[18]All manner of "treasonable" actions of this type come to mind. The French *poilu* who served out his war years as a prisoner in Nazi Germany, and who was farmed out to a village short of males to work on the land, pictured in a film produced by M. Cayette, became a traitor to France. He had become a man of some consequence in the village. They turned to him for advice and help even though he was a prisoner. When he returned to France to join the unemployed at a factory gate, he became one of those faceless ones, a superfluous unemployed worker; he returned to that German village to find a life, and with what thoughts of France, when he heard the *Marseillaise?* Rebecca West has examined, with at least partial success, other forms of treason in her *The New Meaning of Treason.* Margret Boveri (1961) has tried to take a broad view of the shifts in loyalty imposed upon so many in the twentieth century. And in his *Limits of American Capitalism* Robert Heilbroner suggests some of the "treasonable" shifts in loyalty that are required of contemporary intellectuals if we are to avoid cataclysm. Sometimes forces from the dear dead past that the treasonable individual has so successfully killed will rise, unbidden, in a wave of "homesickness" that engulfs him; tears rise unbidden in response to some scene before him. Values that he believed sloughed off literally choke him, as a lump in the throat clutches him like some hand reaching up from an unconscious past.

From resenting her father, this young Nazi went on to resent his values; and, in killing the things she had loved, she also had to destroy something that had been her support, her nexus with others, the very basis of *Gemeinschaftsgefühl*. As a consequence, this insecure adolescent needed the comradeship and affection of her schoolmates, and the approval of her teacher even more. The rituals, the shouts of *Sieg Heil,* the good fellowship of the hike, acquired greater force as the old base withered away. Precisely because old gods are dead, new ones must be found. The dream of the new society became the grand rationalization of her actions. How vigorously she had to purge from her thoughts and feelings the old type of *caritas,* old humilities and compassions and asceticisms that had so long poisoned the German folk-soul; and, especially, how violently did she have to root out whatever remained of Judaism.

The battle within such an individual is not wholly a matter of external pressures from the culture, although we who watch can appreciate their towering force, even from our safe vantage point at this distance. Caught up in the torrent of a revolution, a Dr. Zhivago and his loved ones are like wood chips on the rapids above Niagara, and the pattern of stresses in that human field about them invades the most secret portions of the ego, testing and sometimes breaking its last resistances. Sherrington (1906) described the processes of facilitation, inhibition, and reciprocal innervation in physiological terms appropriate to the spinal dogs that he studied, and the reflex patterns that he observed emerged as the lawful products of the interplay of neural processes. When we face the kind of integrations at work in Bettelheim's illustration, the analogous interplay of forces and the division that develops within the person seem to call for a dramatic kind of language: an internal struggle, moral conflicts, the triumph of a dominant ego over the vestiges of infantile relationships now repressed. In Sherrington's account the antagonists that oppose a now dominant reflex pattern are completely disposed of: the stimuli which call for the dominant pattern also inhibit the antagonists of this pattern (or the kinesthetic return from contracting muscles cancels the last vestige of action in the antagonistic muscles). Even a normal resting tonus is canceled as the stimulus to its antagonists is applied. But in the model of the self-system that Bettelheim is using, the repressed half does not seem to be as completely extinguished: it continues its activities underground. Instead of completely dominating all the processes afoot within the person, the ego controls only a visible outer shell, only a superficial layer, and even this layer is penetrated in the symptoms of the hysterical, when the unconscious reaches up to rob the ego of one of its mechanisms, as in globus hystericus, writer's cramp, or aphonia. (See also Sherrington 1940 and Duycaerts 1954, Chap. 1.)

If we shift from the calm of the physiologist's laboratory, where spinal animals express their reflex capacities in predictable fashion, to the more dramatic scenes that press upon Bettelheim's young woman, we become more aware of the meaning of that need for oneness, closeness, security, affection, as it developed within a personal history, a need that can be especially intense in the close-knit life of a Jewish family and doubly intense in certain natures. It is always the rare spirit who can stand up to the jeers, the threats, the tortures, the dread of the concentration camp and of death itself. Robert Bolt (1966) has chosen such a character for his chief protagonist, and calls him a "man for all seasons": a man for all seasons, yes, but not Everyman. It would be asking a great deal of an uncertain adolescent, still unsure of herself, to demand that she live by an inner standard through all of the fluctuating changes around her, unmoved and sure, anchored in the flinty substance of sacred beliefs. A very friendly fellow who has always leaned rather heavily upon his friends and who is proud to be "a member of the club" could find many reasons for not subjecting his family to the consequences that a too-stubborn clinging to principles would produce.

Analogous problems arise in varying forms all around us. Will the young Air Force cadet "snitch" on his friends who are getting by through cheating in exams? What if the cheater is the captain of the football squad? Will the vice-president in charge of sales refuse to go along when his own superiors and his competitors invite him to join in a plan to fix prices on electrical equipment sold to the government? Will the boy caught in an act of vandalism show what the social worker calls "the right attitude," reveal his accomplices, and thus destroy the gang that alone had furnished him with the very basis of the little order in living that he had found?

It is while a potentially treasonable "infant within us" still craves the feeling of belongingness that the deafening shouts of *Sieg Heil!, Sieg Heil!* arise around her, filling the Nuremberg Square with sound that drowns the still, small voice of the superego. Need we ask why the scruples of good Germans were drowned in that Nazi mixture of terror and brotherhood held out to them? On the one hand, there were threats of loneliness, torture, death; on the other, there on the square, the warm upsurge of the "feeling of union." Even a Jew might say, rationalizing his weakness, "Are not those Jews who are being picked up by the police enemies of order, diseased persons, psychopaths, Communists, vermin?" The human trait of scapegoating tends to intensify the worst features of a few of the "criminals," to generalize these so as to help place a distance between oneself and these who deserve to be crushed. And what a blessed relief comes when the young German joins the colors, puts on the uniform, closes the issues. And so belongingness (so much the cement that underlies our values) validates the new dichotomy that separates society into the pure-blooded Aryans, the loyal ones, on the one hand, and the "outsiders," homosexuals, panderers, loafers, unemployable scum, and the mentally diseased on the other. Cheaters, radicals, Communists, Bohemians, these "others" may have to be eliminated if society is not to become decadent. So the fainthearted find their private ideals fading, changing, under constant attrition, until that point is reached where they no longer feel divided at all; the new selves are made whole by a kind of inner psychosurgery. Only the Nazi half, above the line that screens away the unconscious, looks out to plan, evaluate, and judge the world. There is no longer any guilty association, even in thought, with those who would keep the unconscious half alive.

Perhaps we ought to pause to note what such an unconscious contains in this situation, for it is quite different from what has traditionally been described as the realm of banished impulses. Our thinking started by assuming that social-ization is a process whereby antisocial impulses are repressed. We felt that con-sciousness must represent the good half of the mind, the ethical half. That which had been repressed was a savage little animal within us (as infants): dirty, greedy, soiling, yammering, dependent. In Bettelheim's informant, the unconscious of the new persona, this Nazi-Jewess-psychologist, must contain the memories of the feast of Passover, the lighted candles and the warm family feeling, the tenderness once fused with decency and humanity, the still, small voice of an older conscience, the feeling about a very special form of truth, honesty, goodness. Over and above it has formed a new and different set of standards, a new and dominant *Gemeinschaftsgefühl*, something that was cemented in when the shouts of *Sieg Heil* went up.

Bettelheim's informant commented on the training process that she went through; and her new adult professional interests, as a psychologist, now force her to look at the rituals. Merely offering the outward signs of conformity did not amount to much, at first. But as the terror grew and the threat to existence became real, and as the enormities committed in the name of purifying the race became more obvious, the salute had to cover up and stamp out everything alien to that man whose ravings set the orders of the day. An ever more difficult set of discriminations and an all but impossible logical accommodation had to be made, and that psychosurgery of repression, an unhearing, unseeing stop-page of sensory input and conscious elaboration, had to conceal a half of her.

And so it was that, while attending the *Gymnasium*, she went along with the other girls, rang doorbells, took the census, asked the questions about aspects of family life that (she knew) terrified her Jewish respondents. And as she stood in the doorway, knowing the attitudes of those who so timidly responded, she felt herself becoming the living symbol of Nazidom now come to torment them. She knew how they hated her and, almost reflexively, she hated back. Tempted to sympathize with them, but fearful of the consequences of such a betrayal of something within her, she learned to suppress these feelings. So a social-psychiatric caseworker is tempted to deal with persons, not clients, but finds the process too exhausting, too conflictful, too threatening, and succumbs to become a "case-hardened" professional.

How, we ask, does the spirit so divided ever become whole again? The cleavages which were prompted by forces out there, in society, have penetrated the heart of the family, and have become, finally, a cleft within the self. Does one achieve unity by killing the old superego and washing one's hands of much that was formerly valued? Or by becoming one of the "new men," safely located within a comradely circle? Or by developing a new conscience?

In the first days of the terror, this young Nazi assumed an outward pose that warded off criticism. But as the terror mounted, her participation in the life of the *Gymnasium* forced her into a more and more complete unity with her peers. The doubleness she had felt at first was gradually replaced by a new sense of unity; the regnancy, the regulative self, had changed flags. Suppression had slipped into repression. The old self disappeared into the unconscious. To make the picture complete, we should have some account of the way her sleep was then troubled, for it is said that prisoners still dream of scenes back home, not of the prison camp itself. And we should expect that at an unguarded moment, even while she was awake, impulses from the past would start up, unbidden.

If we should say that such a young Nazi was living a lie at the beginning, how shall we describe the structure of her action at the end, when she began to share the grand illusion of National Socialism and to participate in the persecution of her former coreligionists? Her new illusions, we might say, had come to possess her. They had become a new sacred reality, literally a bloody reality. Completed, this new unity would function to encode her daily experiences in the Nazi manner, and she would lose all consciousness of living a lie. Instead, she would feel that she is on the side of history, making the future come true. It is even possible that her unconscious will finally begin to operate on the Nazi plan. Automatically, almost reflexively, she will respond in the new manner.

What shall we say now in response to Henri Ey's description of a psychosis as a "reality disease"?[19] Is our young Nazi fully adjusted or completely psychotic? Is this a sickness of a society, and she merely a "healthy' belonging member? "To thine own self be true" is a slogan that will be read by such a convinced Nazi as a command to eliminate from his very being any vestige of that older, sickly, humanitarian, Christian, socialistic, Jewish society. It will mean "Let the pure German blood that is in your veins speak." The structure of action and the function of language, shaped by this need for *Gemeinschaftsgefühl* (and by fear), produce new beliefs, new "truths," new reality, new individuals—and a new framework, let us add, within which to diagnose and interpret neuroses.

Gemeinschaftsgefühl and a Young Journalist

It is somehow appropriate that Alfred Adler, a Jew, should have been the one who elevated this concept of "the social feeling" to an important role in the formation of the personality (1927). The chronic and pervasive anti-Semitism that confronts the Jew on every side, today as it has for so many centuries, makes it difficult for him to feel like an accepted brother, or like that chosen one which his religion and a tightly knit in-group tell him he really is. Instead, he discovers that he is one apart, the poor relation, the despised one; and this discovery intensifies his need and increases his sensitivity at the same time. He reacts instantly, touched to the quick, when a group of players put on *The Merchant of Venice* in some summer theater under public auspices. "Why perpetuate the image of Shylock?" he asks. He senses a fresh wave of anti-Semitism in Moscow when other observers merely read of the conviction of two Jews for embezzlement of the funds of a collective. He is suspicious when his son's application to a college is turned down. Or he learns that

---

[19]Ey observes (1960, p. 5): "That which hides from the eyes of patient and physician the structure of mental disease can only issue from that same structure. We must indeed grasp it for what it is—namely, a pathology of reality."

this tavern, that exclusive club, those professional roles, that political office, are —if not absolutely closed to him—nonetheless relatively difficult for him to enter. So he carries with him a constantly reinforced burden of anxiety, as though the tenuous fabric of belongingness were about to give way, leaving him isolated and without support, and so his need for acceptance, for that oneness of *Gemeinschaftsgefühl,* is the greater.

There are sometimes objective events in his personal history, in addition to that collective experience of his people, to justify a certain catastrophic quality in his moods. Gentiles make it easy for him to play the role that André Schwartz-Bart described so vividly in *The Last of the Just.* He, if anyone, should know the meaning of that "abyss" the existentialist refers to. It is not simply that some minor disappointment will overtake him: his whole world can collapse, *he knows,* and his life and the lives of his loved ones can be crushed under that seemingly inexhaustible, relentless, and unreasonable hate which has pursued the Jew for centuries. Only on ritual occasions, within the family circle, so tight and so warm, so firmly welded in bands stronger than steel, can he relax completely and, for a moment, experience the full flavor of *Gemeinschaftsgefühl.*

Even this family fortress is not impregnable. He has other needs, which open him to the appeals and evaluations of that outer, threatening world; and when the class attitudes of those who are higher in the social hierarchy betray their contempt for the ethnic group that has furnished the basis of his confidence, his loyalties are challenged, particularly if he is an insecure Jewish youth on the make. His inner conflict is not unlike that in the man who has married above his station and now has to bring his mother to meet the mother of the bride. He hates "those snobs" who, he knows, are looking down their noses at her, and he is ashamed of his own mother and of himself for his shame.

In an autobiographical fragment dealing with one of his experiences in the 1930's, Alfred Kazin (1962) tells of an evening when he had invited Otis Ferguson of *The New Republic* to his home. He tells of his own treasonable feelings toward his family when he suddenly saw his family circle as it most probably looked to this respected stranger. Loyalty to his family, shame for their embarrassing ways, a snobbish affiliation with his superior, an adolescent's willingness to cut off the social liabilities in his family, a still boyish feeling toward his mother, perhaps a touch of shame toward himself that even the telling does not purge: this complex of painful feelings must arise as he tells the story, along with a touch of nostalgia.

Now one of the ranking literary critics of America, Kazin was then a green young graduate of the College of the City of New York, with a briefcase full of essays and a head full of ideals, but without a job to give him any certainty about who he really was. He could scarcely believe his good fortune when John Chamberlain of the *New York Times* heard him out in an interview, and wrote a note to Malcolm Cowley, who promptly gave him a job of book reviewing for *The New Republic.* The "transference relationship" that developed between the cub reviewer and his new mentors, the eagerness with which he listened to their dicta (both political and literary), is still apparent in the lines he writes almost thirty years later. When, after many importunings and many postponements, Otis Ferguson agreed to come to his home for dinner, it was a strange mixture of anxiety and delight that excited the youth when he accompanied his guest to the home in the Brownsville section of Brooklyn where he lived.

He found himself looking out upon his grubby surroundings with a new curiosity and mockery, and wondering how it looked to Ferguson. He saw the "immigrants" on Union Square that he passed on the way home, and he wondered how Ferguson would accept a family that looked like these people. As he brought this visitor (who had the exalted position of reviewer of jazz music) over the subway route he had traveled for years unseeing, all these surroundings suddenly seemed unendurable. He had accepted it all until that moment, as the Arab accepts his Sahara, as one accepts unchanging and immutable facts of life. Now he was anxious lest Ferguson be bored. (He seems to have shifted the base of his *Gemeinschaftsgefühl,* as adolescents do.)

The dinner his mother served was a complete failure, he was sure. Flustered and anxious, his poor mother kept urging meatballs and chicken and cabbage and meatloaf on "poor Ferguson." Slave to the household as she had always been, she did not sit with the family at table. She would eat after the others had finished, sitting down to the leavings. Why did she have to be so insistent, thrusting on the guest food he obviously did not want? Kazin reports that he talked excitedly through the meal, desperately striving to distract his guest with his chatter. Poor Ferguson! Having to dine among the frantic and frightened lower classes! He will be miserable, Kazin thought, "if I do not keep him amused, show him that there is some culture here." (And perhaps he thought, too, what a tale he is going to tell back at the office!)

Now that Kazin was moving among the literary elite, he began to feel that his own life and his own home were "just the opposite of what literature was for." True, poverty was literature in those years of the depression. But not this kind of poverty! "How dreary everything was, how impossibly provincial." And his guest asked Kazin dryly, on the way back to the subway, "What was so exotic about it?"; for Kazin had promised him cooking that would be unusual, something he would not find elsewhere in New York. Poor Mom. Poor Dad. How they had suddenly grown small, weak, odd. Now that this success-bound CCNY graduate had become an affiliate of that brilliant group who surrounded Malcolm Cowley (who knew when the Revolution would come, and how), how could he ever have taken guidance and counsel from such a miserable Brownsville home, or looked to it for his basis of security?

"Who am I?" such an adolescent can ask, for in this "moment of truth" when two identities are in conflict, he is discovering that he is not what his parents have told him he is, and that the world is not the one he learned to look on through his parents' eyes. He looks down on the old one from that immense height where his new superiors live; he is ready to write off the past, or to conceal his affiliation to it and to its ideals, to crush something within him, and to despise what he had hitherto valued and taken for granted. A youth like Kazin who felt drawn to the new socialist-humanist world of Hicks, Cowley, Farrell, Dahlberg, Algren, Dos Passos had so much to unlearn, to repress, to deny, to forget, to put out of his life, including a great deal that had rationalized a childhood morality. And what will he do with that ethnic

Gemeinschaftsgefühl which was so intensified by those Friday evening rituals in the family circle?

Motion across ethnic barriers, climbing the social ladder, crossing national borders involve the individual in a massive restructuring of habits, beliefs, feelings. Parents who have struggled to launch their sons into a new and strange environment which they do not understand too well, sometimes discover that they have lost a son: the more successful the launching, the more complete the loss, especially if he marries "across the border."

I am not trying to raise the question, for the moment, about whether the new values are better or not, trying to choose illustrations that will make us hate the socially mobile, or choose my facts to show that our social structure *causes* mental illness. When the facts show how social mobility leads to inner conflict and can provide a content for psychobiological tensions, they also show that a personal-social history (in addition to an evaluation of the genetic factor) is required in the assessment of a "case." For when pressures of this type become more intense than can be borne without symptoms, when the "solutions" the person has attempted also initiate vicious cycles that ultimately become pathogenic, or when an unusual personal history makes an individual especially vulnerable to such pressures, then the social framework can become causal. But this same social structure, this same type of mobility, also permits four out of five to adjust without noteworthy symptoms.

A GIRL'S REVOLT AGAINST HER SEX ROLE

A culture is a relatively stable thing. It outlasts the individuals who move through the roles it designs for them. Class attitudes, sex attitudes, diversified roles of the vocations are all transmitted in the course of socialization. A process of mimesis, of imitation, of social drill teaches the individual to conform to the design, as though the individual were born upon a piece of tapestry at a particular point and were made to fit just that part of the design.[20] Usually, this world he never made shapes the individual to fit into an appropriate social niche. Even the Marxian analysis of historical changes leans heavily on the concept of a class consciousness that is shaped by the individual's role in a system of ownership and production. Before we begin to think about the society around us, these regularities in our attitudes have assumed their fateful shape.

There are individuals, however, who do not take on the expected class ways, who rebel against their sex roles, who violate our anticipations. Simone de Beauvoir (1956) has described her own adolescent experiences and her intense hatred for that kind of attractive, middle-class woman her mother and father expected her to become. And in her *The Second Sex* (1949) she has tried to draw a generalized portrait of a process that is, even now she believes, alienat-

---

[20]Mimesis, as used by Toynbee, is a kind of social drill, a set of cultural exercises which train the young in the accepted ways. But transmission also takes place by tales told around the campfire, by funeral orations in praise of the dead, by morality plays and epic poems, by every device which emphasizes the values of a culture.

ing the majority of women from the kind of self-actualization they might achieve. (Perhaps we should note that in her opinion the majority *should* feel alienated, since she is undoubtedly generalizing from her own experience and attempting to stare down "the peasants and contented cows" who, in turn, disapprove of her ways.)

Describing the first separation from the breast and from the mother's warm and protective embrace, she notes how the little girl's struggle to get back to this primal *Gemeinschaftsgefühl* can subject her to a kind of *seduction*. A conditional love (granted or withheld according to whether she fulfills certain requirements) can force the girl to pretend to be the little angel that she is not, to hide a welter of impulses whose expression would endanger the very foundation of her security and prevent the expressions of affection she craves. Or (and Mme. de Beauvoir confesses that by the time her own adolescence came along a violent revolt was her own way of meeting the issue), she may rebel against every restraint, display disgust at every seductive touch. To save herself she may avoid shaking hands, refuse to smile, reject the dresses that would make her attractive to boys. All that the family offers to her is responded to as though it were something dishonest, restrictive, castrating.

In her own words:

"I wanted to go to the Polytechnique, to study math and science. 'What a pity,' my father said, 'Simone wasn't a boy.'...My sex debarred me from such lofty ambitions....I found smiling difficult. I couldn't turn on the charm. Girls were to strive to become brilliant ornaments. I got the reputation of being a monster of incivility. I hardly ever brushed my teeth, and never cleaned my nails. My father... gave up in disgust."

Writing about a friend who planned to marry and settle down, Mme. de Beauvoir observes: "She was clearly abdicating her individuality." And although her own rebellion made her feel terribly alone, she wanted to be different. She would rise above bourgeois mediocrity. "I will always be ostracized."

She rejected the goals which her father seemed to be following, believing that his main aim in life was "to keep out of trouble and enjoy life." And his attitude toward women troubled her deeply. In more general terms, she writes: "Everyone has the right to bring to fulfillment what I called their eternal essence....I had to save myself from them....I found it exhausting to be fabricating masks ceaselessly."

And in her rebellion, she embraced "the principles of immoralism....Doing wrong was the most uncompromising way of repudiating all connections with respectable people....I wished that I could vomit up my heart." And then, somewhat plaintively she adds, "I needed something to believe in." She wanted to communicate all this in some relation of complete intimacy, but the thought of marriage was revolting: "A personal mutilation."

Despising all that was smug and respectable (bourgeois, in her vocabulary) she sought out companions who were also different. "Together we hated the Sunday crowds, the ladies and gentlemen who were conducting themselves so properly, the stuffy and oppressive solitude of the province, the families, the children, and all the oppressive humanism of propriety." And so she haunted the cafés, rubbed elbows with prostitutes and demimondaines, sought out interesting nonconformist characters in that society where "birds of a feather flock together" and create their own *Gemeinschaftsgefühl* far from the despised roles of middle-class propriety. She even felt certain that any *authentic* person was bound to be different; and her active imagination promptly wove a certain mystical aura about those whom she loved and respected, that is to say, about those who, like herself, were walking on the wild side, on the sincere side, for these were obviously ones who would make no compromises. Honesty? Within the middle class? Impossible![21]

Thus the mature Mme. de Beauvoir gives her considered opinion of that adolescent girl who was angry, confused, ready to snap at every hand that would domesticate her, and not always clear about what she was going to be *for*. To accept the normal ways of married life struck her as a complete capitulation (she called it castration); and yet in defending herself she arrived at something less than full womanhood. "I will wipe out every vestige of the simple-sweet-and-girlish in my nature. I will have no children. I will stamp out those instinctive claims that would use me, enslave me, and make me serve the race instead of my own essential self." How vulgar, how very ordinary, to carry out a merely animal mission. "A peasant could do it as well as I, or better. Or still better, a cat: for she has a litter at a time."

Long before she had freed herself from the home, she knew how deep the sigh of relief would be when she had a room of her own, with no one to watch her going or coming. The pure ozone of the streets of Paris would give her that heady sense of freedom she needed. She could study all night and sleep all day, if she chose. She could eat what she liked and forget about food for a day or two if she wanted to. She could dress in her own odd style, half nun, half demimondaine, with a touch of the ascetic male athlete added, defying the mode with her bold swish of independence.[22]

All of this rebellion can be described in the abstract language of existentialism (which Mme. de Beauvoir later adopted). The individual can claim for it the highest of moral sanctions, appealing to his own elite circle for confirmation. The mother who wanted to seduce her can be converted, in the daughter's thought, into a Mata Hari, an enemy of her own sex, while the father, of course, symbolizes the enemy of all self-actualizing women.

All of this, again, can occur "without symptoms" (unless, following the Soviet pattern, the whole complex of attitudes is viewed as a symptom). Or it can give both form and content to a mental illness, and include with these attitudes vicious cycles that lead to serious abnormalities (such as narcotic addiction). The differentiating process can produce not only a complete rejection of the easier conformist role but also an adoption of some of the

---

[21]Like some of our contemporary beatniks, Simone de Beauvoir knew almost instinctively what she was against. She confessed her need to believe in something, but this proved to be more difficult, although Sartre was of some assistance to her.

[22]Perhaps this kind of adolescent drama has something to do with some of those facts Dr. Hare reported in his study of the relationship between the concentration of single-person dwelling units and schizophrenia.

abnormalities that are found in greater frequency among these enclaves of "outsiders."

Such a case history, drawn up as an interpersonal discourse, presents a drama, a struggle, an individual's response to the challenge of conventions. The neural circuits, the genetic susceptibilities, the physiology of muscles and glands are all left out of the account. We may as well admit that the interpersonal data could not have been predicted from the physiological traits of an organism, that some of the psychobiological data might be secondary to the course of interpersonal exchanges. The primacy of this drama is intuitively grasped. A description such as that of Mme. de Beauvoir (or of some clinician with an imaginative grasp of a patient's struggle) can be accepted for the same reason: it arouses an echo within us. A clinician, we conclude, can "make a history" in the way a poem is made; his sensitivity is disciplined both by his personal experience and by such "histories" as the one Mme. de Beauvoir tells, rather than by the sciences which form the backbone of his medical and psychological training. Santayana, trying to assess the relative merits of a scientific and a literary psychology, once suggested that to the former belong all the facts, to the latter all that matters.[23]

Gemeinschaftsgefühl: A Summary

Social feelings can operate to keep us within the bounds of ordinance. They can be supportive, strength-giving, sthenic in their influence. Our three examples also show us how they can lead an individual into social conflicts when the structure of the social field manages to alienate him from his kind. There is every reason to include such conflicts in our account of pathology.

If man could design a culture in which all values would operate in perfect harmony, how different it would be from the one we live in! This is the dream of the utopians, the theme of Plato's *Republic*. In the open-ended[24] society, with its ambiguous future and its opposed tensions in the here and now, *Gemeinschaftsgefühl* is itself divided, and the seam separates two kinds of truth, of beauty, and of goodness.

---

[23]Santayana (1923, pp. 252-61): "Scientific psychology is a part of physics, or the study of nature; it is the record of how animals act. Literary psychology is the art of imagining how they feel and think." To Santayana's evaluation we could add that of Archibald MacLeish (1961): "When the fact is disassociated from the feel of the fact in the minds of an entire people—in the common mind of a civilization—that people, that civilization, is in danger." Grisly, impersonal, scientific, our industrial society seems to push us into calling a man a complex physical object that moves through a world of physical energies, only this and nothing more. So the primrose at the river's brim becomes a botanical specimen. Copulation is studied with parallel records of respiration and circulation, with EEGs of cortical action. And so, complains Joseph Wood Krutch (1929), we witness the decline of love as a value.

[24]A society is open-ended when the thought-stopping word "sacred!" is not posted over traditional ways, or when the "ultimate and last things" are regarded as something to be given final formulation later, as more wisdom is achieved. Its arteries have not yet hardened to the point where a mental sclerosis has also set in. It does not have the rigidity of a governing class that is "cornered" and regards the slightest difference of opinion as treason.

Consider the dilemma of the military psychiatrist: with compassion for the soldier, he could solve the problem of combat fatigue rather simply, by signing a paper that will give him a berth on the transport bound for home. As his own case load goes up (and battle casualties in general increase) with the intensity of fighting, in order to maintain the strength of combat units and to support morale he must urge his patients to contain their tensions and go back to the battlefront. Were he to excuse the tired and exhausted, others would too soon reach the end of their powers. The officer has to do all he can to win the war, to maintain the fighting strength, and if something has to give, it may very well be the tissues of the soldier, as evidenced by some psychosomatic illness. Treatment of a gunshot wound or an ulcer, the command of a line officer or a military psychiatrist, are alike determined by that main objective, not by the health of the soldier or the peace of mind that could be purchased by defeat.

The priest, as spiritual guide, is interested, according to Monsignor Sheen (1949), in his parishioner's peace of soul, not merely in his peace of mind, and to achieve his purposes he may use a confessional and a ritual that would make an agnostic psychiatrist shudder. On the other hand, he possesses a means of bringing absolution and freedom from guilt to his clients that the agnostic psychiatrist cannot use without violating his conception of professional ethics and those other standards of truth that he learned as a medical student. Again, by conforming to a milieu that violates the standards of a humanistic tradition, the citizen of a dictatorship may achieve health and peace of mind, purchasing a behavioral and organic integrity at the sacrifice of other values.

The price we are willing to pay for the values we promote is one measure of their worth. The martyr is a *witness* to something he holds dearer than life. The counselor who puts a symptom-free life first may work to undermine his patient's conscience. A politician who is primarily interested in holding power or in building a strong state may be willing to use a form of terror and propaganda that destroys health and runs counter to every other value.

A great deal of confusion would be avoided if we kept a few of these distinctions clear. Then we would not be tempted to make all anxiety the consequence of some moral lapse. We would not deny the relevance of ethical conflicts in the pathogenesis of mental illness. We would not attribute all mental illnesses to cultural causes when, in fact, so much of it is caused by individuals who put certain private values first. We would not seek to describe all illness in purely biochemical terms when, of all creatures, the human being assumes his stance in a field of inter*personal* forces. We would not blame the milieu for a constitutionally based disorder when it is primarily the *content* of a patient's delusions that has been provided by social meanings. The facts have a way of eluding the rigid system maker; they call for a flexibility that will test any clinician's wit. As protean as life itself, mental illness requires an understanding like that of the artist, but of a very special type of artist, whose imagination is also disciplined in the sciences.

EXCEPTIONAL CASES OF SOCIAL PRESSURE

Steadily enduring social pressures of low intensity may operate in a hidden fashion to produce an annual quota of suicides, mental illnesses, character disorders, and sudden unexplained deaths. These factors can be buried among other, more obvious "natural" causes, so that they do not catch the eye of the observer; when they are not easily measured, they are not likely to appear in any statistical analysis. Only in their extreme forms, when abrupt or massive changes call them to our attention, are they likely to provide those convincing concomitant variations that suggest live hypotheses to the scientist.

Sudden Death and Morale

The feeling of belonging, produced by the warm, supporting milieu whose sensed presence gives us confidence and peace of mind, the strength that arises from membership in a group with high morale—these protect the individual from discouragement and give him the courage for persistent striving. His personal morale is then as good as that of his community and its leadership. Observers on the Western Front and in Okinawa, in World War II, reported fewer cases of combat fatigue in units with high morale and during times of military success.

Sometimes an enthusiast sees a low rate of neuropsychiatric casualties as a direct proof of the values of an ideology. Wilder Penfield, the distinguished American neurosurgeon, serving on a delegation to the USSR in World War II, spoke of the high morale of the Russian troops: "The percentage of neuroses is minimal, because they have provided the perfect antidote, good morale." The Russian press, in picking up his comment, added: "The protection against mental illness consists essentially in the suppression of the conditions which bring about mental illness, in improving the conditions of work and of existence, as is possible in the USSR on a scale that is virtually without limit" (see Wortis 1950).

Morale was also attributed to religious faith, in a breakfast speech to the National Council of Catholic Youth, by Attorney General Robert Kennedy, who was disturbed by reports that "one out of ten Americans captured in Korea turned informer." He attributed the high fatality rate among American prisoners in Korea to the fact that they were thinking more of themselves than of their fellow wounded, and had no belief in anything, and added, "If it is not done by you it will not be done at all" (UP dispatch, Nov. 11, 1961). Belief shapes opinion; opinion unsupported by facts further strengthens belief; and the solidarity of the group within which such self-reinforcing cycles circulate produces a kind of "truth."

When an individual loses this social support, or when there is a disintegration of the structure of a group (for groups also have their periods of health and of decline), these changes may actually spell the difference between life and death, particularly for that individual who has been clinging to a marginal existence.

Consider the very special case of the aging patient whose aorta wall has slowly narrowed the opening for free passage of blood to 0.2 cm. Emergencies that call for increased blood flow and oxygen force the heart rate to double (from 72 to 144 beats per minute) and respiration to triple (from 17 to 51 breaths per minute), and also stimulate contraction in the muscular lining of the aorta. At a peak demand, the opening can close completely, causing sudden death; the occasion could be an altercation between this aging patient and his son. (See Isberg 1956.)

There are other cases of "sudden death" which highlight broader social aspects of the problem. Consider the hopelessness of the Australian tribesman who is undergoing a ritual punishment for the violation of a taboo (Warner 1941):

"If all of a man's near kin, his father, mother, brothers and sisters, wife, children, business associates, friends and all other members of the society should suddenly withdraw themselves because of some dramatic circumstance, refusing to take any attitude but one of taboo and looking at the man as one already dead, and then after some little time perform over him a sacred ceremony which is believed with certainty to guide him out of the land of the living into that of the dead, the enormous suggestive power of this two-fold movement of the community, after it has had its attitudes crystallized, can be somewhat understood by ourselves."

Biological and social factors, such as we have been describing, may have to combine to produce this type of exceptional event. The aging process that narrows the lumen of the aorta may have taken twenty years: the father could have withstood the quarrel at age forty. The emergency that terminates a life could as well be a call for lifesaving action in time of flood. Sometimes the approach of such critical junctures, first sensed as a mere shortness of breath, may itself provide a surge of anxiety that thus anticipates and hastens the catastrophic event. The progressive worsening of a person's situation may produce a mixture of anger, guilt, and fear that mounts to the point where he will actually choose some stressful action that will liquidate the exhausting tension, putting an end to it all. Although the medical verdict will then be "arterial stenosis," the patient's voluntary action (a long walk in the cold, chopping wood, a wild drive in traffic) can be as suicidal as if he had chosen to shoot himself.

EXPERIMENTAL STUDIES OF DEATH

Cannon, Richter, and others, not content with descriptions at the social level, have looked down among the tissues for other physiological processes that might contribute to these sudden deaths. Speculating about the vulnerable sectors in the body's homeostatic defenses, Cannon (1957) has suggested that an emotional stress might induce a disastrous *fall* in blood pressure and an increase in blood volume circulating through the capillaries, the joint action of adrenaline and sympathin creating a state of shock.

Richter (1957) offered another description based on his observations of gray rats forced to swim to the point of exhaustion. He found that death arrived as a parasympathetic action, as the vagus nerve became dominant.

The records of the drowning animals showed a slowing of the heart, a slowing of respiration, and a lowering of bodily temperature. In the first responses of the animals to handling (lifting from the cages, cutting off vibrissae, immersion in water of varying temperatures), the sympathetic branch of the autonomic system dominated (accelerating heart rate and respiration). Prolonged immersion in the water was followed by parasympathetic dominance, until a point was reached in which the animals rather suddenly "gave up." He found that this "giving-up point" varied with the water temperature.

Richter also discovered that animals that had been "rescued" before they had reached this exhaustion point swam longer on subsequent trials; by a gradual extension of this "period of hope," he managed to extend the endurance of the animal. Living in an extended life-span (should we call it a life-space-time?), the human being depends even more on the strength-giving bonds with family and friends, and on that hope in the future into which our lives must reach. Excommunicated, abandoned, rejected by others, the individual's "psychological strength" runs out. Looked at as broadly as possible, the total exhaustion of morale must be described as a psychophysiological affair. Using parallel levels of description, a clinician might be forced to include, among those coacting causes of death (or mental illness): anomie, lowered psychological tension, loss of hope, the lumen of the aorta, a tension-produced tonus in the artery walls, the life emergencies confronting the individual, divorce, ethical conflict and guilt, unjust accusations, or the death of a beloved leader.

The clinical eclecticism that mixes languages in this fashion, languages which are appropriate enough when used in a single level of discourse, produces case histories that are the despair of the logician and the system builder. There is a mixture of "apples, pears, and conscious needs"; and to millimeters of aorta opening, multiplied by anxiety or level of arousal, is added a bit of psychological stress, or of structural weakness in the adrenal glands. Each language may suggest working hypotheses; what the system maker gains by a meticulous exclusion of every factor that cannot be described in his preferred language, a clinician loses because of the resultant impoverishment of his imagination.

The "Sensitive" and His Milieu

The relationships we have been discussing are complicated still further by the existence of those individuals so roughly described by the term "sensitives." They have sometimes been described as hystericals, another term so loosely used as to become an epithet more closely related to something in the physician-patient rapport than to any precise "mechanism" within the individual. Or we call them "suggestibles," since they are the ones who first show exaggerated emotional expressions in the crowd, who first respond to the demagogue's use of bludgeon words. They are the ones who trigger the panic in a fire. When the mob in Nuremberg Square sent up its shout of *Sieg Heil!* they were the ones who felt the wave of excitement spreading to the tips of their fingers and to the base of their spinal cords. Among this vaguely defined group of sensitive persons, there will be one who will experience an epileptic attack, a second who will lose control of his bladder, a third who will suffer a heart attack, a fourth whose nitrogen excretion from the kidney will be disturbed.

The quality (or content) of these occasions seems to be of less importance than the intensity of the involvement and the location of the most vulnerable parts of a psychobiological system. The occasion could just as well be the press at the doors of the Vatican when some saint is about to be elevated to a new level of beatitude; the coacting stimuli which overexcite the sensitive organism will then include the peal of the organ, the cries of *"Pape, Pape,"* and the pressure of the bodies of jostling worshippers. Or it could be the actions of a lynching mob, or a group in the Louisiana swamp performing voodoo rites, or a healing ritual at Lourdes. Those who are acting beside these "sensitives," praying, singing, shouting, shoving, weeping, can sweep one of them off his feet, and can on occasion, instead of healing him or validating his new ideology, murder him. The least stable member of such groups is the first to become deregulated, the first to ascend into an "O Altitude" of ecstasy, or to pass into an epileptic coma, or to undergo an LSD experience when only a placebo has been administered, or to die.

WARS, DEPRESSIONS, AND CONCENTRATION CAMPS

Anyone who has lived through wars and depressions knows of the suffering, anxieties, and death threats these catastrophic upheavals produce; from his own memory there emerge remembrances (with somatic accompaniment) that are still disturbing. He will not be too impressed when statisticians show that, by their measures, there has been no change in the rates of mental illness. One study, for example, may show that the suicide rate actually falls in wartime, another that the first-admission rates to mental hospitals are the same in the years just before, during, and just after a war or a depression. The issue is confused when other studies show that a massive national effort to alleviate the worst effects of unemployment actually lifts the level of consumption in some marginal groups in our society.[25]

And while the combat neuroses are going up in the thick of the fighting, the potentially suicidal in the civilian population have something to think about besides their own troubles. Since the first-admission rates bear an unknown relation to the actual mental illness existing in the society, since unrecorded or privately treated cases are not included in such statistics, we are left in considerable doubt. (See Landis and Page 1938, pp. 137-50; Dublin 1963; Dayton 1940; Whitehorn 1956.)

More important than these considerations is the fact that both of these social crises produce consequences that may not reach the attention of

---

[25]At least 40 per cent of the Negro population of Chicago had been living on less than the standard set by the WPA for a manual worker with two children ($973 per year); as conditions worsened, these families experienced an improvement in their condition (Drake and Cayton 1945, p. 517).

physicians in the form of mental illness until more than twenty years have passed. A commission studying the postwar careers of Norwegian concentration-camp survivors (Eitinger 1962) found that new aftereffects were still emerging fifteen years after their imprisonment and suffering. Eighty-seven out of a hundred who were selected for study had returned to employment and were fully occupied within a year of their return to civilian life. They and their physicians were ready to say, at that time, that the aftereffects of their war experiences were not going to be severe. As the years passed, the "scarring" has become increasingly clear (in both physiological and psychological systems). Only four out of the hundred studied were free from symptoms in 1960. In eighty-four, who felt they were coping with their work satisfactorily, the physicians turned up evidence indicating that, in fact, they were functioning close to the limit of their capacities; they had to lie down after work, exhausted, and they seemed to live within a very narrow margin of safety. Their symptoms ranged through increased susceptibility to fatigue, reduced power of concentration, increased irritability, emotional instability, severe weight losses, disturbed sleep (with nightmares), anxiety symptoms, and recurrent associations with the death camps. Seeing a person stretch his arms upward reminded one survivor of fellow prisoners hung up by their arms as a part of torture. Seeing an avenue of trees made another visualize a long row of gallows, with swinging corpses. Children playing peacefully in the street called up the image of other children they had seen in death camp: emaciated, tortured, murdered.

In another study (Edwards and Acker 1962) the galvanic skin reflexes were used to measure the responses of naval veterans to the "battle stations" signal. Those who had experienced the signal under combat conditions gave significantly larger responses than a control group, even when 15 to 20 years had elapsed since their original service-connected "conditioning" took place.

In addition to these easily measured aftereffects there were others more difficult to appraise. The disruption of family life, the effects on infants who are without fathers may continue to ricochet down the years, cropping up in the next generation and not measured in any admission-rate figures taken in the immediate postwar years. Like the imported spirochetes of syphilis, which return with the troops, and whose ultimate effects on rates for syphilis of the central nervous system (general paresis) will be slow to mature, the ultimate costs in human suffering accumulate slowly. We do not know the precise effects of a trained capacity to kill (the enemy, of course) without compunction, or if this capacity has generalized to produce more crimes of violence in the postwar society.

THERAPIST AND PATIENT IN TIMES OF CRISIS

Sometimes a brief sketch will carry more conviction than a mass of figures; questionable as it may be as scientific datum, it moves us. Psychotherapists are capable of being moved too. Consider the following sketch of military psychiatry, drawn by a participant observer (Wagner 1946) who makes no effort to mask his feelings:

"At one of the reception centers back of the battle lines in World War II, a military psychiatrist observed the men entering the clearing station. Having reached the end of their resources (and morale) and having been 'whipped' and cursed by their platoon leader who called them yellow when they refused to fight any further, and having been told 'to get the hell out of this outfit,' the men seemed to drag their bodies into the tent. Glassy-eyed, apathetic, they sat in the midst of a noisy, grousing, disturbed group of men. The doctors who had processed them by the hundreds sometimes used methods that are hard to relate to any peace-time psychiatric principles.

"There were moments when spontaneous displays of admiration, enthusiasm, outrage, indignation, solicitude, affection, sympathy, or encouragement shook the receiving tent with unabashed spirited fervor. Psychiatrists would provoke such display of feeling for the patient's benefit and perhaps their own relief of tension. Thus, one would pound the table, shout with admiration, and lean toward a colleague to say: 'Hey, Major, here's a real soldier for you. Forty days on the line, knocked on his can by an '88, and he wants to go back and give those bastards some more!' Whereupon all the psychiatrists would turn around, beam, and shout approval. Or, another would shout: 'What an outfit the X-regiment is, by God, keep them on their feet long enough and they'll take the Goddam German Army themselves!' whereupon a chorus of approbation and solemn nods would prevail throughout the receiving tent.... There was no place for sensitivity on the line, nor could the military psychiatrist expect any nursing of his patients once they were marked fit for duty."

There is another war that goes on, even in peacetime, a war with poverty and unemployment. Millions of marginal workers lose their battle when, in a depression such as America experienced in the 1930's, the boxcar loadings fall, the public relief load mounts, and between ten and twenty million formerly self-supporting persons depend on others for their bare maintenance. It was during these years that the following case report (Richards 1934) was published from the Johns Hopkins Hospital outpatient services.

"Earl H., aged 32, a worker of the Bethlehem Steel Company was referred to our psychiatric dispensary. One morning, several weeks before, he ran into the accident room of our hospital in an attack of belching, palpitation, dyspnea, and apprehensiveness.

"The present illness began in September, 1932. From that time until he came into our accident room he was under almost continuous treatment from a gastro-intestinal standpoint. All the examinations were negative. He was tried on belladonna and diets and bromides and other nerve medicine; every time this therapy failed he became even more panicky and upset than before. Within two weeks time his sick benefit would have expired.

"In the background of the condition we find a man who had worked regularly for the Bethlehem Steel Company since twenty years of age. He is a skilled workman. Last June, by reason of two cuts he was unable to keep up the payment on a home which he had been trying to buy during the last three years, and to which he and his family were much attached. All summer they looked for quarters, and in the fall they found a broken-down shack of a place which they were able to get for very little rent because the owner could find nothing else to do with it. A friend of the family who had always paid board until this time lost his job in September, 1932, and Mr. H. felt that he should keep him. The patient did not complain of any of these circumstances that I have mentioned. His complaint was of his stomach and the palpitations. When asked in general about worries and cares he denied the same in a cheerful way, saying, 'We all have our troubles and mine were no worse than anybody else's, I guess. If I were feeling well, I would not mind anything.' This man was put directly back on his job, being told that he would feel badly, that he would have more attacks, but if he would see it through he would not regret the effort it took to break up these nervous habits. He returned to work five days after his condition was explained to him and has not lost a day since then. . . .

"Of 232 cases [treated] 65% responded in a matter of weeks or a month or two to the treatment procedures I have outlined. The remaining 35% fell into the groupings of *unmodifiable human material.*"[26]

In this peacetime "war" the line officers also have to buck up the soldiers and send them back to the firing line. Those who, unlike the case reported, do not respond, who do not "show the right attitude," or who show symptoms that progress to those of a psychosis present a problem to their physicians, and occasionally the diagnosis "hysterical" conceals the low opinion that the examiner has of what he views as "poor human material." (Kurt Schneider has recommended the term be dropped, since it has become vague and charged with moral overtones.) Obviously, with ten million unemployed it would not be possible to provide analytic couches for all who develop anxiety over unpaid bills, loss of home, lack of access to medical services, and so on. The daily fifty-minute interviews, the sensitive probing to unearth early childhood experiences, ingenious interpretations of dreams, will therefore not be used for those who are submerged in the events of a depression (or for Appalachia, or for the "lower lowers" in the class structure of America). Fatigue, anxiety, sleeplessness, apathy, psychosomatic symptoms, and morose inaction may spread like an epidemic. If there is a hardening of class attitudes, it may very well result in the physician's loss of sympathy for the malcontented, shiftless, poor, helpless, weak patients who show up in the clinic.

It was in this setting that Dr. Richards outlined her "rough and ready" therapy for these cases:

"The best educational process is sending such a patient right straight back to work, or to send him into crowds, or whatever else he is afraid of, telling him that he is quite likely to have other seizures, that he will feel wretchedly apprehensive, but if he will stick it out he will cure his fear, and he alone can do the trick. Years ago when we had horses and steam rollers, the same sort of educational process worked in getting the horse over being afraid of this terrifying object in the road.

---

[26]Dr. Richards explains this phrase as "cases in which the symptoms reported are prodromal manifestations of some major psychosis or of a psychopathic personality picture." In light of Dr. Richards's account of a relatively brief and simple therapy that proved to be successful in two-thirds of the cases, her judgment of the remaining 35 per cent may be questioned. Given by a physician responsible for treatment it could become self-validating, in which case some of the difficulties in the unmodifiables might even be iatrogenic.

One drove him close to it, let him shake and tremble and jump, and eventually he became so used to the engine that he did not even shy. Change of scene with its diversions merely postpones the day when the patient must face the situation which gave rise to his fears. Moreover, one must remember that he takes his personality and biology with him to Atlantic City or Europe."

When Hollingshead and Redlich (1958) returned to this problem of doctor-patient relationships thirty years later, equipped with the caste-and-class concepts of Lloyd Warner, they added a new dimension to our understanding of social factors in treatment. Their views might be summarized, briefly, in the following six points:

1. There are today too few trained counselors and psychiatrists to handle the mass of existing mental illness, at least by those methods that would be chosen for paying patients who deserve the very best possible therapy. Mental health is purchasable, but the poor can't pay for it.

2. Economic factors and the lack of staff conspire to give the lowest socio-economic groups custodial care and physical therapies, such as electroshock, chemical therapy, and psychosurgery.

3. Even when therapy is made available to the poor, there remains a barrier between physician and patient, attitudes which block rapport. Insight therapy requires a certain level of education and understanding on the part of the patient, and the interpretations of his counselor may provoke rather than assist the patient. The two worlds are foreign to each other; poverty has its own culture (see Harrington 1962 and O. Lewis 1965).

4. The duration of hospitalization and treatment is longer for the two upper classes.

5. By spreading the work of the experts thin, by using psychiatrists as consultants for "lay counselors," by using group therapy, innovators are attempting to reach that inaccessible lower stratum which contains the greatest number of cases needing therapy.

6. The conception of therapy and the level of expectation of patients vary from social stratum to social stratum.

The difficulties (as found in the New Haven area) that put a strain upon doctor-patient relationships are intensified when therapy has to bridge the gap between a Harvard-trained psychiatrist and the depressed mountaineer who was born on a hillside in western Carolina or Tennessee. Race or caste provides an additional barrier; the attitudes that have arisen during the recent years of civil-rights struggle have been so much in the public press as to need no documentation.

A SOCIOLOGIST STUDIES A THEORY OF MENTAL ILLNESS

We have seen that differences in class membership enter into the relationships between physician and patient. They affect the proportions of the mentally ill under treatment, as well as the kinds of treatment offered. In addition to these concrete findings, there are other aspects of a theory, such as the one associated with the name of Freud, that need to be considered.

Launched at the turn of the century, psychoanalysis has gradually become one of the leading theories of mental illness, if not the foremost one. As it has been diffused through our culture, it has affected books, plays, scholarly essays, criticisms of society, theories of politics, explanations of juvenile delinquency, attitudes toward human growth and development. Even the man on the street who pretends to little education knows something about it: "Freudianism? Isn't that all about sex?" As such a theory is spread, it is also altered, distorted, popularized, bowdlerized; it is both used and abused. Like other symbolic constructions, it could be said to have a life of its own. When it is widely "understood," it may even be incorporated by a patient, so that the one who is experiencing a neurosis comes to his physician with a self-diagnosis expressed in psychoanalytic terms and expecting a certain type of therapy.[27] Or it may get a bad name, be viewed as a force subverting the American character, and so lead a potential patient to resist any treatment that he identifies as psychoanalytic. Or it may be viewed as a huge joke, a matter for the cartoonist and for the manufacturer of "sick" jokes; those who subscribe to this view will greet any attempt to use psychoanalytic concepts seriously with laughter, as the height of the absurd.

Serge Moscovici (1960) has made a serious attempt to discover attitudes toward psychoanalysis, using as his respondents samples of a French urban population. Such an inquiry, conducted by questionnaires and interviews, can be carried on with a reasonable objectivity, and with all effort to persuade or evaluate kept out of the search for facts. The theory is simply taken as any other object to be studied, and an ecological map of attitudes can be constructed.

Briefly summarized, Moscovici's study reported that it was the younger subject, the worker, the uneducated, the women, the economically disadvantaged, who believed that psychoanalysis was capable of producing changes, for the better, in the human personality. He discovered that among the journals of opinion, those controlled by the French Communist party were the most hostile. Catholics, who had at first looked upon psychoanalysis as a dangerous invasion of the priest's province (especially the confessional), tended to follow the Pope, who in 1952 sent a special message to an assembly of psychiatrists, commenting on psychoanalysis as a useful method of treating neuroses.[28]

In the hard core of Communist resistance to psychoanalytic theory, there has been an impression that Freudianism is (1) not for the working class; (2) a typical American outlook on man and life; (3) a Hollywood version of therapy; (4) a means of diverting the minds of workers away from the class struggle and toward a life of licentious pleasure; (5) an ideological defense of the con-

---

[27] Dr. Sclare, writing from England (1953) of his experiences in an American clinical setting, tells of a woman who interrupted him during her third interview with: "You haven't asked me anything about sex yet—I thought psychiatrists believe it's at the root of everything."

[28] Provided that there is no attempt to bring the material of the confessional into the analytic hour, and provided that there is no attempt to pass judgment on the wisdom of the confessor's recommendations. Best of all is the arrangement between a Catholic psychiatrist and a priest where each agrees to respect the territory of the other.

servative bourgeoisie which finds the explanation of neurosis in the inner conflicts of the individual rather than in the capitalist mode of production; (6)
a form of brainwashing that, applied on a massive scale, could create a new
type of father image for immature voters, and could utilize infantile dependent
needs and other human frailties as a weapon against the proletariat. That the
working-class sample endorsed psychoanalysis as a force which could change
the human personality for the better is an interesting comment on the prestige
and power of these "hard-core" leaders and their journals of opinion.

Other interesting items included in Moscovici's summary raise questions that
call for a much more extensive documentation. For example, students were
more favorable to the theory than their professors, whether in the medical
school, the *lycée,* or the engineering school. Adolescents are much more certain
of its power and value than older persons. One adolescent explained why he
knew it was an important form of therapy:

"In my own case, I had the temerity to take over the spiritual guidance of a
young lycéenne. I found her depressed. The young man she had lovd from afar
had disappeared, and she had gone through a period in which painful dreams,
dreams of jealousy and deception, and finally olfactory hallucinations haunted her.
It seems that she had prayed to St. Theresa to guide her, and to show her by some
sign, say a pleasant odor, as had happened to one of her ancestors, if she should
see this youth again. And a few days thereafter the noticed the fragrance of some
mild tobacco—and there was no material cause present—and she had been very
deeply impressed. Indeed she had fainted. Now this girl is a very stable and normal
girl, apart from this episode, sensitive but in no sense 'exalted' [i.e., given to
mystical experiences]. She asked herself, 'Had St. Theresa actually intervened?' ...
Once I furnished her with the true explanation, based on the idea of sexual repression (for she had struggled to put her thoughts about this young man out of her
head), she was at first astonished, then quite satisfied with the idea, and in the
end she had no further suffering from this source and turned toward the future
with a calm confidence that things would work out satisfactorily."

Another respondent, a mother, replied to the investigator's query with:

"I have never tried to apply psychoanalysis in order to understand myself or
others. ... Everyone is doing it, around me, even the young ones (my sons, espe-
ecially, seem interested in it). They have read a whole shelf of books on psychoanalysis, and they try to understand the behavior of their younger sister in this
way. They blame me, too, for not having known how to bring them up, and for
having given them complexes. I believe that one ought to put a little manual in
the hands of every mother of a family, with all of the principles revealed by
psychoanalysis, if only to save her from the later reproaches of her children, when
they become adolescents."

Moscovici advances a tentative hypothesis to explain some of his facts. He
suggests that the higher social and educational categories are more comfortably
installed in their social roles, more conservative in their social outlook, less
in need of a change in either their lives, their capabilities, or their social roles.
The young, the uncertain, the marginal worker, the unfulfilled have the vague

feeling that there is or ought to be some therapy which would release their powers, help them win friends and influence people, clarify their confused and disappointed attitudes toward themselves and toward their society. In short, Moscovici is offering a type of wish-fulfillment explanation for his findings, a view that is itself not wholly unrelated to psychoanalysis. He adds, however, that to judge by his sample of replies, those who have the least familiarity with the theory in question, who lack the education required to understand it, are the most certain that it works, and that its effects are on the whole good.

Moscovici asks: "Why shouldn't psychoanalysis be the theory par excellence for the adolescent period?" He points out that it is a theory of the personality and of the self's attitudes toward the self, the guilty self, the inferior self, the greedy, impulsive, gluttonous, sexual self that has not yet achieved full self-mastery and is in full revolt against society and all authority figures. Traditional psychology had forgotten this adolescent self, he thinks; its accounts of life had been written by psychologists and medical men who had put away (or repressed or forgotten) their own adolescent problems. Freud's theories, on the contrary, are designed to catch the interest of personalities in formation, give them a vocabulary that will enable them to wrestle with the chimeras that haunt them, and, in particular, enable them to come to terms with their sexuality and that problem of love, half myth, half physiology, half sacred, half taboo. This theory is particularly apt for any adolescent who has not yet found his way to a conventional sex role: young males not sure of their masculinity, young high-school girls experiencing a crush on an older girl or teacher. The enormous curiosity that drives an adolescent to find out something about his world, that requires him to appear much more sophisticated than in fact he is, will be rewarded by these books that make him the most sophisticated, the most knowledgable, the most familiar with "the latest word." An adolescent can read them secretly in order to be able to toss off his "clinical opinion" when his chums next provide him with the opportunity. If he receives reinforcement and "acceptance" through his wisdom, he may discover that he is, in fact, a psychoanalyst (as in the case cited above).

In the end, the figures are ambiguous, and will remain so until subsequent follow-up studies show, for example, that the young students become less convinced of the efficacy of the theory as they acquire experience equal to that of their skeptical professors. It may turn out, however, that subsequent studies will show that the new "older" generation will be convinced of the truth of psychoanalysis, and that the weapons it provides will have been turned against another adolescent group, who then will be hostile to a theory that will have become "old hat."

SOCIALLY AGREED-ON INTERPRETATIONS OF DREAMING

When dreams have become embedded in social practices and have been given a special significance, their form as well as the frequency with which they are reported and given emphasis will be altered. Anthropologists report that dreaming often is given a practical role by primitive peoples. A similar role has been assigned to dreams and related phenomena by various religious groups, particularly those of mystical inclination. Since Freud, many psychotherapists—notably members of the psychoanalytical schools—have found use for dreams in diagnosis and treatment.

The primitive medicine man believed that man in his dreams approached the spirit world, the kingdom of the dead. Spirits of the dead were believed to be moving among the tribesmen during the daytime, but until sleep removed the barriers that blinded the eyes during the day, man could not see these spirits clearly. Maintaining contact with the spirit world, and especially with each tribesman's personal spirit guide, was an essential preparation for the future; where hunters or war parties dreamed of game or of victory over an enemy, they sallied forth armed with confidence. And fasts, suffering, isolation, exposure were used to coerce dreaming. The anthropologist Lowie has described the fixed ritual of the Crow Indians:

"A would-be visionary would go to a lonely spot, preferably the summit of a mountain. Naked except for a breechclout and the buffalo robe to cover him at night, he abstained from food and drink for four days or more if necessary, wailing and invoking the spirits. Usually some form of bodily torture or disfigurement was practiced as an offering to the supernatural beings."

The modern coercers of dreams, the cultists who use mescaline, LSD-25, psilocybin, peyote buttons, hashish, marijuana, sacred mushrooms, morning-glory seeds, or any one of a number of new synthetic "tranquilizers," are the successors of these primitive tribesmen. Though the contents of their dreams have changed, along with their supporting rationalizations and beliefs, there is a basic similarity of attitudes.

As for more modern types of religious mysticism, as well as Freudian and neo-Freudian psychoanalysis, they also carry a metapsychology with them—a set of preconceptions into which they fit the facts about dreaming. According to Freud's theory, the dream has a double function: it expresses, ventilates, and at least symbolically gratifies instinctual forces; and it conceals and gives a half-reasonable order to what would otherwise confuse, shock, and waken an ego. Before a dream is visible, there has been "dream work," a process that shapes the action. Widely ramifying and often contradictory tendencies are condensed into some single act or object; for instance, important impulses may be disguised, toned down, reduced to a minor role, while relatively unimportant characters are moved into the principal roles, or the opposite of the real (latent) theme may be shown in the foreground (manifest content), as when an act of saving a life is permitted to symbolize a murderous wish. What the dream work does, then, is to mediate between an ego (and its conscience, the superego) and that mass of repressed impulses that each of us carries out of sight. To undo the dream work, an analyst needs the willing assistance of the dreamer through many hours of unraveling the association chains that dangle from each part of the manifest dream. Freud's metapsychology, briefly summarized here, has been applied in thousands of cases—and completely validated in none.

EPILOG

The evidence we have reviewed shows that the incidence of both treated and existing mental illness is greatest in the lowest socioeconomic groups. The attitudes of psychiatrists, most of whom were born in higher-status positions, affect their understanding of those whom they treat; wherever interpretation of life-history data is important for treatment, this handicap can interfere with therapy. The proportion of the total potential case load that is treated is smaller in these lower socioeconomic groups; and those who come to therapy bring a more serious illness (psychotic) rather than the neurosis most of the upper-class ill bring. There is every reason to suspect that the therapy provided for the lower groups is of an inferior type. Even the theory of mental illness adopted by the patient and his physician can be affected by the status factor, thus corrupting some of our published data at their source.

While conservative physicians in America are interpreting these findings in terms of social drift, endowing the poor with unfortunate personality character-istics[29] as well as an equally unfavorable genetic constitution, their professional counterparts in the Soviet Union look on our published data as evidence of the depressing consequences of the capitalist mode of production. Although the population of the USSR is larger than ours, and their percentage of doctors and total hospital bed space not far from ours, they can boast of having only 100,000 beds earmarked for the treatment of the mentally ill (Wortis 1950, p. 60); such a provision of bed space by *one* of the states of our union would mark that state, in our medical opinion, as backward. It may be difficult to discover mental illness in the Soviet Union.

The optimists among us look forward to the time when the war against poverty will have eliminated all the slum conditions which *produce* twisted minds. Our pessimists call for a greater effort and an improvement of morale in those who "just don't want to get ahead."

In the USSR a therapist is likely to recommend an objective kind of recon-ditioning, or some form of work therapy that will reintegrate the patient with the Communist system of production. Meaningful work will provide the tonic for his musculature and restore his sense of social significance. In America the patient who can afford it will be given a highly personalized treatment, and an exploration of his inner conflicts and of his life history will try to provide him with insight that will neutralize these inner conflicts.

In his discussion of medical utopias, René Dubos (1961) observes that with advances in medical knowledge "we can indeed expect a 'new chapter in the

---

[29]Among the traits Harrington (1962) ascribes to the poor are that they: are "rigid" and suspi-cious; have a fatalistic outlook on life, and so do not plan ahead; are prone to depression; have feelings of futility; lack feelings of belongingness, friendliness, and trust in others; are not joiners and doers in community work, such as Civil Defense; are less competent, less educated, and less articulate than the middle classes; are pessimistic about both politics and their personal future; have a poor family life, and a special kind of sophisticated ignorance about sex (and more illegitimate births); they not only, as families, fail to supervise adolescents, but provide delinquent patterns for the latter to copy. In his chapter on "The Twisted Spirit" (pp. 119-35), it is clear that Harrington believes these traits are forced on those "who cannot run any faster."

history of medicine' but the chapter is likely to be as full of diseases as its predecessors: the diseases will only be different from those in the past." He points out that, with maximum effort, we are more likely to alter the forms of mental illness and our understanding of it. If our efforts greatly prolong human life, we may expect that the sanitoria of the future will contain only the aged, who will possibly have certain new syndromes, and the psychiatrists by that time will all have to specialize in geriatrics. Many physicians, especially those of a conservative turn of mind, will rise to hail Dr. Dubos as a realist.

Chapter 4 • Parents and Children

For more than a half-century there have been intensive efforts to study the early relationships between mother and child. Freud was partly responsible, inasmuch as he made the Oedipus complex, with its theme of incestuous affection, central to his doctrine of repression. The behaviorists also did their part, as they attempted to show that many animal choices could be better explained by early conditioning than by the never too satisfactory concept of instinct. Whitman's studies of the sex choices of pigeons (1919) had shown how nest habits changed instinctual patterns so that carrier pigeons would mate with ring-necked doves. Lorenz returned to the theme of "imprinting" in his *King Solomon's Ring* (1952). From the insect to the chimpanzee, the comparative studies had explored these parent-child relationships, while clinical studies that traced the distorted behavior patterns of mentally ill adults back to early infantile experiences and faulty parental care were multiplying. Social workers were talking about the broken homes and the parental rejection that produce deviant behavior, and courses labeled "The Family" became a standard offering in the college curriculum.

During the prenatal period of the human species, the bond between mother and child is so symbiotic as to make this twosome a single biological unity: deficits in the one may be compensated for by the other—as when the hypothyroid mother borrows the hormone from the maturing gland of the foetus—and surpluses in the "host" are matched by compensating subnormal outputs in the "parasite." Even as the two bodies become separated, the child carries a kind of dynamic biological imprint of the mother. Still dependent upon her for his very life in the early months, his first steps toward autonomy, the little orientation flights about an apartment or play yard, are made with one eye on the mother and with a constant readiness to return to that base of security. Bold in her arms, timid when he confronts novelty alone, his courage to be has to be built by trials with successes until he has mastered a wider life-space. She could keep him a "knee baby," tied to her apron strings, if she would (or if she were the only one involved); the father sometimes has to interfere when her anxieties over her as yet helpless infant bar him from normal learning. Before we develop a myth about anxious mothers and courage-demanding fathers, we should mark the infinite variety of relationships that can surround the infant: often it is the mother who is the bold one; sometimes a real handicap in the child complicates the situation; broken homes can distort the relationship. It is not surprising that the therapist, bent on diagnosing and treating the later stages of pathological developments, should be anxious to get all the information he can about his patient's infancy; if he has strong theoretical convictions, the body of data he builds may demonstrate his own bias rather than provide the proofs of cause and effect a science of development must achieve. That the World Health Organization should have devoted two volumes of its reports to summaries of studies of the relationship between mental health and maternal care suggests that we may now have arrived at some general consensus (see Bowlby 1952, Ainsworth *et al.* 1962).

Studies of the role of the mother have shown us that it will be equally important to study the role of the father. The mother is only one of the nurturant agents. Even if she is in fact the most important one in the early months, if she is to function well, her own relationship with the father, as well as her role in the larger society, must be good. It is all too easy for her to pass some of her own tensions onto the child. While the clinician is helping set up an "ideal pattern" for mother-and-child relationships, there are social changes on foot that are carrying this mother into factories, offices, professions. Whether she is glad to relinquish her old role in the family or not, new patterns of nurturant care are developing, and with them, no doubt, new consequences for mental health. Kibbutz, crèche, day-care center, are developing new pathways to autonomy and dependence which we shall need to study in the days to come.

Although in our culture we have made the mother the principal agent in the life of the child, we now know enough about the varieties of maternal care not to count on some magical wellspring of instinctual force that will carry her through her tasks properly in spite of everything. The "maternal instinct," we now know, is a name that covers every variety of mothering: possessive, seductive, rejecting, cruel, overconcerned, overprotective, affectionate, infantilizing, dependent. However, the clinical literature reveals a surfeit of interpretations which insist that the mother is always the focus of the abnormality, that place a greater burden on her shoulders than the facts warrant. Such an Oedipus-complex and "mother-hating" pattern in clinicians is comparable to certain patterns in their neurotic clients; and so sticky has the "tender, loving care" patter of our social workers become that, almost in protest, we shout "Love is not enough!"[1]

---

[1] This was the title that Bettelheim chose for his study (1950) of seriously disorganized children who were treated in the Orthogenic School that he directs. This slogan could mean: "There must be some common sense, too; there must be a permissive but firm discipline that will help the child establish boundaries; there are other organic and physiological problems that mere tender, loving care does not touch."

De Grazia (1952) points to "the mother-hating tendencies of modern psychotherapy."

IDEAL PARENTHOOD: MYTH AND REALITY

Who is this mother whose failure to be all that she might have been now makes her the target of so many psychiatric diagnoses (and reproaches)? In his little book, *In Defense of Mothers,* Leo Kanner summed it all up: "a good and competent mother is a good and competent person." But to spell out precisely what this definition means for those very specific interchanges between mother and child, interchanges that must alter with each stage of development, is not easy. The woman who was a rather poor nurse for a small infant may prove later to be an excellent support for the young professional man about to undertake his first crucial tests as a lawyer; conversely, a wonderful mother for an infant may fail him completely at adolescence. Just as a schoolteacher, happy with her third-graders, becomes terribly unhappy when she is promoted to take charge of a junior-high group (as if they reminded her of problems of her own adolescent years, problems that were never completely resolved), so a mother may be much more successful for a certain early period, and a very bad influence later. The good mother of the psychiatrist's fantasies will be that "woman for all seasons" whose own well-grounded maturity has the confidence and wisdom to confront each of the stages from infancy to maturity, when, let us hope, her child can confront life on his own.

Such a paragon of strength and virtue is a kind of ego-ideal that would make a sensitive mother flinch as she faced the implied responsibilities. Every mother carries her own version of this ego-ideal: it is one of the "gifts" that our culture bestows upon her (see de Beauvoir 1949, vol. I, and Deutsch 1944, vol. II). When her version is also solidly fused with common sense (as Kanner hopes it will be), she will not be swept off her feet by each new enthusiasm that spreads among those who can read, as some clinician discovers some new distortion of nursing, toilet training, demand schedules, bodily contact, or permissive discipline. She will be so well-anchored in her own sense of what life is about, in her natural feelings about people, that she will not need detailed instruction in these matters. As a result she will know when she is too close, too protective, too quick in cutting off her encouragement and support, and can "play by ear," steer her course flexibly, respect the responses of her child which tell her unmistakably when she is off-center. Autonomous youths have been launched, after all, for a long time.

Such a mother would not assign herself the impossible task of keeping her child happy. Instead, she will aim at a much more difficult goal: to teach him how to find his own happiness in productive activities and in good human relationships. She would certainly avoid being autocratic, which is a poor way to govern a household, a self, or a state, and a poor example for a child. She would not need to be a devouring and absorbing mother, for her own life

---

He describes the extent to which some psychotherapists are aligning themselves with their neurotic subjects against "the mothers"; they are described as saying, in effect, "She was a witch, wasn't she? I can be a better parent to you. I will understand you better, permit you the kinds of gratifications she denied, forgive your trespasses, and free you from guilt."

would have its fulfillment outside of those her children bring. Neither will she allow herself to become the slave who, like all who allow themselves to be imposed on, comes to feel a simmering hostility toward those who exploit her.[2]

Such a good and competent woman will be able to help, support, counsel, at every stage of her child's development, but in such a way as to release her child to a freedom and responsibility in which she plays a progressively smaller role. The normal mother-child pair passes through three stages: (1) at first there is a symbiosis in which the mother is both protective and regulative; (2) differentiation emerges and an independent ego develops in the child, who still remains partially dependent on the mother's encapsulating affection and concern until a clash of wills develops and finally resolves itself; (3) the child is released to form a succession of new relationships with others in an ever-widening series of friendly competitions, of giving and receiving, of new freedoms and new responsibilities. As her child grows, such a woman becomes something more and other than a protector and regulator; she stimulates him, disciplines him, makes enough demands on him to teach him the blessings of giving as well as of receiving, of obedience as well as of unconditional immediate satisfactions, and increases his burdens according to his strength and capacity. Almost without intending it, she will become a goal-setter, stimulating him by her own enthusiasms and rewarding him by her praise, even when his goals do not match hers.

Not excessively anxious herself, this good and competent person Kanner describes does not fill her child with a fear of the world or a fear for his own future, whereas it is difficult for a neurotic mother, who is also anxious and depressed, not to fill her child with fears, since the child first sees the world through her eyes. Steering her course between helping and hovering, the competent mother supports his learning while giving him enough latitude to learn from his own experience, some of which will be, no doubt, painful and disgraceful. Will he not have to form judgments of his own, finally? Such a mother must be ready to receive her child's confidences without requiring him to divulge what he ought to retain in privacy, that is to say, without invading something that should remain inviolable.[3]

---

[2]It is interesting to see how many clinicians diagnose a case as "overconcerned and overprotective mother who conceals an unconscious hostility toward her child." This theme is repeated, for example, in Levy's studies of maternal overprotection (1943), in Bruch's studies of obese children, and in Helene Deutsch's sketch of motherhood (1944). See also Cole 1953, especially Chaps. 4 and 8. This diagnosis is most often made by physicians trained in psychoanalytic practices, which can best be used with the upper and upper-middle classes of our society, where neuroses are treated. Neuroses may exist in the lower classes, but, except for the exceptional forms that are referred to clinics by court officers or social workers, they go undiagnosed, untreated, and unreported (except by researchers, such as Srole and his associates). Allison Davis (1943) has shown that child-training methods differ in the lower third of the class structure, and, as Davis and Havighurst (1946, 1947) have pointed out in their studies of character training, the pressures on the child are different. We should be on guard against assuming that a life-style common in one social class is something universal. (See also Whiting and Child 1953, and Orlansky 1949.)

[3]Easy to state in abstract terms, her course must obviously steer its way between opposites;

MOTHERS PLUS FATHERS

A mother, of course, does not exist alone, but shares her responsibilities with a father. The kinds of triangles that develop have infinite variations; each variant creates forces to which the child must adjust and which, in turn, affect the internal regulator (the self) that is taking shape within him. While imagining a good mother, we ought to place beside her a reasonable facsimile of a good father, toward whom psychiatrists (most of whom are males) seem to have turned their blind spot. For many years his portrait was vague. No doubt he is, in fact, a less important figure in the early months, when the mother is so completely in charge. Perhaps there is even a grain of truth in Parrinder's notion that the witch is usually female because this is a male-dominated world. Certainly in a nineteenth-century world, where it was the father who went out to earn the daily bread while the wife remained by the fireside to superintend the kitchen, the nursery, and the household, the woman was supposed to be somehow more concerned with and more gifted in handling the personal and emotional life of the family, and in looking out for the psychological well-being of her child. It may have been in such a society, predominantly agricultural, that our myths took shape.[4]

This father, who goes outside of the home to fend for his family in factory, marketplace, or professional life, can get so engrossed that he forgets that he has a family, at times; he becomes a weekend visitor, an evening playmate that the children see for an hour or so at most, or a Saturday afternoon guest who is preoccupied with the football game on television. Occasionally he is converted into an ogre called on to dispense even-handed justice to all small fry who have misbehaved. Because he is not also engaged in the daily feeding, cleaning, nose-wiping, or toilet training (which are regarded as women's work), and because he disappears into a mysterious outside world (or brings home work that is *important*), he can become a bit strange, distant, fearsome, aweful. He symbolizes outside reality, the marketplace, the law of the land, the important affairs of the world.

A father is also something special to his son, in the way of "copy." He knows how to fish, hunt, build rabbit pens, and do a thousand other things a boy wants to do. And what better place is there to learn about women (well, roughly) than to watch how a father treats the one woman who is so important to the child? If the father "cuts her down" or "lords it over her," the budding masculine ego can see that, before long, he will not need to take

---

the principles she must respect are in fact contradictory. It is this harmony of opposites that the obsessive mother cannot manage; just as she orders her own household so much that its precision interferes with the lives of her spouse and children, she finds difficulty in harmonizing the rest of these opposites. The Supreme Court, too, has to steer its course between respect for the individual and respect for society.

[4]Just as we have not reshaped religious truths to fit the modern secular city, we may have been sluggish in reformulating clear interpersonal relationships for the new home, or in training males for new roles to compensate for the changes in women's status.

any sass from his mother. If, on the other hand, the father treats his wife with tenderness and respect, and with a gentleness that she deserves, his son can internalize and incorporate some of the traits of the "gentle man" as a part of his own nature. The son will also see other aspects of masculinity at close hand. Unhappy the boy who sees a weak father, a poor figure of a man who does not know enough to come in out of the rain, who cannot assert himself against his wife. Such a son would see maleness as a dangerous position, might become a woman hater as he seeks to escape his father's fate, or might even identify himself with women, who seem to have the best of everything. A female-dominated household, like a male-dominated one, is skewed, distorts those roles that sons and daughters inevitably use for copy. It may even warp their life goals.

To his daughter the father is a "sample copy" of the heterosexual partner that hopefully she can one day adore; now as a little female she can study the sample at close hand. And what a mixture he is, of tenderness and terrifying might, of dressed-up grandeur at times, but at others, what an example of disheveled vulgarity! His belches disgust her; his tenderness melts her. He is wonderful, terrible, revolting, frightening; yet, strangely enough, most daughters manage to accept, respect, and even love such mixtures. Succeeding in this task of incorporation, they sally forth into the zoological garden ready to contract an enduring (more or less) relationship with another member of this sex.

Both fathers and mothers are something more than other organisms, more than protectors, punishers, rewarders. They are storytellers, dream merchants. Peter Rabbit, Uncle Remus, Tennyson, Homer; the stories may have originated in faraway places, but as they are told the myths of the culture are filtered to the child. The strange world not only comes alive, but acquires unusual auras: there are castles in Spain, triumphs where little Davids slay mighty Goliaths, great adventures that lie ahead, explorations, voyages, constructions, scientific discoveries. Both the sense of a tough matter-of-fact world and the sense of that more fluid and sometimes utopian world-to-come add meanings to all the internalized values, and are communicated to these small and immature specimens before parents release them, only half-shaped, to the world that gives their egos the finishing touches.[5]

---

[5]Of the autistic dreamer who remains enthralled in a fantasy world, and whom we sometimes call a visionary (and sometimes respect as an artist), we could say that adult reality has never managed to reshape that inner world so that a close fit develops. Angus Wilson suggests that this gap between the two worlds may be, indeed, the mainspring of artistic talent. Commenting on Zola, Wilson (1952) observes: "The form in which an artist's creative impulses are ultimately expressed is frequently moulded by the stresses placed upon his emotions in childhood and early adolescence; stresses produced by the gradual realization of the dreadful gulf that lies between his fantasy world, often protected and nurtured by parental affection, and the vast, uncomforting desert of the society in which he must live. Artistic creation, it would seem, represents such fragments of this fantasy world as he is able to retain and impose upon society." André Maurois, describing (1965) how Balzac developed that richly populated world of La Comédie Humaine, noted: "He might seem graceless and heedless in the real world; but he was all tenderness and passion in his own, the only world in which he truly believed, and in which his heart and spirit were actively and intensely engaged."

To the mother and to the father these small charges are also important factors in their own maturing. The small daughter who looks up into her father's eyes with a sweet innocence helps restore and keep alive a tenderness and humaneness that has sometimes been forced beneath the surface as he struggles to take his place among competitive males. An infant daughter provides an experience that is the reciprocal of the one the father experienced when, as an infant son, he lay in his mother's arms. The male adult can now learn the other side of the coin, a little, as he holds her. Life becomes a bit gentler and more beautiful to him because there are daughters. They complete his maturing as a male, restoring a portion that had been curbed in his adolescence.

Fathers, like mothers, are also tempted to see in the helplessness of their children, and in a daughter especially, a need for complete protection. Paternal overprotection is a chapter that Dr. Levy did not write, but it is as much needed as the one on maternal overprotection. Some fathers, we discover, have to supervise the dressing of their daughters, select their shoes and accessories, even in postadolescent years. More important still, some are inclined to try to select their mates. Who could be more jealous of that young buck, not yet dry behind the ears, or more suspicious of his motives, than the father, who knows from the inside what he has on his mind?

Kanner concludes his defense of mothers by noting that his ideal mother is

"... tender, self-possessed, informed, understanding ... a real builder of man, a solid pillar of true democracy, an object lesson in the art of preserving the integrity of family life at a time when so many families crumble and dissolve. It matters little that, being human and therefore fallible, she makes an occasional mistake, errs in some unessential detail. She can well afford to make mistakes, for they usually serve her as constructive experiences. Her personality and attitude will always keep her on the right track, steering competently through prosperity, calamity, and the many contingencies of life.... It is undoubtedly of such a mother that King Lemuel said in the last chapter of Proverbs: 'Her children arise up and call her blessed: her husband also, and he praiseth her. Many daughters have done virtuously, but thou excellest them all.'"

Among the testimonials that have been circulated in our own time, we might add the phrases (from Puner 1947, p. 162) of Sigmund Freud, who paused at one point to note:

"The only thing that brings a mother undiluted satisfaction is her relation to a son; it is quite the most complete relationship between human beings, and the one that is the most free of ambivalence.... A man who has been the undisputed favorite of the mother keeps for life the feeling of a conqueror, that confidence of success that frequently induces real success."[6]

---

[6]What renders the relationship so full of psychological dynamite, he believed, is the fact that the libido knows nothing about social taboos: suckling, dependence, affection grow apace and overshoot the mark until the mother becomes the primary sexual object. Then the conflict emerges that ends in repression, a repression that can be successful or disastrous but which in any case leaves its mark in ambivalence and as that sunken cathedral of fantasy which exists in our unconscious.

THE TOO-PERFECT MOTHER

The very effort to portray the ideal parent carries us into dangerous territory. What Freud called "undiluted satisfaction for the mother" and a ground for complete confidence and expectation of success in the son—namely, her devotion and adoration—can hypertrophy into something monstrous on both sides: the "doormat mother" and the supreme egotist son. There is need of balance: a mother can be too, too perfect, and a son needs even-handed justice rather than the unconditional love that he sometimes fantasies. Both Marcel Proust and Baudelaire have celebrated such mothers, and the images of these first love objects seem to have haunted these artist sons throughout their lives. Instead of creating the basis of a normal masculine confidence, the mothers became part of the now notorious failure of these sons to achieve masculine maturity. A hundred years before Freud, Stendhal wrote (1890, p. 22) of his own mother, as he looked back at his own six-year-old performance:

"I wanted to cover my mother with kisses, and for her to have no clothes on. She loved me passionately and kissed me often. I returned her kisses with such ardor that she was sometimes obliged to run away. I abhorred my father when he came to interrupt our kisses. I always wanted to kiss her bosom. You must remember that I lost my mother in childhood when I was barely seven."

A too-perfect relationship can leave the psychological umbilical cord unsevered. When we see Proust, aged 34 at the time of his mother's death, withdrawing from society and literally climbing into bed, there to try to recapture his own past, the beautiful relationship and the view of life he had developed as he watched the world through his mother's eyes, we are witnessing a strange commingling of pathology and artistic endeavor. Philip Kolb, the editor of a collection (1953) of letters which Proust had written to his mother, observes:

"Proust here addresses the person that he loved above all others in this world: his own mother. With her, never a reticence in expressing his most intimate thoughts. Never an inhibition in voicing his honest opinion about any person or event. Here at last is Marcel Proust himself, free from excessive politeness or his characteristic 'gentillesse,' from all affectation."

Making due allowance for the enthusiasm of an editor (the biographies of Proust suggest that there were indeed many things which he never shared with her), the image of the mother that emerges from this correspondence is not only that of a woman who was at one with her son, who gave generously of herself, but also that of a woman who demanded, constricted, struggled, to possess her son, *psychologically.* Proust emerges as incompletely differentiated from his mother, as physically male, but with the essential male psychology missing. We could say, using Freud's figurative language, "He was psychologically castrated by this too, too good mother." The metaphor has some truth, but like all metaphors it also distorts the facts. In an obscure and complex manner, Proust remained fixated at an immature level of development (in one aspect of his life); we wonder, did the normally intruding male parent, whom Stendhal vividly describes, fail somehow to do his duty? Was he preoccupied elsewhere, in his business or profession or sport, or in one of those liaisons that a complacent society seemed almost to expect, since truly romantic love was sought outside the marriage relationship? Perhaps enough is suggested, here, to point up the importance of the severance of that original symbiotic tie, of a "going beyond momma" that is as important as cutting one's teeth or as the descent of a male child's testicles, especially if she is a near-perfect mother.

THE BATTERED-CHILD SYNDROME

Such refined, yet constrictive, bonds are only half the story. At the other end of a continuum that contains every degree of indifference, rejection, and finally cruelty are found parents who savagely assault and even kill their offspring. Every day hospitals are asked to patch up the bodies of infants, less than three years of age, who have been beaten, burned, stabbed, exposed to cold, and so on. Mysterious drownings, suffocations, accidents are now discussed at medical symposiums under some curious heading such as "the battered-child syndrome." If all the existing cases could be identified and reported, suggest the experts, the number would far surpass our traffic deaths. Between this almost unbelievable extreme of cruelty and the milder but equally pathogenic "overprotection fused with hostility," which also distorts and retards development, a hundred varieties of distorted parental behavior exist. Sometimes it is just the harshness of a father's criticism that manages to "cut the son down to size" and make him hate both himself and his father. Sometimes it is the overconcern of the mother that keeps her son away from the swimming pool *and by her side.* The subtler forms masquerade, of course, as something for her child's good, something that requires of the mother an unusual sacrifice, a giving up of her own interests for the child.

Another fact should also remind us that not all infants enter the world to be cherished by fond parents. Consider the figures for abortions, the true volume of which we can discover only in those countries where the practice is both legalized and accepted as a preferred method of contraception. In such countries the number of abortions often equals or exceeds the number of natural births (including those that are illegitimate). Japan is reported to have the highest abortion rate in the world (although accurate comparative figures are unobtainable). There, observers report, it is indeed the preferred method of contraception. Where, as in our own country, it is illegal and frowned upon, we can easily imagine that some unwanted children enter the world with the psychological cards stacked against them, especially when they are born after futile attempts at abortion, guided by an ignorant folklore, have failed (see Hecht and Chasteland 1960).

SIMPLE DEPRIVATION: MOTHERING INTERRUPTED

Mothering can be abruptly interrupted, as when a mother dies or is removed to the hospital, and the institutional or personal substitutes for it may be altogether inadequate, even though physical care is good enough to keep the child alive and growing. Sometimes the child's disturbance at separation from the mother prevents him from accepting what would otherwise be adequate substitutes; sometimes the substitutes are so poor that normal growth and differentiation are arrested. If one could plot the child's development on a curve that would make his progress visible, a sharp "notch" would show the traumatic effect of the separation. Like the tree rings that show what the rainfall was in the early years of growth, the smaller increments of skills show that something essential was missing at these periods of deprivation and disturbance. Even when growth is resumed, we suspect that the deep scar in those sensitive early months where "imprinting" occurs may produce a greater vulnerability to stress in some later "time of troubles." In a few children the results are apparent at once: they have to be hospitalized for incorrigible or schizoid symptoms. Just as the bodies of battered children give visible evidence of mishandling by parents, some of whom may be mentally ill, the selves that emerge from defective, distorted, or traumatic mothering bear less visible but no less fateful psychological scars, as their subsequent behavior shows.

The Case of Desperate Desmond

Instead of statistically impressive evidence, let us note a single case (Bowlby 1953b) that was presented by the psychiatrist who made the first study of the relationships between maternal care and mental health for the World Health Organization. Reported from a child-guidance clinic in England, the case of Desmond illustrates how an early break in the mother-child relationship can lead to a series of events, each compounding the ill effects of preceding ones until another "social problem" is produced. Although Desmond was only followed as far as his adolescent years, we can already see the poor socialization, the defective "conscience," and the behavior problems that some may want to label "psychopathic personality."

When Desmond first came to the clinic, he was 11 years old, and seemed so fixed in his nature and so difficult to reach that no one seemed optimistic about the outlook. Neither the family nor the school could bring him into line with his age peers; he was not going to be an ordinary English schoolboy. His teachers were primarily concerned about his truancy, his petty stealing, his lack of friends, his restlessness, and his lack of any constructive interests.

His family admitted that he was almost a stranger to them, although he lived under the same roof: he was cold, secretive, aloof. When, rarely, he chose to play with other children, it was usually with girls or younger children, and each companion in turn seemed to bore him. He had struck up an acquaintance recently with an older man (an undesirable type, according to the family), and this new friend worried his parents even more than the boy's solitude. The social worker who reported to the clinic what she had seen in the home described his aging father as a truckdriver who seemed completely baffled by his son. Sympathetic enough, in a vague and helpless way, he never spent much time with the boy. He could not even talk with him. The stepmother, his father's second wife, did not always handle the boy right, the father thought; she nagged him. Desmond was just as puzzling to the stepmother. He was a "cool number," hard to reach. She had never won his affection, though she had tried to be a good mother. As an American might have put it, she had undertaken her task with "two strikes against her."

Desmond's own mother had developed cancer of the breast soon after his birth; his nursing was disturbed and she had to be taken to hospital. She died when Desmond was 15 months old, at which age a child has strong preferences for the mother, as a person; Desmond not only showed that he missed her, but refused all substitutes. A maternal aunt was pressed into service for a year; a second aunt relieved her during the second year. Three mothers and three "desertions" had occurred before Desmond was three and a half years old. While other children were learning to creep, walk, and control bladder and bowel sphincters, Desmond proved to be a "problem," a slow learner. The countermeasures taken by his substitute mothers struck the social worker as strict to the point of cruelty. The fourth mother-substitute, a paternal aunt, who filled in until the stepmother appeared on the scene, was a slight improvement, but she was scarcely established in the household before Desmond was again "deserted." A series of "battles," frustrating experiences, and disappointments of this sort would scarcely prepare a boy to expect much from his new mother. How could he have any clear idea of or craving for a firm and affectionate relationship when he had never formed any such bond with the others?

We could speak a word in defense of these substitute mothers. Some of them had to interrupt their lives, spread the love for their own children to this waif belonging to others, and when it is a Desmond who resists and rejects them, who rebels at their training, who shows not the slightest gratitude, their countermeasures are understandable. They are inexpert, determined to do with discipline what has obviously not been done by affection; they have no more than their limited share of maternal affection to give in a setting duty compels them to enter, somewhat unwillingly. One could understand the various methods such a substitute mother might use: bribery, severity, cold indifference, tight-lipped martyrdom, anger, and brutality. And would there not be, for each of these, corresponding "answers" on the part of the child: sullen silence, withdrawal, rebellion, the timidity of a wild and frightened animal? These are all *possibilities;* and as the dialogue develops (wordless or with shouting), the reciprocal postures of the protagonists will develop into set styles of life. That precise mixture of discipline, understanding, affection that will both warm the child to life and give it shape was not provided by these "antagonists" who got off on the wrong foot.

By the time the social worker or the clinical psychologist entered the scene (at eleven years in this case), the child had become a puzzle to his parents, unmanageable both at home and in school. Those who tried to penetrate his defenses found him hard to reach, without feeling, hard, not quite human. He seemed to have no conscience, little feeling, no need for affection, and no capacity to respond with affection. All concerned began to think about some place, some school, some kind of a military boarding school where the authorities would have complete control and could hammer some sense into this flinty personality. In this British clinic they began to speculate about a constitutional psychopathic personality structure and to group the boy with those others that they had come to call "affectionless thieves."

Such diagnostic classifications are themselves fraught with dangers, for they can mean to a case worker: "No use wasting a great deal of staff time on this one; here is another one of those who do not profit from experience." Nonetheless, therapy was undertaken. Suspicious and aloof at first, Desmond was soon expressing to his counselor his needs and fears. "I would like to be liked; they do like me when I'm a good boy, but I cannot be a good boy, not very often, anyhow. I am getting worried about it. I better keep out." When the therapist had to be absent over a holiday, Desmond reacted with an outburst of physical aggression, which at the clinic they took to be a sign of his need, although its form was poorly calculated to win friends. He was jealous of the other clients his counselor saw, and jealous in advance of the child his stepmother was now expecting. Sometimes wistful and pleading, he could turn violent; he tried to set the therapist's chair on fire, to burn her hair and her stockings, and, once, to strangle her. While throwing sand about, he shouted, "That's for you, for Mummy, for the baby, and for Daddy. I'll kill you all with bombs!"

Operating upon her certainty (or faith?) that the child's greatest need was for a stable, understanding, and affectionate relationship that he could count on, his counselor persisted through all of Desmond's "testing." And when this eleven-year-old began writing "mash notes" (after an Easter holiday during which she had been away), she felt a certain sense of triumph:

> Oh my little darling I love you,
> Oh my little darling I don't believe you do.
> If you really loved me as you do
> You would not go to America and leave me at the Zoo.

Other poor poetry followed, and he continued to write to her after he had been sent away to a "training school" by the family. Returning after a lapse of a year, he visited his therapist: "You always knew when I was unhappy." And asking for a pencil, he wrote, "Pugno et amo." It was not only a demonstration of what he had learned, but, the counselor thought, a kind of vague foreshadowing of the formula that his future love objects would have to find the answer for: fighting fused with loving, expressions which would test each of these partners. After all, he had been deserted, repeatedly. Even at eleven he was again being sent away from home.

The predictions for such as Desmond are uncertain. Everything will depend on "what happens when," on his acts and their consequences, and on the counteractions and responses of those around him. It would seem much too mechanical to emphasize any particular period or any particular phase of training (nursing, toilet training, punishment for masturbation, deprivation of mothering, absence of the father from the home). Issue after issue gets "settled," and effects cumulate until they become extremely difficult to reverse or penetrate. Plasticity runs out, in time, declines steadily month by month. What is so startling in Desmond's case is to see the wrong direction taken and the cumulative compounding of effects begun so very early. Once started, the series of consequences begins to generate pathogenic situations; the dialogue grows less and less reversible. Behavior that society calls criminal or pathological could thus become the last stage in this "conversation," this series of blunders.

Looking at the earliest stages, as he saw it in the clinic, Bowlby thought that children affected by such interruptions of mothering passed through three stages, the first being a phase of protest, tears, anger, fretfulness, crying, whining, sobbing. Sometimes those around the child interpret his reactions as anger (no substitutes wanted!) or as simply a restless and fearful search for the lost mother. This first phase is followed by a phase of quiet despair. And lastly a phase of detachment follows, in which the demand and search for the mother are given up, sealed over by a cool indifference. These phases are sometimes accompanied by a refusal to eat (which sometimes swings to an exaggerated appetite), a subdued withdrawal, thumb-sucking, dreamy solitary play, and a quiet and depressed mood. (See Bowlby 1952, 1953a; Yudkin and Holme 1963; Ainsworth *et al.* 1962.)

In the final phase he is no longer interested; if and when his mother returns she may be greeted as a stranger, or he may turn away from her with a burst of tears or an unusually intense bout of bad behavior. Somewhere between the sixth and eighteenth months these separation reactions seem to be most acute; by this time the child knows what he wants. His need for the mother is still great, and so specific that substitutes cannot be "palmed off" as easily as with the smaller infant. It requires an increasing amount of "cozening" to penetrate his defenses.

If the separation is prolonged, and if the substitute-mothering is of poor quality, the developmental quotients—based on such standard measures as the Gesell tests—will register the degree of arrest in each dimension of growth: locomotion, manual dexterity, language expression, social reactions, rate at which new learning takes place, and so on (see Aubry 1955 for a specific and quantitative expression of these "arrests"). Limited studies—such as Aubry's—suggest that even small improvements in nursing care are registered in improved growth; a few hours per week of a more personalized handling of the child arrested these declines in developmental quotients in one orphanage. Return to the mother, or prompt placement in good foster homes, can restore growth to its former pace, but delays, it is believed, will result in residual deficiencies in language and possibly in some other, less easily observed, and as yet difficult to measure weaknesses in interpersonal and affectional relationships. Even where the recovery seems to be complete, a child's reaction to subsequent separations (on entering school, at the loss of a parent at adolescence, or at the loss of a spouse at maturity) may reveal the presence of the earlier "scars" in the form of exaggerated mourning. Such long-delayed effects are difficult to establish either experimentally or statistically with human subjects. Readiness (including my own) to make inferences in this area represents a conviction rather than a scientifically validated conclusion (see

Bowlby 1961a, Barry and Lindemann 1960, Barry 1949, and F. Brown 1961).[7]

In the present state of our knowledge, such permanent residues have to be described as hypothetical, inferred for the most part. Where the statistical evidence supports these inferences, there are usually other, coacting causes that make the results ambiguous. Moreover, some of the statistical evidence seems to reduce this maternal-deprivation factor to one among many others, and even to suggest that its role is a minor one *in treated forms of psychopathology*. For example, when the case records of older delinquents, depressives, and schizophrenics are compared with the records of normal controls (who have been neither referred to clinics nor treated for "problems"), the loss of a mother prior to the fifth year is significantly higher in the abnormal ones, yet not high enough to support the kind of certitude many clinicians seem to be ready to express. In a study of 947 cases that had been diagnosed as neuroses or as psychosomatic illnesses, Barry and Lindemann (1960) found that 4.12 per cent of the patients and 1.18 per cent of the controls suffered such a loss. The most critical age for the little girls who later developed neuroses fell between birth and the end of the second year.[8] Barry and Lindemann add this terse note of caution: "At least 85% of the psychoneurotic patients in the present series had *not* lost their mothers prior to their 21st birthday. There are causes of neuroses other than parental separation."

The efforts of other workers to locate the most sensitive period approximate the one just quoted: somewhere between the sixth and eighteenth months is a common clinical appraisal.[9] Summarizing more than a hundred studies that appeared in the decade since the first W.H.O. report (Bowlby 1952) on the question of maternal care, Ainsworth suggests (in Ainsworth *et al.* 1962) that when deprivation occurs early in the first year, subsequent recovery

---

[7]Convictions can form the basis of a policy, which in turn may produce the data that future studies will reveal. The results of the Head Start program show the problem: the improvement in the learning of the underprivileged child under the new advantages supplied by the program can be measured, but unfortunately, when the child is returned to his usual home and classroom environment, the gains rapidly disappear. One group will hold that, with additional effort, these gains might be consolidated. The other will conclude that (a) the program was obviously of no use; (b) such well-intentioned efforts will never alter a genetically caused limitation in the capacities of these disadvantaged ones; and (c) the funds which might be allocated to those who profit least from their training are more wisely spent to enrich the educational experiences of those who will profit most (and permanently). Schoolboards are now debating these policy suggestions.

[8]Interestingly enough, these workers found no statistical evidence to indicate any similar effects from a father's death, which showed up in the records no more frequently for patients than for samples of the general population.

[9]If we were dealing with experimental animals, we could arrange for groups with a similar genetic endowment to be separated according to a precisely spaced set of intervals, and thus establish a precise critical point, as Seitz (1959) did for kittens. With varying post-separation experiences and a continuous testing program, we could show the precise degree to which the effects are reversible. Harlow (1960, 1963; see also 1958) was able to show that the sexual behavior of monkeys who had suffered early maternal deprivation was abnormal at maturity, and that their mothering of their own offspring was so ineffective as to initiate a new set of pathological effects in the next generation.

is the more complete the earlier the deprivation, and that, once the first year is over, the later it occurs the more readily reversible the effects will be. The impact of separation is probably greatest on just those functions nascent at the time of separation. Aubry (1955) also noted that a child just beginning to walk at the time of separation suddenly showed an inability to walk. Perhaps we should say he would not try, or could not try, or lacked confidence. Or perhaps walking is affected by some much more general volitional factor, which we describe roughly as the "willingness to put forth effort." The nascent patterns suddenly collapse, whether we speak of arrest, inhibition, or loss of motivation; locomotion, verbal expression, interpersonal actions, manual skills, can all be affected.

Similarly, the child's response when mothering is resumed will differ with the phase of development reached, as well as with the skill of the mother (or substitute mother) in restoring the supporting relationship. He may show an angry, resentful, rebellious pattern, or an anxious clinging and "mummy-ishness" as though afraid of losing her once more. His apathy and withdrawal, his quiet and depressed mood (if this is the pattern), may test the mother's resources most of all, especially if she in turn happens to have schizoid, depressive, or hostile-aggressive tendencies. Then her own responses can deepen and fixate a gulf between them until it is difficult for either to cross it. These consequences may be negotiable and modifiable, but they also demand skill, persistence, flexibility, and a strong and enduring affection on the part of the older and presumably more stable partner in the transactions.

The study by Goldfarb (1943) in particular deserves special comment. It has been given a central position in both of the W.H.O. reports, and has been displayed as representing the ideal in experimental design. Since it extended over more than a decade and involved an intensive program of measuring two matched (for heredity, according to the experimenter) groups of child subjects, we can see why there are so few comparable studies.

Goldfarb compared children who had passed through an orphanage and had been quickly placed in foster homes with a second group that had spent the crucial interval from their sixth month to their third year within the institution before being placed. This particular institution, Goldfarb pointed out, was above criticism as far as the physical care of the children was concerned, but infants under nine months were confined within little cubicles ("to prevent the spread of infection"). Apart from the brief contacts involved in feeding and in keeping them clean, they were kept in a kind of solitary confinement, healthy organisms in clean pens. There was a minimum of interaction between the children. Whether we regard it as cold, impersonal, lacking in mothering and affection (emphasizing the human factor's absence), or simply look on it, as some behaviorists might, as a setting with a very low level of arousal (and therefore as one brand of stimulus deprivation), it proved to be a barren environment for the developing children; it did not stimulate the growth of either skills, language, or interpersonal bonds of affection (or *need* for affection).

TABLE 5. *A Comparison of Test Scores of Children Adopted after Their Third Year with Those of Children Placed Very Quickly.* (From Goldfarb 1943.)

Function Tested or Rated	Rating Method	Result Expressed as	Results	
			Institutionalized Group (N = 15)	Control Group (N = 15)
Intelligence	Wechsler test	Mean IQ	72.4	95.4
Ability to conceptualize	Weigl test	Mean score	2.4	6.8
	Vigotsky test	Mean score	0.5	4.7
Reading	Standard tests	Mean score (yrs)	5.1	6.8
Arithmetic	Standard tests	Mean score (yrs)	4.7	6.7
Social maturity	Vineland scale	Mean social quotient	79.0	98.8
Ability to keep rules	Frustration experiment	Number of children	3	12
Guilt on breaking rules	Frustration experiment	Number of children	2	11
Capacity for relationship	Case worker's rating	Number of children judged as normal	2	15
Speech	Case worker's rating	Number of children judged as average	3	14

As the months went by, the institutionalized infants were formed into groups of 15 or 20 under the supervision of a single nurse. Since these nurse-mothers were changed from time to time, there was little opportunity for those person-to-person bonds that are developed in normal mothering. In short, separation was made a repeated feature of their lives. When the children were finally placed in foster homes after their third year, the investigator continued to follow their progress and to compare their performance with that of the children who had been promptly placed in foster homes. Final comparisons were made when the ages of the two groups ranged from ten to fourteen years. Goldfarb considered that the foster homes of the two groups were similar in all measurable criteria; if anything, the institutionalized groups were placed in homes in which the mother's occupational, educational, and mental status was slightly superior to that of the mothers in the homes provided for the other group.

From Table 5, which summarizes Goldfarb's findings, we can see that the development of the institutionalized children was retarded in intellectual, social, and emotional facets alike. The children of the institutionalized group did not abide by the rules of the game in their play; the case workers found them slow to form relationships with others; and their IQ's, school work, and performance in tests of abstract thinking were all below par.

Although Goldfarb felt that he had selected samples similar in heredity, his critics have pointed out possible constitutional differences. Pasamanick and Knoblock (1961) have indicated that some of the institutionalized group in Goldfarb's study were brain-damaged or grossly defective. If the differences which were measured, and which persisted through the years in the foster homes, were founded upon such constitutional factors, the results would of course have no bearing upon the maternal-deprivation question. These critics have also suggested that the presence of such defects may explain why the orphanage could not place the children promptly. If such an organic factor had been at work in determining which children would be in the two groups (and not some scheme such as selecting every other admission to the orphanage for the experimental group and placing the child for adoption or for retention in the institution according to his admission number), the final differences cannot be attributed to the impoverishment in mothering provided by the institution.

Both Ainsworth and Bowlby have summarized the mass of studies on maternal deprivation as "confirming and supporting each other." Overlooking the numerous contradictions, they emerge from their studies with the conviction shared by so many: "What each individual piece of work lacks in thoroughness, scientific reliability, or precision, is largely made good by the concordance of the whole" (Ainsworth *et al.* 1962, p. 97). Such an affirmation of faith (in spite of the evidence) reminds us of some reviews of experiments on extrasensory perception in which, after consideration of the confusing data, a belief in telepathy is reaffirmed. Other investigators, with other biases, are less certain; certainly a thousand studies, each of low validity, would testify to little more than that some community of opinion or enthusiasm has prompted certain research workers. The fact is that the exponents of "environmentalism" and intensive mothering can be matched by equally enthusiastic organicists who see constitutional and genetic factors as the primary causes of deviations in development. The one group abides by the wisdom of grandmothers, who have always known that every child needs a discipline that balances wholesome and affectionate support with proper constraints, generous gratifications with a prudent and conditional withholding, such as is normally provided by a close bond with a nonneurotic mother. The other group, focusing on a neurobiological maturation process that goes on down among the cells pretty much at its own pace, is more impersonal in outlook and (its defenders would add) more realistic. This second group is inclined to expect no more than minor modulations in the curves of growth when there are changes in mothering; this view demands less from parents, relying as it does more on a physiological maturation.

In sum, the effects of separation from the mother can be observed on the spot, *especially in some children.* They are to be seen wherever clinics deal with children whose mothers die, enter a hospital, or for one reason or another have had to desert their children. The effects are so varied, from child to child, that preseparation differences (either in constitution or in earlier sensitizing experiences) have to be invoked to account for the diversity. The effects of such separation are usually reversible, although some residual effects may persist, especially if the ties to the child's own or substitute mother are not resumed in a prompt and skillful fashion. Language development and the affectional life appear to be the most vulnerable. The long-term effects of early separation have a minor role in the total array of causes that produce adult mental disorders, as we discover when we note that only 4 per cent of adult neurotic patients studied have experienced such early separation.

One qualification might be appended to this conclusion, which seems to violate so much clinical opinion. Although we no longer send children under ten to work in offices, stores, and factories these days, a century and a half since Robert Owen introduced his reforms, we seem to have been busy in recent decades in inducing their mothers to take their places. One-third of our labor force is composed of women; one-half of these women are married. Approximately one-half of the married women who are employed have children under 15 years of age. Within the lowest socioeconomic groups, where the need for the mother's wages is greatest, the provisions for substitute mothering (day-care centers for infants and children) are the least satisfactory. If mothering is important, the march of social change pays no attention to the fact; and mothers, balancing the gains in standard of living and in personal freedom, have often decided, as their actions show, that any possible loss is a minor one. Should mothering prove to be more important than the studies have shown it to be, the present decline in mothering may show up in future studies of the incidence of neurosis in the lower socioeconomic third of our population.[10]

Deprivation of Mothering without Separation

What is it that is interrupted when mother and child are separated? Is it something that is always present when the two are physically near? If we could be more specific about the transactions which normally occur, perhaps we could identify types of deprivation that occur even in her presence.

There are two *functions* which come to mind in addition to the education of affection which the psychoanalyst stresses: the mother has to serve as *buffer* and as *regulator*. Consider the way in which the mere presence of the good mother reassures an infant. She carries a kind of *mana*, like that of the shaman or medicine man, or of the physician, whose entry into the sickroom makes his patient relax even before he has diagnosed and prescribed for an illness. The buffering mother intuitively holds her small offspring while she shows him the dog, or the even stranger "bossy," or the unfamiliar creatures of the zoo, for the

---

[10]Figures released by the Labor Department (AP dispatch, Nov. 20, 1966) show that this migration of mothers out of the home affects college graduates too, not merely the mothers in the lower classes. More than half of a group of 6,000 college women who graduated in 1957 were still employed in 1964, though their age group was then at the peak of child-rearing and family responsibility. An earlier report, made six months after this group of women had graduated, showed that 85 per cent were or had been married, and 66 per cent were mothers. Whatever their college courses taught them about mothering had not altered their choices to any great extent.

first time. He in turn, protected, is willing to point or lean toward the animal as long as she holds him, and even to go farther when his first contacts come off well. The mere presence of the mother provides a protective aura, and through its effects the child learns to accept and approach novelty that otherwise might prove too much for him.

When Liddell (1956) shocked young twin lambs, following a dimming of the lights in his animal laboratory, he found that the presence of their mother acted as a protective barrier. Left with its mother, the lamb subjected to the stimulus changes ran to her side. The other lamb, isolated from the mother, became sluggish (as evidenced by failure to react to nearly half the signals in one experimental test) and showed increasing lethargy as the training sessions were extended over a 24-day period. The separated animals were described as "lacking in the muscular tonus necessary to be on the alert for slight environmental changes. Their vigilance had become blunted." The lambs protected by the mother in the early training did not show this deterioration in responsiveness. Her ministrations, from the moment of the birth of the animal, had made the mere sight of her a signal for relaxation, a signal that all is well. The isolated lambs were traumatized by the training series, whose long-enduring aftereffects showed up again the moment testing was resumed, even after full maturity. The twin, who may have been "troubled" by the training, could nonetheless, in the supporting presence of the mother, tolerate the stresses, which did not produce the residual effects shown in the separated twins at maturity. By the time the lambs were three months old, the training series, even in isolation, had lost its traumatic quality.

Greenberg (1962) offers an illustration of the interchanges between the human mother and her child that we might call *regulative* when they go well. That they can also be disruptive, we shall soon see:

"An infant is observed lying supine in its crib, crying, kicking about, and seemingly hungry, since he has not been fed for about three hours or so and seems in need of some intervention. The mother approaches her infant and rearranges its garments as she lifts him from the crib, placing him on her shoulder, patting gently in the process as she walks to a chair where she then sits to feed the neonate. In the lifting-holding activity the infant eased its crying but began to sob and remained fussy. As he was cradled in his mother's arms, his crying ceased altogether, and it seemed that his extremities were less active and there was a reduction in body tonicity. The mother gently directed a bottle towards the infant's mouth, and as his lips were brushed by the nipple, he began to roll his head from side to side in a most active fashion. The mother seemed a bit disconcerted by this behavior which delayed his sucking, and she began to shift about; she introduced the nipple directly into the infant's mouth and appeared more tense, until finally the infant's mouth clamped about the nipple and began sucking; but as he did, his fists clenched, the lower extremities tensed, and the arms and forearms were brought to a 'midline clutch' which remained in this fixed position. The mother remained very attentive, but it was only after some three or four minutes of fairly continuous feeding that she appeared more relaxed and a more flaccid state developed in the infant as he entered into drowsiness. Had measures of heart rate and muscle tone been performed during the feeding, we might have noticed that the onset of sucking was accompanied by an elevation of heart rate which attained a certain level, remained constant throughout sucking, but dropping whenever sucking ceased, even for a few seconds. With this, our electromyographic measures might reflect an increase in tonicity of various muscle groups, e.g. palmar musculature during sucking, with the level gradually reducing over the period of feeding. The sucking-feeding initially seemed to induce generalized increments of muscle tension, a rather different instance than a vociferously crying infant, who, when given a nipple to suck on, ceases to cry and shows a marked drop in heart rate and decrease in muscle tone."

Even though as many as half the infants in a maternity ward may need some assistance in getting the nursing activity started, this is rarely a matter of any great concern. However, in a few infants the reflex mechanism seems weak; and some mothers have inverted nipples that are difficult for the child to grasp, or may hold the child unskillfully, so that mouth and breast are not in proper apposition. These factors can make this simple task a source of confusion and anxiety, both for the mother and for the child. Ribble (1944), commenting on the problem, suggests a third factor in one of her cases: "conscious or unconscious hostility was apparently communicated to the child in some way, for a poor sucking response appeared invariably in the unwanted infant." Omitting for the moment any comment on this rather hasty generalization, we should note how these first confused transactions can develop: "if their primary sucking was not made easy and satisfying, their sucking activities gradually diminished, and they became either stuporous or resistive." We can easily imagine such a mother, discussing the experience later as the clinician probes for the beginning of a neurotic relationship: "He was different from the very beginning. He was difficult to feed. He rejected me."

Cuddling, rocking, patting, humming to him, offering her breast or a bottle, a mother may use a wide variety of methods of restoring her fretful child to that optimum level of arousal that she likes to see, to a condition in which he can go forward, learn, tolerate the necessary stresses. We take her triumph for granted, and, on the other hand, look in amazement at the mature woman who allows herself to be baffled by an infant, who recoils from the task, who converts a normally gratifying feeding period into a frustrating and unhappy experience for both mother and infant, or who can only interact with a child that is playful, smiling, and acting "cute." Such an atypical mother may react to the restless and resistive child with responses that reinforce and intensify his anger and frustration; the observer will be hard put to decide the question, "Who rejected whom first of all?" A mother can suddenly feel herself to be a destructive, defective female, when the child refuses to eat, and feel—in response to her own infant as to her extended family—unloved, rejected, and unworthy. If she also did not want a child and tried some futile method (an automobile journey over rough terrain) to produce a miscarriage, she would also have reasons for imagining that her child must hate her, reasons which she may not tell her physician.

In the light of such observations it is easy to believe that the infant who is calmly confident in the face of novelty and who can pitch into new experiences with eagerness and curiosity may very well owe his poise to a mother who knew how to control her infant's tensions. Such a child has an autonomic background that smoothly supports his striped-muscle activity: no excesses, no deficits. His interests are directed boldly outward, and he looks ahead rather than backward; as a result, he is ready to learn to perceive, to manipulate, and to approach life directly. I do not mean to imply here that genetic differences do not exist. The same mother, employing—as far as she can determine —the same methods of handling and training her child, responding in her usual way to his protests, and displaying equal affection for him, will discover that one child does not emerge as balanced as her other children have.

THE MATERNAL-DEPRIVATION HYPOTHESIS IN THE CLINIC

EARLY INFANTILE AUTISM

In 1943 Leo Kanner described a remarkable form of developmental arrest. His clear delineation of the syndrome was accompanied by a vivid description of the family environment, and he emphasized the rather cold, detached, and obsessively perfectionistic mothering that he observed in most of his case studies. His term, "emotional refrigerators," is such a vivid metaphor that, almost in sympathy with the infant, we shrink a little and are half-convinced that he has indeed identified the cause. Of higher than average intelligence, the parents struck Kanner as lacking in warmth and in ability to give the affection an infant needs. Although he was careful to insist that he had not noted any signs of parental neglect or cruelty, he wrote, a decade later: "It is difficult to escape the conclusion that this emotional configuration in the home plays a dynamic role in the genesis of autism."[11]

At the same time, Kanner expressed the opinion that these children had been "different from the beginning of their extrauterine existence." Since the pattern was not clearly identified until well into the third quarter of the first year, a variety of emphases has emerged. A few observers looked for evidence

---

[11]Kanner's pioneer study (1943) was based on eleven cases seen in the Phipps Clinic of Child Psychiatry at Johns Hopkins Hospital in Baltimore over a period of years. Denis de Rougemont (1963, p. 24) speaks of a "tremendous tidal wave rising from the collective soul," referring to a chorus of critics protesting against censorship, repression, and even the most elementary forms of educative discipline. What the Aldriches (1938) were urging on the positive side (a respect for the child's needs, demand schedules, an easy and permissive atmosphere for growth), Eisenberg and Kanner (1956) support by showing the extremely unfortunate aspects of the opposite type of discipline. The historian of culture is moved to conclude that the middle class, the bearers of Puritan and Christian values, had run out of steam and was now under attack. The words "commercial," "virtuous," "will power," "discipline," "puritanical," "mid-Victorian," "prudent," "prudish," "virgin," the whole vocabulary rooted in a self-regulative pattern that nineteenth-century parents had been proud to teach, had acquired a pejorative value. Eroticism erupted everywhere. And the clinical evaluations of mental illness also changed. (See also Whiting and Child 1953, and Orlansky 1949.)

of a genetic factor, others for birth injuries and brain damage. Kanner thought that these children had suffered a deprivation of normal mothering in the very earliest stages of development.

The Autistic Child Described

There has been little difference of opinion about the observable facts. Others agree with Kanner (1949) in his emphasis on the following traits:

"A profound withdrawal from contact with people, an obsessive desire for the preservation of sameness, a skillful and even affectionate relation to objects, the retention of an intelligent and pensive physiognomy, and either mutism or the kind of language which does not seem intended to serve the purpose of interpersonal communication. An analysis of this language has revealed a peculiar reversal of pronouns, neologisms, metaphors, and apparently irrelevant utterances which become meaningful to the extent to which they can be traced to the patient's experiences and their emotional implications."

"Islands" of verbal-symbolic or manipulative skill are often preserved, and are so well-developed that the children do not fit the concept of any general intellectual retardation, of feeblemindedness. Their mutism is not like any ordinary aphasia. One five-year-old who had never been heard to produce articulate speech suddenly cried out, "Take it out of there!" when he became distressed at a bit of prune skin that had stuck to his palate. The children seem isolated from the surrounding interpersonal world. They are very disturbed when their routines are interrupted. There is a great deal of rhythmic, repetitive play: head-banging (both in the crib and in the arms of the adult holding him), rocking, jouncing, turning lights off and on, opening and shutting doors. The uncanny preoccupation with things (flashlights, vacuum cleaners, light sockets, blocks, tops) recurs in these case histories. Feeding problems and toilet training do not represent a simple incapacity to learn, for some of these children can remember names, tell time, read maps, recite dates, give the names of presidents and vice-presidents in the proper order, repeat nursery rhymes, or answer 25 questions on the Presbyterian catechism.

The lack of normal affective contact struck Kanner: they did not respond to the approach of people; they never made any anticipatory movement to meet half-way those who were about to pick them up, nor did they adjust their postures to the bodies of the persons holding them. Those physically near or in actual contact with them either did not penetrate a shell of indifference or were actively shut out, rejected. Some of the children seemed extraordinarily sensitive to noises, moving objects, to any change in their food or their surroundings. Others were so unresponsive to the efforts made to gain their attention that their families worried about the child's hearing; it was sometimes a parent's fear of the possibility of deafness that had brought some of these children to the clinic.

Looking at the children from a purely physical-physiological point of view, Kanner was impressed with their health: there had been no unusual history of diseases, of encephalitis, or of endocrine malfunction, no bodily abnormalities, no clear-cut signs of neuropathology. They were, on the contrary, well-formed, well-developed, slender, attractive children, and had no history of allergies, asthma, eczema, or urticaria to link them with those adult cases we classify as psychosomatic.[12]

The Parental Matrix: Families in Which Autism Develops

Aware of the interest in any evidence of hereditary factors in schizophrenic patients, Kanner explored the histories of parents and relatives. He found that, with the exception of one paternal aunt of one of the children, there had been no history of psychosis in any antecedent. Their ancestry, in fact, resembled that of Terman's geniuses. The fathers had been business executives, artists, clergymen, scientists, physicians, college professors. The mothers also showed educational and professional attainments that placed them in one of the higher socioeconomic groups. "My search for autistic children of unsophisticated parents has remained unsuccessful to date," Kanner noted, leaving us to puzzle out whether early infantile autism passes unnoticed in humbler households, or is there treated as a simple retardation about which nothing can be done, or is something that is produced by a mixture of high expectations, unusual advantages, and an unusual kind of disability. We are tempted to join other "enemies of the middle class" in charging these parents with preoccupation with professional success, intellectual and artistic accomplishments, business competition, to such a degree that they provide too cold a climate for the affectional needs of a child. Successful in a socioeconomic sense, the parents, in particular the mothers, have not provided an emotional warmth that would permit small egos to develop in proper fashion, have not "buffered and regulated" them into a confident autonomy that, in turn, reaches out with warmth and affection to its personal milieu.[13]

As Kanner observed these parents of autistic children more closely, he was struck by their narrow margin of tolerance for social life: they were not comfortable in the presence of people. Instead, they chose to read, write,

---

[12]Although early infantile autism is often classed as a form of childhood schizophrenia, in this freedom from any physiological or psychosomatic involvement Kanner's group is radically different from the studies of Bender (1956), Terry and Rennie (1938), and others who find the childhood histories of their schizophrenic patients spotted with unusually many physiological disturbances. It is also different from those more general findings of the Leightons, who showed a high correlation between multiple physical symptoms and the presence of neurotic trends. Kanner found no evidence of the general autonomic instability Bender found in her schizophrenic children, and no noteworthy frequency of night terrors, stammering, difficulties in bladder and bowel control, of the type found by Terry and Rennie in the early histories of older schizophrenics.

[13]Eisenberg and Kanner (1956) present an analysis of 100 autistic children and their 200 parents. The educational and occupational histories of these parents identify them as members of a certain social class. Kanner checked his impression of the high educational attainments of the parents by comparing them with parents of nonautistic cases selected at random from the clinic files. Neither the high educational nor the high professional attainments were found among the latter parents, nor was there evidence for the detachment, obsessiveness, and coldness that was almost uniformly present in the parents of the autistic group.

paint, make music or listen to it, or "just think." The few who described themselves as socially inclined were quick to assure Kanner that they did not like simple chitchat: theirs was a social life with a purpose. He described these parents as serious, polite, dignified, aloof, superior, withdrawn, and disdainful of all that was frivolous. If there were components in these personalities of that erotic, impish, sensual, lazy, pleasure-seeking libido which others posit as at the core of our nature, it had been so pruned, inhibited, and hidden that the clinician could not note its presence, so sublimated that it took these "cultivated" and "proper" forms, which, Kanner seems to imply, did not draw out and develop the normal traits in their children. Montaigne's insistence that "supercelestial thoughts" usually coexist with "subterranean conduct" expresses the common man's fear of any design for life that departs too far from the average. The hypocrisy and cruelty of the middle classes (their detractors might insist) is nowhere more brilliantly identified than in the acts of these parents of autistic children, in their coldness toward their offspring.

Kanner's inquiry into the nature of the marital relationships among the parents convinced him that the bonds were firm (there were far fewer divorces than a random sample would show), but there seemed less of that warmth, spontaneity, and impulsiveness that, in other couples, make married life both unpredictable and exciting, and occasionally tempestuous. He judged them to be undemonstrative, practical, reasonable, formal, cool, prudent. Glamour, romance, passion, and "foolishness" had been replaced by a kind of self-regulation that makes the "dance of life" more like a Bach fugue than a Stravinsky ballet.[14]

Kanner felt that the mother's lack of warmth could be spotted before she entered the office:

"As they come up the stairs, the child trails forlornly behind the mother, who does not bother to look back. The mother accepts the invitation to sit down in the waiting room, while the child sits, stands, or wanders about at a distance. Neither makes a move toward the other. Later, in the office, when the mother is asked under some pretext to take the child on her lap, she usually does so in a dutiful, stilted manner, holding the child upright and using her arms solely for the mechanical purpose of maintaining him in his position."

This relationship was by now reciprocal, whichever one of the partners had been responsible for initiating it. Had an unresponsive mother educated a "cool" child? Or had a child who could not utilize normal mothering educated these mothers to expect rejection, educated them to a controlled indifference? The children did not hold up their arms when the mother bent to

---

[14]Another study (Hamilton and Mann 1954) of an entirely different patient group identifies this same quality of life-style. The patients were cases diagnosed as involutional psychosis, and their own rigidity and emotional impoverishment were being described. The wife of a patient described her husband: "He did everything according to a rigid schedule. I got kissed three times every morning and twice every night. We had sexual relations at 10 P.M. on Saturday nights." The physicians were discussing the prepsychotic personality of patients. In Kanner's study the parents were unusually free from certifiable mental illness, as we also noted in the studies of the upper economic groups by Srole, Hollingshead and Redlich, Rennie, and others.

pick them up, and were lifted passively, like little bags of meal. Their "loppish" postures did not adjust to the body of the mother, but assumed limp and awkward patterns as they hung within supporting arms. In short, the children did not "snuggle" and the mothers did not "hug." If we remember the three phases of mother-child relationships, in which the earliest symbiosis is gradually replaced by autonomy, we see that these twosomes had achieved a premature autonomy that showed no trace of any stage of close interdependence. "I saw only one mother of an autistic child who proceeded to embrace him warmly and bring her face close to him," Kanner observes. The coldly correct and proper relationship between the parents had its counterpart in the pattern he observed between mother and child. Kanner found it easy to pass from observations of this sort to an implication: it is this coldness, operating at an early phase of development when a personality first receives the imprint of the world about it, that *creates* this premature autonomy. The child does not develop the kind of outreaching affection that anticipates good reciprocal responses, because there was no warmth to imprint itself during the primary exchanges between mother and child. In the place of an easy and affectionate flexibility between the two, there has developed a cool and anxiety-laden distance which is self-maintaining. Once this foundation had been established, a later approach by some person determined to impart warmth affects the child as something threatening, invasive, something that must be repelled.

The perfectionism in these parents was revealed, Kanner felt, by the completeness of their records of the child's growth and development. They had kept a complete baby book: the first tooth, the first word, the nursery rhymes learned, every utterance and every illness, the successive changes in height and weight. In a sense they knew the *data* about their child's development better than they knew their *child;* they seemed, to Kanner, to be intent on producing a perfect product rather than enjoying the product as a person; they were a little anxious to hurry the development, to perform the complete experiment, and to produce the perfect child.[15]

One parent had purchased an encyclopedia for his two-year-old; another had tried to accelerate walking by exercises initiated in the infant's third

---

[15]We might note that where families are small, and children highly valued, and where the aspirations for a child are high, as in an upward-mobile middle-class family, such records must be common. If the mothers have studied in college the course of human growth and development, and have learned how to use, for example, one of the Yale charts as reference point, they will have reason to keep detailed records, since the child is not only father to the man, but a fair basis for predicting what the man can become. Does not his "developmental quotient" tell the clinic whether the infant will be good college material at age 17, even as early as his fourth year? Perhaps Dr. Kanner may have been unwittingly sampling one aspect of class culture that is much more widespread than early infantile autism, and thus describing factors that may also apply to any child, autistic or otherwise, that happens to be born in one of these ambitious, upward-mobile, well-organized, middle-class homes, which are in fact less likely to have deviant children than homes below them in the socioeconomic scale. Kanner's study deals with identified, referred, and treated early infantile autism, not with all cases that exist, and with a patient sample that is possibly not representative either of the total autistic population or of the total population of upward, mobile middle-class society.

month. These children did not suffer from parental indifference or neglect. We can call the children well-conditioned; the histories have some qualities of an experiment in accelerated growth. Such training, the clinician is apt to insist, is not an incidental outgrowth of the free and flexible gift of love, and not too well-suited to the needs and interests of the child.[16]

The Fathers of Autistic Children

Kanner found that the fathers too were remote, aloof from the child and from the family, married to their work rather than to a wife, and scarcely acquainted with their own autistic offspring. We would do well to remember that we may again be touching upon something that is more widespread than autism. In our haste, before we have control studies of representative samples of the normal population, we are likely to describe as the cause of autism something that is generally distributed throughout a class position. When Hollingshead and Redlich use the phrase "do not care for anyone but themselves and their goals" in describing their "unpleasant" but upward-mobile patients, they are pointing to qualities Kanner isolated in his fathers of autistic children.[17] Often hard-driving, trying to live up to their own perfectionistic standards, the fathers of autistic children concentrate on special skills in their effort to achieve personal security rather than on ways of achieving reciprocal affection or erotic gratification.

One of the fathers, described by Eisenberg (1957), might symbolize the group. Of a hundred fathers, Eisenberg found 15 who might be counted "normal"; the rest were obsessive, humorless, detached, well-educated, perfectionist, preoccupied with minutiae, relatively unaware of the larger human and social field in which they lived, more interested in the *performance* (adequacy) of their children than in their happiness, and strict in their demands for conformity, gave precedence to work rather than to family life, and looked on the intrusion of day-to-day family problems into their preoccupations as something unwarranted.

"Doctor R. was a caricature of the...psychiatric stereotype of a surgeon. He boasted that he never 'wasted' time talking to his patients or their families. When feasible, his first transaction with the patient took place with a draped and disinfected torso prepared for the surgical incision. He conscientiously supervised

---

[16]If we are, in fact, worshippers of Eros whether we are aware of it or not, as de Rougemont insists, any sensitive mother of an autistic child who reads Kanner's discussion will respond as to a most damaging criticism. What is intended as an objective description is thus converted, by the mother and by the clinician's choice of words (which convey *his* values) into a moral judgment.

[17]In contrast, compare the words Oscar Lewis (1965) used in describing the Puerto Rican lower-lowers: "Money and material possessions, although important, do not motivate their major decisions. Their deepest need is for love, and their life is a relentless search for it." Unfortunately, these lower-lowers seem neither able to give nor able to receive a very stable form of love, and the high rates of pathology among them do not make their "warmth" seem to be a very potent hygienic force.

details of postoperative care, but through his assistants. He dealt with infected gall bladders, diseased bowels, or tumors, with little or no curiosity about the person in whom these anatomical problems were housed. His day was thoroughly organized from the first surgical scrub to the last journal he might glance through while preparing for bed. The work he accomplished was prodigious and had earned him a position of considerable solidity in the professional community. Family life was the one item for which his schedule had no provision, not because of an inability to fit it in, but rather because of no perceived need for it. There were, of course, contacts with wife and children but these were kept to the unavoidable minimum inescapable at meals and bedtime. It was not that he could not see the need for relaxation; on the contrary, with each week's schedule was a half day for fishing or hunting, alone; each quarter there was a long vacation trip, alone.

"His wife was well provided for. She could spend what she chose. A mink coat was far more easily obtained than a discussion. If she were to bring up details of family living when they were together, she would draw a reproving look, a contemptuous dismissal of the problem as too petty to trouble him, and cold silence as he returned to his scheduled activity. Insecure, frightened by his cold and unaffectionate manner, and unable to express her overwhelming resentment, she grew less and less able to bring any matters to his attention. Intelligent and attractive when they married, she became progressively more of a slavey to the household and presented an incongruous appearance for the wife of a leading professional man.

"Distressed by her son's problems—the third of her children to show emotional difficulties—she at length had the temerity to suggest that a psychiatric consultation was indicated. Her husband's reply was a gruff statement that the boy would 'outgrow this nonsense,' but he was quite willing to displace the responsibility onto another and agreed to allow her to make the appointment. Mrs. R.'s account of her marital situation was indeed pathetic. Her husband had no apparent need for social life himself. As for her friends, 'He doesn't care for them. He says they talk too much.' He displayed affection neither toward her nor [toward] the children and had succeeded in isolating her from any possible satisfactions outside of her immediate family. He was himself the youngest of eleven siblings and by far the most successful in terms of money and prestige. He boasted—with justification—that he had achieved what he had on his own and with no dependence on others. All the less could he comprehend her feelings of inadequacy and self-pity.

"He agreed to come in to review the situation with the psychiatrist. He arrived on the scheduled moment prepared to deal with the problem in a forthright and business-like manner. He discussed the child's symptoms in an 'objective' and detached fashion. Once he had assured himself, through discreet inquiry, of the psychiatrist's competence, he was willing to accept the diagnosis and its full implications. He felt that the child had had 'something basically wrong with him from the beginning.' That there might be any connection between the child's difficulties and his (the father's) role in the family was a completely foreign notion, intellectually and emotionally alien to him. When, in an effort to provoke some feeling on his part, the question was posed as to whether he would recognize the child if he met him on the street, he gave the matter a moment of deliberation, answered 'objectively' that he was not entirely sure that he would, and gave no evidence of resentment of its obvious implications. Once the diagnosis had been decided, the issue was to determine with dispatch what course of action should be followed. The possibility of placement with affectionate and relaxed foster parents was mentioned. Almost at once he proposed two families in his own kinship and was prepared to terminate the interview, the problem in his view having been resolved. The possibility that either or both might find it impossible or undesirable to go along with the plan was simply beyond comprehension.

"This rather grim account had a happier issue than its own logic suggests, for the mother was helped to rouse herself from her torpor and to take the child on as her own responsibility, with a remarkable flowering on his part. The accomplishment was one of main force, stemming from untapped resources within the mother, with the father, all along and to the present, remaining as a barrier to be overcome."[18]

A Follow-Up of Autistic Children

Kanner and his associates were able to follow 63 of their autistic children for an average of nine years. Of 50 boys and 13 girls (this ratio of sexes has been reported by others), only three were classified as well-adjusted when seen at adolescence, either academically or socially. Another 46 were judged to be poorly adjusted, as not yet emerged from their earlier autistic patterns; in spite of "islands" of special skills, their general level of school performance was at a level expected of children of subnormal intelligence. Fourteen were described as functioning at a fair level; they attended regular school classes and could do work roughly commensurate with their age, but their contacts with people were still limited. They were aloof, schizoid, introverted. One factor in the development of these children seemed to have a prognostic value: the child that had failed to acquire a spoken language by age five had about one chance in 30 of reaching this middle category of fair adjustments. All three of the well-adjusted children had acquired speech early.[19]

In these cases followed to adolescence, the records show that the whole

---

[18]Among the questions that trouble the author (and reader) of de Rougemont's *Myths of Love* are "Where do these myths come from?" and "How and where are they taught, transmitted?" Are they Platonic ideas that exist independently in some circumambient ether above our lives, but influence the forms of our thought? Are they archetypal patterns, such as Jung proposed, arising out of our individual (or generic racial) unconscious to assume visible form in each generation? Are they taught, preached, reinforced by some drill or mimesis, dramatized in mystery plays that have to be written for each new generation, or in novels that spell out what is so difficult to put in words? Do clinical reports and psychiatric theories give concrete shape to that ancient phrase, "and the greatest of these is love"? Love takes innumerable forms, it seems: love of self, of professional success, of the precisely executed surgical procedure, of order, efficiency, and time that is never wasted. It may have innumerable expressions in a man such as Doctor R. and still lack the one dimension that makes a difference for a little son. This we can *feel*, and in feeling it so keenly express the fact that we, too, are bearers of the "myth of love." We can become passionate in our plea for Eros, and for the child. The scientific question remains: Is such passion relevant to the problem at hand, the autistic child? Poor parental love has many consequences, but is autism one of them?

[19]The persistent speech impairment might indicate a degree of social isolation, the kind of mother-child relationship emphasized by Kanner, or some obscure but fundamental neurological difficulty that had passed unnoticed. In any case, the impairment operates as a cause for the

armamentarium of therapy had been tried: electroshock, psychotherapy, carbon-dioxide therapy, foster-home placement, placement in special schools for disturbed children. A few had been given special instruction (by Montessori methods). One had a play group specially constructed and designed for the child. One had had "paid companions." Perhaps the very difficulty in inducing any positive improvement in these children accounts for the fact that comparatively sophisticated parents had sought so persistently to test all of the therapeutic possibilities. Surveying the meager results, Kanner could find little relationship between the kinds of therapy used, the intensity of effort, and the gains which were reported.

One case, followed over a twenty-eight-year period, has been reported by Darr and Worden (1951). The behavior of this girl, first seen in 1917, before clinicians had been alerted to the pattern named by Kanner, now seems to have belonged in the autistic syndrome. By the time she was finally hospitalized, she was expressing paranoid delusions about poisoned medicine and about urinating cider, and had become so unmanageable that she had to be placed in the disturbed ward. At the end of her career, her physicians were speculating about the possible advantages of using insulin shock, topectomy, electroshock. Her tantrums, spastic speech, disorganized behavior, shuffling gait suggested to them that a general deterioration had occurred. First described at two years of age, she behaved like one of Kanner's autistic children; at thirty she was classified schizophrenic. Seen in the best clinics, placed in a psychiatrist's home, provided with play groups and a Montessori teacher, attended by "paid companions" who looked out for her in a "home away from home," placed in special schools, the very best that could be purchased for her ended in a complete therapeutic failure.

Alternative Hypotheses

Even in the reports of Kanner and Eisenberg, who stress the importance of the "family climate," there emerges a doubt: the parents frequently insist "This child was *different from the others from the start.*" Moreover, we have been centering on the personality of the cold, detached, and obsessively perfectionist mother, and have failed to emphasize two important features of these records: there are a few cases of autism in which neither the mother nor the father fit the pattern; and there are normal siblings that are successfully reared by these same mothers. Of 131 siblings of his first 100 cases of autism, only three were regarded as "possibly autistic." Some brothers and sisters of autistic children were selected by their teachers for programs designed for the specially gifted.

A logically precise study would begin with the parents. If we were to select a group of these so-called "refrigerator parents," locating them in the same social classes from which Kanner's patients came (mostly upper-middle and

---

cumulative retardation, since this is the channel through which our rich social surplus filters down to the child.

lower-upper, with very few lower-lower cases),[20] it is highly probable that (1) the rates for mental illness in their offspring would not markedly exceed those for this class position in general, and (2) that those children who would be classed as emotionally disturbed would show every type of neurosis, character disorder, and psychosis, in addition to the autistic patterns identified by Kanner. If upper-middle-class parents (and patients in general) of this personality type, who have not endeared themselves to psychiatrists, were statistically more common, we would be faced with an interesting problem, for the rates for mental illness are lower at this socioeconomic level than for the classes below. Since the studies reported in the literature have originated within patient groups (*treated* disorders), we have a limited knowledge of existing cases: we need evidence to complete the design. That there is another type of home, in which parents are warm, friendly, and indulgent to the point of neglecting essential disciplines has been pointed out in one study; and their children at adolescence are emotionally insecure and lacking in motivation.[21]

These considerations have led some clinicians to look on the child's lack of response to the mother as due to some genetic or constitutional factor within the child. The factors that have been proposed have ranged from birth injuries and special sensitivities (genetically determined) to special traumatic experiences that have produced abnormal responses to essentially normal types of mothering.

One case, reported by Ross (1959), had been studied at autopsy; and extensive brain damage was revealed. This possibility had been overlooked in spite of a series of neurological examinations that had produced only negative findings; in short, the child's behavior had been a better index of his neurological status than the clinician's "signs." The child conformed to the autistic pattern; her parents were also within that range described by Kanner. The clinicians (conforming to the "myth of love") had described the child as "a product of an unsympathetic, nonunderstanding family situation." The prolonged efforts at psychotherapy based on this interpretation, the stigma placed on the parents by this type of evaluative diagnosis, can of course produce its own pathology, in addition to whatever else is at work in a case. Rimland (1964, pp. 110-11) has described one mother who had made a 320-mile

---

[20]Bender and Grugett (1956) found that schizophrenic children seen in the Bellevue service in New York City were from homes slightly higher in socioeconomic status than the homes of other types of "problem children." Parents, friends, rabbis, physicians, aware of a service in which specialists were carrying on research with schizophrenic children, may have referred a sample different from the sample schoolteacher, police, and social agencies would refer in dealing with delinquents, firebugs, sex offenders, and truants.

[21]See Baldwin, Kalhorn, and Huffman (1945), who stress "There are parents whose general adjustment is adequate, but whose insight into children's needs is not." Dorothea Leighton makes a similar point (in a speech reported in the *Chapel Hill Weekly,* Dec. 4, 1966): "Neurotic children do not necessarily have neurotic parents or vice versa. . . . Parents who show no evidence of stress themselves can produce stress in their children. . . . Poor homes, and poor communities, that are well-integrated have a higher level of mental health than well-to-do communities that are disorganized."

trip twice a week to get her child to a university clinic over a period of 18 months. Sensitive parents who have had an autistic child and who have experienced the devastating effects of this type of clinical diagnosis will understand what was motivating the mother, and the kind of penance she felt was being exacted.

Hyperoxia

Retrolental fibroplasia, a destruction of newly forming and incompletely vascularized retinal tissue, can produce blindness in premature children who are given too much oxygen. When the case reports include such features as head-banging, rocking, musical interests, and the typical autistic language difficulties, there is some reason to speculate that some pervasive neurological damage, possibly involving the reticular network, which is so important for the arousal and encoding of perceptions, may also be involved. Blindness produced by damage to the optic tracts alone does not have such associated traits. Gathering his evidence from many sources, Rimland (1964) suggests that either hyperoxia or a hypersensitivity to even normal concentrations of oxygen may cause a defective development of the central nervous system, with resultant neural processes that produce the typical autistic pattern, and that these causes may account for some of the cases of autism now appearing in pediatric clinics.[22]

Unusual Sensitivities

Among the children classified as cases of "early infantile autism," there are some who show exaggerated reactions to minimal stresses, who are excessively sensitive to any "hurt," and who seem to have abnormally strong reactions to special sensory modalities. The comparative psychologist has alerted us to genetically determined differences of this nature. Even the mild tension induced by the light of a 200-watt bulb hanging over a strange open field will differentiate the members of a rat colony. The tensions, betrayed by excessive urinating and defecating and a refusal to eat, normally subside in four days of testing, but a few animals will be disturbed for eight days or more. Selecting the "sensitives" and the "tough" by picking and mating animals at the extremes of this distribution, Hall (1941) succeeded in breeding two strains of animals, one of which he called "emotionals" because of their low tolerance for this stress. The animals of the other strain seemed somehow to be tougher, more aggressive, less fearful, less sensitive. In the same fashion the biologists at the Jackson Memorial Laboratory have bred audiogenic-seizure-susceptible animals. In other laboratories breeding experiments have produced a colony of animals that are especially vulnerable to experimental-neurosis training.

---

[22]Some observers have reported more prematurity (12 per cent) in their series of autistic children than in the general population (7 per cent). Other research points ot the greater vulnerability of multiple births to hyperoxia, as measured by their susceptibility to retrolental fibroplasia.

Liddell (1956), and Anderson and Parmenter (1941) at Cornell, learned very early that they could best produce a "breakdown" by special conditioning procedures if they selected their animals from a certain "jittery" breed of Cheviots, rather than from other, more stolid and phlegmatic types of sheep, such as the Shropshire.

Such differential susceptibilities also exist in children, some of whom show an abnormally high frustration tolerance (analogous to that of the placid Basset hound), others of whom are sensitive, emotional, skittish, easily disturbed. Bergman and Escalona (1949; see also Escalona 1948) have suggested that some of the sensitive children who appear in the clinic lack the normal "protective barrier" that prevents excessive reactions to disturbing situations; they believe that this special susceptibility may be responsible for some cases of autism, especially when this sensitivity is combined with atypical patterns of mothering. Certainly any mother of a child with this exaggerated sensibility will be called upon to exert better than average "buffering" and "regulating," since the child's genetic endowment will multiply each of her errors.

A group of five children studied by Bergman and Escalona showed a wide variety of sensitivities. One boy behaved much like Klüver's monkey (see Klüver and Bucy 1939), in which an agnosia had developed as a result of a temporal-lobe extirpation, smelling everything that he came into contact with, as though—lacking the normal neural mechanisms for encoding stimuli —he could not perceive an object through other sensory channels (he did not lack visual sensitivity). To the sound of voices the child responded with fear, but he was fascinated by classical music. Many autistic children show an abnormally low tolerance for sounds, some of them responding to the ordinary noises of household appliances—the mixer, the vacuum, the dishwasher— with an almost catastrophic terror. Abnormal sensitivities to touch appeared in one child, who would laugh at the touch of velvet, but reject or withdraw from any woolly surface with considerable feeling. They showed strong preferences for colors, lights, "sad music," along with intense preoccupation with mechanical objects, or with a fascination with symphonic music, or with a photophobia. The same kinds of rocking or repetitive movements that Kanner observed were also noted in these "sensitives" whom other clinicians could easily have classified as autistic. Four of the five later became psychotic (see Rimland 1964, p. 101).

When these differential sensitivities emerge in the first year and persist throughout development, they may form the basis for precocious islands of skill in listening, touching, handling, viewing, discriminating, modeling, dancing; they can also be the nucleus of phobias and obsessive-compulsive concerns. Frequently both aspects of development proceed pari passu, and can create an acute problem for a mother, a camp counselor, a "house mother." This child cannot learn, concentrate, or endure under conditions that are scarcely noticed by other children. Excessively vulnerable to emotional hurt, they do not easily and naturally acquire skills in regulating the social tensions.

Referring to this type of constitutional predisposition, Mahler (1952) observed:

"There are infants with an inherently defective tension-regulating apparatus which probably cannot be adequately complemented by either the most quantitatively or qualitatively efficient mothering. It seems that there are infants with an inherent ego deficiency which from the very beginning—that is to say, from...the undifferentiated phase—predisposes them to remain or to become alienated from reality; there are others whose precarious reality-adherence depends on delusional symbiotic fusion with the mother image."[23]

This lack of a protective barrier seems to point to some sort of inner buffering process in the normal. Like the new hearing aids which have a built-in "buffer" to protect the wearer from abnormal surges of sound, the normal nervous system can dampen sensory surges, so that they are well-received and accurately discriminated. The sensitive is still disturbed by the mere reception of the stimuli which the normal is tolerating, investigating, becoming adapted to, discriminating between, and using to manipulate the objects of his environment. The mothers of these sensitives are required to do a qualitatively superior job; they must be attentive and flexible, sensitive to the nuances in the child's behavior, playing by ear, yet not permitting the child's special exaggerated receptivity to stand in the way of his learning (and his "toughening"). We can easily imagine the consequences which would accrue from these transactions if the mother were (1) too aggressively maternal, invasive, overstimulating; (2) lacking in sensitivity yet determined to accelerate the growth of an intelligent child; (3) unusually secure in her own hearty approach to life and correspondingly annoyed at all of the finicky sensitivity that, she is certain, her child will outgrow if she is firm in her methods; (4) indifferent or busily preoccupied and unable to deal patiently and insightfully with a sensitive child who is unusually hard to draw out and even more difficult to launch as an autonomous individual; (5) anxious and fearful, not only aware of all of the difficulties in adjustment that await her child, but feeling rebuffed and rejected by her child's response; (6) forced to work, so that the child has to be separated from her and placed in an inferior type of day-care center.

Since there is no guarantee as to what type of maternal competence one of the sensitive children will draw in the lottery of birth, all manner of transactions can contribute to a variety of destinies, each cumulatively constructed on the basis of this original sensitivity. It is the opinion of Escalona that:

"...the more one studies the early life history of psychotic children, the more one is impressed with the atypical and pathological reaction of the children to

---

[23]I will translate Mahler's special vocabulary into the simple message to mothers it is intended to be: You should not accept the responsibility so many counselors are ready to lay on your shoulders. There are children for whom the best of mothers could not provide the "buffering and regulating" that would make them well-integrated with social reality, with good social coping mechanisms, at peace with themselves and with others. An ego is not implanted, preformed. It develops in time. But these "sensitives" do not take on the well-balanced ego in spite of what looks like a most normal mothering.

perfectly ordinary maternal attitudes and to inevitable daily routines.... Therapeutic programs might at times be modified if these early developmental disturbances were regarded as arising in large measure from the pathology within the child rather than from parental attitudes per se."

It is clear that the sensitivities here described could easily convert a training procedure that is good enough for the normal child into an increasingly traumatic experience for both child and mother.

Along with a progressive deterioration in the mother-child transactions, the mother may become increasingly anxious, oversolicitous, overconcerned, filled with a feeling of helplessness. Or she may become hostile, rejecting, retaliatory, projecting her irritations upon the child and reading into his behavior a "meanness" that she then tries to correct. In a few mothers the child's reactions will intensify maternal feelings and lead her to redouble her effort to protect and regulate; in thus compensating for the child's special weakness, she can develop additional incapacities as she intensifies the symbiotic bonds and makes her child more and more dependent. All the dangers of "maternal overprotection" that Levy described will then flourish in this situation, and when a mother is also a "sensitive," her identification with the child intensifies the problem.

As this mother-child bond grows, it may hinder growth at each point where the mother attempts to withdraw her support and to "launch" the child on his own. The degree of infantilization and the intensity of the symbiotic needs will appear absurd to all those outside the family, who may produce friction between the mother and the father, who may be less involved. The mother who is still buttering her son's bread, unbuttoning his pants, carrying him to school, sleeping with him at night, at an age when other mothers are freed from such constant claims, may feel greatly "put upon," yet prove unequal to the task of breaking the vicious circle. Both mother and child will face problems at each transitional point: going to school, going away to camp, leaving for college, entering boot camp, taking the first job, becoming engaged, getting married, having a first child. Not only are these transitions difficult, they raise the question, "Who has failed?" Recriminations often ricochet among child, father, mother, and counselors.

A common consequence of such an excessively prolonged symbiosis is an atypical pattern of growth. Many of these children are "split growers," to borrow Willard Olsen's term (1943); they are low in autonomy and in social skills, sometimes very high in mechanical skills and in fantasy. These odd growers, with islands of precocity and large swamplands of retardation, do not show the even and well-rounded progression in growth that we count normal.[24]

When this sensory selectivity and exaggerated symbiotic tie are in force early enough and consistently enough, and when the transactions between mother and child fail to cope with these fragile organisms, the child can be-

---

[24]One of the children studied by Bergman and Escalona showed this pattern of "split growth" in the early months. Fish *et al.* (1965) believe that potential schizophrenics can be spotted within the first 12 or 18 months if the clinician pays serious attention to irregular and atypical patterns of growth.

come autistic, nonsocial, nonspeaking, involved in a private world of mechanical, repetitive, imaginary, noncommunicative activities. The milder form of neurotic anxiety that occurs at each threat of separation intensifies the problems of vocational and social adjustment that go with maturing. The "sensitives" want to be alone, to work at their own pace, yet they are deeply in need of a supporting relationship on which they can depend. They resent "invaders" and at the same time suffer from their own solitude.

What Bergman and Escalona call premature ego-formation (the autistic pattern) is an early structuring of life without people. The incorporation of parental "images" and the relationships with other significant persons do not take place normally. Normal emancipation from the parents does not develop. Some have systematically "cooled" their relationships with those whom others count significant; others both cling and rebel. Either the regulator-buffers are reduced to "nothings" or these immature ones place impossible demands upon them, or both. At adolescence theirs could be called not so much an "identity crisis" as a struggle to prevent any autonomous and responsible identity from emerging.[25] Other types of deviations emerge from such faulty mother-child transactions: vagrants, firebugs, affectionless thieves, aggressive and uninhibited antisocial types.[26]

If such a "sensitive" becomes in his turn a parent, he can set a new cycle of pathogenic processes in motion. Many of the ineffectual and withdrawn fathers who were highly successful within the narrow island of their special skills (as described in the Kanner-Eisenberg studies) behave toward their own children in such a way as to intensify the pathogenic quality in the transactions between mother and child. Their own ineffectuality as fathers and as social beings, their lack of normal interpersonal bonds, can facilitate their selection of a spouse who also does not seek too intimate a bond. Such "cold climates" thus tend to reproduce themselves, even apart from or in addition to any genetic transmission.

From the clinicians' descriptions one might conclude that there are two ways of being autistic, and of expressing a lack of consideration for or involvement with others. Overtly aggressive, some autistic personalities behave as though they look upon other persons as objects to be manipulated, used up, wrung dry, exploited, flung aside. They want a kind of relationship, but no involvement, no responsibilities, no tomorrows. Others seem to retreat within a shell of indifference or of fear, repelling all "invaders" and seeking a kind of self-encapsulated autonomy. Fear, apathy, and rebellion might conceivably stem from a single root. Apart from possible genetic dosages of "aggressiveness"

---

[25]The young schizophrenics whom Hare (1956) observed entering hospital from single-person households (away from the family) showed this same lack of identification with and futile rebellion against their "home folks."

[26]In a 30-year follow-up study of children seen in child-guidance clinics and who later became schizophrenic, O'Neal and Robins (1958) reported that the most frequent antisocial symptoms in the group were physical and nonphysical aggression, incorrigibility, vagrancy, running away, and pathological lying.

or "emotionality," which some breeders of animals are certain are inherited (see Scott 1958, Lorenz 1963), the particular direction which autism takes will be determined by the cumulative transactions we have been describing.

Compensatory efforts to recreate the symbiotic attachment, which once served so well to reduce anxiety, may appear in a marriage to a "substitute mother," in a flight into "the mother church" or some other "buffer institution," or in rejection of the role of a mature sexuality. The monastery cell, the niche in the organization, the mechanically repetitive and impersonal task (with a supervisor who is responsible for all decisions) can serve the needs of the sensitive, who is so quickly overwhelmed by any confusion or competition, by any invasive "closeness." A research worker's laboratory or a bibliophile's cubicle also may attract such a person, as does even gardening, since the plants do not talk back.

Another outcome is that chronic need for guidance with which so many counselors have to deal. The inability to assume a firm stance in a confusing and disorganizing world, to make a field and plot a future, to withstand the pressures of barriers and distractions while working persistently toward a goal, is a later version of that "inherent ego deficiency" referred to above. These are the ones who find it difficult to live among men and demand respect for themselves while collaborating with others and respecting *their* uniqueness.

Not all the outcomes achieved by these sensitive "split growers" (some of whom are also autistic) fall into the debit column. We would have to name the poems of Baudelaire, efforts of Proust to recapture his past, the sentimental journeys of Flaubert, the scientific discoveries of Willard Gibbs, the prose of André Gide, Ernest Renan's *Life of Jesus,* the paintings of Van Gogh, if we were to accept the accounts of biographers, who, let us admit, are also under the influence of our current psychiatric conception of infancy. In the personal lives of such men, we discover much pain and neuroticism, along with precocious flowerings of talent, special "islands" in which the very highest capacities to perceive and create have developed; their products have delighted, mystified, and entertained the rest of mankind, and a few have contributed, notably, to that mastery of nature that makes us an affluent society. Along with their gifts, a few of them have been notably perverse, rebellious, odd, crotchety, sensitive, complex, difficult to know, and so unhappy in their interpersonal relationships that we have to call them "geniuses in spite of themselves."

A Schematic Summary of Complementary Hypotheses

Garcia and Sarvis (1964) have presented a diagrammatic summary (see Fig. 2) of what they call a "multifactorial approach" to the problem of early infantile autism. The factors which they include range from "unconscious needs of the parents," which direct their interactions with the child in such a way as to reinforce the quiet, withdrawn behavior, to that inborn "thin protective barrier" that Bergman and Escalona emphasized. They look on autism as a reaction to an assault endured at a vulnerable stage of development, and they see the child as interpreting his stress "as if the mother were persecuting him." From this point on, interactions between mother and child will deter-

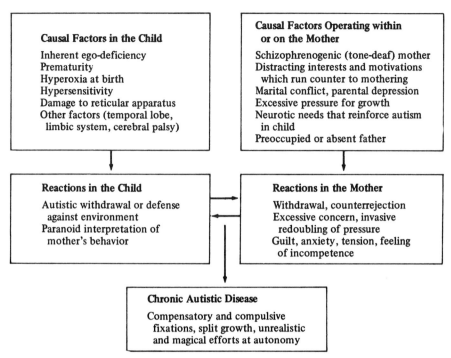

FIGURE 2. THE AUTISTIC DISTURBANCE IN MOTHER-CHILD RELATIONSHIPS. (After Garcia and Sarvis 1964.)

mine whether the response is deepened and made chronic, or reversed. As a corrective to what has undoubtedly been an overemphasis on the mother's role, these authors suggest that: "Although some authors seem to feel that parents should always be able to make up for the child's lack of modulated defenses and be able to provide alternatives for behavior or promote sublimations, we feel this demands a degree of parental omnipotence which is not consistent with human capacity." In other words, parents are people, not gods. Clinicians expect too much of them.

This view makes the paranoid rejection of the parent by the child the primary factor. Neither the parent, who is the target for this reaction, nor the child, who is so immature at this early point in his development, can work through to a solution of this conflict easily. The clinician who automatically (and erroneously) assumes that interpersonal family psychopathology is the primary and principal causal factor only reinforces paranoid distortions. On the other hand, to automatically (and equally erroneously) assume that the family has no role whatever in the causation, that it is basically organic, is to encourage a heedless policy that would miss important therapeutic possibilities.

EXTREMES OF MOTHERING IN SCHIZOPHRENICS

In many respects the schizophrenias tell us little we can be sure of about the relationships between mothering patterns and mental illness. Most schizophrenics are admitted into hospital between the ages of 17 and 40 (with a peak at 25), and their earliest experiences have to be reconstructed from hearsay evidence. Not only are these psychotic patients themselves poor witnesses, since they live in a world so distorted that we cannot trust any testimony that comes from their lips, but many of the facts about their earliest experiences with mothering, which some are ready to insist are so important for early infantile autism, are not open to recall by any adult. Their mothers, and the other adults in the family, are known to be poor sources even for their medical histories (see Wheeler *et al.* 1950). Since some of the probing is carried on by physicians who have preconceived notions about the mother's guilt, we can understand how a mother might have to be excused as a hostile witness (she has no Fifth Amendment for mothers to plead, no higher court). Occasionally, as in infantile autism and childhood schizophrenia, mothers and patients can be observed and treated together, and their interrelations can be observed on the spot, even though, as Garcia and Sarvis noted, they are not easy to interpret.

Seven Subtypes

There is an additional reason why schizophrenia offers special difficulties. Schizophrenia should still be called a "psychosis of unknown origin," and as many as 22 varieties of it have been identified (see Stephens and Astrup 1963). Standing by itself, the diagnosis is somewhat like the diagnosis attached to soldiers on the Flanders front in World War I: they were running a fever under conditions where no laboratory studies could be made, so their medical officers hastily wrote their diagnosis as "P.U.O." and evacuated them to base hospitals. There, hopefully, the "pyrexia of unknown origin" could be classified according to its causes: bladder infection, tuberculosis, hepatitis, or that still obscure category, influenza. It has been a hundred years since Morel (1809-1873) identified the form of dementia praecox that Bleuler later renamed schizophrenia. This latter name now includes such a variety of forms that it needs a more refined definition. Today schizophrenia does not always mean a deteriorating dementia, and its forms can strike at any age from three to sixty. Its course is varied, and is sometimes interrupted by a complete and permanent remission; about one-fourth of the cases proceed to a rut formation with mental deterioration. Not only does it assume varied forms—catatonic, paranoid, hebephrenic, pseudoneurotic, and so on—but sometimes several of these forms may be displayed in succession, by a single patient in the course of his illness. The early infantile autism identified by Kanner, which many have hesitated to call schizophrenia, can in fact develop into an adult form of this psychosis. Its symptoms appear in every dimension of behavior that we can measure: some observers see the essential defect as a *thinking disorder;* others stress the incongruity between *emotional life* and speech or action; still others sense the patient's failure in practical action, and especially his loss of a vital interest in reality, as a part of a basic *volitional defect.*

Individual profiles of disability vary so widely that some clinicians have questioned whether there is in fact any unitary process underlying the symptoms.[27] Even the much more strictly delimited area of childhood schizophrenia has been broken up into more than a half-dozen subtypes. When these subtypes are examined more closely, they turn out to be concrete clusters of symptoms. Frequently the cluster is given a name by an enthusiastic investigator who believes that he can impart order by some causal hypothesis. We have almost arrived at the point of speaking of schizophrenia Kanner, or schizophrenia Mahler, or schizophrenia Bleuler.

Consider a representative classification of the subtypes (Hirschberg and Bryant 1956):

1. A "nuclear" group who show disorganization in every level of maturation: autonomic functions, locomotion and basic motor skills, speech, perceiving and thinking, and social-emotional integrations. This group was first identified by Lauretta Bender, whose view of the illness makes the faulty maturation a process that is in turn explained by a faulty inheritance. The *homes* of these children were judged to be slightly above those of the other Bellevue Hospital mental cases, but their family histories showed many psychotic ancestors. In Bender's interpretation of her findings the deviant examples of mothering are regarded as merely contributory factors, secondary to a basic developmental weakness of genetic origin. (See Bender 1956, Bender and Grugett 1956, Bender and Helme 1953.)

2. The early infantile autism of Kanner, Garcia and Sarvis, and others that is described above. Although Kanner views it as almost uniformly associated with a mothering that lacks normal flexibility and warmth, others are more inclined to think it has multiple causes. The existence of normal siblings in these same families should make the diagnostician hesitate to attribute the symptoms wholly to the personality of the mother.

3. A group described by Mahler (1952) as suffering from a symbiotic psychosis and composed of children who failed to achieve normal differentiation of their egos from the mother's by the usual date. As a consequence the child remains "regressively fused" with the mother. Any threat to his possession of and power over the mother precipitates panic and stress, making the progress beyond this point of arrest difficult. Besides this notion of differentiation which has to be completed at a normal period, Mahler posits an inherent deficiency in the tension-regulating apparatus. Centering her attention upon the progression from symbiosis to normal autonomy, Mahler envisaged a variety of causal relations. Among her cases she identified some children who had been given normal mothering but whose *inherent* weakness left them irreparably warped, unstructured, narcissistically vulnerable; in other cases the overactive mother seems to have attempted to compensate for such weakness.

4. A group of very young and extremely sensitive children who are excessively vulnerable to emotional hurt. Occasionally they are gifted with special

---

[27]"No one can cure a 'spectre' like schizophrenia," wrote Karl Menninger (*National Observer,* Feb. 11, 1963). Reichard's study (1956) of some of Freud's patients who had been labeled hysterics indicated to him that the hysteric of one generation may be called hypochondriac, or schizophrenic, in the next. And Dr. Szasz (1961) would undoubtedly classify them as simply "persons with problems in living."

powers of discrimination and patterning. These are the "sensitives" of Bergman and Escalona (1949); the anxiety and overprotectiveness of their mothers are seen as a reaction to unusual children.

5. A group of children with a variety of organic brain syndromes. Their behavior makes them difficult to distinguish from the second category mentioned above. They, too, develop defensive and paranoid distortions of reality, a reality that is rendered even more difficult by the counterpressures for growth, the guilt feelings of parents (often enhanced by some pernicious certainties of clinicians), and the cognitive-perceptive difficulties which block normal learning in the child. As a result the arrests of growth are difficult to "unfix" and require expert professional intervention.

6. A borderline group that may contain admixtures of each of the above groups but which can shift from normal functioning to psychotic functioning when stress is suddenly increased. Described as "attempts to master anxiety," these regressions to a disordered level of functioning in fact master nothing, and so are not reinforced by successes. Some psychotherapists have found that, by skillfully entering such a child's symbolically represented conflicts, they can assist the child to master them and thus to return to a normal conception of reality. This category is created by a clinician's interpretation of the purpose of the symptoms and by the pragmatic value of the therapy founded upon such interpretation. (See Ekstein 1954, 1962.)

7. A group called pseudoschizophrenic that shows transient regressions to schizophrenic behavior, with the entire range of symptoms described above. When this regression is closely related to a severe emotional stress, and when therapy, which includes removal from the stress situation, restores normal functioning, the pattern is considered *reactive* (symptomatic of extreme stress) instead of—as Bender had viewed the symptoms of her group—the result of a genetically determined "process" that produces a faulty maturation.

The Seventh Category Explored

Within this seventh group we might place a series of cases that come from the most traumatic and distorted forms of mothering. In presenting a few of these children, Bettelheim (1956) interpreted their paranoid resistance to all therapeutic efforts as founded on their experience with a brutal reality: the child had concluded that he was "totally at the mercy of irrational forces which were bent upon using him for their goals, irrespective of his." The extreme situations from which these children had emerged had overpowered and crushed whatever tension-regulating potentiality they may have had. Comparing them to the concentration-camp victims, who had lived in an unpredictable and catastrophic world run by a group of homicidal psychopaths, Bettelheim asks, in effect: "If adults who have already achieved a reasonably stable and mature ego can collapse under the extremes of torture, why should we not find parallels in the lives of children who are still in a vulnerable phase of development?" In the death camp where Bettelheim had himself experienced some of these same extreme pressures, he had seen prisoners unable to sleep and eat, men experiencing hallucinations, men filled with paranoid delusions that exceeded the horrors of reality, with ideas that they were being mentally influenced. He saw the normal controls of reason and conscience break down, revealing a deteriorated and degraded set of impulses; he watched the disorganization spread downward from the highest functions through apathy and anomie, until the simplest autonomic controls and the inhibitions of bladder and bowel sphincters had been lost. These disorganized prisoners also lost their memories; they grew suicidal; their capacity for a full and affective response disappeared (their emotions, we could say, had been bleached); some sat in a catatonic-like stupor.

Now, we may ask, what kind of homes could Bettelheim possibly be referring to? One child, referred to the Orthogenic School supervised by Bettelheim, was only five years old, yet he seemed to be in continuous and dreadful fear for his life. None of the therapist's efforts succeeded in unearthing his secret until an interview with a former servant gave a clue. It seems that the mother had been discovered *in flagrante delicto* by her three-year-old son, and had thereafter repeatedly threatened to kill the child if he ever told anyone; before the child was five she had deserted him.

Other clinicians have described other types of "pressure." Tietze (1949) described the mother of a 36-year-old woman who had been schizophrenic for 16 years:

From her interviews with the mother, Tietze discovered that when the daughter was only a year and a half old, the mother had made a heroic struggle against the girl's attempts to masturbate. On her first contact with the physician the mother had brought up this problem; she seemed preoccupied with it. Twice she had persuaded a surgeon to operate upon the girl's clitoris (prior to age three), and for several years thereafter, on the advice of her physician, she had examined the girl's genitalia every night. If the labia were found irritated, the child was spanked. This vein of punitive concern permeated other aspects of the girl's psychosexual development. Competing with the daughter for the attention of the young men the girl brought home, she tried to "outshine" the daughter. But she warned the girl against any physical familiarities.

Tietze described a more subtle form of dominance in a mother who would take to her bed whenever her daughters planned to go to a party, and demand that they stay home to care for her. The daughters resolved their difficulties by never planning to go out. In her own eyes this mother was a devoted mother and wife who had never raised her voice at husband or children. When her feelings were hurt, she wept and took to bed with a sick headache. In their efforts to achieve some autonomy her daughters literally "made her sick." But she won, at the expense of the health of her daughters, one of whom had to be hospitalized for schizophrenia.

To return to Bettelheim, once more, consider the child who carried the following traumatic memory dating from age three:

From an older brother of the patient, his counselor learned about a hanging game in which the small boy had been the victim. "The rope had cut off the child's breathing and he was only revived after artificial respiration had been applied. Dreading that the boy might tell, the older ones established a regime of terror. Repeatedly and severely they beat up this youngster, threatening even worse tortures if he should ever reveal the story. In order to make the threat more effective, they repeatedly locked him up in a dark and inaccessible excavation and kept him there for prolonged periods despite his terrified screaming. Although this boy revealed fantasies of being locked up in dark rooms, he had given no direct evidence of the core secret, the hanging episode, to his counselor.

Another child, believed to be feebleminded, seemed so stupid to his parents that they felt free to discuss him in his presence, revealing their intention to put him away, as well as their wish that he had never been born. His autistic withdrawal resulted in his being placed in an institution for the feebleminded, where he was badly neglected. Punished by having his meals withheld, he interpreted it all as a part of his parents' plot to kill him by starvation. His own fantasies, revealed to his counselor at the Orthogenic School, had to do with his own desire to torture and kill others before they could kill him.

Sometimes the child's experiences that result in a combination of autistic withdrawal and paranoid hostility contain numerous contacts with the psychiatric profession. Treatment which involves electroshock, tranquilizing drugs, lobotomy, can result in a psychosis that is properly called *iatrogenic*. In a paper charged with considerable emotion, Hilde Mosse (1958) describes one of her boys seen at the Lafargue Clinic:

"Seven year old Bernard is representative of the many cases where unnecessary hospitalization and harmful treatment followed this wrong diagnosis (schizophrenia). His mother took him out of the hospital and brought him to the clinic. She said, 'He had only six shock treatments, not the full 20. He had forgotten even our dog's name when he came home, and he had known him since the dog was a puppy. It was just like he had to learn all over again. It seemed like he was in a daze most of the time.' Clinical tests, examinations, play-group observation showed no evidence of schizophrenia.... The boy recovered with group and individual therapy."

A Statistical Study of Mothers of Schizophrenics

One of the few studies that have published figures for controls comes from Denmark. Yrjö Alanen (1958), a young Danish psychiatrist, studied the mothers of 100 schizophrenic patients, and matched them with the mothers of 20 neurotics and the mothers of 20 "normals." Although we can gather "testimonials" and persuasive evidence from interviews with the mothers of schizophrenic patients, we seldom get data obtained by comparable methods from the mothers of normal subjects. We have little to balance the possible subjective factors or methodological biases of the particular physicians reporting.

The most striking fact in Alanen's study is the heavier loading of pathology in the mothers of the schizophrenics (see Table 6). As a group, they had many psychosomatic complaints, were insecure, full of anxiety, and given to dereistic thinking, and showed limited capacity for warm human ties. They were not the kind of mothers who could form easy and empathic relationships with children, or allow the child to be himself. In looking back upon their own childhoods, they complained that their own mothers had somehow failed them; certainly the grandmothers of the patients had failed to give their daughters the "feel" of good mothering, if one can judge by the behavior of the mothers of the patients. Their marriages had been stable enough, divorce

TABLE 6. *A Study of Mothers of Schizophrenic, Neurotic, and Normal Subjects.* (From Alanen 1958.)

Clinical Estimate of the Status of the Mothers	Schizophrenic Patients (N=100)	Neurotic Patients (N=20)	Normal Subjects (N=20)
Mothers with manifest psychosis	12%	0	0
Mothers with weak ego, showing intolerable anxiety, classed as pseudoneurotic schizophrenia or borderline schizophrenia (with evidence of dereistic thinking)	11%	5%	0
Mothers with illness surpassing the usual neurotic categories (classed as schizoid types with character neuroses)	40%	5%	5%
Mothers with neurotic illness, and with a degree of poverty of affect	21%	35%	25%
Normal (or near-normal) mothers	16%	55%	70%

being rare, but there had been a great deal of conflict and disharmony (25 per cent of the fathers were judged to be alcoholic, and 12 per cent were reported to be pathologically jealous). Sexual relationships between the parents were notably poor.

Attempting to evaluate the relationships between these mothers and their schizophrenic offspring, Alanen felt that the traits of the mothers (anxiety, depression, overconcern) had not prevented them from giving adequate physical care, but they had reacted to their children with aggression, possessiveness, overprotection, rigidity, and indifference, rather than with a warm and flexible mixture of affection and discipline. They tended to act possessively toward their sons, and with hostility and ambivalence toward their daughters; where the ties were unusually "close," the psychosis tended to appear earlier.

Looking into these extended backgrounds, Alanen suggests that a psychosis may require two generations to develop. Just as it requires generations of "good breeding" to raise the gentleman who knows intuitively how to behave, it seems to require two or three generations to prepare the groundwork for these psychotic breaks with reality. But whether this is a cumulating and compounding process (involving mate-selection and the assorting of genes) that is mainly *biological,* or whether it corresponds to the accumulation of a *tradition* of behavior, such a statistical study cannot show us. The study does indicate that approximately a sixth (16 per cent) of the cases of schizophrenia emerge from families in which there has been a normal mothering.

Clinical Bias against "Schizophrenogenic" Mothers

This sixth with normal mothers is important, since such cases tend to be swallowed up and hidden by the cases that emphasize bad mothering. Hill (1955), writing in defense of his patients, is bitter in his attack on "schizophrenogenic" mothers, convicting them by naming as he presents a composite portrait.[28] Many others (e. g., Rosen 1953, Tietze 1949, Reichard and Tillman 1950, Lidz *et al.* 1958) who have offered their opinions about these mothers have not presented systematic studies of the mothers of normals, or of the mothers of other types of mental patients. Taken as a group, such mothers present an impressive amount of pathology: they manage to violate about every dimension of that ideal of the good mother so deeply embedded in our values. Instead of the Biblical "the wages of sin is death," they seem to suggest "the wages of abnormal mothering is psychotic behavior in the child." The whole notion has a certain vague fitness: surely evil things come out of evil things. But its very fitness should alert us.

One can understand, as one reads the case reports, how a clinician can develop a stereotype of "the abnormal mother." She is the one who objects to the counselor's prying questions, who fights to withdraw her child from the hospital when it is the considered judgment of the staff that the child should not return to the home, who seems unable to hear or accept formulations that are offered to her, and her marital conflicts and her own pathology (many such mothers are ambulatory schizophrenics themselves) help convince the physician that she is, in fact, schizophreno*genic*. Hill is most frank: "Psychiatrists do not generally like or have sympathy for or understand the mothers of schizophrenic patients."

As his stereotype forms, the clinician tends to lapse into inclusive generalizations about *"All* of the mothers...." For example:

"All mothers were overanxious and obsessive, all were domineering—ten more overtly and fifteen in a more subtle fashion. All mothers were found to be restrictive with regard to the libidinal gratification of their children" (Tietze 1949, pp. 64-65).

"Not a single family was reasonably well integrated, but it requires illustrative material to convey properly how seriously disorganized or aberrant these families were" (Lidz and Fleck 1960, p. 332).

"From the description of the parent-child relationships reviewed in this paper it is clear that none of these patients received genuine love: a minority of them received virtually no love at all; the others received pseudo-love. In a few cases their needs were fairly well met by their mothers at the suckling stage, but the inflexibility of the love-attitudes of these mothers made them progressively less able to meet the needs of their growing children. In no case did we find a proper respect for the individual's needs to be himself, and an acceptance of him in his own right." (Reichard and Tillman 1950, p. 247).

---

[28]Hill supplies no statistics, selects cases to make a point, paints a composite portrait in ugly colors: a formidable person for the mother of a schizophrenic child to meet! These mothers, he notes (p. 123), are in need of treatment. Their children have as "one of their major preoccupations . . . the preservation of their ideal mother and her ideals. On the one hand, the patient sees her as domineering, all-powerful, immortal, not in any way to be resisted or opposed. On the other, and with equal intensity, the patients repeatedly . . . report that their mothers are weak, sick, poorly put together, and on the verge of impending mental or physical dissolution."

Three facts prevent us from agreeing with such a position. The first one, made abundantly clear in the painstaking research of Lidz and his associates, is that every type of abnormal mother-child relationship is found: there is no single form that appears consistently throughout the series. The second, underscored by Lidz again, is that the abnormal behavior of the parent may be an expression of genetic weaknesses that are passed on to the children via the DNA substance rather than by way of faulty conditioning of the children. The third has haunted all these discussions since Kanner first pointed out the statistics for the siblings of his autistic children: there are too many normal brothers and sisters in these same families for us to rest easily in the conviction that it is the personality and mothering pattern of the parent that is schizophrenogenic (see Fleck, Lidz, and Cornelison 1963, Lu 1962, Lidz and Fleck 1960).[29]

Theory and Therapy: Process and Nonprocess Schizophrenia

We have pursued a roundabout course only to validate little more than we knew at the outset: *of course* mothering (and fathering, too) are important! Parents transmit values and the basic beliefs of the culture; as agents of the culture they fit a young *socius* for life with others. They support, regulate, and direct the actions of their offspring until the latter become autonomous, once they have internalized these powers and are ready to assume responsibility for their own acts—more or less autonomous, that is, and with a new and more widely extended dependence and responsibility. Everyone knows this.

We went beyond this, however, to ask: "Can a pattern of mothering also lay the groundwork for mental illness? And can it be present in such limited amount, or in such distorted and traumatic forms as to *produce* the symptoms of a psychosis?" In the course of our excursion we have uncovered a wide consensus that would answer "Yes" to such questions, that would go further, to point to the early months (when imprinting is so potent) as the critical ones. But we have also discovered that this consensus tends to overlook many facts. Utilizing the schizophrenias both of childhood and adulthood as our measuring stick, we have identified some of these missing considerations; we have also discovered that schizophrenia (and early infantile autism) are categories that contain groups of disorders so varied in form and in causation that any simple generalization is impossible. We discover that the consensus can distort the facts that must be found by exploring or imputing events to an infancy that is no longer open to recall. Where a psychosis is in fact a disorder of unknown origin, we have been put on notice to be alert wherever a physician's convictions and prejudices run as far ahead of the facts as they do in these areas.

If the physician or counselor places mothering at the center of etiology,

---

[29]I should also note here that there is some evidence that hebephrenia might be caused by hypothalamic lesions, that is, might have a cause other than the psychogenic ones that have dominated the discussions of this chapter. Such a schizophrenia does not arise out of the transactions between a child and his mother. It must be based on a developmental arrest and involution, a disease process, some toxins with an affinity for a particular center in the diencephalon. Its causes are as impersonal as those of Huntington's chorea or phenylpyruvic oligophrenia.

he is likely to seek ways of making up for the mothering deficit, to undo maternally produced traumata, to provide permissive and security-bringing substitute mothers; he may, through psychoanalytic methods, try to explore the residues of distorted mothering in the unconscious of the patient, bringing to light what has too long inhibited his growth and providing an insightful basis for fresh progress. Using an institutional form of mothering, in his Orthogenic School, Bettelheim observes that it takes his children as long to get on their feet (whatever their age) as it takes the normal child, only, in addition to unlearning the old ways, these children have to accomplish this growth at a later period. Slowly his "truants from life" have to be wooed back to vital relationships from which they have been excluded or that they themselves have rejected.

Some of these clinical "substitute mothers" look on the schizophrenic child as an appendage of the mother; in treatment they sometimes concentrate on *her* problems, hoping to free her to do the job that has hitherto been left undone. Others, like Bettelheim (with children) or John Rosen (with adults), feel that they must operate much more directly on the patient. Some try to de-repress, to release unconscious forces by a prudent and planned regression that will enable the patient to work through and assimilate much of what he had laid away prematurely, but others (like Federn 1952) feel that the patients must be assisted to repress and organize what has obviously gotten out of hand. What we might call the "therapeutic posture" of the clinician seems to be based on hunches about early childhood experiences, few of which can be directly validated.

In addition to the difficulties inherent in validating any therapy's effectiveness by any controlled method of testing, there is the fact that schizophrenia is not a unitary process, is not the same on every occasion the diagnostic term is used, is not clearly either present or absent, is not a disease with a predictable course and outcome. From 10 to 30 per cent of the cases so diagnosed show spontaneous arrests, remissions, and complete recovery, *for no known reasons.* Another 25 per cent proceed to a deteriorated chronic dementia in spite of persistent and sometimes heroic efforts at therapy.

It is this latter form that so often breaks the hypothetical lance of the clinician who starts out with an easy confidence in a psychogenic etiology that can be corrected by a specific psychotherapy. It has led some clinicians (see Langfeldt 1959, Ey 1959, Redlich 1952a) to make a distinction between a nuclear form called "process schizophrenia" and a nonprocess or reactive type (sometimes referred to as "schizophreniform") that is more likely to respond to any therapy. In the former class they would put the schizophrenias that have a constitutional basis (including some with a disorder visible from the early months of childhood), in which there seems to be a large organic component (revealed in atypical maturation, abnormal biochemical exchanges), or that have a family background which would support the notion of a genetic basis for the illnesses. In the other class they would place those symptom clusters that, in spite of some resemblance to the nuclear type, arise out of

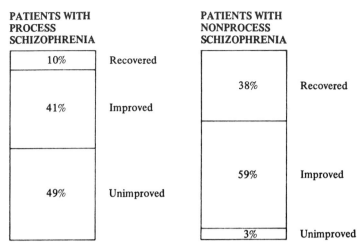

PATIENTS WITH
PROCESS
SCHIZOPHRENIA

10%	Recovered
41%	Improved
49%	Unimproved

PATIENTS WITH
NONPROCESS
SCHIZOPHRENIA

38%	Recovered
59%	Improved
3%	Unimproved

Recovered = employed or doing housework, and with no residual symptoms.

Improved = no longer overtly psychotic, employed or working at home, but with some residual signs of former illness.

Unimproved = in hospital or committable.

FIGURE 3. CONDITION OF 143 PATIENTS AFTER FROM FIVE TO THIRTEEN YEARS. (from Stephens and Astrup 1963.)

experiences, mother-child transactions, external stresses, intrapsychic conflicts.

Such considerations lead to a serious practical problem. If there are types of schizophrenia that respond to psychotherapy, and others that do not, can we identify the hopeful ones? Are the criteria for selecting them so certain that, in turning our attention away from the more resistant forms of "process schizophrenia," we do not validate our guesses about the latter form by our neglect? Can we evaluate any therapy until we have samples of cases that are matched for the presence of the "easy" and "resistant" forms?

A study by Stephens and Astrup (1963) approached this problem, utilizing the case records of 178 patients that had been treated in the Henry Phipps Psychiatric Clinic. Of these, 143 were followed for from five to thirteen years and their status reassessed (see Fig. 3). Their course in hospital had been followed closely, since they had been a part of a study evaluating various types of therapy, and the staff had carefully evaluated their status and progress at the time of their discharge from hospital.

From the rich mine of data in their records, Stephens and Astrup reclassified the patients into some 20 subgroups of schizophrenia, using a descriptive-classificatory system that had been published by Leonard (1957, 1961). Leonard's schema contained thirteen forms of process schizophrenia and nine nonprocess (or reactive) forms. The outcomes of these two groups are shown in Figure 3. These facts indicate that, whatever the nature of the unknown, endogenous, constitutional, or genetic factors may be, there are identifiable characteristics that enable clinicians to predict outcomes *for groups,* with better than chance accuracy. Unfortunately, within the process group the ones who went on to deterioration could not be discriminated from those who improved.

In an effort to identify the two groups more precisely, these authors note the following traits that appeared more frequently in the "process group": the onset of the illness was insidious (rather than florid, sudden); the pre-psychotic personality was introverted, schizoid; near relatives had been hos-pitalized for schizophrenia; poor social adjustment, work habits, and sexual adjustment were the rule; pressures from the environment, physical illnesses, and external precipitating factors were minimal or absent altogether; the symp-toms that were observed bore no clear and understandable relationship to past conflicts; emotional reactions were blanched or blunted, even beyond the gen-eral defect in interests and the lack of initiative; fantastic, bizarre, and cosmic delusions, with little rationale or interrelatedness, were observed; halluci-nations (auditory, tactile, visual) were frequently so bizarre that physicians had difficulty in understanding what the patients were experiencing; massive experiences of passivity and feelings of influence were clearly apprehended (but not discarded as unreasonable); silly and senseless behavior blocked com-munication; neologisms, perseveration, echolalia made their speech something quite different from communication; defects in perception, in reasoning, and in higher ethical and social feelings marked a real change from the prepsy-chotic personalities.

Such a checklist of "bad signs" has been suggested by others: Bellak, Sulli-van, Terry and Rennie. The lists do not coincide; there are contradictions from author to author; and, as we have noted, the list of Stephens and Astrup does not enable them to predict the course of the disorder with more than a very limited accuracy. What the study does show, however, is the fact that any unselected group of patients called schizophrenic according to current diag-nostic practices will contain such diverse specimens that, without some further effort to refine diagnosis and to classify the members of the group so that matched samples can be studied by other investigators of this disorder, any generalizations about etiology or the effectiveness of therapies are open to ques-tion. The relevance of the "mothering hypothesis" and any therapies based upon it can probably not be established until these refinements are made.

Because we are dealing with such an extensive territory, which has vague limits and unknown etiological factors at work, schizophrenia has taught us a lesson that might be valuable when we approach other categories of mental illness. There may very well be "process" forms of neurasthenia, psychopathic personality, compulsive neuroses, depressions, hysteria—forms that resist psy-chotherapy and have endogenous and constitutional causes. As we approach these illnesses, and again when we return to a more detailed study of schizo-phrenia itself, we shall be alerted to this possibility.

SEPARATION ANXIETY

Separation anxiety is an especially good example for those who push the "mothering hypothesis," for this group of symptoms frequently emerges as the child enters school and the mother makes an effort to launch him into the world outside the home. Among the group first entering school, an observer will note one child who clings to his mother sobbing and retching, another who will quietly and fearfully withdraw and become so inhibited that he can neither participate nor learn. A few will quickly transfer an anxious and clinging dependence to the teacher, seeking her attention, sitting beside her when the reading group is formed, laying a hand on the teacher's arm, waiting anxiously for her return to the classroom when she is called away for a few minutes. (One of these "clinging vines" who insistently appealed for his teacher's affection and interest was selected for special study. The home visit revealed that the mother, abandoned by the father and forced to work to support the child, was leaving the child with the grandmother, who was all too often at the corner tavern when the child came home from school. Small wonder, the teacher thought, that the little one reached out for some stable anchorage in a world that was so preoccupied elsewhere.)

If some of these children, so anxious on entry into the strange world of the school, come from unstable and indifferent homes, others enter from especially good homes, where relationships are close (too close, we might easily conclude) and where the child has been isolated not only from the germs other children carry but also from their bad language and improper behavior, and so from the types of learning that would long ago have extinguished the anxiety that arises in the presence of strange children. Consider the case of George:

> A four-year-old now, he still clings to his mother. An only child who has been the center of attention of his parents, he clings to her hand, follows her in the supermarket and on her visits in the neighborhood. He will not leave her to join the other children in the primary class in Sunday school; he protests so violently when a babysitter replaces the mother that she has restricted her social life. We feel that we can almost predict how he will react when he meets the little band of Indians that will form a circle around him in the play yard at school, particularly if, in the transition, he clings to the teacher, knows all the answers, and becomes her ally as she (for whatever personal reasons) responds with a reciprocal affection.[30]

Some of the "separation-anxiety children" will resemble the autistic ones that Kanner identified, who were disturbed by every change, even those within their own household. The schizoid child, whom teachers and nurses frequently

---

[30]Having watched a number of "Georges" make the transition from "hothouse" homes into the school and finally into the marketplace, I can only confess that their behavior is difficult to predict. One became a museum curator, a highly introverted specialist in the field of archaeology: his effeminate speech, his glasses, his obvious relief when visitors leave his cubicle, all suggest that he never made the normal transitions. Another George was soon resentful of his mother, and asked her (before the year was over, when she came to visit the first grade at the invitation of the teacher), "What are you doing here?" The gang became his new mother before he entered adolescence, and the political manipulation of the affairs of his ward from behind the bar of his own tavern was his "vocation" as an adult. On the other hand, one George who almost flunked out of college, because of his inability to function outside a very supportive family, later served in the Navy, completed medical school, and became a successful allergist.

find so appealing, and who so obviously needs human affection, commonly finds it difficult to accept and adjust to the affection that is offered, finding it too invasive, demanding, threatening.[31]

Separation anxiety, however, is not limited to the child entering school. It is found among the older boys who enter their first summer camp, in the teenagers who have been "sent away to prep school" (sometimes as a solution to the problems created when parents are about to be divorced). It is found in late life, in any group of depressed widows (or widowers), some of whom fall ill at the death of a spouse. In a quite different form it is found in the newly retired who, at age 65, are suddenly separated from the job that had long been too exclusive a reason for living.

In discussing the schizophrenias that emerge for the first time in old age, Kay and Roth (1961) point out that social isolation is prominent in the case histories. They found isolation due to deafness, isolation enforced through loss of relatives, social transplantation, or failure to marry. It is a nice question, in some of these cases, whether the isolation is a primary factor or is actually secondary to a self-isolating process that utilizes some of these "occasions" in the basic effort to repel "invaders."

To identify a case of pathological anxiety as "separation anxiety" is to classify it and prejudge its nature. The inner consistencies of a patient's life history, and the success of a rough-and-ready therapy, may provide a kind of validation for such prejudgment. But we have not learned the lessons implicit in our study of mothering if we begin to generalize, as though, having had one success, we are now ready to handle all forms of anxiety by similar procedures, and as though, having found one family structure at the root of a youth's difficulties, we expected to find duplicate patterns at the root of all adolescent anxieties.

An Anxiety of Cycloid Type

Consider the following account of one of Leonard's case studies (1961):

"Wolfgang Sch. was born in 1932. He was a baker and confectioner by trade. There was no family history of mental illness. According to his mother he was always very anxious as a child and was easily upset. When the other children hit him he did not hit back. On his first day of school he was extremely anxious, so much so that he threw himself on the floor and screamed. Only after some days did he go to school. He also suffered very much from anxiety in later life. However, he could be contented, happy and well balanced. On the whole he was very energetic in spite of his mood changes."

---

[31]The "computerized typewriter" and some adaptions of the Skinner-box (designed for the instrumental learning of rats) have been suggested as ways to capitalize on the autistic child's fascination with mechanical objects, and to avoid the more direct and "personalized" type of instruction (or play therapy). The hearty clinician who looks on any kind of "cubicle" treatment as a regressive movement away from the socialization that the child needs might tolerate such regression if he could also see it as a first step in establishing a useful mastery over the environment for a child who finds the human environment unpleasant and forbidding.

The mood changes ebbed and flowed in Wolfgang's life. He seemed capable of at least three levels of functioning: (1) a level of calm confidence and normal efficiency; (2) a level of acute anxiety which on one occasion was diagnosed schizophrenia; and (3) a level of excited euphoria in which he had grandiose plans for the salvation of man and looked on himself as greater than Marx, Stalin, or Lenin, and as a redeemer sent to save the world. Up and down he fluctuated, from one level to another, as though obscure, endogenous "tides of life" were regulating some psychobiological shifting of gear mechanisms. He was three different kinds of person as he moved from one level to the next. The shifts were not always independent of his life experiences: one of his anxious phases began at the death of his wife. He was first married on one of his upswings, when he was just completing his training and his future seemed bright. The anxious, screaming fit that occurred on his first day in public school was initiated by that separation experience, and was controlled, temporarily, by withdrawing him from school. At times no visible precipitating factor for the shifts could be seen; the hypothetical "endogenous process" quiets the concern the clinician feels when he has no ready reason to explain his client's actions. The gear shift might carry Wolfgang upward to a level where he was filled with an afflatus, a readiness for new projects and new learnings, or it might carry him downward into an entirely different kind of learning, where he seemed to generate poor integrations with his environment and to develop the kind of symptoms that carried him, eventually, into hospital. A cyclic illness produced three types of integrations with his environment, only a few of which seemed to be accounted for by the external challenges and stresses.[32]

Two characteristics of these "illnesses" are worth special emphasis. The first is created by our temptation to formulate a psychogenic interpretation and to relate a life style to the earliest shaping of a child's character by the mother. The stubborn clinician can find himself in an embarrassing theoretical trap when one of these cycloid psychoses "shifts gear," after he has explained the pattern by an infancy which, now over, has to remain ever the same. "One cannot explain how a personality development, which began many years before, can lead to the sudden appearance of a psychosis which then remits and recurs without obvious reasons" by reference to a specific set of psychogenic causes now long past. When the next clinician sees one of these Wolfgangs in a quite different phase, he will be tempted to imagine a quite different kind of mothering. Which one of Wolfgang's three characters should be traced to his infancy: the calm, efficient, and confident Wolfgang I? the anxious and disorganized Wolfgang II? the euphoric world reformer Wolfgang III?

The second emphasis that differentiates these cyclic psychoses from a "deteriorating process schizophrenia" is the completeness of the recovery once the period of extreme mood shift has passed. In the midst of his motility psychosis, the patient resembles the catatonic: he sits motionless, mute, unrespond-

---

[32]Leonard identified three types of cycloid changes: (1) a motility psychosis that swings from hyperkinetic extremes to an akinetic apathy with poverty of movement, emotional expressions, and reactions to challenges; (2) a confusion psychosis with excited phases of euphoria and grandeur and with an opposite swing into a perplexed and stuporous condition; and (3) anxiety-elation swings.

ing. Yet when such a patient recovers to dance with grace, to speak with lively expressiveness, or, as Wolfgang did on one of his upswings, to direct a hostel and found a new home with much courage and initiative, after having spent months in the depths of a kind of "pan-anxiety," our confidence in the "psychogenic theory" is shaken.

Leonard's study is a useful reminder that anxiety is not a unitary phenomenon, and that our diagnosis "separation anxiety" can so prejudge the phenomena that we are led to a fruitless collection of irrelevant data about mothers and fathers when we should be entertaining alternate hypotheses. We shall have occasion in discussing neuroses and depressions in later chapters to reexamine the concepts of both separation and anxiety.

EPILOG

Two major points are suggested by this review of the role of nurturant care: (1) we are trying to grapple with this relationship between mother and child at the very point in history when it is undergoing rapid changes; and (2) the evidence is not in. The attempt to grapple involves many of those who gather and interpret the data in a passionate defense or attack that sometimes seems to corrupt both evidence and theory at the source. A few clinicians seem so passionate in their defense of their patients that one is sometimes led to wonder whether these physicians have resolved their own mother-hating tendencies; they can be balanced by those who, in their defense of mothers, look on the constitutional and genetically caused incapacities of children as something no mother should be asked to compensate for.

The most serious charges that can be leveled at some of the clinicians who have studied mothering are that they have selected cases to prove their points, have never given a statistical account of the range and variety of the diagnosed disorders, and have never given comparable control data. The tendency to form stereotypes that correspond to the names of illnesses is understandable, but when the words "all," "invariably," and "commonly" are not backed up, and when other studies show a wide variety of types and numerous exceptions to their generalizations, we must learn to discount the prejudices of the stereotypers. In the study of anxiety, autism, and childhood schizophrenia, we seem to be ready to go beyond our present position, but still lack the definitive studies.

Where mothering is charged with being the cause of a particular deviation, detailed analyses of the data have tended to reduce the mother's role and to make the hasty conclusions of many clinicians appear to be passionate polemics rather than objective and impartial science. The limited success of therapy based on the "mothering hypothesis" (as in the case of autistic children) tends to reduce our certainty, as do studies of the patients' siblings who develop normally. The division of these illnesses into process and nonprocess forms that respond quite differently to therapy may produce higher validity in our formulations, but we still have a long distance to go.

Where the evidence points most clearly to faulty mothering, we discover that, for a particular disorder, every form of deviant mothering appears in the histories, and that, for a particular form of mothering, a wide variety of unfortunate effects are found. The relationship between mother and child is not such that specific patterns of mothering and specific patterns of response by the child can be identified. Findings such as those of Alanen (1958) and Brown (1961) clearly indicate that we should not rest content with single-factor explanations: there are normal mothers among the parents of the most severely disturbed patients.

Intensifying the study of facts about mothering, examining the mothers' relations with their own mothers, looking at every detail of the mother-child transactions—the efforts extend our understanding and complicate our analyses (quite properly), but also tend to create a somewhat neurotic climate of opinion, blowing up minor features of mothering until they are much too heavily laden with a threat of pathology. The "whole transaction" is not that difficult, and mothers should not become frightened by this enthusiasm of the research worker.

The passions which sometimes show through a scientific report sometimes emerge at scientific meetings, with such white heat that one fears for the whole process of data collecting and interpretation, which is never too objective at best. Where class attitudes corrupted the findings discussed in Chapter 3, feminism and its counterparts, mother-hating and mother-defending, have affected those discussed in this chapter, and not in overly subtle ways. Hatred of the schizophrenogenic mother (which may result from contacts with women who are themselves borderline psychotics) makes many case studies shed more heat than light. Both the organicists and the psychoanalysts who stress mothering think their viewpoints the only truly humane ones, but the facts seem to point to such a diversity of relationships and causes that both houses have to be put in order. Given our present state of knowledge, eclecticism not only best serves the needs of a developing science, but also preserves us from the worst therapeutic errors and is the best defense of mothers.

Chapter 5 • Neurasthenia: Exaggerated Fatigue and Hypochondria

Neurasthenia was an American discovery. Some of our contemporaries regard the term as an American "mistake," and would like to see it dropped from the literature altogether. For one thing, the name implies some underlying biochemical change in the nerve tissues, and patient search, from the time (1867) when this classification first came into use to the present, has failed to identify such change. "Nervous exhaustion," "brain fag," "a depletion of nervous energy," all point to some process in the central nervous system, and these implications were taken quite literally by earlier investigators. For example, one team, seeking an explanation for the "shell shock" seen among American soldiers in World War I, made a careful study of microscopic slides prepared from the brain tissues of experimental animals that had been kept awake for days and then subjected to high explosives. The "nerve weakness" implied in the name of the disorder was still under scrutiny in 1918. (See Beard 1869, 1880a, 1880b; Deschamps 1908, 1919.)

Those who were soon to develop "a more dynamic description of mental illness," which would stress the history of mental conflicts that sometimes originated in infantile traumata, in repression, or in the Oedipus conflict, thought this hypothesis of changes in cellular physiology too static, too simple, too far from the real causal factors. The hypothesis of some vague neural change did not help one understand how the bodily complaints of these patients were actually made to conceal problems that should have been faced, or how hostilities, family conflicts, and failures in adjustment could produce the bodily complaints or the exaggerated feelings of fatigue of which these patients complained. Many clinicians began to feel that their patients needed more a new design for living, a new way of coming to terms with life, than the rest and the escape from the demands of living that they seemed to claim. Freud himself was soon left behind by his pupils, for he also originally saw a simple material cause for the state. He had suggested that there could be a toxin in the blood stream caused by frustrated sexuality. Since a hypothetical toxin was the probable cause, not some mental conflict leading to repression,

158

he believed that these *actual neuroses* (in contradistinction to the *psychoneuroses* originating in mental conflict and repression) could be dealt with by common-sense procedures. He did not count them of any great psychiatric significance.[1]

While Europeans were calling neurasthenia "the American disease" (or Americanitis) and attributing it, as Beard had done, to the breathless pace of living in the new American cities and to the stresses of business competition, Pierre Janet was identifying what he believed to be a constitutional type. This type, so fatigable, emphasized for the clinician a set of exhausting actions, difficult for everyone but excessively so for these "sensitives." Their defect called Janet's attention to a force or power that, in the normal individual, carries him through these difficult tasks; Janet called it *psychological tension.* This tautness, or elasticity, is the very opposite of the *asthenia* that troubled these patients. Because it enables a person to live up to the role he has selected as his vocation, to meet the demands others make of him, it could almost be called a *moral force.* As difficult to define as "integrity," this power to integrate a good life (without symptoms) suffered attrition from many sources. As Janet reviewed the cases he had treated, he found such diverse causes as a brain injury, a loss of blood, a siege of typhoid fever, a failure in examinations, a loss of love, and mounting external pressures. Whatever lowers this psychological tension releases neurasthenic symptoms; less and less able to make a good life, the patients focused on such "issues" as eyestrain, headaches, paresthesias, and digestive disturbances, and especially on a tense fatigue. This fatigue seemed to be a fatigue of interests, or higher-level action systems rather than of organs, a faltering of the will of the man as a whole rather than some local change in nerve fibers; the global qualities of action showed the changes of fatigue before the separate muscle groups. Holistic in nature, Janet's theory attempted an objective description of changes in the behavior of the man, rather than in the tissues, although Janet was eclectic enough to include the toxins, the genetic weaknesses, the early training, and the local failures in living among his causes. Like some cost accountant called in as a consultant for a business threatened with bankruptcy, Janet attempted to put his patient's house in order, using therapies that ranged all the way from hypnosis and reeducation to moral suasion. (See Janet 1924.)

With interpretations changing, with therapies being redesigned to fit each new explanation of the symptoms, only the cluster of symptoms and complaints has remained constant. More recently, portions of this symptom cluster have been distributed among other disease categories. Some cases have been placed with a larger group of psychosomatic disorders, in which the bodily symptoms are more pronounced and more resistant to therapy (e.g., migraine,

---

[1]If the "gastric neurosis" that produces peptic ulcer turned out to be caused by an excess of fried food, and if the ulcer were to disappear with an appropriately bland diet, a physician would see no point in analyzing an "oral character" or in tracing eating difficulties back to a primal feeding frustration. Similarly, the lung cancer produced by excessive smoking of cigarettes would not require, for its explanation, treatment, or prevention, an analysis of the oral craving that is gratified by smoking (unless the habit proved to be impossible to break, of inexplicable force).

gastric ulcers, neurocirculatory asthenia). Other symptoms have been grouped with anxiety attacks, neurotic depressions, or schizophrenic delusions. Indeed, in their milder manifestations and in the early phases of most mental illnesses, many patients do show symptoms that resemble those of the neurasthenic. A patient may suffer a single brief episode of short duration, or the pattern may recur throughout his life, responding each time to one of the variants of therapy, only to recur after symptom-free intervals. It may run its own brief course to arrive at its own self-limited terminus with no therapy whatsoever. Four out of five who consult their counselors for this cluster of symptoms are reported as cured *for the episode.*

SOME ILLUSTRATIVE CASE HISTORIES

It is often hard for a clinician or physician to grasp the concept of neurasthenia as a specific form of illness. It is even harder for anyone else, especially for the well-integrated person who is making a success of his life. It would therefore be useful here, before we get into theories of causation and therapy for neurasthenia, to present some cases that will help establish the contour of this disorder.

MAINE DE BIRAN

Just to indicate how very out of date the writings of Maine de Biran are, we might describe this philosopher-statesman as "the man who restored the will to a central position in French philosophy." But Maine de Biran, the mentor whom Janet was still quoting in the late 1920's, was also a "sensitive," a man who sought an anchorage in that *Au Delà* which lies out there, beyond the horizon of our thought. He was not at home in Paris, in the Chamber of Deputies, nor at his country home, Perigord, nor even in his study, where, wrapped in his thoughts, he penned out the pages of his journal. He was a restless spirit, rarely at one with himself, and upset by the weather, diplomatic tasks, metaphysical questions.

The perfect anchorage beyond the sky, the perfect relationship with his God, seems to be almost as unattainable for such a sensitive person as is a robust and happy relationship with this world. If he is full of plaints about the weather or about his own too-sensitive carcass, this is merely a somatic phase of a global process that seeks restlessly to find the perfect expression for his discontent with social life and with his own imperfections. He is full of yearning for inner peace and wholeness, a harmony within and without; the other side of this yearning is a constant sense of his own imperfection or incompleteness, a trait Janet was to emphasize when he described the psychasthenic.

The troubles that continually agitate society, Naville (1857) comments, have a way of converting public affairs, the tasks of government, the struggle for power into ultimate concerns, whereas they should normally be treated lightly, as means only. Whereas some men grow ever more deeply attached to the means, and more and more confident in their employment, the Maine de Birans of this world tend to remain detached. A few become more and more repelled by the very thought of serious involvement. Out of their feelings they produce statements in that mood of Ecclesiastes, or in the manner of Thomas à Kempis. The interactions between such a self and his environment arrive at quite different degrees of involvement and detachment. A true "sensitive" tends to withdraw from life in bad times, and then to return to integrate with men and affairs when things clear up. A tougher realist is able to remain involved to the hilt, even in bad times, struggling uphill while keeping his eyes steadily on the whole scene, while the psychasthenic, tiring more easily, begins to sigh, "Vanity of vanities, all is vanity." The man and his times, always interacting, take a course that depends, at each stage, on how the dialogue is developed. If Maine de Biran had been more successful, in repose at Perigord, in making his peace with himself, his work, and his Deity, and if he had consistently sought this peace of his countryside or his study, instead of promptly turning his thoughts back to Paris as soon as he had established himself there, we might be more certain as to where to place the emphasis. As it was, once in Paris, he yearned for Perigord, and, back in Perigord, for Paris.

The stable anchorage that this philosopher-statesman sought in the *Au Delà*, one might have hoped, would have finally given him the inner peace he sought, but the God that he wanted, far above all temporal turmoil, was equally elusive. He had an idea he was never able to actualize, and it kept churning within him. Though he lived reasonably well, outwardly—and his contemporaries who heaped honors on him seemed to feel that he functioned very well indeed—he did not feel at home in his world. In the midst of diplomatic successes he felt detached, unsatisfied—at least, so he confided to his journal.

By all of the principles of a "gratification psychology," where simple pleasures and palatabilities are supposed to organize behavior into harmonious sequences, Maine de Biran's "successes" should have been "reinforcing," and he should have grown content. He was the successful man, by all external standards: he lived at the center of things, moved among those at the seat of power, and was praised and honored. But he remained unhappy, detached, aloof, always searching for some attachment somewhere beyond the world of common actions and those simple, sensory delights, beyond the approval of his fellow men. While he was living in the midst of Parisian social, intellectual, and political life, he turned in that inner self to that Beyond. Like a disappointed bride, he seemed to ask himself, "Is this all?"

All this man had to do was to drop the word to the electors of Perigord, and his bondage to the Parisian life he complained about so often to his journal would have ceased. But, as Naville notes, "This word...was never given." Is all his breast-beating about the pressures of Parisian life then a sham, the listing of symptoms a form of malingering before his conscience? Would he have been better off if, like Spinoza, he had chosen some humble work like lens-grinding, freed from every excessive claim upon his time, able to devote himself wholly to philosophy? What produced this strange incongruence in the parts of this man, one half of whom yearned for the repose of the rural philosopher, while the other half turned back to the world of affairs, dutifully, even eagerly, and who suffered from neurasthenic symptoms all the while, both in Perigord and in Paris?

ALICE JAMES

Alice James, the sister of the famous Harvard psychologist, William James, suffered her first nervous breakdown at age 19, just when the ideas of Beard were becoming popular on both sides of the Atlantic, and was from then until her death at age 42 (from cancer of the breast) virtually a prisoner in her sickroom, from which she ruled her tiny kingdom imperiously, at the price of a resistance to, and withdrawal from, life. (See Matthiessen 1947, pp. 276-84.) Diagnosed variously as suffering from neurasthenia, hysteria, rheumatic gout, spinal neurosis, and nervous hyperesthesia, she enjoyed the attention of the best experts money could buy. The attempted cures included rest cures, hypnosis, morphia, and bromides, but none produced any relief from her symptoms. Her "nervous prostration" was as complete a state of nonfeasance as if she had spent ninety days in the trenches. A visitor would "prostrate" her, and she would faint. Like a frightened bird whose protective "death feint" puts it *hors de combat,* she had to live outside any field where a drastic call for energies would produce this radical form of inhibition. Even a visit from her brother, unannounced, would be too much; the way had to be paved. She had to adjust in advance, with ample quiet time to face up to even this small emergency. Such collapses, after a severe bout of pneumonia or typhoid fever, when the person is extremely weak, we can understand. When there has been no overwork, no fever, no prolonged emotional strain that we know of, the disorder takes on a mysterious quality. It becomes a "purely mental" fatigue, that is, a fatigue of unknown origin.

Alice wrote of her condition:

"Owing to some physical weakness, excess of nervous susceptibility, the moral power *pauses,* as it were, for a moment, and refuses to maintain muscular sanity, worn out with the strain of constabulary functions. As I used to sit, immovable, reading in the library, with waves of violent inclination suddenly invading my muscles, taking some one of their varied forms, such as throwing myself out of the window or knocking off the head of the benignant Pater, as he sat, with his silver locks, writing at his table, it used to seem to me that the only difference between me and the insane was that I had not only all the horrors and suffering of insanity, but the duties of doctor, nurse, and strait-jacket imposed upon me.... Conceive of never being without the sense that if you let yourself go for a moment, your mechanism will fall into pie, and that at some given moment you must abandon it all, let the dikes break and the flood sweep in, acknowledging yourself abjectly impotent before the immutable laws."

CHARLES DARWIN

Consider the situation of the student whose family has designed a career for him, encouraged him, provided the funds for his education, selected his college. It was such a set of enveloping concerns that made Charles Darwin feel so guilty about his nonfeasance as a college student. Everyone who looked at his father, or at that famous grandfather who had written *Zoonomia,* expected that Charles would turn to medicine as a profession or to one of the other "respectable" roles. Yet there he was, spending his nights out with his cronies, his days in sleeping off the nights before, and his schooldays were slipping by. He wrote of himself, "I was a sport, a rat-catcher, a card-player, fit for the life of a gentleman tramp." The family was concerned, wondering what he could possibly do that would not be disgraceful. Would he have to turn to the ministry, as a last resort, and take some easy appointment to some distant parish? Charles himself was bored. He suffered from a variety of bodily complaints. Kempf (1921a, p. 251), studying the biographic data, suggested as a diagnostic classification "anxiety neurosis." Whatever name is applied, it lasted over forty years, and involved an "inability to adjust to excitement, anticipations, changes of heat or cold, cardiac palpitation and vasomotor flushing, indigestion, nausea, vomiting, violent tremors, insomnia, persistent thoughts, inability to criticise, or to endure social contact or worry."[2] Yet when he became excited about his evolutionary hypothesis, he worked day in and day out for over twenty years before he published his findings and gained recognition.

THE BEARD-MITCHELL CONCEPT

In the early days after Beard's identification and description of this form of "irritable weakness with tension and fatigue," neurasthenia became one of the most popular clinical diagnoses. The symptoms reported were varied, and the notion grew that each organ had its peculiar kind of weakness. Along with the tension and fatigue which have remained at the center of the symptom cluster, patients reported insomnia, photophobia, exaggerated sensitivity to noises, headaches, pains in the joints, paresthesias (tingling, burning, feeling of something crawling), palpitation, ringing in the ears. The major systems of digestion, respiration, and circulation are affected; there are fluctuations in appetite, difficulties in digestion and elimination, cold extremities, thread-like pulse, flushing of skin surfaces, difficulties in breathing. Some patients complained of a loss of sexual potency; others spoke of an inability to feel anything or to maintain an interest in living. The "emptiness" from which

---

[2]Kempf's analysis might be called "psychoanalysis at a distance," a speculative interpretation of causes that rivals Freud's analysis of Woodrow Wilson in its readiness to inject interpretation without the validating presence of the patient. If, as Kempf believed, Darwin's great scientific achievements were related to his neurosis, we may have to accept some of these neurotic sufferers with a kind of gratitude (and natural piety) as we note how much good can come out of so much misery. A man, we would be forced to conclude, can be very sick and at the same time one of the greatest contributors to our human tradition. There will be some, like Edmund Bergler (1946), who believe that it is the sickness that is, in fact, responsible for their becoming painters, writers, scientists. How fateful for the rest of us if some traveling analyst were to suddenly remove—with one insight-giving word—the core of a complex that would have otherwise driven the individual to paint the *Mona Lisa,* to write the *Origin of Species,* or to write a novel such as Gide's *The Counterfeiters.*

some patients suffered made them feel like automata: they could act if forced to, but lacked both purpose and the feeling of ownership of the actions they performed. In the place of a wholesome and vital interest in life, these neurasthenics were peevish and hypochondriacal. They suffered from a strange kind of "psychological poverty," lacking the force to initiate and liquidate actions. They seemed equally unable to rest. The insomnia which frequently accompanied this pattern helped to complete a vicious cycle: too exhausted to sleep, and unable to rest, they became chronically exhausted.

Beard's theory of the disorder was that impulses were radiating from an exhausted reflex center of the brain to all parts of the body. This hypothesis, invented to account for the many symptoms the patients presented, did not suggest any very clear-cut therapy. He tried sedatives, tonics, rest, isolation, in those cases where he judged that his tense patients were overdriven; in others he encouraged work, activity, new interests. On a few he used poultices that produced blisters. Whatever he tried seemed to be of help. Strong in his convictions, he gave his patients a rationale for living, an explanation of their symptoms; this "understanding," together with his own capacity to support, reassure, and stimulate them, seemed to produce excellent results.[3]

Silas Weir Mitchell (1829-1914) carried Beard's notion a stage farther. In 1877 he was writing *Fat and Blood,* developing a theory that the exhaustion of the nervous system was based on deficient lipoids, and designing a treatment that combined absolute rest with a high-calorie diet. The patients were isolated from all visitors, the shades drawn. They were not even allowed to rise to care for bladder and bowel needs, as though the least ounce of effort would be too costly for their already exhausted nerve centers. Moving little, conversing only when absolutely necessary (and then with physician and nurse), these patients were subjected to conditions approaching the type of "sensory deprivation" that has been so closely observed in recent years. Following similar routines with a hundred consecutive cases, one of Mitchell's followers (Ross 1938, p. 7) reported that his patients showed an average weight gain of 22 pounds in six weeks.[4]

---

[3]Then, as now, many clinicians were ready to describe these neurasthenics as "bad patients." Frequently their physicians could find nothing organically wrong, and, even when there was some basis for a complaint, the patient seemed to them to exaggerate. The patient in the bed next to the neurasthenic, down with a serious illness for which the physician had a ready treatment, seemed to him to complain less. One clinician described a neurasthenic patient as "contented never to know a well day in his life" (Richards 1919). Noyes and Kolb (1963, p. 412) note: "Asthenic patients are often critical, whining, dissatisfied, envious, resentful. A tendency to projection is not uncommon. Some patients develop a complaining attitude and may appear to take pleasure in finding fault with and annoying others." When observations of this type are multiplied, one gains the impression that the very diagnosis carries with it a note of reproach.

[4]It is interesting to think what this theory must have meant to the patient. The elaborate rituals of rest must have made the latter regard every occasion that called for decisive action with dread. Balzac once portrayed this dread of decision in *Peau de Chagrin,* whose protagonist thought that every thrust of his will depleted an already exhausted reservoir of force; as Mitchell's patients must have done, he tried to cultivate an "educated passivity." It was almost as though the doctor expected his human Leyden jars to remain wholly inactive in order to accumulate a fresh charge.

As Beard had done, Mitchell reported great success in curing neurasthenia. This form of cure became as fashionable as psychoanalysis did in the more recent past. As time elapsed, and records accumulated, clinicians found many patients who did not improve under the regimen, or who, having just recently been cured, had to return for another round of "rest." After half a dozen rounds, both patient and physician began to enter such therapy with less enthusiasm and certainty. Mitchell finally abandoned it, and his contemporaries, each for himself, chose new explanations and designed new therapies. The historian of this period is apt to attribute the successes of Beard and Mitchell to their personal gifts. Their enthusiasm was infectious, and it may have been the valuable thing for patients who were in need of assurance, excitation, strong suggestions, active interest and support. Reviewing Mitchell's work, Adolf Meyer (Winters 1951, II, 6) observes tersely: "He possessed a wealth of common sense not absorbed in his science and in anything that could be called communicable psychiatry."[5]

A Case from the Mitchell Period

Ross (1938, pp. 42-45) describes a woman of 45 who complained of extreme fatigue: she could scarcely walk across the bedroom. She felt empty-headed and worthless, was unable to concentrate, and had bilious attacks with difficulties in digestion and elimination. This cluster of complaints had recurred periodically over 22 years. Six formal rest cures had restored her to near-normal living, although the last two had been less successful.

An illness, diagnosed as influenza, had left this woman exhausted, nervous. She did not recuperate normally. When she was accepted as a neurasthenic and put through the rest cure, she recovered. Reviewing her history later, Ross doubted that this had been a genuine influenza, for there had been no elevation of temper-

---

[5]Such "powers" are not wholly unlike those possessed by our contemporaries in Ghana, the medicine men who also produce cures. Some suggest that it is the power of suggestion which goes with any lively, commanding figure who is enthusiastic about his therapeutic rituals. A few have suggested that the rest cure succeeded because, in the end, its extreme form of solitary confinement grew more and more irksome with each day of treatment, until the patient began to wish to get well as the only means of escape. Others have seen a clue in the common sense of the physician, in his ability to give simple and direct advice in the business of living.

A recent example of theory and therapy for these symptoms has been reported from Nigeria. A syndrome, there diagnosed as "brain fag," has appeared among students who are being rapidly inducted into Western ways of living and study. The patients complain of mental fatigue, of inability to concentrate, of headache and of pains in the neck region, and of a "sensory impairment" that is not so much sensory as perceptual. They can see, but they cannot see to read or study. They can hear, but they cannot listen attentively to a lecture. In short, it is a type of "I-can't-study-any-more" syndrome.

Brought into a European type of school, called upon to achieve *as individuals,* and intensely desiring the status of an educated person, these students find they cannot "make the grade." Raymond Prince (1960) believes that the family and tribal background, where everything is done together and where the responsibilities are carried by the collective strength of the group, have not prepared these young people for the degree of autonomy that is suddenly thrust upon them. He proposes a type of group learning as a kind of prophylaxis until the new ways of socializing a child can lay the proper groundwork for competitive individuation. In the meantime, these patients were treated with chlorpromazine hydrochloride and reassurance (easy substitutes for individual psychotherapy), with considerable success.

ature, and there were other circumstances surrounding her first illness that may have contributed to her feeling of exhaustion. She had been worrying over a projected engagement. Her own father had previously committed suicide. "Did this mean," she asked herself, "that with such a 'taint' I should not marry or have children?" As she entered the cure she seemed to lay the burden of all decisions on her physician and on the outcome of the treatment. Like other psychasthenics who are always making "pacts," she told herself, "If I recover it will mean that I can marry." She did recover, the doctor supported her decision, and she married.

Another epidemic of influenza was the occasion for her second attack. Another "chute" followed the suicide of her brother. In her last reported illness, Ross drew out some of her secret worries, including scruples about having children, and he undertook to give her some very direct guidance in a few brief interviews, without the elaborate ritual of the rest cure. Once more she rapidly lost her fatigue, and, although she could not navigate the length of her bedroom during her attack of "pernicious fatigue," was soon walking the fifteen or twenty miles that, as a seasoned hiker, she was accustomed to do in a day.

Although, from Ross's account, we can see that the elaborate ritual of the rest cure was not an essential element in this neurasthenic's recovery, we need not conclude that neurasthenia is a kind of paper tiger that can be brushed away by a few words of advice or a strong dosage of common sense. The "neurasthenia" that afflicted Alice James endured from age 19 to her death at 42, and it had received the attention of the most skilled therapists of the time. Yet Ross's case responded, without the use of drugs, without the high-calorie diet and the ritual of rest, without any deep probing into hidden or unconscious causes or any review of possible early infantile experiences; a fatherly kind of direction enabled her to resume her normal life. One never knows, of course, just how long such a case will continue to function well. Perhaps a seventh round of psychophysiological complaints will later appear on the record of some subsequent clinical visit, and a fresh diagnosis, a "better understanding," and an "improved dynamic therapy" will once more restore her to "enthusiastic living."

LESSONS LEARNED FROM THE BEARD-MITCHELL CONCEPT

From the findings of Beard, Mitchell, Ross and others, certain emphases seem clear:

1. The symptoms that constitute a disorder of this type challenge the clinician to develop a theory and a therapy. The symptom cluster has seemed to persist, while both the theory and the therapies have undergone changes.

2. A wide variety of therapies produce favorable outcomes. These have included suggestion and reassurance, chlorpromazine hydrochloride, high-calorie diets, work, rest, blisters, supportive care, and brief hospitalization.

3. The novelty of a therapy and the enthusiasm of both client and clinician seem to be factors in the success of the therapies.

4. It is much easier to remove a cluster of symptoms than it is to alter that basic susceptibility to neurasthenic attacks, whatever the nature of this latter state (or capacity) may be.

Writing about what he called *la misère psychologique* (as he called this poverty of moral force, this lack of the power to synthesize), Janet (1889, p. 156) observed, "As soon as you discover that you can cure a person by suggestion, you may rest assured that you are dealing with a person who is ill."[6] This illness, in Ross's case, would consist in the persisting condition that makes a person susceptible to recurrent bouts of neurasthenic symptoms whenever difficulties in living mount beyond a certain level.

JANET'S APPROACH

It is difficult to present Janet's view of any mental illness without pausing to develop his central concept of *psychological tension*. The concept is, in essence, very simple: some persons have the strength to integrate their lives in a purposive and realistic fashion, and some do not.[7] Most of us have more of this strength at some times than at others. Although rather wide fluctuations in this "power to integrate," to deal effectively with novelties and frustrations, may still leave the individual within that range of performance we count normal, the moment it falls below a certain level the typical symptoms of neurasthenia emerge. His behavior takes on a certain automatic "feel"; the "vital quality" in his relations with the real and with those who surround him fades; and a taut and reflective kind of thinking is replaced by a slightly delusional form. In the neurasthenic a tense fatigue (Janet called it a "morose inaction") replaces normal volition. Attention, instead of being focused on an interesting future, is absorbed in bodily complaints. (Or should we say that his consciousness is invaded by symptoms that force themselves on his attention?) And whereas some of us seem to have inherited this kind of "psychological poverty," others have it thrust upon them.

Usually our morale rises with successes and triumphs. Failures and frustrations weaken this power. In some the decline seems caused by an unrealistic form of striving, by vague and inappropriate aims. Can a marksman learn from shooting at a target so dimly seen that he can neither correct his aim nor estimate his failures? Our integrative power can be weakened by accidents,

---

[6]Janet's *L'Automatisme Psychologique*, first published in 1889, when Bernheim's therapy through suggestion was beginning to catch on and when the popularity of Mitchell's rest cure was at its height, called attention to the "weakness" that made the individual dependent on external sources, susceptible to "talking cures" and to the pressures of living that others bore without symptoms. For his own discussion of the rest-and-isolation therapy, one of the best summaries of the method found in English, see Janet 1919, I, 372-588.

[7]One is tempted to add, "without external supports," although the moment one thinks of drawing the line the problem becomes difficult. In our *addicted society* we need the supports of central heating, prepared foods, comfortable clothing, alcoholic beverages, soporifics, tranquilizers, mind-expanding drugs. From hearing aids to aids to elimination, we seem to require a corps of assistants, along with those who entertain us via the "idiot box" or night clubs. I believe that Janet was speaking as a clinician, about those who can manage without the support of the "specialist in integration." It was Epictetus who counseled his young followers against becoming bound fast to so many things that they would become burdened by them and dragged down. "Ask yourself, 'What is mine, and what is not mine?'" Janet, whether from reading or temperament, was one of the Stoics; he had a strong appetite for autonomy, which made him speak at times like one of our "rugged individualists."

diseases, by the loss of loved ones, and by the sheer weight of circumstances too crushing to bear. If it is the affection and support of those close to us that normally buoy us up, their rejection or indifference will leave us lonely, poorer in spirit, and more vulnerable to every pressure. Now and then some vital threat will set us to vibrating emotionally, and in the process release energies for major effort. There are other occasions when emotions disorganize us and exhaust our forces, when our skills, the very means for coping with life, are disrupted and our psychological tension is lowered. There is such a thing as "fatigue of the spirit," and it can progress to the very edge of collapse. Thus, rising and falling, this integrative strength spells the difference between sickness and mental health.[8]

In neurasthenia, where a "tense fatigue" is at the center of the symptom cluster, we are tempted to search for the *work* that has tired these patients, and to construct our account of the disorder on the analogy with physical fatigue, in which carbon dioxide, lactic acid, and other fatigue products reduce the contractile power of any group of muscles; this fatigue is a local, peripheral process, within the muscle itself (although it can be transported to adjacent tissues, or into another body, by transfusion). Anyone who has ever trimmed the edge of his lawn with a grass clipper knows that the fatigue is there, in his right forearm; for he can avoid it by shifting the clipper to the other hand, and go on working.[9] In the "mental" fatigue of the neurasthenic, it is the man who is bored and exhausted, and not some peripheral group of muscles. Although, in general, Janet decried the habit of inventing a pseudoneurology to explain this type of holistic fatigue, he, like Beard and Mitchell before him, was not above referring to excessive "brain work" as a cause of the symptoms; yet there were times when he planned tasks for his patients that would "make them work with their brains" *(travailler cérébralement)*, as though he hoped to rouse some of these cells from their numbness. These were patients who were *afraid to work* lest numbness descend. His measures proved exciting to

---

[8]The materially minded will be quick to point out that the "weight of circumstances" that bear down on the poor should keep this level of psychological tension chronically low. As Srole *et al.* (1962) point out, among the poor the "stress factors" are most numerous: broken homes; unemployment; poor living conditions; depressing neighborhoods full of "poor copy" provided by vice, crime, quarrels, shouting, crowding; all the supporting factors of good medical care, adequate food, shelter, clothing, and so on, in short supply. Maine de Biran, Alice James, all the "upper-upper" neurasthenics, do not suffer from these sources. The material processess which they cannot integrate are of another sort. To speak of a "fatigue of the *spirit*" in these cases does not imply that their conflicts are any less material, or that "good spirits" are something more and other than an integration of the common, everyday, garden variety of impulses. A spirited person, in contrast to the neurasthenic, is imaginative. He does not give up easily. His tolerance for stress includes an elasticity and flexibility that, compromising here, giving way there, can still press toward goals that he constructs and chooses. Resilient, creative, with the toughness of a Damascus blade, the spirited one cuts through difficulties without serious loss of integrative forces. A "fatigue of the spirit" means, therefore, a loss of precise qualities like these.

[9]The statistician can shift his work to the larger muscles; the novelist who has spent the morning writing may be ready to attack his woodpile or walk five miles into the country, with enjoyment and vigor. In general, shifting from difficult and confining work, from painful discriminations, to easy and automatic movements, reveals a lower level of action-potential that is yet untapped.

them as they discovered that they still possessed their powers. Here, the "fatigue" was anticipatory, and exaggerated (a fear of *becoming* fatigued). By and large, however, Janet's theories were theories of behavior, of action, and they were not formulated in physiological terms. Typically he spoke of the fatigue of *tendencies*, and his treatment was planned to arouse the person rather than some muscle group or some cerebral center.

FATIGUE BEHAVIOR

To identify fatigue as the essential core of the neurasthenic's complaints can divert our attention from some of the root causes of the illness, for fatigue is so common an experience that each of us has his own simple recipes for dealing with it. Overwork, exhaustion, poor spacing of work and leisure call for simple and direct measures. But the problem for the neurasthenic is not always as simple as common sense would have it. He seems to get tired *before* he works, to initiate rest behavior when the spurt of work is called for. Yet he learned his rest behavior in the same school as the rest of us, and so it may be instructive to look more closely at the simpler forms of fatigue that we do know how to handle.

Let us begin by distinguishing two levels of description: (1) a chemical and physiological level, with interest centering on the contraction of muscle fibers, and (2) a behavioral or psychological level, with interest centering on the action of a person. The first level would involve us in a study of energy exchanges, of the production, transportation, and reabsorption of fatigue products, and of the minute changes in muscle-fibril responses that occur as these inhibitory substances are produced. The second level of description would force us to keep our eyes on the performer as a whole: we note changes in his powers of attending, in his sensory thresholds and his reaction times, in his powers of discrimination, and in the organization of his action. Learned responses of avoidance-in-advance appear, as do skillful ways of preventing the onset of fatigue (rest behavior); rarely, we may note that fatigue has gone so far that the person cannot initiate action.

At the first level of description, the muscle can be viewed as an engine for converting the chemical energies stored within it (and brought by the blood) into a shortening of the fibers that move the body's levers. Extracted from the food we eat and the air we breathe, these chemicals are stored in our tissues and circulate freely in the blood stream. Every shortening of a muscle fiber uses some of these energies. Like the spark that fires the gas in the cylinder of our auto engine, the motor nerve's impulse explodes them. Each contraction creates breakdown products, some of which are carried away from the muscle by the circulating blood, ultimately to be excreted (via lungs, kidneys, intestines) or to be resynthesized into compounds which can be used over again.

If one contraction is crowded on the heels of a preceding one, with insufficient time for recovery of the original excitable state, the muscle's stores may be depleted, the breakdown products will accumulate, and the muscle will grow sluggish, unresponsive. This choking down of contractions is accelerated if a tourniquet cuts off the muscle's supply of fresh blood. If, for example, an experimenter records a series of contractions made by a subject who is lifting a weight, or squeezing a dynamometer, and if the subject is required to keep pace with a metronome which beats 100 times per minute, he will note that the contractions at first improve in vigor for a brief warming-up period. Soon, however, the contractions will grow weaker, and a point will be reached where their appearance is irregular, faltering; finally, the subject will report that he cannot move the member. We can see him moving the muscles of his neck and shoulder girdle, in time with the metronome, like the pianist who nods "commands" to his forearm muscles. And no movements come forth. On the other hand, if the contractions are spaced, to allow recovery between strokes, the decline in their force will occur more slowly. Exhaustion can be postponed beyond the limits of any ordinary experimental period.

If one is interested in maintaining the efficiency of both work and recovery processes, these rest pauses must be introduced before severe depletion has developed; for once exhaustion occurs, recovery is slower and, within moderate recovery times, less complete. In terms of bookkeeping analogy, persistent and unspaced energy expenditures can create debts; when these are large enough, their "carrying charges" impair the recovery process itself. The actor behaves as though some slow leak, comparable to the interest on a debt, were continuing the expenditures in the rest pause. At another level of description, we might speak of an individual who is so tired that he cannot rest properly, remembering that one of the symptoms of the tense fatigue of neurasthenia is insomnia.

If one were an efficiency expert, interested in pacing the work of some employee on a production line in such fashion that a maximum output could be maintained, it would be necessary to find the precise placement and duration of rest pauses that would allow muscle contractions to be made at an optimal level. The pauses would have to be introduced early enough, at such points, and in such amounts that recoveries could occur rapidly and completely; their pacing would undoubtedly have to vary with the advance of the work day, and be "computer-adjusted" to some average constants that represent the central tendency of the production line. For the employer who is buying a workman's time, and who must pay for the rest pauses as well as the working periods, there is a neat problem of calculation involved; since each type of task and each individual will produce unique work curves, any type of skilled teamwork will call for an elaborate program of testing and computation with such compromises as are necessary to fit the schedule to the central tendencies of outputs.[10]

---

[10]In our imagined 1984 for workers on the production line, we have been considering limited muscle groups, and have given no thought to the man as a whole, but it is he who first shows the signs of neurasthenia proper: boredom, restlessness, lack of interest, inability to force attention on a task that has become utterly mechanical. Good for machines, the perfect timing of automation can be deadly for the men. As we eliminate the "challenges," the "novelties," and all of the "inefficiencies" of the older, independent artisan workshop, we create a new environment ill-suited for men, whose perplexity was comically portrayed by Chaplin in his *Modern Times*.

As for the debts which are created when work is pushed beyond the point where the recovery process can balance the expenditures (and in all bursts of strenuous effort such debts pile up), repayment has to be promptly made if efficiency is to be restored. We can witness such a repayment process at work as we watch the labored breathing of the quarter-miler at the end of his race. His heart and lungs continue to work to pay off the oxygen debt that his muscles have created, for he not only used up the supplies readily available, but also borrowed from tissue reserves, and now these other tissues are putting in a claim which has to be met by the laboring chest muscles and heart. He will be paying off the full debt for several hours, and if his coach permits him to run again before the debt is fully liquidated, his performance will show this effect of impaired reserves. He will fatigue more rapidly, run a slower race, and his style of delivery will deteriorate. He is somewhat like the neurasthenic in this respect, for the latter is also a fatigable who acts as though he had lived too long in a monotonous sort of unpunctuated living, never fully recuperated, never able to summon his resources for the race.[11]

Anything which interferes with a muscle's recovery process will cause a more rapid decline in the work curve. Thus, the tourniquet placed around the working arm, cutting off the flow of blood to and from the contracting fibrils, will deprive them of the needed energies and at the same time prevent the removal of the breakdown products which must be excreted or reconverted to usable energies elsewhere. Anything which interferes with breathing, heart action, or proper relaxation during the rest pauses will likewise hamper this recovery process. Any disease process or toxic condition which attacks the basic energy-maintaining mechanisms may create or facilitate the development of a state of chronic fatigue, in which the person is incapable of sustained effort. In these cases, even minor tasks may induce a rapid and complete exhaustion from which there is a slow and incomplete recovery. The person not only feels tired most of the time, but reacts to minor calls for effort with breathlessness, palpitation, excessive perspiration, that is, with reactions more appropriate to an enormous outlay of effort. Although he has spent little energy, he complains of great fatigue. If the condition becomes chronic, he spends time resting in preparing for action that he never gets around to.

This "psychological fatigue" impresses the observer as exaggerated, as he thinks of what any standard man should be able to do. One is even tempted to speak, as Janet did, of a delirium of fatigue, or of an "objectless fatigue." For

---

[11]There is another source of "brain drain" on the poorly scheduled life. Too many distracting stimuli, too many projects started and left incomplete, more things than we can properly use, more appeals from advertisers than our budget could ever permit us to respond to, more toys than our children can enjoy, more gadgets in our homes than we know how to repair, so many energy savers that our energies are consumed in caring for them: all of this cries out for some simplification in life. In the midst of life, choked, with affluence, a Buddha-like person can suddenly feel, "These are not of me," and literally walk out on these demands. The neurasthenic is far less drastic: he merely withdraws his investment of interest, claims to be bored, replaces effort by rest behavior. We have a central and finite store of integrative force; it can be used up, dispersed, depleted until what we call "creativity" is at a low ebb. Too many and too inferior investments have drained our sources of integrative energy.

how can the fatigue products, the real causes of the rest behavior, be there
when the effort has never been made, the contractions never commanded? Are
there hallucinations in this realm, just as there are when voices are heard in
schizophrenia or "thoughts materialized" when no speaker is present? Should
we speak of a "conditioned fatigue," once appropriate to a genuine exhaustion
and now aroused by "signs," conditioned stimuli, the very *thought* of effort?
Such a chronic withdrawal from effort in advance, a persistent rest maneuver,
can come, we know, to replace the normal cycle of effort, work, fatigue,
recovery. An "invalid reaction" can become stabilized and persist—say, from
age 19 to age 42—so that all activities are maintained far below the level
that would seem physiologically and behaviorally appropriate for a "standard
man."

Recurrent fatigue not only alters thresholds of arousal at the level of the
muscles, but can also become associated with cues, so that in the place of effort
a defensive rest maneuver is put forth.[12] Painful fatigue that has been experienced earlier, and the consequent serious disorganization of action, might
"instruct" the person to rest in advance. We know that this has happened in
the case of the old-timer on the logging crew: knowing what the long day's
work will require, he adjusts his pace to the total task, and smiles at the novice
who pitches in with unrestrained enthusiasm, knowing that the youth will be
"poohed out" before the day is done. In the same way the experienced hiker
will adjust his pace to the long climb ahead of him, and take a reasonable pace
long before his muscles raise any kinesthetic complaint at the impact of the
slope. Our neurasthenic seems to have adjusted in advance, too, but his exaggerated fatigue behavior has become chronic and has no visible and adequate
physiological or behavioral cause.

Fatigue and Skill Disorganization

A more careful inspection of any performance that is pushed to the point
of fatigue shows that more is involved than any mere decline in the force of
the movements, more than a raising of the threshold of arousal. The more
skilled the performance, the more this difference is apparent. The pianist who
has practiced too long begins to make errors; the muscles around his shoulder
girdle and in his arms and forearms grow tense. This should warn him that
it is time to stop, but these signals are often unheeded when the drive for
accomplishment is strong. The conscientious student may even feel that he
is "being good" as he pushes his practice to this tensing point. The muscles
have announced that they are ready to quit, but the pianist has not responded

---

[12]It is difficult to draw the line between the automatic conditioned rest behavior and the
voluntary maneuver. This distinction has plagued the discussions of the psychoneuroses for
more than a hundred years. Hysteria was long regarded as "an act" by a mischievous malingerer.
Whether it begins as an automatic action that is later discovered to be useful, or as a voluntary
maneuver that becomes automatic and uncontrolled, is a nice question. It may even be "automatic" (outside all efforts or intents on the part of the person) from beginning to end. Like
the voices of St. Joan, it may have been summoned by genuine motivations whose sources lie
beneath that level of personal control we call consciousness.

to their message. A truly ambitious student can push his practice to the point where a persistent and painful cramp develops. Such an unpunctuated period of intense effort can produce "piano arm," or "writer's cramp," or the "aphonia" of the lecturer who cannot manage to speak any louder than a whisper. Such occupational cramps may require more than complete rest. A slow period of reeducation of his working posture and movements may be called for, lest the resumption of work reinstate the same exaggerated contractions early in the return to effort.

A stammerer who is making some progress in overcoming his speech difficulty may find that involuntary muscle contractions (in the intercostals and larynx) may block his speech whenever he grows emotionally tense or is overtired. The housewife, besieged by the demands of her small children, may find them just too annoying at the end of the day and, in spite of her resolutions, will shift gear into that shouting-scolding-spanking pattern that marks a complete disorganization of her skill in dealing with them. In the morning she can be cheerful, speak in the low voice, manage with a gentle pat or a playful tug, but by nightfall her diplomacy and tact have flown. In the factory the accident curve rises in the last quarter of the shift; after a rest pause (the lunch hour) it will drop again. Examples could be multiplied to illustrate this one principle: with the onset of fatigue, output declines both in quantity and in quality. This principle becomes of the greatest practical importance in any training program where a high degree of skill is required. More rapid gains are made when the practice periods are shortened to such a point that no disorganization is introduced by fatigue. Practice beyond this point risks a fixation of disorganized behavior. Stated somewhat differently, a training program managed by a tyrant with an obsessive conscience will automatically eliminate all of the pupils whose resistance to his methods is insufficient. They will react emotionally, develop piano arm (or ballet leg), fixate clumsy errors, and so on. Their teacher may comfort himself by the phrase: "They lack the talent."[13]

Even as simple a skill as that involved in gripping a dynamometer undergoes deterioration as fatigue sets in. For one thing, the fatigued muscle does not fully relax in the period between strokes. In the rested state the two sets of muscle contractions involved in opening and closing the hand keep out of each other's way: when the flexors close the hand, the extensors on the back of the forearm are relaxed, and when the hand is opened, the flexors let go abruptly and thus get out of the way of their antagonists. Thus, one muscle group never pulls against its antagonist group; the movements are free strokes, in the sense that they are freed of opposition. The strokes in golf, billiards, tennis, typing, are of this same free character (or should be); the moving members can thus be flung at the target (they are, literally, *thrown* move-

---

[13]The entrance of an emotional component into the behavior of the exhausted person should not trap us into viewing the disorganization as caused by the emotion. Rather, the irruption of these reflex-like and explosive responses should be viewed as a part of an over-all disorganization of the man-in-action. Those who urge us to "trust our emotions" overlook the extent to which emotions represent an "escape from control" that is on a par with the uncontrolled twitching of the eyelid (or the restlessness) of the tired brainworker.

ments), and no energy is wasted in overcoming correction movements or opposing contractions in their course. For this reason such movements have been described as ballistic. We have already noted that, as fatigue sets in, there is an overlapping of the contractions: fibrils on the opposite sides of the limb are contracting at the same time. Such a pattern of opposed contractions produces a stiffening of the forearm muscles and of the wrist, and a fall in the dynamometer output. At the end-stage where movements can scarcely be made at all, random and independent firing of the fibers of both muscle groups is continuous, and the muscles exert a slight and steady pull on their tendons. The subject can feel this pull as a stiffness and a discomfort. While the fibers are thus firing at random, the subject cannot produce the response that depends on their synchronous and independent contraction, nor can he relax the forearm muscles by any fiat of will. The separate muscle fibrils, whose actions can be viewed on an oscilloscope, are in the meantime "milling about," like the men of a military company who have fallen out and who in their disorganized actions are in no position to respond to their commander. Head and shoulders of the person may still beat out the rhythm of the metronome, but the forearm has become detached from them, and cannot follow the pattern. The fibrils are acting spontaneously, on their own. (See Stetson and Bouman 1935.)

This behavior of the fatigued muscle reminds us of the overtired person who cannot voluntarily "go to sleep," or relax, and who is also unable to make his body act as he wishes. The disappearance of synchrony in the contractions, with relaxation in the intervals, reminds us of the neurasthenic who is dopey in the daytime and wakeful and restless at night. He can no longer command his musculature directly. His eyelid twitches on its own, and other processes will react spontaneously. He cannot find a comfortable position, and the relaxed posture that can "hold still" is quite beyond him. He cannot even bring his two eyes to fixate together as accurately and promptly as he wishes. Spoonerisms creep into his speech. Even his thought is cluttered up with side-issues, klang associations, irrelevant puns. At such times his emergency emotions lie much nearer the surface, ready for slight triggerings. In a slight dosage, this kind of fatigue is sometimes experienced as a "richness in ideas." A shade more of it and it becomes an annoying, distracting irrelevance. Still more of it, and the person will begin to feel obsessed by what he cannot control.

Sir Frances Galton once described the person who struggles to remain alert and attentive while the lecturer drones on: the fatigued (and bored) listener yawns, grows restless, shifts his posture, contracts his facial muscles in strange grimaces. The schoolteacher can see the same signals in the class when the hour is late or the matter very difficult (or very "dry"): the students begin squirming, wriggling, nodding, sniffing, scratching, doodling on the margin of the notebook; he seems to have lost them, and they, in turn, have "lost control." The movement of sitting attentively is a positive accomplishment that requires practice, discipline, and the integrative power that knows how to withstand fatigue.

The Psychological Factor in Fatigue

When the tired troops have marched until their dragging feet seem too heavy to lift, when each marcher is wondering if he can go another quarter-mile before he will have to fall out, when slogging marchers seem to have borrowed the last ounces of energy from available stores, a curious fact emerges. Let the regimental band strike up "From the Halls of Montezuma," or let the marchers suddenly round a bend beyond which, on the plain below them, their base camp lies in full view, and their pace will quicken and they will even find energy for a shout, a song. Pulse and respiration accelerate, packs are shifted, the pace improves, and faces suddenly lose their lackluster expressions; the men begin to think of the hot shower, the good meal, the evening in town, instead of their aches and the possibility of finding a soft ditch in which to rest. Even the spleen participates in the recovery, pouring forth a fresh supply of red corpuscles to carry oxygen reserves to the tired muscles. The whole pattern of action has shifted: an orientation to a near and inviting future comes alive, and replaces "rest behavior."

The new stimuli have released energies that had been present all the time, but in a hidden, untapped, hoarded form. If we attribute the change to the shift in attention to the new prospects of release (and away from the heavy packs and the endless marching), we imply that a prudent and all but automatic restraint of action had been operating up to this point, and that the men had somehow lost sight of their goal or had somehow ceased to believe in what was in store for them. The situation reminds one of the cautious commander who is in charge of a long-beleaguered garrison: when he receives the news of an approaching relief column, he orders his men to break open the stores he had been so carefully guarding and rationing until then.

In the case of the fatigued marchers, we need not describe their fatigue as *"purely* psychological" merely because the sudden release of action reveals that adequate physiological reserves were there all along (the old malingering argument, the answer to which is that the decrement in output is *both* psychological and physiological).[14] Nor could we expect to produce such effects

---

[14]Ross (1938) takes a somewhat different position: "We cannot conceive that the band could act as a restorer of energy if treatment of this sort can make men, who were apparently exhausted, do more work; the exhaustion in question must have been *wholly* psychological" (my italics). Perhaps we have to recapture the old certitudes that underlie a complete dualism if we want to make this argument have any meaning. If the distinction between a psychological and a physiological fatigue seemed clear at one point (the former dealing with an exhaustion of higher-level tendencies of the man as a whole, the latter dealing with muscle groups and basic energy supplies), it grows less easy to maintain as we continue to push the analysis. Perhaps there is a "physiology" that is pertinent to each level of integration, a physiology that will eventually cope with the problem of psychological fatigue. We would have to study the "physiology" of these higher levels of integration, learn the precise nature and location of the inhibitory substances. But so far the techniques of the physiologist have not proved too helpful.

One aspect of the problem should not be overlooked. As we feel that our integrative powers are slipping, one of the devices we learn to employ is that of restricting the field voluntarily. We consciously shift gears, "pull in our horns," select a smaller area to work in or some simpler level of work, one that our attention can encompass easily. One of the barriers to more creative types of adjustment in the aged is increasing awareness of the terminal state that lies not too far ahead: "It would not pay to start anything as complex as that now."

repeatedly by military music and promises of rest that lead to no genuine pause in the marching with opportunity for rest and recovery. The illustration does point up the fact, however, that a morale component may be operative at the same time that real exhaustion is taking place, and reminds us that human action is typically adjusted to a field whose structure and extent affect this ability to put forth effort.

A second type of situation seems to call for a slightly different explanation. Take the case of the woman who cannot manage to give an hour's lesson to her children. She is too tired; it would completely exhaust her. Nevertheless she can read on, in her novel, for another three hours. Or consider the man who is too exhausted to ride to *work* on the subway, yet who can walk miles into the countryside. We have heard of students who fall asleep if they try to study in the afternoon, yet who seem to possess sufficient reserves of energy on the playing field. Ross (1938, p. 31) tells of a patient who was utterly fatigued by washing her niece's hair, but who could ride her bicycle twenty miles without trouble.

A simple biochemical conception of "fatigue products circulating in the blood stream and inhibiting contraction of muscle fibrils" does not explain why the inhibition is so selective or why certain actions are so much more difficult, so much more vulnerable than others. And how does a chemical differentiate so quickly between the movements of work and play? How does the factor of interest and motivation fit into this complex of action and non-feasance? Should we say, "The woman could wash her niece's hair without fatigue *if she really wanted to*"? Could the student study, brain fag or no brain fag, if he were really *committed* to his task? Do the actions which fail belong to some higher level in an action hierarchy that has its own peculiar biochemistry? And do these actions-at-the-top which fail actually cost the person a degree of effort and require a higher level of integrative power that the fatigued cannot expend? If so, we are confronted with a special form of deficit, and we shall be forced to make discriminations between easy actions that require only a simple form of physical energy and a more costly type of action that requires another and "more costly" organization of these energies. It also appears that this higher form has its own rate of exhaustion. Indeed, this higher form is the one that is especially vulnerable in the neurasthenic.

Conditions Altering Psychological Fatigue

When our activities are unrewarding, when we cannot see that we are "getting anywhere," our performance declines even though energies are still available. The power of the incentives, the summons to action, the cues which originally beckoned us, is extinguished (as for the boy who called "Wolf!" too often). The comparative psychologist, studying the spider's reactions to tones, notes that the insect drops from its web when a tuning fork sets the web vibrating, as if from a potential danger. When no danger ensues, the reflex decreases in force on subsequent soundings: the spider does not drop as far; each time its drop is shorter; but it has plenty of energy left for other movements (Peckham and Peckham 1887). In Pavlov's language, we could speak of hypothetical inhibitory substances accumulating on the synaptic junctions across which the impulses have to pass. Thus the psychological and physiological consequences of "actions without consequence" are blended.

However, when we follow the Pavlovian technique in establishing a conditioned salivation, the buzzer-salivation "connection" is not maintained if the buzzer is sounded repeatedly without the food reinforcement. The food must follow the buzzer occasionally, or the reaction will be extinguished: the flow of saliva grows sluggish, and finally ceases. We could, by analogy, look on the plotted values for this salivation reaction as a "fatigue curve," and we could speak of the "exhaustion" of a reaction tendency, although the "chemical depletion" has to remain purely hypothetical.

The boredom that numbs our faculties when we enter a repeatedly unrewarding situation could be described as a similar *inhibition of responsiveness,* which tends to become generalized, attaching itself to all cues in the setting, and to affect all of the "higher" reaction tendencies required for the setting.[15] The entrance into the social group of the bore produces a special type of fatigue in all those who sigh as they know they will have to listen to him. They grow restless, plan escape, or, if he is so distinguished that they must stay and be polite, they fight sleep, yawning as though their oxygen supply were really running low, and acting as if their blood streams were actually clogged with the breakdown products of strenuous work. Yet the moment they are released from such unrewarding situations, they behave like schoolboys released from the classroom. The bell that releases the nodding children transforms them into shouting, tussling, racing young animals, highly responsive to the new stimuli. To call their previous inattentiveness a "psychological fatigue" does not make that fatigue any less real, any less physiological; but we are dealing with what must be considered a "state of inhibition" rather than some simple depletion or exhaustion. If the physiologist explains this "inhibition of integrations" by referring to a "central fatigue" or to some hypothetical central inhibitory substance, we know the kind of thing that he is looking for even though he cannot identify it.[16] In this context, to call the fatigue *psychological*

---

[15] Oddly enough, it spares these impish tendencies that set our thoughts to commenting on the absurdities in dress and manners of those about us, or to drawing cartoons on the margin of the church service's program. We escape from boredom into the comical and absurd (or into the disruptive); we vent our hostility toward the dull speaker by making him into a Chadband, a stuffed shirt. A political regime, always sensitive to the disaffection of the artists and novelists (who sometimes make a similar flight, lampooning those in authority), retorts by calling them irresponsible beatniks, and, in the dictatorships, punishes their "dangerous thoughts" with imprisonment or worse. At the fringe of every social group there will be "fatigables," who take the social disciplines with resistance, rebellion, and boredom; like the neurasthenics in school and marching squad, they are the first "dropouts."

[16] Some theorists have postulated brain centers which accumulate and store energy with a sthenogenic function (see Deschamps 1919), and some have described the neurasthenic as constitutionally weak in this function (see Janet 1919, I, 378). To date no such theories have been confirmed.

emphasizes that it is experience-determined, that it is the product of the patterning and sequential ordering of stimulation rather than of actual exhaustion of energy stores, and that new arrangements and new learnings can restore the individual to responsiveness. If we call the fatigue situational, interpersonal, holistic, we begin to put a strain upon our now inadequate physiological concepts. What is the physiological consequence of *action that is unrewarding to the person?*

Contrast the unmotivated student or routine worker with the professional person who finds novelty, challenge, satisfaction in his work, or with the entrepreneur and the promoter whose enterprises are as exciting to them as gambling. The latter can work long hours, experience little fatigue, and never feel bored. Some of these interested ones even consume their "free time" in work-related activities. When their interest drives them to the point where the normal warnings of a genuine fatigue are disregarded, they can borrow too heavily against their reserves; at this point the rewarding activities in the narrow zone of keen interest begin to defeat the goals of the person.[17]

Some psychological fatigue, we conclude, is simple anticipation. Just as the sight of a cocktail is nauseating to the patient who has been given conditioned-response therapy (in which emetine is mixed with his drink), a person's mere *entrance* into any behavior cycle that has regularly proved to be too long, too arduous, and fatiguing in the end will induce *in advance* many of the responses (including the "rest behavior") which originally did not emerge until late in the cycle. His actions have simply moved forward into the cycle; he prepares for the exhaustion-to-come, either by a defensive slowing down of movements, or by the restless, yawning, fidgety, crotchety, bored attitude. His behavior undergoes some of the disorganization characteristic of exhaustion, with the release of part-processes from control and the intrusion of irrelevant thoughts, in advance of those original causes. We imagine that we understand such advance adjustments in the fearful person who gets ready for threats-to-come by quickening pulse, secretion of adrenaline, tensing of muscles, accelerated breathing. These part-processes fit into the general adaptation to stress with which we are familiar. Now we are invited to look at the adjustment to fatigue-to-come as types of rest behavior (or disorganization of skills) that are characteristic of all humdrum, exhausting, unmotivated, coerced actions. The slowing of our pace and the withdrawal from effort in advance has a corresponding adjustive quality, even though it may not be adaptive in the role we have selected to play.

Finally, we can see that having no clearly formulated goals at all may contribute to ennui, for where there are no exciting goals, no deep-seated

---

[17]Compare the penetrating and witty discussion of these problems in de Grazia (1962). Ironically, in spite of their shorter "work week," a close study of their schedules shows that Americans are prone to consume their "free time" in work-related activities. Always ready to buy a "time-saving gadget," many find themselves so busy getting the money to buy the gadget to save the time that they have no free time left. And some would not know what to do with their leisure if they were to discover it.

needs to be gratified, no important meanings unfolding in our actions, how can there be rewards, or anticipated jubilations, or reinforcements? There is nothing but the small palatability, the simple pleasures of sense, along with the irritations, the disgusts, the part-processes. Behavior comes in short spurts, impulsive actions, self-limited cycles. Each short cycle is as meaningless as its predecessor, and the whole takes on a gray sameness, grows weary, stale, flat, and unprofitable. Those who live always in an immediate present resemble the frontal-lobe patient, even though they do not suffer from his neurological handicap. Without an inviting "beyond," without a lively future to shape the present, action is replaced by mere movement. Whether we describe the condition as a lack of imagination, or a lack in motivation, or—as Viktor Frankl names it—a *noogenic neurosis,* it is a structure of action conducive to fatigue. Like the frontal-lobe patient, who also can enjoy the simple palatabilities and pleasures, this type of person can chatter but has little to say; he can react to present stimuli but no larger field "engages" him.

Consider the young man who gets things too easily, is bored with them, behaves irresponsibly, and feels ashamed. His state might be described as a conflict between that layer of habits where good intentions are easily verbalized and where an ego-ideal has developed (an image of that admirable creature he is to become), and that second layer of real actions where deeds are delivered and stubborn and persistent effort has to be applied. Robert Ort (1952) has described the problem as though it were a social-class matter: a study of two samples of high-school students drawn from different social classes showed that such conflicts were less acute in lower-class boys, who were prone to "do what comes naturally" and to strike out for very immediate types of gratifications, whereas the middle-class boys had taken on goals and tasks (nonpleasurable work) and assumed an orientation toward a higher social status that required them to act repeatedly "against nature."[18] In every dimension of our striving, this two-layered conflict develops, whether it is a matter of business success, ethical and moral progress, aesthetic standards, or the achievement of a good marriage. Only where the "poverty of culture" makes the superego structure so weak and thin that it has no great pressure to exert upon the individual are these "gaps" absent.[19] Perhaps we should accept that gap between expectations, goals, and the actual delivery of accomplishments as *natural* in any creature with imagination. We find our pleasures under diffi-

---

[18]Sometimes our sociologists seem to suggest that it is unnatural to be ambitious, and that, conversely, it is both easier and more hygienic to take a regressive course back to the level of the noble savage. The greater frequency of mental illness in the lower strata and our study of the mental health among the upward-mobile should remind us, however, that it is not *successful* and vigorous upward striving that makes a youth fall ill, or show the symptoms of neurasthenia.

[19]Esmeralda (Lewis 1965, p. xxvi) voices her freedom from guilt: "I never look back." Of the Rios family, Lewis writes, "They tend to accept themselves as they are, and do not indulge in soul-searching or introspection." And this is the bottom of the social barrel, where something of the sociopath is in most of the characters.

culties, make progress at the cost of effort, and never *quite* accept the bargains we make as the best possible ones, that is, where there is not too great a "poverty of culture." The neurasthenic blows up this gap, feels the complaints of his body, and sometimes hides behind its nonfeasance as a relatively inferior way of preserving his self-respect.

The Noogenic Neurosis: Frankl's Boast

Any extended discussion of Frankl's concept of the noogenic neurosis would carry us beyond our present purpose. We have set out to discuss the problem of fatigue as a prelude to a discussion of Janet's notions about neurasthenia. In the course of our discussion, we noted that when a muscle is fatigued, its fibrils begin to act independently. While the "dynamometer-measured output" is gradually falling, the "pieces of the movement of contraction" act out of phase with the main movement. It is tempting to extend this notion, and to anticipate that when the man as a whole is fatigued, his habit systems begin to operate on their own. What the Nigerians call "brain fag" and others call mental fatigue, Janet wanted to describe as a lowering of psychological tension. Objectively described, the lowering of tension involves a restriction of the field, a tendency to react to more immediate and pressing stimuli, the emergence of conflict and stress between the parts of the system. In our imagination we might consider a hierarchical order of response systems, arranged in loopline circuits, so that as the highest integrations are inhibited, the lower circuits begin to act independently, to escape from control.

Such a concept of a hierarchy of actions, with the top-level organization holding the subordinate systems under control, raises knotty problems about the relationship between the "higher" and "lower" functions, questions as old as the mind-body problem, as old as the conflict between authoritarian and democratic forms of political organization. In discussing Frankl's views briefly, we can note Janet's notion of a behavior hierarchy, and contrast his own answer to the problem with that of Frankl.

Growing out of his experiences in a concentration camp, where he arrived at the conviction that only those prisoners who managed to find some meaning in their existence could survive, Frankl developed a form of therapy that focuses on this restoration of meaning (see Frankl 1956, 1959, 1960). This search for meaning in one's life is, he believes, the primary motivational force in man. Nevertheless, some men "get lost," and, blown about like chaff in a high wind, they are not able to stand up to pressures; the little palatabilities and pleasures are not a secure anchorage.

In Frankl's case the extreme pressures of the death camp generated an extreme counter-affirmation, taught him what he really did believe, and this affirmation brought strength to him in a time of troubles.

"Man is free. He can transcend the biological, social, and psychological determinants either by conquering and shaping them, or by deliberately submitting to them. The mind is free, and also rational.... Even though conditions such as lack of sleep, insufficient food, and various mental stresses may suggest that the inmates were bound to react in certain ways, in the final analysis it becomes clear that the sort of person the prisoner became was the result of an inner decision, and not the result of camp influences alone" (1959, p. 22).

This free agent, who possesses that meaning-given strength, can face all manner of adversities. St. Ignatius Loyola faced the experience of a shattered limb that swept away his life plans; others face blindness, wasting diseases, stifling environments. But though these conditions are given, the responses are not. The man must still choose what he will do, and when he can find (or create) the proper meaning (or plan), it will absorb and utilize his predicament.

This boast, which defies all that fate can bring, is so extreme that those of us who have not undergone such tests as those of the death camp and emerged triumphant may hesitate before this proud description of the human being's powers in the face of extreme stress. The genetically minded will stress that each individual has his "cutting point," a constitutionally determined stress tolerance.

Both psychoanalysts and behaviorists have been inclined to look on this "cutting point" as a modifiable one; resistance to stress can be built up by dosages of stress that can be endured and finally surmounted, and by carefully calculated dosages of "support." The analyst likes to point to a lowering of stress tolerance by types of mothering; he believes that he can demonstrate an increase in such tolerance after insight therapy has been successfully applied. Both the analyst and the behaviorist introduce new dimensions of determinism, however, and neither counts on any hypothetical freedom, or upon any absolute power of transcending through choice.

Others look on chronic and extreme present pressures (and losses of support) as factors which sensitize the individual to the next application of force and reduce his power of integrating, coping, resisting. From brainwashing techniques to the use of drugs, from water torture to the lash, men in our time have been systematically seeking ways of undermining their victim's grip on reality, his determination to resist, and all too successfully. Under the death-camp tortures, some who were not as tough as Frankl developed depressive, paranoid, and suicidal types of thinking. These stresses made it increasingly difficult for them to discriminate between real and near-real, between what is promised and threatened and what is most probable. The stresses that turn up in clinical records (and that have undermined sanity and the rational pattern of living) are seldom like those of the death camps, but they include tuberculosis, approaching death, anoxia, general paralysis, tumors of the frontal lobe, toxic conditions brought on by drugs, prolonged isolation, chronic interpersonal conflict, and abandonment by friends and loved ones. These stresses seem to have a way of attacking that very citadel of the proud self that is so free to boast that no circumstances are insurmountable. So viewed, the ego, with its willful plans, the spirit that gives or withholds consent, the grasp of the field that organizes action into one coherent whole so that living has a meaning, becomes something finite, limited, frangible.

To these considerations we can add another simple observation which most of us have experienced. In the course of acquiring a new set of habits, such as that of speaking a foreign language, we acquire both simple associations and higher units. There are the separate words which we begin to catch, here and there, as we hear the foreign phrases spoken, and the larger rhythms and phrases that give the drift and intent of thought. Working late at night on a passage of text in this new language, the student may grow fatigued, and he discovers that suddenly he can no longer read the larger meanings. The words are there, and can be pronounced and defined, but the higher units do not leap forth. Janet (1928, p. 254) quotes the observation of a French mine inspector who had been working underground all day. As fatigue set in, he found himself unable to carry on a conversation with his German colleague, a task that had been easy in the forenoon. Imagine, if you will, the visiting school inspector who has spent a long and busy day inspecting classes and who, speaking late at night after a dinner and a too-long introduction, looks down at his notes only to find that, while the words are legible, the meaning they were intended to signal simply does not gel.

Similar facts emerge in those situations that produce regression. The three-year-old who has finally learned bladder and bowel control and is "a big boy now" sometimes regresses to soiling, crying, negativism, when his mother brings the new baby brother home from the hospital. Occasionally such a child will peer up into his mother's face to ask, "Mommy, do you still love me?" The more vulnerable portions of his habit system seem to lie at some higher level, of a big little man among his peers, along with the other latest acquisitions.

A Hierarchy of Motives

These notions have led some students of motivation to arrange human motives in a hierarchy, with the earliest, most primitive, and least expendable actions placed at the base of the pyramid. (A man must eat, and drink, and rest occasionally.) Such "first requirements" would include physiological needs, security needs, sexual needs, Maslow (1954) believes.[20] Above them, once the simplest needs are gratified and made secure, there will develop second-order needs as socialization proceeds: needs for esteem, needs for *Gemeinschaftsgefühl*. And if, at last, with the first and second stories of this many-layered hierarchy made secure, the individual gropes for something we might call self-actualization, there will appear such needs as are gratified by truth,

---

[20]The Catholic celibate will, of course, challenge the necessity for sexual expression. Some of the clergy who wish to modify the rules about marriage seem to have come around to the position that very few have the "grace" necessary for a truly celibate existence. Others will argue that the socialist's effort to produce a truly collective society violates "the instinct of property" and the territorial imperative that some animals place above all other needs. These others try to restore an *essential* part of human nature by naming it an *instinct;* political purposes may enter here.

beauty, justice. But these, one can see, will be the most vulnerable of all: the last to develop, the first to collapse when life grows too difficult.[21]

Janet also tried his hand at a hierarchy of actions, quite different from Maslow's, yet containing a similar notion. He used this hierarchy as he described those changes which come about as psychological tension is lowered. In his discussions (1903) of the obsessions and of psychasthenia, he offered a fivefold classification of actions:

1. *The function of the real.* Effective action within a field of shared reality, especially where novel actions are required and where the sharing requires sensitivity to the beliefs and intentions of others (with negotiations, compromise, exhortation necessary), represents the most severe demand on our attention and our integrative forces. At this level we sense the ownership of our actions and decisions, take full responsibility for them, remain alert and vigilant toward the field about us, even searching out the meanings that are hidden behind the words and facial masks of others. Creative and insightful action is required rather than routine, passive, mechanical compliance. When the function of the real is in full operation, an alert child would know and assent to the purposes of his conditioners; an alert patient would have to "go along with" his therapist, assenting to what he is trying to do; a citizen, able to see through the slogans of advertisers and political leaders, would cease to be suggestible. This would require the working Communist to be as familiar with his Machiavelli as was Stalin, who kept a copy on his bedside table.

2. *Disinterested activity.* More or less automatic habits, conditioned responses, mechanical skills, can be performed with a very limited amount of feeling, without "regulative effort." Vigilant action that has to be continually corrected belongs at a higher level. Eliminate this component, and the feeling of a lively and interesting present disappears, and with it the sense of personal ownership of action. Thus purely disinterested activity has an unreal quality. As we approach the passive and mechanical form of action (which some forms of behaviorism seem to consider typical), nothing "matters" very much. The ego is not involved and the evaluating-interpreting process is in abeyance.

3. *The image function.* At this level an automatic and purely representative memory takes place: images arise under their own power and develop independently of any control, regardless of how they fit a well-grasped present field. Here, too, belong forms of abstract reasoning and revery that are also divorced from any lively context. Hypnagogic images represent one of the pure forms of the image function (see Fig. 5, Chapter 6). The person acts as a voyeur, watching the waxing and waning of these visual (or auditory)

---

[21]Only when we realize how vulnerable, how contingent they are, will we be able to safeguard them, not by making them the most essential, the most basic, the most ineradicable. Justice? Hasn't it always been hard to secure? sometimes difficult to discriminate and define, even? Self-actualization? What is that? a basic instinct? or the most vulnerable claim of an ego never too sure that it can survive, even? Ask, rather, What parts of the self deserve to be actualized? or, Whose self?

forms, and is unable to summon them or direct the changes (save at that point where an aroused ego wakens and they vanish).

4. *Emotional reactions.* Janet uses the term *emotion* in a special sense at this point. He refers to those explosive, reflex-like actions that function outside the control of the higher units. Tantrums triggered by frustration would be an example of this type of response. The diffuse reverberations that spread to every cell of the body may express, in part, the force of the stimulus that evoked them (as in the startle to a pistol shot), but they are not canalized and directed in such a way as to cope with the precise nature, meaning, and location of the stimulus. What we might call a "reaction with feeling" is quite a different type of emotion.

5. *Automatic movements.* Reflex in character, irrelevant to any purposes of the person as a whole, these responses express the neuromuscular arrangements in our tissues rather than the working out of some realistic intention (as in type 1, above). In the half of the body below a severed spinal cord these automatic movements, which can still be evoked by stimuli, function without any regulation from the higher looplines, and certainly without the participation of the man himself (as when, in an operation with spinal anesthesia, the patient is an onlooker unable to interfere with what goes on below the chemical block). The reflex eye-wink, the reflexes of swallowing and of peristalsis, the constriction of the arterioles of the face in a cold wind would be examples of this fifth type.

Coupled with this conception of a hierarchy of actions is the added notion of an "escape from control" which the neurologist Hughlings Jackson contributed to our vocabulary. The lower loopline activities escape to function autonomously, when the higher levels fail, as with the decerebrate rigidity that follows a cerebral lesion. Janet reminds us that a wide range of factors can weaken the higher elements in the hierarchy. Whatever lowers psychological tension (or integrative force) weakens the higher level of action first of all. That very level of action which Frankl, in his theory of logotherapy, depends on as the essential human motive, which he would activate and utilize in therapy, which would stall off disorganization and disintegration, is here viewed as the most vulnerable level.[22] The neurotic complaint, "I am just a machine," is voiced by a man who has lost the top of the loopline system, the power to grasp life meaningfully and to act on this grasp of things. The last to disappear are the automatic actions; even the deteriorated schizophrenic sits endlessly repeating what once may have been a symbolic movement, but is now just an automatic contraction. In this logic the bodily

---

[22]"You must renew your faith," the religious healer is apt to counsel the neurotic, the obsessive, the depressed. Yet it is precisely in this higher level of action that self-confidence and a global faith in a benevolent universe dwell. The obsessive's doubts about his intelligence, his appearance, his ability to win friends spread to produce religious doubts. As his motivation runs thin, so does his faith. When depression strikes the devout, it seems to the patient that the Lord, too, has turned his face away from such a guilty, worthless creature. With the return of health and the functioning of the higher loopline systems, the patient smiles at his period of doubt (self-doubt, world-doubt, God-doubt).

complaints, the independent action of part-processes, that we see in the neurasthenic represent one form of this "escape from control."

Up to a point Janet, Frankl, and Maslow agree. Each one senses, in his own style, the existence of a hierarchy of functions. Each places at the top of the hierarchy those functions which he counts uniquely human, the essential mark of the genus *homo sapiens* when he is functioning at his best. Regressions, exhaustions, injuries to the central nervous system, toxins, fatigue shift action into the lower looplines and categories. But where Maslow and Janet would trace the descent to the conditions, Frankl seems to want to affirm that it is a matter of choice. Meaning can be and is lost deliberately. On such occasions a man hides from his responsibilities and seeks diversions (in pleasures, palatibilities, the illness game, or schizophrenic double-talk). Here the psychiatrist is tempted to join the moralist, the disciplinarian. Frankl speaks in a langauge similar to that of Pascal and of all those who, in their thinking, set the spirit against the flesh while affirming the spirit's full responsibility to overcome the latter.[23] To the physician or counselor who follows the determinism of either psychoanalysis or behaviorism or genetics, Frankl seems to be saying in effect: Doctor, your theories of neurosis are themselves neurotic. Behaviorism is a disease, and it produces a paralysis of will. Psychoanalysis mirrors the neurotic patient's regressive search for security and for the "lesser pleasures."

Between the absolutes of freedom and determinism lies the area in which a clinician must work. In practice he is forced to estimate the integrative powers of his client. His therapy may resemble that of the morale officer who orders the regimental band to strike up "The Halls of Montezuma." He may try to stimulate, arouse, enthuse, "emotionize," all in the effort to impart new forces and new meanings to lives that seem to have run aground, that have become lost. Courageous, sincere, enthusiastic, impressive, therapists of the makeup of S. Weir Mitchell or Frankl may literally lift the neurasthenic to one of his better levels of functioning. The ultimate meanings employed by the healer have varied (while achieving approximately the same degree

---

[23]The patients described by Ludwig and Farrelly (1966) seem to be able to "turn on" a typical schizophrenic performance whenever they consider it necessary to convince their physician that they are not ready for discharge from hospital. Their deliberate loss of control can be checked, these authors believe, by a kind of ward management planned according to a mixture of good reinforcement principles and group discipline directed at breaking "the code of chronicity" and calculated to establish a kind of "collective responsibility" for these infractions of rational conduct. Whether the "descent" below the level of meaningful action and communication is conscious and voluntary, at the start, or not (the old debate about mental illness as malingering), these authors *intend to make it so*. One is reminded of Wagner-Jauregg's electrical treatment of war neuroses, instituted in the Austrian army in World War I. Shocks described as excruciatingly painful were used to demonstrate to the shell-shocked soldier that his malingering would prove unprofitable, with the result that the number reporting sick was decreased, while the number hospitalized for more serious forms of psychosis was increased. (See Jones 1957, pp. 21-24; Zabriskie and Brush 1941; *Brit. Med. J.* 1916). Zabriskie's terse summary runs: "The results were poor, 40 per cent were unfit for further service and 20 per cent had to be discharged to other hospitals or asylums." Voluntary or involuntary, the illness pattern has behind it forces that are not deterred by rather severe "reinforcement" schedules.

of success). Buddhists, Mohammedans, Catholics, Christian Scientists, existentialists, and the proprietors of sanitoria in which the rest cure is used have developed diverse procedures to restore "meaning." Typically, each has insisted that there is but one meaning behind the world of appearances, one "best" plan that will properly subordinate the aberrant part-systems so as to restore a wholeness that has been lost.[24]

In contrast to these optimists who are certain that the patient can operate at higher levels of psychological tension, a clinician may conclude that, in fact, his patient's forces are distinctly limited. From the days of Mitchell, who thought of the neurasthenic's problem as created by a deficiency in blood lipoids, there have been many who have chosen to "work from below." That is, they have sought to improve the conditions down among the cells, to strengthen the part-systems, to teach relaxation of the musculature, to assist a client to find one or another of those basic gratifications which, he is sure, will lift the spirit. Then, and only then, this type of clinician would argue, can the patient risk any grand attempts. Only after the parts are strengthened can they fit together into those so-called higher, or essential, human powers.[25]

A Summary

Although we began our discussion with a description of fatigue, our analysis has forced us to go much further, even to face the ultimate question of human freedom. We have encountered certain ambiguities among which there are a few guidelines worth emphasis.

Proud as Dr. Frankl's boast sounds, and flattering to our ego as it is in inviting us to assume a grand posture of defiance, the facts point to some very sharp limits to the freedom of those who succumb to the strains of everyday

---

[24]When Denis de Rougemont describes *Gauloiserie* as a kind of voluntary escape from the *serious* form of love, he makes a similar voluntary-purposive analysis. When we explain clowning as an effort to keep from crying, we imply a tragic meaning too painful to remember. In *explanations* of this type we assume the freedom to choose and seek to indicate *what the choice is for*. Looking at the wide variety of healing systems that work, one can see that there are many beliefs that provide "the one true religion" for those in serious need of some orienting philosophy. Since there are multitudes of men who stay out of hospital and avoid incapacitating neuroses in spite of the fact that they have scarcely a shoestring of orienting belief, a vague and seldom invoked Grand Plan, it may very well be that those who both seek and respond to this type of "belief therapy" constitute a special case, or a special class of patients. Janet thought that his psychasthenics (of whom the neurasthenics form one subclass) were, as a group, *"terrible metaphysicians"*: weighing the pros and cons, doubting, in need of a belief that would resolve all conflicts, that would enable them to make decisions, restore their will, explain to them precisely "who they are."

[25]Edmund Jacobson (1929), who directs his patients to attend to the low-grade tensions within their musculature, to practice relaxation exercises calculated to eliminate them, is attacking the signs of anxiety in piecemeal fashion. Under the guise of contemplation and a kind of "communion with Nature," Joseph Wood Krutch (1956) recommends life at the edge of the desert. Others such as Solomon and Leary (1964) recommend the states induced by LSD as a way of pulling oneself together. And while the initiates of contemplation, with or without assistance from drugs, are speaking of the search for an ultimate meaning, their opposite numbers will be noting that the states they use also lower the level of arousal, reduce the sensory input. These critics are apt to define the condition in need of correction as "sensory surfeit," and the therapy as a form of sensory deprivation.

living. Man is neither wholly free nor wholly determined. He is an agent, creating his future, creating something new with each of his decisions. It is true that his life is no eternal recurrence, predetermined: its march is within his hands, *to a degree.* He is as strong in transcending stresses *as he is,* as free in actualizing the best within him *as the conditions permit.* Within his limits a man can be held responsible for his neuroses, his poor choices, his avoidance of meaning, but only within these limits.

He can become lost because of events over which he has no control, and with which he possesses neither the means nor the power of coping. Each one of us can reach that "cutting point" beyond which effective and creative action is impossible. Savonarola was broken by the Pope's torturers, though he was a strong-willed and committed man, not lacking an ultimate meaning for his existence. General James Dean, faced with an extended stay in a Korean prison, toyed with the thought of suicide as he felt himself succumbing to the conditions of the prison. He feared to pass beyond that point where he could live according to the code of honor of a soldier, a code dearer than life.

Now this "cutting point" is where it is. One recruit will bellyache in boot training, filled with neurasthenic complaints or manifesting hysterical symptoms (and for the good of the service the military may treat him as a malingerer). His comrade may postpone his collapse until the beachhead landing (just before going ashore). A third soldier may endure until sixty days of unrelieved combat have passed, breaking only when an extreme physical exhaustion suddenly makes him "blow his top." At each of these points an observer could raise the question about the one who breaks: Could he not have gone further? Are there not still deeper levels of energy that some morale officer or logotherapist could have tapped, appealing to his pride, restoring to him the "lost meaning" of the battle? Perhaps if such a thought had not haunted Richter, he would not have tried to extend the swimming times of his drowning rats by introducing "rescues" before they broke.[26]

For a human being, facing a crisis on his own, a "do-it-yourself" job of therapy is often bungled. Life and its tasks may not reveal to the individual precisely what kinds of burden he can safely assume, with his devices. Perhaps Dr. Frankl has a point: our constant tendency, in psychology, to locate the full set of factors that determine the cutting point *outside the self* creates the delusion that someone knows enough to predict the strength of a particular individual. Frankl's emphasis invites us to look on an individual's area of freedom as something other than a simple outcropping of a calculable, inherited toughness and an objective and measurable external stress. Even when we add those factors that provide a background of preconditioning, we still have little more than a very rough approximation on which to base our predictions.

---

[26]Sometimes there is a touch of the absurd in the stories of the men who broke. "I stood it O.K. until they made me dig up the strawberry patch that the Frogs had planted. And just for a latrine!" It was too much for a farm boy who knew how much work was involved in getting a good bed of strawberry plants established. The last straw for another soldier came as the wallet of his prisoner fell out, spilling photographs of a wife and a child. *The enemy was a human being!*

Moreover, the extent of this area of freedom is always changing, our range of choices extended or restricted as a result of our choices and of the changing conditions. In any given case, the judgment of the clinician is both arbitrary and loaded with consequences. He may say, in effect, "You can do better if you will. Let me encourage you. Let us try." Or his words and his recommendations may say all too clearly: "You have not been able to help yourself. We might as well enter into a planned relation of dependence, a calculated regression. You are going to need a long period of support." These clinical decisions will affect the patient's integrative powers, opening up areas of autonomy or dependency or discouragement. There is a form of determinism that is created by these decisions. Even entrance into therapy is a decision which the patient must make, with trust in another person, confessing his own weakness. Thus the estimate of a man's capacities can itself inhibit or release his striving. Let us make these abstractions a little more concrete by describing how a psychiatrist with Janet's outlook actually handled individual neurasthenics.

JANET'S APPLICATION OF THEORY

The case study with which Janet opened his volume of case studies of psychasthenia (1903, II, 4) has a touch of the absurd about it, yet it is instructive. It highlights one of the contrasts between the theories of Freud and those of Janet and provides at least one concrete meaning for that concept of psychological tension so central to the latter's thinking. In this brief sketch we can also sense that relationship between a busy and sucessful clinician and his humble client.

The Case of Ron

Ron was a youth of 17, rather thin in face and body, with hands that were blue, cold to the touch. He perspired freely. His nose and his ears were redder than they should have been, his tongue coated. He complained of poor digestion, of constipation, and of occasional bouts of diarrhea. He suffered from hemorrhoids. He was not an impressive figure of a man. Sitting there, in the patient's chair opposite the ruddy and hearty physician who was so full of assurance, his complaints took on a pathetic quality. Had he complained of inferiority feelings, the physician might have thought, to himself: "I can well understand."

Ron had a voracious appetite: sometimes bizarre, his tastes could have been described as "faddish." They ran now to sweets, now to proteins, and so on. He was concerned about food. Overeating, he never felt satisfied. He ate to relieve his stomach discomfort, and then his eating made him feel bloated, stuffed, and the acid contents of his stomach rose in his throat to produce a slight nausea. Overeating, vomiting, he remained thin.

Ron suffered from frequent headaches, and there was a constant prickling sensation at the crown of his head. These paresthesias gave him the impression of "something going on up there in the skin of his cranium"; yet examination revealed no local basis for these sensations. Janet may have asked himself: "Does this youth lack normal absorbing interests that would keep bodily sensations in the background? Have these sensory tracts been freed from the normal inhibitory control of the rest of the integrative system that is normally fully employed? Are there actually operating, in this poorly integrated nervous system, streams of pain impulses that provide a real basis for these complaints? Or is this youth's imagination making use of some 'remembered pain'?"

Ron also spoke to the doctor about recurrent nocturnal emissions. This not too unusual adolescent concern seems to be constructed, in part, out of the threats and admonitions that parents have used in controlling the first body explorations. There is a folklore that has existed from the time of those ancient Hebraic injunctions against casting one's seed upon the ground, a lore that couples strength with sexuality under control. Ron's questions may have been searching out answers for (and concealing his interest in) the problem of masturbation. He asked specifically, "Are these emissions of sexual fluid the cause of my enormous feeling of fatigue?"

When Janet tested Ron's strength with the dynamometer, he found a 30-kg. index on the right, 25 kg. on the left, but Ron could not produce these scores a second time. Harnessed in the ergograph, so that his movements would inscribe a "fatigue curve" on the kymograph, Ron showed a surprisingly rapid decline in his power to respond in pace with the metronome. He insisted that he could not work the lever after four trials. He was a "fatigable," and so radically fatigable that he seemed to have convinced himself that his reservoir of energy was completely empty. He gave the observer the impression that, if sharply commanded, he might be able to make the ergograph work, but if such an outside press could produce contractions in his muscles, Ron's puny volition could not put out the effort. If this rapid fatigue symbolized the state of a youth's will, then his power to insert his private plans and hopes into a world he never made and to cope with occasional jeers and contempt must have been poor. *"Maladie de la volonté,"* Ribot (1914) was to call it: a will sickness.

A patient of this type poses an interesting problem for the busy clinician. Busy from his first early appointment (made for some worker at 7:30 A.M. and before his usual office hours), he may have been running his appointments, a new case every half hour, for seven hours. And then there enters this poor, limp, weak Ron. His very posture, as he oozes into the chair, or squirms restlessly in his tense fatigue (that permits him neither to rest nor to play nor to work) is irritating. When other patients that the physician has seen have had organic difficulties for which his skills provide clear-cut remedies, the very vagueness of this tired youth's fatigue tests his patience and understanding; for there is nothing wrong with the heart, kidneys, lungs, except the way they function together in action. Yet, in one sense, Ron's illness is more severe than that of some of the others. Impaired merely in a single organ, the selves of the organically ill patients were still tough and resilient. (A sixteen-year-old schoolgirl with a broken back, who had to be trussed up in a special bed that rotated her on her body axis, still managed to go on with her schoolwork and, in addition, to cheer up her wardmates with her humorous quips.) Ron seemed to suffer from some failure of nerve, some basic lack of moral force, some weakness in *integrative* strength, some lack of motivation. His physician was strongly tempted to sermonize, moralize, shock, emotionize, discipline him. Anything that would stimulate this fretful person into productive action and get him out of his preoccupations with bodily complaints would be good therapy.

Such a neurasthenic gives the impression of being a "body without its full quota of spirit," as though whatever it is that vitally engages the surrounding field has somehow run down. He acts as though inhibitions had accumulated until the normal impulses to act were neutralized by some biochemical state. For a person such as Ron, life often seems monotonous, unpunctuated, boring. Instead of flowing out into gratifying action, his weak impulses merely tense his musculature, produce a restless and agitated shifting of posture. The separate physiological systems act on their own initiative: the blood vessels that supply the tip of his nose run their own way; whimsical appetite runs counter to his true homeostatic needs. He gulps his food and then regurgitates it. All the while his "I dare not" seems to inhibit his "I would." Ron does not act as one piece, as a person; his impulses are poorly integrated (like the fibrils of the fatigued muscle). Even those homeostatic mechanisms that are supposedly basic to life do not act as a part of a single organismic unit. If it were true, as the Sophists once argued, that the dog goes where its legs carry it, this particular dog seems to be running off in several directions at once. This "fatigue" of the central regulative network, whatever its ultimate nature turns out to be, provides a concrete instance of what Janet meant by his concept of "lowered psychological tension."[27]

The occasional bursts of accelerated heart beat, the palpitations of which such a patient will complain, suggest a chronic readiness for emotional responses that is similar to the symptoms found in that state of weakness which follows any fever, when the patient finds the slightest exertion too much, and little things cause a "spill-over" into a fretful emotionality.[28] Janet noted that there is also a proneness to muscular cramps in these psychasthenics:

---

[27]We do not like to use the word "will" in modern psychology. In American textbooks, the chapter on the will was dropped with William James's *Principles of Psychology*. Traditionally described as free, and therefore something that lies outside the kingdom of prediction and control, its injection into any psychological discussion was regarded as disruptive. We conceal the problem under the term *motivation*, occasionally. However we name it, the form of action that we once referred to as voluntary continues to plague us. Paradoxically, as soon as we identify it, we ask, "What are the conditions that govern this type of action?" That is, we seek to reduce it to the status of a determined thing. Such a determinism would be very helpful for the clinician who wishes to put a patient like Ron "on his feet," particularly if a manipulation of "the conditions" could give Ron what he lacks and thereby make him less dependent on the clinician's manipulation of *external* conditions.

Commenting on the English therapist who used avoidance conditioning to correct his client's tendencies toward infidelity, one observer asks plaintively, "Are we not going to be able to learn anything for ourselves, by experience, any more? Must we be 'learned' by someone else?" The temptation to become Big Brother haunts clinical work (as well as politics); the temptation is intensified by the existence of many patients who are all too eager to thrust this role upon their counselors. To say that these are persons of "low psychological tension" is almost a euphemism for "weak-willed."

[28]See the discussion of the "effort syndrome," the "soldier's heart," and the disorder known as neurocirculatory asthenia (Chapter 7). What makes the symptom a puzzle to the clinician is that he can frequently identify no adequate cause for any emotion that would rationalize the autonomic changes, no weakness in the personality makeup that would warrant speaking of "low psychological tension." A person of courage, whose life is well-ordered, may show this type of vulnerability in a single sector (e.g., in heart action). The proof of the pudding lies in the manner in which he "carries on" in spite of his local handicap.

spasms of contraction which occur spontaneously or in connection with minor bursts of effort, and which endure beyond any usefulness. In less susceptible subjects, such cramps arise only after extreme exertions, but these asthenic patients, we remember, are easily fatigued.

Nonetheless, such a patient may keep his job, more easily, perhaps, if his work is relatively routine, and if some supervisor makes all of the decisions, yet of all work this type is most apt to induce fatigue, and boredom. While a patient such as Ron will show none of the obsessions and hallucinations or the compulsive habits that mark the more deeply involved person, the beginnings are here. His recurrent vomiting to clear his stomach of its distressful contents and his concerns about eating and elimination approach the obsessive-compulsive pattern. Because he has the natural need to make his actions appear reasonable, his symptoms and his preoccupations get woven into a mildly delusional system. His intestinal tract, he says, does not function properly. He is losing his strength through nocturnal emissions. He would be the first to understand what the advertiser means when he suggests, "You may have tired blood!" We wonder: "Is this a simple somatopsychic problem that will clear up the moment we can correct the organic basis?" Or are his concerns just so many rationalizations of his more general personal nonfeasance? Should attention be directed toward the "weakness in the man as a whole," a weakness that may have to be traced back to the training of early infancy? Is it an expression of his current inability to find a suitable identity in the world, a life with a meaning?[29]

In Janet's analyses of cases of this sort, he frequently explained them by "a general asthenia of the nervous system," a kind of "irritable weakness" of the integrative mechanism.[30] Such an interpretation influenced what he did, as therapist, and limited the range of his inquiries and analyses. He advised Ron to change his absurd eating habits: to eat less, to avoid meat, to eat plenty of milk, eggs, cereal, green vegetables, and cooked fruits, and to eliminate all wine and alcohol. For good measure, he prescribed thyroid capsules (as though to provide an endocrine "jolt" for this hypoactive organism). He made no extended analysis of childhood experiences, made no attempt to restore and liquidate traumatic memories, did not use hypnosis to explore a

---

[29]Ron's behavior, let us underscore it, is ambiguous! If we ask, "Is it due to genetic endowment, or to some current press, or to some early phase of life history, or to a present organic condition, or to interpersonal relationships, or to the broader social setting?" the answer for each of these questions ought to be "Yes." Yes, it may involve any one or any combination of these causes. It may be due to all of these, and to some that we have not yet guessed. It usually is not one *or* the other.

[30]When these words are interpreted literally, as a "weakness in the nerves," we are explaining what we see by something we know little about. When in addition we proceed to treat the nerves chemically instead of canvassing all possibilities, we narrow the therapy and avoid the difficulty of confronting a disorder of the personality. The clinician who prescribes benzedrine for the child with a behavior problem (suspecting the consequences of encephalitis) and the physician who prescribes dilantin as a means of controlling attacks of *petit mal*, illustrate other direct attacks on the nervous system. The more this logic is extended so that it covers all forms of "inability to integrate a good life," the more we shall deserve the epithet "an addicted society" and the more our physicians become simpleminded materialists.

possible inhibiting past that had been forgotten, and did not advise a rest cure (Ron was no millionaire of the pocketbook, either). Furthermore, he did not attempt to work out with Ron a better plan of living, or to retrain or reeducate him as a person. Janet leaves the method by which he reassured Ron about his "nocturnal emissions" largely to our imagination. (We have only his terse phrase, commenting on the patient's concern: "He exaggerated their importance.") Perhaps his voice and his gesture of medical authority were all that was needed.

And the result? A rapid recovery. Vomiting ceased, Ron's appearance improved, his mood lifted, he became more alert, and on the dynamometer his tests gave normal indices. Janet, in a brief aside, suggested that with a forthcoming visit to the country, where an outdoor life and considerable exercise could further strengthen his sluggish system, continued gains could be expected. So the case of Ron was closed, marked "cured."

One has to remember that the Salpêtrière clinic where Janet worked was a busy one in Paris, where working-class patients were referred from other services. Such a clinic, often clogged with more "untreatable" than its staff could care for, may drift into treating the symptoms that can be handled easily and quickly. It will seldom aim at producing fundamental changes in personality structure, the achievement of full social and psychological maturity, the goals of maximal productivity, strength, and happiness. It aims rather at removing symptoms, restoring workers to their jobs and mothers to their families. In our own time such clinics are resorting to group therapy, a device for spreading the expert's effort over more patients, for socializing the therapeutic process, and for allowing patients to help one another and themselves.

Those who work in such centers come to accept the existence of many weak, immature, dependent persons as one of the hard facts of life. These patients seem to lack the force needed to meet effectively all the demanding and frustrating situations that life thrusts on them. Their original constitutions, the kinds of education and character training their families have provided, the extremes of pressure that they have met have resulted in a type of weakness that is expressed in symptoms, in their inability to put forth effort, as well as in their inadequate and vague life plans, many of which are altogether inappropriate for their circumstances and capacities. In the face of this tide of "Mr. Notquites," so full of feelings of inferiority and incompleteness, the clinician who chooses to treat symptoms only can be pardoned. Reorganizing and reeducating these "weak" selves would take so much longer that, under present conditions, it cannot be achieved, except in rare cases, especially with the very young.

A thoroughgoing therapy for Ron would involve a painstaking review of his assets and liabilities, an attempt to work with his family or any other significant persons who are interested, until all of his basic developmental tasks had been faced and worked through, and until his potential strength and capacity had been fully exploited. Like a concerned parent, such a clinician would have to give, out of his own certitudes and strengths, the force to shape and energize another life.

Janet found himself caught up in this problem in his work at the Sal-pêtrière. On one occasion, lecturing at the College de France, he offered the judgment that many a neurotic or borderline schizophrenic could manage very well if he but had sufficient means to pay for the efforts of others that he cannot make for himself. There are servants who can smooth the way for the psychasthenic who, put on his own, would find the burden of life too great. (See Janet 1932, p. 258.)

The Case of Marceline

It was Janet's Marceline, whom he described at great length (1893, pp. 690 ff), who first enforced this view on him. This poor working girl who had to run back to Janet about every two weeks "to get her battery charged" might have made a go of it if, like some other patients, she had been a young woman of means. "She was one of these persons who would have appeared normal if she had had sufficient means so that she did not have to go to work and could have, on the contrary, been surrounded by a continuous care from an entourage."

Treating Marceline at intervals (spaced sometimes by two weeks and sometimes by six), Janet observed his patient improve under his efforts; then as she returned to work, facing conflict, reprimands, and constant effort, her energies would subside, a serious disorganization would set in, and, full of symptoms, she had to return to him for another "booster shot" of psychotherapy. On several occasions she remained in fairly good health for months. His contact with Marceline extended from the woman's seventeenth year to her thirty-fifth year, when she finally lapsed into the terminal phase of tuberculosis.

Throughout Janet's account one senses a certain querulous note, almost as though he was irked (and guilty) because of his inability to make Marceline eat, work, sleep properly and to give her that kind of internal regulator that could do without so much "battery charging" from without. He had other tasks. He never seemed to be able to consolidate the gains in a new autonomy, although his hypnotic sessions produced an almost magical change in her behavior. Supported and "rewound" periodically, this strange biological clock could run for a week or two, and then she had to be given his attention again: persuaded, cajoled, hypnotized, set right. He had gradually become a kind of built-in adjunct to the life of this woman, a service station for replenishing her energies. Worse (and no doubt because Janet felt a certain guilt), as soon as he withdrew his support, attempted to see her less often, her eating, her sleeping, her work, her very life and spirit would descend to a lower level of functioning. She knew what she needed: Janet called it a "trance need," although it was something much more complex, much more human than that.

The Case of Mary Lackwill

Whatever her real name may have been, the central factors of inertia and fatigue justify her pseudonym. Mary's neurasthenia was more severe than

Ron's, and the phobias and obsessions of the more severe forms of psychasthenia had begun to appear (see Janet 1903, II, 18 ff).

This patient, 37 years old at the time of her study, reported that she had had convulsions in her first year of life. She had always been prone to depressed moods and to boredom. Her interests were tenuous, and often ran aground, as though insufficiently charged with energy. A serious attack of depression had occurred at 20, when she was first faced with the problems of marriage. Instead of finding new energies in the excitement of the life opening up to her then, she became so exhausted that she could scarcely get out of bed; she wept endlessly, and a cloud of gloom settled down upon her. Instead of formulating a clear course of action, her mind became involved in a tangle of ruminations, in a welter of thoughts that she could not resolve. What might fairly be called "a fear of life" did not crystallize into specific phobias, however, and after about six months the attack subsided.

This was not a new pattern for this family. Her mother had had a similar illness following the weaning of a sibling of the patient. The mother's illness, too, was self-terminating, coming to an end spontaneously after a few months, but a year later the mother committed suicide.

The patient married, and two children were born without unusual incident. It was not until she was 32 that the neurotic pattern reappeared. The family had changed their residence and style of living, and had opened a store that she and her husband managed. Her mild depression, now seemingly precipitated by the new responsibilities and extra work, lasted this time for a year. Then at 37, a bout of neurasthenia was precipitated by financial losses which took away their business and left her husband without work.

Radical changes, new responsibilities, sudden losses and worries, seemed to be more than this person could cope with. At the beginning of her present illness, her symptoms and complaints centered about her digestion, but as her depression deepened, her mental symptoms moved into the foreground, and she ceased to complain about her stomach. Instead she began to overeat, to complain of head pains, aching eyes, back pain, pains in all her joints, and she suffered from a painful fatigue. Although it seemed exaggerated, in view of the very little work she accomplished, it was very real to her. Her "failure of nerve," if this is what it amounted to, had left her with ruminations, preoccupations, and an inability to will. In place of productive action, her attention centered on her symptoms. She hesitated to undertake anything, as though sure that her strength would be inadequate. Her fatigue had now become chronic, a perpetual withdrawal from work in advance, a fear of action, and a vague "What's the use?" attitude.

The patient could not reach decisions in simple things. Going to bed was postponed. Going to sleep was too decisive an action; she suffered from insomnia, lying awake in futile rumination. Her immediate memory was also clouded; she became unsure of what had just happened. This was not too surprising, since she paid such poor attention to the events around her. Her poor grasp of reality, her lack of lively plans, left her feeling empty. Her mind seemed to lack both structure and significant content. Her conversation was affected: there were breaks in her thought, gaps in her memory. Events seemed to enter awareness and to leave after having made little trace. She complained: "I no longer know how to cry." Things did not move her as before. Curiously, her skin was dry, and her mouth and nose as well. If she was sensitive, it was to her neurasthenic aches and pains, rather than to the life going on about her.

Mary's neurasthenic depression lasted this time for two and a half years. In the last year there was some improvement, but most of the symptoms persisted. Her complete cure occurred in a manner that was highly unusual. One evening the patient found herself alone with a niece who was approaching the end of confinement. When the niece began to feel the labor pains, Mary went out in search of a midwife. Failing to find one, she rushed back to the house to find herself confronted with a birth in progress. Life did not adjust itself to her neurasthenic needs, and her numbed lack of emotionality now suddenly gave way before the crisis. She did what had to be done, by herself, and the excitement, and possibly the jubilation at her power to deliver a healthy baby boy, neutralized whatever inhibitions had clouded her mind before. She said afterward, "I could feel something change in my head," and she pronounced herself cured. She came to visit the clinic the following day and gave her version of her cure, and she remained symptom-free for two years.

Janet, who often pointed to his patients' emotions as the factors which had exhausted their energies and left them with a lowered psychological tension, was forced to admit that some emotional states are *sthenic*: they not only lift our level of functioning while they last, but leave behind them a higher and enduring level of integrative power. Although few clinicians will be able to command the precise emotional crises that will rouse their benumbed neurasthenics, it is well to remember that there are means, quite apart from the talking cures or insight therapy, that can alter the depressed functioning of such patients.[31]

JANET'S THERAPY

What Janet did about these cases of neurasthenia gives concrete meaning to his notion that the disorder involves a lowering of psychological tension. In Ron's case we are moved to conclude that the disorder is a mild one if it improves under such minimal therapy, a dietary reform and the positive suggestions implicit in the therapeutic interviews. In the case of Mary, the rut formation of depression lifted in response to a sudden, exciting crisis; by implication, the screen of inhibition that was swept away was a set of generalized failure responses, a fear of action. These accounts make neurasthenia appear to be a disorganization of integrated striving, rather than a true physical exhaustion; although the symptoms center around fatigue, it is a curious kind of "learned fatigue," a *maneuver* that checks action, and a pattern that can be displaced. These cases alone, however, do not do justice to the complexity of Janet's thinking. At least five types of therapy are described for this type of illness, and a brief characterization of each will help fill out his conception of the nature of the neurosis.

---

[31]Manfred Bleuler (1931) describes an experience of his father when the latter was a director of a mental hospital in the Swiss countryside. Neither telegraph nor railroad facilities existed at the time, and the director could not obtain the nursing help that he needed at once to meet an epidemic of typhoid that had broken out. He was forced to assign nursing duties and responsibilities to schizophrenic patients, and he found that many could assume these duties as normal people would, while the emergency lasted. When the trained nurses finally arrived, the majority of the patients fell back into their customary psychotic state, but a few utilized the gains from the experience and proceeded toward a stabilized improvement.

1. Suggestion and Hypnosis

Janet did not hesitate to use hypnosis to induce an anorexic girl to eat, to restore memories that had been lost, to increase the sensibility of a hysterical who had become anesthetic over some bodily surface, to convince a hysterical paralytic that he could walk. Like many of his contemporaries, he believed that there was something inherently tonic about hypnosis, something that "boosted" a patient and restored his run-down energies; he cited many instances in which a cluster of neurasthenic symptoms disappeared after a single hypnotic session. He also used this suggestible state to restore lost functions, since he found that, with this type of support, a patient could perform in a way he could not when normally alert. In addition to this kind of reeducation, he used to restore memories and then, by posthypnotic suggestions, to keep them alive in the waking state. When the rest cure was at the height of its popularity, he occasionally used a prolonged hypnosis that extended the relaxed state over several days as a means of restoring the exhausted integrative powers.

2. Simplification of Life

Energizing a run-down system is only half the story. The neurasthenic who has a limited store of integrative force can frequently function without symptoms when his responsibilities are reduced, when he assumes a simpler role. The rest cure represents an exaggerated form of such simplification. Janet believed that his neurasthenics needed "activity budgets" and some training in living within their psychological resources. Poor in spirit, they had to learn to spend less. "Restrict investments, call in some of your poor loans, spend prudently so that your effort will bring in income, maintain a reasonable reserve." Janet spoke to them like an investment counselor addressing a person forced to live on a small pension. At other times he resorted to a military analogy: "Make a concentrated attack on a limited sector; achieve a local victory; take care how your troops are deployed." A counselor might say, to a distraught mother of four, "Put away at least half of their playthings; they will use the remainder more constructively." Perhaps the same holds for adults in an affluent society who have more than they can use or "own" in any psychological fashion.

There was a double concern that shaped Janet's thinking at this point: (1) He wanted to restore the individual's power to act, for in the rewards of successful action lies that sthenic influence that keeps an individual strong. (2) He wanted to keep the undertakings within the limit that could be handled by a person with limited powers.

3. Liquidation of Unfinished Business

One of the most important ways of simplifying life and of stopping the slow leaks that deplete our energies is the habit of constantly liquidating unfinished business. Write the letter, pay the bill, complete the term paper, finish spading the garden, see the importunate committee, terminate the contract negotiation that has been hanging fire for weeks. Each one of our projects requires a certain investment of energy, and this energy remains tied up until the project is finished; then the "charge" of energy (that bit of "vigilance" that keeps it alive) can be withdrawn, and the revenues of satisfaction in accomplishment can be enjoyed. Even the sharp loss of energies from a project that is definitely abandoned may be less than the slow drain of continuing false hope. In life, as in any business, we dare not invest in too many projects, carry on too many operations at the same time, distribute all of our working capital, for the call of some important but unplanned outlay will find us bankrupt (and in the neurasthenic this spells "symptoms"). The unfinished bits of business that we carry about are not just dormant traces: they are partially active, they irrupt into other actions, they continue to influence our choices, and they keep gnawing away at our energy stores. With too many of these on board, our conscious and voluntary functioning becomes inadequate. A clinician may find that, to cure his patient's inability to generate and regulate a normal field of action, he may have to study his schedules of action, searching out those unfinished projects that rob new trajectories of action of their force. In contrast to Freud, who had rather specific kinds of unfinished business in mind as he explored the unconscious of his patients, Janet assumed that any type of preoccupation could function in this fashion, and did not expect to find any automatic increase in the subject's coping powers with the discovery of the leak. A change in action, a new way of distributing and liquidating energies, had to occur.

4. Reeducation

Aside from the general effort to correct a faulty character formation, which would require a therapist to do what the family and a lifetime of experience have not done, there are sometimes specific and relatively minor jobs of reeducation that need to be carried through. For example: (1) a student may not know how to study; (2) a youth may not know how to choose a reasonable diet; (3) a girl may not know how to hold a simple conversation; (4) a housewife may not know how to plan her twenty-four hours a day; (5) a young wife may not know what is expected of her in the marriage bed; (6) a boy can lack all knowledge of guns, games, and sports.

The list of possible skills that could be important to a neurasthenic's progress would be long. Strange lacunae in training are reported as existing beside the most highly developed talents. Janet's Nadia could compose and play beautiful music, read seven languages and converse in five, and had a keen appreciation of literary values, yet she could not go down town alone, bargain with a storekeeper, plan a week's menus, give orders to a servant, do the simple chores about a household. The very thought of a child near her made her shudder, and she could not meet strangers or endure the presence of another person in her household, with the single exception of an old and faithful servant.

Thus reeducation can reach all the way from imparting information to moral suasion, scolding, and cajoling; and from nondirective counseling, in which the counselor seems little more than a good listener, to an active reconditioning in the face of settings which have proved disorganizing. Sometimes this is an uphill job, against all the patient's inclinations. Like the child who does not want to like spinach, the psychasthenic who shrinks from people does not want to become "intolerably extroverted." A counselor's approach has to be flexible, and he has to learn to "play by ear."

5. Raising the Level of Psychological Tension

Throughout his experience as a therapist, Janet struggled with the one problem that was inherent in his own theory of mental illness: how to make the psychologically impoverished rich. When the cause of mental illness is defined as a weakness in integrative strength (by whatever name), the therapeutic effort must attack this deficiency, finally. Even in those who are limited by their genetic endowment and by irreversible constitutional "scars" left by physical illness and psychological traumata, there is still some scope for a therapy that improves and consolidates the level at which they function. Even with a limited ceiling to effort, psychological tension can be seen to rise and fall with every success and failure, with every turn in health and in physical well-being.

What a "total push" this calls for! Physical therapy, hydrotherapy, baths, massage, diet, improved regimen of work and play, and even the restoration of the normal functioning of a sensory surface (through hypnotic treatment) lifted this level of functioning. In Janet's time physicians were also using electrical stimulation and massage, as though to enliven a central neural mechanism by the currents and manipulations. Janet also used exercises, drill, games, whatever would require the interested and concerned attention of the patients. The latter had to "go to school" under a taskmaster who tried to excite, arouse, exhort, encourage, and test their performances, announcing their improvement when it occurred and lending his approval to their efforts.

Moving from the simpler physical and intellectual exercises, he encouraged his neurasthenics to enter into social activities. He urged them to participate in games, such as billiards or bridge, involving the individual in a limited group. He urged some of them to give a tea, plan a dinner or picnic, trying to get them involved in planning, making social arrangements, asking for help and risking refusals, participating in the mild clash of personalities, for all of these activities entail a certain "cost," a spending of psychological energies.

If therapy for the neurasthenic begins with rest, a restriction and simplification of life, it must end in planned risks, in tasks that will call for more and more serious involvement of the person in testing and defining reality, in goal-setting and discharging of responsibilities.[32] Finally *real work* must be

---

[32]In his account of the methods he used at Silver Hill Sanatorium with phobics, William Terhune (1949) describes such simple tasks as going into town on a shopping expedition, going unaccompanied to a movie, and so on. Planned beforehand, discussed afterwards, these tasks, absurdly easy for the normal person, were used to demonstrate powers that the patients believed they did not have, and to train them in structuring and discharging actions until more difficult ones could be managed.

introduced, and those roles that are required of the responsible man who can decide, plan his actions, and liquidate his own unfinished business. The therapist who would advise such a patient has to estimate the costs of each of these outlays, the possibilities of success, the risks that are involved.

The first rule of these investments, in the case of bankrupt personalities, is "The action must succeed." Beginning, therefore, with tasks that are easy, he tries to prove to the patient that he has the capacity for successful action. As the patient is guided from easy to more difficult tasks, the therapist hopes finally, with occasional spaced interviews and fewer contacts, to make the patient capable of acting as his own mentor and guide. Thus the second rule is "A therapist must begin a planned retreat as soon as he can safely withdraw his guidance." The aim of therapy is to make the therapist unnecessary. The extreme of complete guidance might be symbolized by the animal in a harness. When such a technique is used to eliminate the taste for alcohol (by substituting a mild nausea at the mere sight of a cocktail for the impulse to drink), the part-process can be eliminated rather quickly. Cured, the patient's integrative level and self-regulation are pretty much at their old levels.[33] The more serious problem is to correct the weakness that required alcohol as a crutch.

The sensitive one, the person who lacks some of the force required to integrate his needs in a changing and sometimes difficult human environment, seems to have been brought to a halt at the threshold of his tasks. Tired, tense, exhausted, a mixture of heavy-lidded numbness and restlessness has settled down upon him. To break this vicious cycle of fatigue, tension, and failure in advance, Janet tried to exhort, to build him up physically, to suggest, to reeducate, to emotionize him, to give him a plan and an organization of action that would both conserve his limited forces and direct him toward further growth in that essential integrative power.[34]

The modern emphasis that has turned the attention of so many students of the abnormal toward the period of infancy, as though in that period all our inadequacies were first nurtured, would involve a therapist in much more questioning about this period than Janet attempted. Although he sometimes mentions this aspect of his patients' lives, it was not his central concern, to judge by the hundreds of case histories he published. He does not ask, "Was this an apprehensive, sensitive child who was not protected as he should have

---

[33]Reacting against this form of passivity in the patient, as well as against the directive aspects of psychoanalysis and of moral suasion, the "nondirective" school has fled to the opposite extreme. Oddly enough, as De Grazia (1952) points out, at the end of twenty counseling sessions, the nondirective therapist's clients have acquired a common vocabulary and a common philosophy of self-regulation. They have been directed, in a nondirective sort of way.

[34]Although this plan of treatment was designed for a group that Janet felt was constitutionally weak, reflection suggests that his devices fit every man, in some degree. For each of us has limits that he must discover, and each must wage a constant battle to maintain or exceed his "area of freedom." We observe, in the child who is just emerging from dependence, an "I want to do it myself" stage. In the adolescent this "appetite for autonomy" grows intense. Why, we ask, should Dostoevsky make his cynical Grand Inquisitor so sure that the appetite for such autonomy with responsibility is so weak in the average *adult?*

been, not loved enough?" Or "Was he, on the other hand, loved too much, and not too wisely?" Occasionally he stopped to describe an authoritarian mother who has produced a daughter who is hesitant, scrupulous, full of doubt and indecision, and in need of excessive direction. He also described a kind of hothouse education that kept a youth from mingling with his peers, from learning how to box, swim, dive, sail, ski, shoot, fish, fight, and feel confident and at home in a world of men. He did speak about a training that is required if the child is to be adjusted, not merely to his family but to the people next door. There have to be risks. The growing youngster has to stay away from home overnight, for a week, for a month in the summer. He has to learn to speak in public, to dance, to date a girl, to work, to wait, to promise and deliver, to finish his tasks. He has to experience a bit of that Spartan's training, to become inured to cold, wet, unpleasantness, arduous work, and rough commands, to get dead tired and still keep going, to control the complaints that rise to his lips, to meet his personal crises with his own devices and to take the consequences of failure, to work with and for strangers who will not defend or excuse his whims as the family did, and to develop something that we call character, which the soft and the immature do not have. Otherwise he will behave, from time to time, as a neurasthenic, and release rest behavior and other defensive maneuvers when effort is called for.

The full-scale therapy described in Janet's *Psychological Healing* requires a degree of effort and concern from an expert that few can purchase or command. The cases of Ron, Marceline, and Mary Lackwill received something less.

FREUD'S THEORY

While his contemporaries were experimenting with various methods of treating this "nerve weakness," Sigmund Freud was arriving at a quite different conclusion. Compounded from ancient folklore and backstairs gossip, from ancient Mosaic law and Hebraic hygiene, from religious teachings and the practices of asceticism, there was a tradition, half-explicit and half-hidden by a sense of guilt, waiting for someone to apply it to the problem of psychoneuroses. If it existed in the private knowledge of many medical practitioners, it had not had public and official sanction in high places. It was something of a shock to Freud to hear Charcot remark, in private conversation, that there is always a sexual cause in the neuroses, for the great teacher had never incorporated this theory in his writings or in his public lectures.[35] Freud was ready to develop this notion, even if it caused a scandal.

---

[35]A group gathered around Charcot were discussing a case of Brouardel's in which a wife suffered from symptoms, a husband from impotence. The phrase Freud remembered from Charcot's lips, and recorded in his *History of the Psychoanalytic Movement*, ran: "Mais, dans ces cas pareils, ç'est toujours la chose génital, toujours, toujours, toujours." Ernest Jones, Freud's biographer, describes Brouardel as Charcot's assistant, a medical jurist, and the one in that circle around Charcot who most impressed Freud. Jean Delay (1956b) tells how the young Andre Gide, sent home by a schoolteacher who suspected him of "playing with himself," was suffering from a variety of nervous symptoms and was taken to the great Brouardel. The boy, only nine years old, was shown a glass cabinet in which the doctor kept the surgical instruments that he used to operate on "bad little boys" (*petits garçons vicieux*).

Although both Freud and Janet learned from Charcot, Freud returned to Vienna to develop a theory quite different from that which flourished at the Salpêtrière. He began to analyze the sexual life of his patients, to look for the libidinal-emotional roots of unconscious ideas that had been repressed. He had arrived at his conviction long before the supporting evidence was available, and he set out to demonstrate that there is *no neurosis where there is a normal sexual life.*[36] Neurotic symptoms arose, he thought, because some taboo, some repression, some frustration, prevents this life-giving instinctual force from finding a free and satisfying expression, *free from guilt.* In his letters to Wilhelm Fliess (in Bonaparte, Freud, and Kris 1954), in whom he had found an interested and sympathetic supporter, we can see his ideas taking shape: He had the courage and determination to apply them to himself, to analyze his own dreams, to study the unconscious causes of his own anxiety neurosis there revealed, and to publish both his dreams and his conclusions to all the world.

The neuroses which really interested Freud were the *psycho*neuroses, for in this type the symptoms had a meaning, which an astute analyst might read long before his patient realized what he was revealing in his dreams and free associations. Freud attached great importance to the interpretation of dreams, which he regarded as "the royal road to the unconscious." His cases were as exciting as a new Agatha Christie "whodunit" to the avid reader of detective fiction. Each case presented a special problem in tact and diplomacy as this spelunker of the unconscious found that he had to reveal something to the patient that was often unpleasant and usually shameful. This communication to the patient would, he hoped, result in freeing the patient from the bondage to the repressed materials, a freeing of libidinal energies that no longer had to be restrained. The new insights and the resultant growth would mean "a great leap forward" for the patient, and when psychiatry had assimilated his discoveries, this not always artful art could become scientific.

As his method developed, he found that the occasions where repression had first segregated and checked these vital impulses had to be sought in earlier periods, until he found himself seeking evidence about the early infancy of his patients. If the ego of the adult is weak, he concluded, it is because the energies that should have gone into strengthening its structure had been diverted, constrained, and even turned against the self. Like naughty children, banished to the basement when important guests are expected, these repressed libidinal impulses continue their clamor until the distracted ego can scarcely keep his mind on his conversation. The explanation for the lowered psychological tension that Janet was speaking about must lie in this division of the forces at that early date, in an inner conflict which left

---

[36]Charcot and Janet might have agreed had Freud phrased his generalization as: "It is rare to find a neurotic person leading a normal sex life. His neuroticism will find expression here, as elsewhere." But they would have looked on the sexual factor not as the primary cause, but as a symptom that was not always present. The Salpêtrière group knew as little as Freud about the sexual life of those who are symptom-free.

too little energy free to attack outer tasks or to structure a future in the real world. The energies were still there, within, but locked up.

"ACTUAL NEUROSES" AND PSYCHONEUROSES

As he studied these psychoneuroses and worked out his theories of causation and treatment, Freud became aware of a division within his cases. Although he was still ready to ask each patient the same question, "What about your sexual life?" (if not directly, then indirectly, as he set the patient to giving free associations), he was prepared to find in the answers of one group a rather simple explanation for the illness, an explanation that raised practical (and moral) issues rather than medical and psychological ones calling for skill in depth analysis. This group he called the *actual neuroses,* which were, he thought, as somatic in origin as any neuritis or inflammation of the meninges.

Four characteristics marked the actual neuroses as different from the psychoneuroses: (1) symptoms express physiological effects, anatomical arrangements, not meanings at the psychological level; (2) their cure may not require a psychoanalysis at all; (3) the underlying explanation is biochemical in the same sense that drug effects are chemical; (4) the cause of the symptoms is acting in the present. The three neuroses that he was ready to include in this category were neurasthenia, hypochondria, and anxiety neurosis.

The cause of neurasthenia is masturbation. Freud stated it bluntly (1894, 1926, p. 68). His followers expanded the notion. Regis and Hesnard (1914, p. 200) were to add, "The actual neuroses are secondary to a diffuse and direct intoxication of the organism by poisons resulting from genital disturbances at the physical level." A still later effort to salvage the theory and to put it, at least speculatively, on a believable physiological basis was made by Fenichel (1945, pp. 186-92, 238), who also suggested that some chemical change which occurs when the sexual drive is normally satiated is missing in masturbation, coitus interruptus, or otherwise frustrated sexual excitement, and in consequence, "disturbances in chemistry result. Undischarged excitement and affects mean an abnormal quantity and quality of hormones, and thus alterations in physiological functions." From such a hypothetical abnormal blood chemistry, these revisionists of Freud's doctrine traced such effects as changes in the excitability of the autonomic nervous system, headaches, fatigability, backache, paresthesias, atonic dyspepsia, flatulence, retarded digestion, and sexual impotence.

In spite of these efforts to specify some biochemical change that results from masturbation, no such change has ever been identified. Freud's very positive language has never found confirmation in any careful study that correlates practices and symptoms. Nonetheless, Freud wrote as though he had such evidence: "Neurasthenia in males is acquired at the age of puberty and becomes manifest in the patient's twenties. Its source is masturbation, the frequency of which runs completely parallel with the frequency of neurasthenia in men."[37]

---

[37]Bonaparte, Freud, and Kris 1954, p. 68. This passage is included in a draft of his theory which he sent to Wilhelm Fliess with this notation appended: "You will of course keep the draft away from your young wife."

Freud prepared an answer to the objections which he anticipated, since, even then, it was generally assumed that masturbation was much more widespread than neurasthenia.

"The principal objection to my proposition of a sexual aetiology for the anxiety neurosis will probably run as follows: abnormal conditions in the sexual life of the kind mentioned are found so very frequently that they must must be forthcoming *wherever one looks for them.* Their presence in the cases of anxiety neurosis quoted does not therefore prove that the aetiology of this neurosis is to be found in them. The number of people, moreover, who practise coitus interruptus, is incomparably greater than the number of those afflicted with anxiety neurosis, and the great majority of the former tolerate this unhealthy condition quite well. [Freud also included certain contraceptive practices, such as the use of the condom, among his causative factors.]

"To those I have to reply that we should certainly not be right in expecting to find in the neuroses an aetiological factor of *rare* occurrence, seeing how very great their frequency admittedly is, especially that of anxiety neurosis; also, that it actually fulfils a postulate of pathology if in an aetiological enquiry the aetiological factor is proved to be more frequent than its effect, since for the latter other conditions are also required (disposition, summation of specific conditions, reinforcements by other 'ordinary' injurious factors); and further, that detailed exploration of suitable cases of anxiety neurosis proves beyond question the importance of the sexual factor."

In his case studies and in his correspondence, Freud also expressed convictions that the practice of masturbation need not be continued into the present (as his theory of the actual neuroses elsewhere asserted) to result in neuroses. He describes individuals who had practiced autoeroticism between the years of 12 and 16, and who later, after years of normal sexual relations, had to be treated for neurasthenia or anxiety neurosis. Freud also compared autoerotic habits to other forms of addiction, to alcohol, morphine, or tobacco (see Bonaparte, Freud, and Kris 1954, p. 238). Indeed, he looked upon the other addictions as a "masturbation substitute," autoerotic, oralerotic, and he thought that these other habits advertised their history to any alert clinician. He even thought that autoerotism played a great role in hysteria.

Freud's theory of the actual neuroses has been a source of embarrassment to some of his followers. Dalbiez (1941), who wished to credit Freud with being one of the first to take a stand against "the academic conceptions of the harmfulness of masturbation," implies that, in the end, Freud discounted its pathogenic effects. When Freud spoke on the question before the Vienna Psychoanalytic Society in 1910 (see Jones 1955, p. 301), he seemed ready to admit that the harmful effects were primarily those of the moral conflicts aroused, the persisting guilt feelings, and the tendency for masturbation fantasies to bind the impulse life in such a way as to weaken the interest in any real partner. He stressed its essentially infantile character: it both reactivated and expressed this component. Nevertheless, he was still affirming his belief in its real and physiological aftereffects in 1925, when he wrote:

"I am far from denying the existence of mental conflicts and of neurotic complexes in neurasthenia. All that I am asserting is that the symptoms of these patients are not mentally determined or removable by analysis, and that they must be regarded as direct toxic consequences of disordered sexual processes at the biochemical level." (See Freud 1925, pp. 45-46.)

It is interesting to compare Freud's judgment with that of Kinsey. Investigating the sexual histories of 5,300 males by his interview technique, Kinsey found that 5,100 reported masturbating, and he adds, "It would be difficult to show that masturbatory activities have done measurable damage to any of these individuals, with the very rare exception of the psychotic who is compulsive in his behavior." Kinsey suggests, in fact, that boys who are not psychically disturbed tend to find in masturbation a regular sexual outlet which has "alleviated nervous tensions; and the record is clear in many cases that these boys have on the whole lived more balanced lives than the boys who have been more restrained in their sexual activities.[38]

The history of our attitudes toward masturbation contains some rather depressing chapters, some rather recent; it reveals how deeply rooted a tradition underlies some of the guilt-charged tensions that clinicians have uncovered. Kinsey cites both Jewish and Christian authorities who have condemned the practice, and to a mass of folklore still extant he adds a ruling of the United States Navy Department (1940) to the effect that an examining surgeon who finds evidence of such indulgence in a candidate shall reject him from the list of those eligible for the United States Naval Academy. Folklore attributes a wide variety of failings, from pimples to insanity (and softening of the brain) to this cause. The mothers who threaten their children in order to check the habit appeal to this same folklore as they search for something that will frighten their offspring. According to Mabel Huschka (1938), who had considerable pediatric experience to back up her study, these mothers say: "You can get a blood poison from that, and you can die. Do you want me to take you to a doctor and have him cut it off? You will not grow strong. You will become a cripple. You look so pale! Are you doing things you shouldn't? It will stunt your growth. It will make you very nervous and unable to concentrate. I know two who got crazy and died as a result of masturbation." And to these threats of mothers, Sigmund Freud added his authority: "You may become a neurasthenic!" His followers who speculate about possible chemical factors in the blood stream, or who attempt a neuromuscular theory of the tense fatigue state, compound the folklore with pseudoscientific formulations.

Fenichel tends to place more emphasis on the conflicts that cluster about the practice and to minimize the hypothetical toxins. The chronic fatigue,

---

[38]Kinsey, Pomeroy, and Martin 1948, p. 514. Kinsey's statement is, of course, a judgment. One would search in vain for evidence in his data to support his belief that the boys who masturbated "lived more balanced lives." This may have been clear to Kinsey, but it belongs with other intuitions, beliefs, and opinions. This conflict in the conclusions of the "experts" is instructive in that it warns us of the nature of such beliefs. In order to complete the logically possible opinions, we should quote an *authority* to the effect that masturbation is wholly unrelated to mental health, is neither hygienic nor harmful nor correlated in any way with the symptoms seen by those who treat neurasthenics. But this, too, would probably be an opinion, since the supporting evidence would be most difficult to obtain.

he argues, may very well be due to actual muscular tensions. The frustrated fantasy life, the persistent aftereffects of self-stimulation, the sense of guilt probably produce low-grade and persistent tensions in the musculature. This argument would make the neurasthenic's "nervous tension" basically an affair of the muscles, something that a good workout in the gym and a sound night's sleep could easily correct. But frustrated sexuality is not the only source of tensions of this type. Fenichel's extension of Freud's notion suggests that the clinician would do well to seek out any sort of chronically unsatisfied need or purpose as a potential basis for the symptoms. Thus extended, Freud's interpretation of the disorder would lose its uniqueness. Like any "psychophysiological symptom" that arises out of current stress or frustration, the neurasthenic's symptoms would be *actual,* in Freud's usage, but the symptoms would call for an open mind on the part of the clinician reviewing the status of such a patient. Freud's interpretation now seems narrow, too exclusively preoccupied with a single form of frustration, and based on a hypothetical physiology that has never found supporting evidence.[39]

The housewife who says, "I always give in to my husband; I know it is unfair, but quarrels completely incapacitate me and leave me jittery, drained, and with chronic diarrhea" is not speaking merely about sexual conflicts, but about a cold war of coexistence with threats of passionate explosions in the background. If her suppression of hostile feelings leaves many tensions unreleased, unliquidated, the causes of the "incompleteness" which produces wakefulness, fatigue, and an aching back demand a more general theory and therapy.

It was such an extension of Freud's theory that led Edmund Jacobson (1929) to propose his relaxation-training method of treating psychoneurotics, a treatment which many psychiatrists (analytic and otherwise) regard as too peripheral, too symptomatic. In teaching his patients how to relax chronically tensed muscles, he was aiming at the proximate cause of the subjective symptoms. In general, the more recent recruits to the army that follows Freud have concerned themselves with the broader areas of interpersonal conflict and with the earlier infantile roots, rather than with the peripheral outcomes. Where Freud was willing to dismiss neurasthenia as of no great interest to the psychoanalyst (since, if masturbation and other frustrating practices are stopped, the symptoms disappear), his successors, even those who insist that the cause for the tension will be found in the sexual sphere,

---

[39]While Freud was advancing his notions of neurasthenia in Vienna, the American Adolf Meyer was formulating his notion of the neurasthenic: "The term should be reserved for the cases combining the symptoms of *great exhaustibility* and irritability, depending largely on the mental attitude of lack of repose and of ready recoverability, frequent head pressure, palpitation and uneasiness of the heart, gastric disorders, phosphaturia and oxaluria, and, in men especially, often abnormality of sexual responsiveness. It is necessary to distinguish acute forms following exhaustion or infectious diseases in persons without hereditary or constitutional defect, the subacute and chronic forms or habit neurasthenias frequently without heredity, and the chronic constitutional type, said to be to a large extent familial.... It may be well to specify cerebrasthenia, myelasthenia, gastrointestinal neurasthenia, vasomotor and sexual neurasthenia." A truly eclectic (if not "buckshot") diagnosis (Winters 1951, II, 327).

have wanted to ask: "Why does the individual remain arrested in an infantile or juvenile pattern? Why does he not transform his tensions and drives into a more constructive search for a partner, or into the establishment of a home, or into the life of a couple and the family? Why is he content to find gratification in autoerotic practices instead of learning new adjustments to that real world shared with others, a world in which affection, admiration, and gratification can be earned in a more mature fashion?"

From Beard, via S. Weir Mitchell and Janet, to Freud, there is a continuing tendency to evaluate the neurasthenic as "a man with a weak ego." In the general scheme which psychoanalysts, following Freud, have developed, the weakness of the ego is commonly conceived as arising from the fact that the person is divided against himself, because a half of him that desires, that seeks indulgence and gratification, is condemned by another half that wishes to go beyond these gratifications, that wishes to be mature, to achieve, to merit. If the ego could kill desire, as Buddha preached, or if it could kill that superego which is the mainspring of guilt and of the need to amount to something, the inner war might cease. Ibsen's Peer Gynt and Gide's Ménalque seem to preach the gospel of "gratification in the passing moment." These figures are idealizations of irresponsibility, a kind of adolescent dream. The ascetic, turning against the desires which enslave him, sometimes pushes his struggle to the very edge of extinguishing life itself. The ebb and flow in the divided self, with its rise and fall in integrative force, leaves the person impaired, at times, weakened by attacks of guilt and anxiety, full of restless tension and insomnia, and unable to will. With its energies impaired and the thrust of action pulled back, with interest centered on some organ system that begins to "act up," imaginary concerns and pseudo-explanations help to keep attention deflected from the basic problem of a better organization of living. Where Freud gives a highly simplified account of the neurasthenic's need to readjust, the holistic accounts present a problem that is almost too complex and ambiguous.

JANET AND FREUD CONTRASTED

Between the views of Janet, who dismissed the concerns of Ron about his nocturnal emissions as exaggerated and too unimportant to discuss, and those of Freud, who saw the actual neuroses as caused directly by the toxins created by sexual frustration, there is certainly a contrast in procedure and attitude. Shall we follow Janet and dismiss the problem as a "pseudoproblem" which only foolish adolescents worry about, or listen to Freud as he gives a medical sanction to some very persistent folklore?

Shall we say, with Freud, that this *actual* neurosis forms the core of a set of secondary developments that arise from a primary ego weakness produced by autoerotic practices? In his notes and drafts of a theory of mental depressions, Freud left various schematic drawings (e.g., see Bonaparte, Freud, and Kris 1954, p. 104) that gave explicit form to the folklore and to his private conviction that the dissipation of glandular secretions and seminal fluid weakened both attentive vigilance and voluntary powers. His argument ran: arising from the gonads and genital structures, by way of both chemical and neural transmission, there are influences which energize the highest integrative levels. Alertness, confidence, ego strength, all the integrative functioning of the higher cortical layers are supported by this neurochemical influence so long as a normal rhythm of abstinence and expression, of sex hunger and satiation keeps this supporting stream of energy strong. Excessive expression, frustrated forms of expression, masturbation, coitus interruptus, the use of contraceptives, all sexual actions where the interpersonal relations and attitudes run counter to aesthetic and moral beliefs, weaken this sthenic influence.

There is no question but what this folk wisdom is carried deep within us, and Freud drew on it heavily. If a wisely managed sexuality makes a man strong, so that, like the morning sun emerging from its chamber in the sky, he too is ready to run his race when he wakens, then it follows that mismanaged sexuality produces weakness, both physical and mental. The adolescent male or female who stands, somewhat timid and confused, at the threshold of life, can find a convenient formulation for his general sense of incompleteness in some private version of this particular bit of folk wisdom. Warned by his mother, perhaps too long ago to remember, he may experience a vague sense of guilt, or perhaps he remembers all too well about things that have never been spoken of since, and his "secret practices" then become the Big Cause, uppermost in his mind. If, perchance, he voices his disquietude to a priest or counselor who, in turn, adds the weight of his authority to a youth's concern, the results get built into a vicious cycle of exaggerated concern and guilt, a half of which is iatrogenic.[40]

Spelling out his conclusions, Janet (1903, I, 633) wrote: "In masturbation, in coitus reservatus, and in normal coitus, it is all the same: these individuals could find sufficient satisfaction *if they were normal*." Thus, he counts the concern about the sexual segment of life (important as it may be) as only one of the expressions of a much more general feeling of incompleteness that has multiple causes, that has frequently existed long before puberty, and that continues to exist into the middle years, long after full opportunities for the establishment of normal sexual rhythms have been enjoyed. Contrary to Freud, Janet found the same hypochondrias, anxieties, and signs of neurasthenic fatigue in patients who had no reason to complain of their sexual life. Where some poorly designed form of the sexual life has become the focus of discontent and the source of guilt feelings, the therapist adds to the patient's problems when he acts as if he shares the patient's obsessions. His task is to divert the patient's interest and effort to more important questions, and his questions and interpretations must be designed to desensitize the patient's concerns rather than to reinforce them.

---

[40]One college woman told her counselor that she had suffered from a severe conflict over masturbation in her high-school years. She had also experienced an extremely painful cystitis (bladder infection) and had attributed it to her own practice of masturbation. "Did your physician suggest this as a source of your infection?" she was asked. "No," she replied, "I simply *knew* it."

It is true, if one consults the patients themselves, many neurasthenics testify to a variety of disturbances in their sexual life. But they also have disturbances in their social life, in their capacity to discharge intellectual work. Whatever task is difficult precipitates symptoms; whatever introduces conflict brings doubts, scruples, and indecision. Whatever calls for promises and goal-setting impels them to make drastic pacts. The "golden mean" is difficult for them to find and maintain. To the sexual concerns of adolescence, Janet would add those of the family, of the profession, of citizenship.

As the analysis of neurasthenia is extended, the symptoms begin to express tensions arising from a generally disorganized personality. Centering too exclusively on the sources which Freud emphasized may make it easy to formulate the problem, easy for a physician to give a kind of "absolution." But just as the symptoms may serve the patient as a screen to keep out considerations of the true nature of his difficulties, the sexual theory of neurasthenia can limit the thinking of the physician and block the types of therapeutic action required. The reports of "quick recoveries," whether made by Janet or Freud, whether accomplished by the use of one theory or the other, raise a question. If the broader analysis of interpersonal relations is the correct approach, as we suspect, neurasthenia may turn out to be both more serious than we had suspected and less easily treated. It can prove less serious when it represents merely the psychological "growing pains" of a confused adolescent whom life will shortly teach what a clinician cannot. It will prove more serious when it represents a fundamental weakness in the organization of the personality, something reaching far beyond the narrow limits Freud first suggested, something that requires much more than palliatives. It can persist from adolescence throughout mature life, and it can be the prelude to a progressive disorganization, an early announcement of a psychosis to come.

GANDHI AND FREUD: TWO WHO WERE OBSESSED

From the superior position of the comfortably adjusted adult, who has learned to take things in stride (i.e., in moderation), it is easy to laugh at the logic of confused youths treated by Janet and the early Freudians. In our time, when "the new sexual freedom" and "the erotic revolution" have carried sexual conflicts into a new phase, in which "shame about chastity" has replaced the "shame about impure thoughts" of an earlier generation, it may seem that we are placing too much emphasis on a dear, dead past. Yet that backlog of folk wisdom persists, and although sexual expression is far more free in our time, there is no evidence that psychological conflicts about sexuality are any less intense. The "tired blood" and the "tense depressions" that the advertisers make the target of their daily commercials are still with us; if anything, we are more "obsessed" with the sexual problem than our Victorian ancestors.

One form which the obsession takes is to make sexuality *the* vital force, the source of all creative energies. Aldous Huxley, in his *Ends and Means,* gave considerable space to a doctrine proposed by Unwin (1934), a doctrine close to the central notion behind the Tantrist yoga developed between 400 and 800 A.D. (see Eliade 1954). Mahatma Gandhi and his wife, in mid-life, came to the conclusion that they could not hope to accomplish their life mission unless all sexual relationships ceased. On the basis of this conviction, Gandhi further worked out a scheme of dieting that would reduce sexual desire. The writings and the letters of this saint-reformer-politician show a compulsive concern about food which, in his thinking, was also linked with *brachmacharya,* personal purity, and spiritual power. Even his "love letters" to Miriam Slade (1949) were filled with this obsessive interest in dieting. Food, he reminds her, should be taken as medicine, and in minimal amounts. His *Guide de Santé* is full of ascetic "wisdom." Gandhi is the direct inheritor of Gautama Buddha, who had a similar view of desires.

The obsessive concern with the problem of sexual abstinence is still an obsession with sex. Sexual expression, this perverse saint had come to feel, was worse than a mere temptation: it was a lust-filled trap that can catch and destroy the unwary. It must therefore be fought against, and this fight is best won when it is accompanied by a fight against all other forms of indulgence, for indulgence is one, and all indulgence weakens spiritual power. There is a curious similarity between Freud and Gandhi in this basic fear of sexuality. It is not too startling, therefore, to discover that, like Gandhi, Freud too decided to give up sexual life in his forties.[41]

In his letters we can see Freud trying to find a "golden mean" in which a mixture of gratification and restraint would provide him with that sthenic stream of impulses which would support his cherished "psychic apparatus" and preserve his productivity. Narcissist and Epicurean, he could see how one should fast a little while, in order the better to enjoy the banquet later, and he struggled to find some middle way in which a self-regulation could guarantee optimal pleasure, optimal creative force. Too much self-denial, as he noted when he tried to give up his pacifier, his cigar, had to be corrected: the stress of his ambitious program of work and writing required some interspersed pleasures to tone up that work apparatus. And so he fantasied a schedule of gratification dosage, interspersed with periods of ascetic denial, all aimed at a maximum ego strength.

As one reads the letters of these savants, one is forced to conclude that neither found any great serenity. Each, in his own way, had his sights fixed

---

[41]Observing that a new "religion" appeared in the twentieth century, a religion that often claimed Freud as its patron saint, Gregoire notes that while the religion claims to release us from centuries of inhibition and a false spiritualization of sexuality, the public forgets the capital role that Freud assigned to sublimation. If Freud's personal sexual life was brought to an end voluntarily much earlier than is the case with many men (in his forties), one can estimate the gap between the founder's practices and the popular version of sexual expression the public attributes to him. We might emphasize, here, that those who make a fetish of erotic expression, who see, in the sthenic effects produced by this life force, the source of mental energy and creativity, are as prone to obsessive concerns about sexuality as those who, like Gandhi and the ancient Tantrists, seek to husband these forces like a miser.

upon perfection. Gandhi struggled to achieve *satyagraha,* a perfection in which sublimated love dominated all lustful claims of the body. Freud, with a self-designed role resembling that of Prometheus, the light-bringer, planned to shatter the myths that veiled the eyes of man, to free man for the life of reason, to guide him in his search for maximum impulse strength, with all forces in proper balance. Both men betrayed certain neurotic mechanisms, and both achieved great strength of purpose: one directed the movement that freed India from British control; the other shook the world from its complacent denial of the darker side of our impulse life, refashioning the view of man for the twentieth century. Neither Gandhi nor Freud waited for the patient collection of scientific data to support the conclusions about which they were so certain.

Freud was clear about his purpose, but remained unsure about the attainability of that working sublimation he aimed at. In his own middle years, his letters reveal that he was struggling with neurasthenic symptoms which he had himself diagnosed as originating in autoerotic indulgence. His willingness to interpret the neurasthenia of an adult male as the outgrowth of masturbation in childhood showed his doubt about ever escaping from the aftereffects. No mere *insight* into these relationships could cure an actual neurosis.

Psychoanalysis is still in the process of achieving a mature evaluation of sexuality. As it throws more and more weight on interpersonal elements of sexual love, the id becomes "psychified," more human, less simple, less like an itch or a toxin eliminator. Love becomes a need that requires us to be human, for it needs to be merited if one is to be sure of it, and returned as well as sought. Some of the neurasthenic's concerns suggest that he has not developed to a very mature level of selfhood. His counselor has to raise problems in living so that he may go beyond his concern with symptoms and beyond his self-diagnosis, his self-regulation for the sake of the self and its body. Freud's mechanics of ego strength are scarcely adequate as a theoretical basis for healthful self-regulation; the neurasthenic's deficits are more pervasive than some blood-stream toxin, more difficult to repair than a mere loss of seminal fluid.

THE NEURASTHENIC AND HIS EMOTIONS

Human emotions can be viewed as responses to blows, blows which sometimes strike an organism that is totally unprepared for them and incapable of summoning enough strength and skill to master the novel and massive pressure. A stimulus-response psychology tends to treat certain primitive emotional reactions as reflexes; some theoreticians wish to select the visceral component of the response as the appropriate content for the term *emotion.* When emotions are studied in the laboratory, they are frequently assumed to be just such measurable reflex responses to stimuli. Watson's infants, pinched or rapidly lowered, and responding with a cry or a gasp along with random striped-muscle contractions, offered us an example; so did the subjects of Carney Landis, who were asked to thrust their hands into a bucket (which happened to contain live snakes). The "blow" studied is sometimes a chemical one, as when the responses of Marañon's subjects, who were given injections of adrenalin, were compared with the typical emotional reactions to other kinds of *psychological* stresses.

Developing more slowly, and from less obvious causes, an emotional state may be one of the end-products of accumulating fatigue, or it may depend on some toxic condition that alters the response level (as in a prolonged fever); the changes in behavior may emerge without any clearly organized coping responses of attack or defense. (Peevish and fretful, easily angered or frightened, the patient, we say, "is not himself.") Equally gradual is the development of a feeling of well-being or mastery that comes with good health, balanced living, and a sense of acceptance and belonging among well-loved companions. If we could only stave off the asthenic form of emotion (by well-planned rest pauses, by a design for living that brings satisfaction, and by a direction of efforts on those basic and essential goals of human existence that Angyal repeatedly emphasizes: homonomy and autonomy), we might insure a "sthenic" state. One can readily see why the emotionality that accompanies the chronic neurasthenic state should prompt any clinician to consider the problem of emotional control. The patient himself often "experiments," flirting with Zen Buddhism, or New Thought, or Christian Science, or lysergic acid, or he avidly reads the reports of those who have found a new avenue to mystic experiences. He is vulnerable to the claims of all those who have "the remedy" or the gospel.

The introspective neurasthenic seems to be striving to become "aware of his awareness" so that he can control not only his acts but even his thoughts. As we follow a "genius of introspection" of Amiel's type (Brooks and Brooks, 1935) through the pages of his journal, we become aware that what began as a planned approach to an examined life, as a way of escaping from his feeling of "being lived by life rather than directing it," became in the end an absorbing interest in dissecting experience, a pathway to a deepened consciousness, even a substitute for living. His dissection of experience preoccupied him so excessively that he came to fear it as the destroyer of his will. His examination of his life became a flight from living, and his journal began to run itself on a minimum grist of action. His "method of control" became a chronic introversive maneuver; the manuscript of his unpublished journal ran to 17,000 pages.

Not all of these "self-regulators" plunge inward, away from life; some turn outward instead. They cultivate adventure, excitement, "happenings" that will lift their spirits, and some become manipulators of others, using human beings as one would use a medication.

ADVENTURISM, EXCITEMENT, AND ROMANCE

Whether it is the roller-coaster, gambling, lion-hunting in Africa, riding in the steeplechase, or the pursuit of fair women, adventure and excitement may be sought, not so much in and for themselves as for their effects on the self, for "kicks." This "objective" is more important than the "objects" sought or used, which seldom hold the interest of these essentially self-centered ones. When interests of this type pall, as they are likely to, they are promptly dropped for a fresh source of excitement. The boost to a flagging spirit is the thing. One of Janet's patients, whom he refers to as Ne., fought off a recurrent numbness that kept descending upon her by letting little drops of boiling water fall upon her flesh, drops that produced painful burns where they scalded the tissues, but that also brought a momentary lifting of the lethargy and numbness that she was struggling against (Janet 1903, II, 483).

Others, who seem much more normal to us, seek to dissipate their boredom is a poor one, and the creative energies required for "real actions" are low, by some "happening," the "crazier" the better. When the design for living the appetite for these "happenings" is apt to grow. A bit of shoplifting, conduct that lies just outside the bounds, the excitement of forbidden fruit, a row, something that will get attention or make a stink, an affair, can add the fillip. All this is an answer, or rather an attempted answer, to the boredom, emptiness, gnawing guilt, feelings of worthlessness, but most of all to the numbness and fatigue that are so troublesome to the neurasthenic. Whatever causes the state, *something has to be done.* The neurasthenic's loves will assuredly be evanescent and subject to the *decrystallization* that Stendhal wrote about: his partners in the dance of life have to be changed if interest and potency are to be renewed.

Occasionally these adventurers seem to court disasters. They scale the face of dangerous mountains, and enter into relationships that involve them in desperate issues, as though to force their sluggish livers and torpid hearts to supply their cortical cells with the glycogen and oxygen that would awaken vigilance, make real actions more possible, supply the power of decision. They use their emotions as a fireman would use a forced draft, fanning the fires of vital reserves until the new energies restore that sense of vital engagement with life. What amphetamine does for the weary truck-driver numbed by hours of monotonous driving over the turnpike, these adventures do for the bored, restless, and numbed neurasthenic. The daily round of work and suburban living, the endless mending and cleaning, the church-children-kitchen complex that a peasant might be satisfied with, do not do it: something *exciting* is required. There is even a *nostalgie de la boue,* a yearning to get mucked up a bit, which can drive a bored bank clerk into the Foreign Legion, or off to Tahiti where, like Paul Gauguin, he imagines he will find excitement and time to cultivate the spirit, with no wife, family, or other ponderous responsibilities of a bourgeois existence that "get him down."

Among the solutions which these seekers imagine and plan for, one of the favorite is the romantic adventure. Usually these adventures are entered into with the thought that there will be "no tomorrows," no encumbrances, and no serious commitments. A call girl or a gigolo might do, for a while; these paid entertainers have learned how to simulate real feelings and produce an illusion of affection.[42] But like the kleptomaniac who gets no real kick, finally, out of stealing small articles from the dime store, and who is, therefore, compelled to go on to greater risks, the romantic adventure-seeker who wants a real "boost" will find himself drawn into near-real involvements, real risks.

While it is possible to play at life and love, risking a little involvement at times, the bored neurasthenic faces a dilemma: the more playful his adventures are, the less potent they are in restoring his spirit; the more commitment and risk they involve, the more powerful their effects are, and the more they will call for a large expenditure of the energies and integrative powers he lacks. He intends to arouse emotions that will restore a sense of vitality. He seeks the illusion of potency and charm, vicariously, for he intends to remain aloof, secure, untouched, never trapped.

LOVE ADDICTION

One of Janet's patients, whom he calls Pepita, described herself in these words (Janet 1919, II, 925):

What is the history of my life? All my serious nervous disorders came on during the periods when I was behaving "properly," and I could only get well by doing the other thing. At home I lived most respectably, most decorously; but really I have a taste for debauchery; I love the atmosphere of vice, it intoxicates me and makes me well again. I like to live several lives at once; one life is too monotonous for me. If it were possible, I should like to be sometimes a man and sometimes a woman. Since I cannot manage that, I change my environment, my name, all the external circumstances of my life. I contemplate the strange existence of people who amuse themselves, who engage in conspiracies, who steal; I mingle in their activities. Besides, I think that I have been able to do fine things. I wanted to cure this young fellow, to raise his spirits, to find him a position.

These "love addicts" diagnose their own needs. Perhaps genuine love has little or nothing to do with the case, and perhaps the kind of fidelity and

---

[42]As we try to describe these fringes of life where real emotions are simulated, it is apparent that Freud's concern about masturbation should also have embraced these more elaborate forms of autoeroticism. The immaculate self, keeping aloof from involvement and "playing at life and love," uses others as *things*. Ethically he is operating on the same plane as the youth with his masturbation fantasies, his "pillow books." Or, since his partners may be damaged as he uses them, perhaps his ethical plane is really much lower.

There are many in-between stages in which romantic adventures are just adventures, understood by both parties to be just temporary arrangements. In these adventures the freedom from any long-term involvement or serious consequences is a necessary feature that makes possible a certain ease of action (and action is never easy for the neurasthenic). But excitement without responsibility, and a shallow "play-acting" of affectionate relationships, can easily become boring! The quality we are trying to identify also accounts for some of the difference between play and work, between a private jotting-down of thoughts in a notebook no one will see and the writing of an article for a professional journal or a tale for the public to read, between a serious engagement and a flirtation.

responsibility that Denis de Rougemont writes about lies wholly beyond their ken. Nonetheless, the word "love" is on their lips continuously. If, as Janet implies, the cure comes about because of a kind of excitation that momentarily lifts their level of psychological tension, their partners affect them as a placebo affects the suggestible patient, for a while. The analyst who chooses to diagnose such illnesses as the outcome of some earlier failure in their love life, of some deficit in the affectional ties as a child, can insert his views into their thinking, since he, like the patients, assumes that "love is all." Though they have met with repeated failures, they are sure a perfect love relationship is waiting for them, will come easily and naturally and solve all of their problems. Their husband's inability to satisfy them merely proves that he is not the one. Perhaps there is something about Pepita's bourgeois existence that makes a real love impossible. Both she and Freud seem to fit in with a certain romantic tradition that our novelists have kept alive.[43]

Another incurable romantic reported by Janet had similar experiences. Married to a good fellow who proved dull and unromantic, she required an affair, she was sure, if she was to get out of her doldrums. When her state of emptiness returned on one occasion, she thought that it might be a good thing to give religion a whirl, and she began visiting a certain priest every day. "This was the beginning of fresh intrigue, with renewed 'mysterious' assignations," she told her physician. Her melancholy disappeared. The priest, however, grew uneasy and decided to pull out of the intrigue; when he left the country, she plunged back into her neurasthenic state. Neurasthenia is more than a mood: it reflects the way one is managing one's life.

THE NEUROTIC NEED FOR LOVE INTERPRETED

We accept and understand the organism's need for food; we count the needs for shelter, safety, and security as basic. This is the way living organisms operate, and they either have built-in reflexive-instinctive mechanisms for correcting such deficits, or, as in the higher animals, where these matters are loosely organized, they soon acquire them. In the cases we have been discussing, the person himself defines his troubles as a "need for another," a sexual partner, a lover who will excite, arouse, sympathize, praise, threaten, endanger, and somehow complete that feeling of incompleteness. Such an "addiction" calls for a partner who can awaken, emotionize, give life to, reorganize, give a new center to a life that has run down, grown dull, feels isolated.

---

[43]Oscar Lewis (1965, p. xxx, Introduction) joins this same tradition when he describes the Rios women. "Money and material possessions, although important, do not motivate their major decisions. Their deepest need is for love, and their life is a relentless search for it." With multiple "marriages," many of them never legalized, with an unusually high proportion of them having been prostitutes, they are capable neither of giving their children consistent care nor of giving or exacting fidelity to or from spouses. The *word* is there, but it has a very shallow meaning. This aspect of a "poverty of *culture*" can exist at any social level, even though it seems to be concentrated at the very bottom of the social pyramid and is sometimes misjudged as the "culture of *poverty*."

This "hunger" is obviously more than a simple sex hunger: both Pepita and Janet's other love addict were married. If they experienced a sexual boredom (or frigidity) with their spouses, in all probability they experienced an interpersonal boredom, a work boredom, a life boredom, as well. Shall we say that nature, in designing these reaction systems, did not fit them out with responses that could long endure, or that nurture did not develop within them the resources to transform their life situation into something better? The romantic tradition, especially in those novels so dear to adolescents, would have it that chance, in allotting partners somewhat blindly, aided and abetted by emotions which send shivers down the spine and transform "the other" into a thing of crystalline beauty, also brings about commitments between the "wrong" partners, engagements that simply can never work out well. A de-crystallization process will inevitably begin; little disgusts will come to the surface; hostilities will emerge; soon the partners will begin to bore each other; the marriage bed will become a chore; the excitement will vanish. The partner is not "the right one." Another one, perhaps, will do.

Some of these "seekers" do not define their need as anything more than a simple need for excitement: they need someone to arouse, emotionize, lift them, give them a "charge." If there is a "level of arousal" that is maintained by the action of the cells of the limbic area in front of the hypothalamus, a stream of excitation that keeps the whole reticular-cortical apparatus charged so that the individual is quick to pick up "challenges" and to relate events to his purpose, this limbic area is "fatigued" in these neurasthenic love addicts. Their "engagement" with a sweetheart or with a job is apt to run thin after a short while. The patterns of integration that another might build cumulatively into a solid design of collaborative purposes of a couple tends instead to fall apart, to run down, to leave the individual "out on a limb," isolated.

Among these patients there are a few who define their need differently. What they need, they are sure, is someone with spiritual authority over them, someone to boss them, order their lives, set them back on the track when they deviate, not so much because they do not *know* what they should do (though doubt easily becomes a central feature in the psychasthenic), but chiefly because they lack the staying power and the inner fortitude to put into practice what they know full well they should do, what they really want to do (if we can take their word, in interview). They seem to want to borrow a kind of integrative energy from the guide they are looking for: a new pastor, a new psychiatrist, a new lover-critic-guide.

Such seekers after guidance present us with an interesting question. "How," we ask ourselves, "can a weak, suggestible, distractible, easily fatigable person, who lacks the integrative strength to manage his own affairs, *give to another person the authority to induce these very changes in his conduct that he cannot produce himself?*" "Hypnotize me," he tells his counselor. "I want to stop smoking and you can make me do it if you use hypnosis." Does not the hysterical patient master his paralyzed limb in this special state, with the suggestions of his counselor poured in his ear, while *he is completely relaxed?* He seems to be able to act if he doesn't have to try, if he does not attempt it voluntarily. With this special type of suggestion, with the authority that he has given to the hypnotist, he is now able to carry out a regimen that he cannot impose upon himself. Sometimes the obese patient goes weekly to his physician, just to be weighed and cajoled into another week of dieting, as though he did not know that the excess weight is caused by what goes in through the mouth, as though he could not read the scales, as though *he could not tell himself to eat less.* These patients seem to have to draw upon some socially supported bank account of integrative energies, some faith in others, some belief in the power and authority of the man in the white coat, or some myth about love. We do have a romantic tradition that imputes special powers to a lover, a complete selflessness that makes the needs of the loved one equal to his own.

Such dependence on this "social bank" is not so exceptional, when we stop to think about it. We ask the bank to withhold a monthly allotment for the Christmas fund. We ask Washington to hold out social-security payments that we can collect in our old age, as though we could not manage these things on our own. We buy insurance that prepares us for hospitalization, and pay more for it than we would if we could manage to set such funds aside ourselves.

Sometimes our conservative friends look on this "encroachment" of society on the individual as a process that weakens our individual fortitude and keeps us essentially infantile and lacking in autonomy. What maternal over-protection does for the individual child, government overprotection does for us all, including those business tycoons who connive among themselves to escape from the wear and tear of competition. (Price-fixing might be considered a kind of extension of neurasthenia into the general economy.) Is this impulse, which so many of us share, something much simpler: just an infantile component that is within each one of us, the residue of that early experience when we were the recipients of a generous and unconditional love, a residue that has left needs that we never quite outgrow, and that makes it easy for us to lay our private responsibilities upon the shoulders of another?

To the outsider who watches them, these patients do not seem to have developed a full self-regulative capacity, a capacity strong enough to work out a design for living *and make it work.* A clinician will find that he has to sort out varied types. Sometimes a dependence seems to rest on a constitutional deficit: it begins to be visible in the child and continues throughout life. Though such a person has been assisted to recovery, repeatedly, through some eight or ten rounds of rest cures, electroshock, psychoanalysis, religious healing, Christian Science, or the Norman Vincent Peale correspondence-school form of therapy, he is not guaranteed against the next bout of the same old symptoms. Let a new brand of cure be announced, whether it be existential psychoanalysis, reality therapy, direct analysis, LSD-25 medication, Zen Buddhism, prolonged narcosis, operant conditioning, or conditioned-reflex therapy, and the neurasthenics will show up, hopeful that at last their sense of incompleteness, their doubts, and their fatigue will be understood and removed, once and for all.

Some dependent women find their way into the faculty of a girl's school, the nunnery, or the offices of a corporation that supplies enough fringe benefits (and guidance) to serve as a kind of institutional mother. Their male counterparts can be found in the army, or in a monastery, or in a university. They may even lose their identity (and the need to behave autonomously and with full responsibility for their individual actions) in a militant revolutionary group which provides such a strict discipline that every ambiguity in living is canceled and there is an answer for everything; they have but to follow the party line, or Chairman Mao, or the directive of the central committee. Two qualities in these solutions, present in varied amounts, seem to help some of these patients: (1) On the one hand, the discipline orders, excites, challenges, emotionizes them out of their lethargy, and subjects them to enough novelties, dangers, risks to keep them functioning. (2) The new outer authority orders, regulates, guides them into channels of work and play, a ritual existence with standard coping habits that they could not design for themselves.

There is also a kind of "love addict" who discovers some Dionysian brand of religion, some moist-palmed circle where intimate soul revelations are made, some holy-roller type of revival meeting that provides this combination of fillip and guidance that neurasthenic weakness requires. This is not a new type of discovery: Euripides described scenes in his *Bacchae* (produced in Athens before 405 B.C.) that betrayed his own disturbance as he recognized the terrible import of all this for what one might call the life of reason.

In these seekers, emotions function as blows that set reflex systems reverberating, releasing energies that lift the spirit, for the moment. The ritual relations they enter into *force* a new organization of life and a new level of functioning, so that there is a freedom to act that was lacking. Something like a "wholeness" or unity is felt (even in Nuremberg Square where the shouts of *Sieg Heil!* go up), that unity that had been lost or badly frayed by the daily wear and tear, or submerged under an accumulating cloud of inhibitions. Though we refer to it as a quest, and describe them as seekers, the basic operations involve a certain quality of passivity, a surrender of autonomy and integrity. The desired emotions have to be struck off by the blows that act on the jaded organism's receptors, by the shouts of the coacting crowd of believers. Such operations do not arise in the natural course of autonomous (self-regulated) actions that are well-fitted into the rest of the design for living, springing from within and embedded in a plan for existence that is intrinsically satisfying.

Carved out of the tribal life, the ritual or festival is designed to produce a collective excitement, a daemonic feeling of possession and of oneness. Whether it is the dance of the Bacchae, of the Hopi Katchinas, or of the Shakers, it lifts that "arousal level," cancels all doubts and inhibitions, pulls the "loner" back into the collective life, and lifts his capacity to act. Like the return to his native heath of some wandering farmer, this reentry into the coacting collective is more important than the wine of the ritual, or the peyote buttons, or the psychedelic drug. Individuation, development toward autonomy and toward responsible choices, is painful and exhausting, at times, as the neurasthenic's fatigue suggests. What a range of "addictions" there are to fill this form of emptiness! Soma, hashish, peyote buttons, alcohol, dervish dances, orgiastic rites, fasting, torture, flagellation, Black Masses—all are pathways to a kind of divine madness, and some of the seekers have been unwilling to settle for anything less than ecstasy, or for what they call a "mystic union" that seems to carry them completely outside themselves.

The neurasthenic can remember other days when his mind functioned normally. His unhappy state may arise out of nothing more dramatic (as cause) than the accumulated inhibitions and tensions of daily living. The "Mr. Notquites" who do not see clearly or feel keenly, and who populate our towns (as Thornton Wilder describes them), are pained by their feeling of dullness, frustrated by the invisible "wall" that somehow shuts them away from zestful living. They yearn for a kind of fulfillment or completion, a sharper vision, a keener feeling, even if it should be a painful one. The moralist is sure that it is the poor design for living or an excessive self-centeredness that is at the basis of it all. The geneticist is sure that it is constitutional. Mr. Notquite himself says that it is his dull wife, the routine of his work, the drab and unpunctured existence where nothing ever really happens. Pepita blamed it on the boring monotony of middle-class bourgeois existence. Even Simone de Beauvoir (1963), who tried so desperately to break out of every barrier placed in her path, concluded at age 57: "I have been gypped. It is the role society has designed for this second sex, to which I belong."[44]

Whatever lies near, whatever is striking, whatever has become the mode in social criticism at the time, whatever is the individual's central preoccupation, tends to be woven into the neurasthenic's evaluation of his predicament. Those on the radical left will be sure that the real cause lies in the disintegration of a decaying capitalist society; those on the conservative right will say, "We are getting soft. We are pampered and undisciplined. It is this creeping socialism that is to blame. We need to return to a rugged individualism."

The Pepitas and the Amiels, who feel like prisoners in this world they never made, imagine a future, another life, a more perfect love, a different and fascinating type of life that would wholly enlist every ounce of effort in them, *not this life!* Others who live beside these discontented ones, in a world that is surprisingly similar and with objectively similar sets of

---

[44]Her words are, "J'ai été flouée." Looking at her face in the glass, feeling age and decrepitude creeping up on her, wondering about her choice not to have a family (and to flout all the demands a middle class would impose on a woman), her autobiography seems to end on a note of horror at having to pursue further a life that has become empty of meaning. A model for many young Frenchwomen, Simone de Beauvoir, her reviewer insists, can find an answer to the question on her mind: "What have I done with my freedom?" It would be, "I have given it to others."

"demands" made upon them, manage to create tasks and interpersonal relationships that are exciting, fulfilling, challenging, tasks that call for responsible action and that yield in turn deep gratification for their serious efforts. These others do not need to use human beings in an inhuman fashion, do not fear the "tomorrow" that inevitably follows any commitment, do not approach life as one would approach a steel trap.

In spite of our shortened work-week, in spite of the highest standard of living that any people have hitherto been able to achieve, in spite of a government that is concerned to provide parks, highways, fish hatcheries, and cultural development to fill our leisure, and social security and medicare for old age, the designs for living of millions of Americans seem to leave something to be desired. The theater, sports, and television, and the distillers (who at annual meetings express their disappointment when the annual consumption has not reached the projected quotas), all leave a residue of felt wants, of feelings of incompleteness, of widespread boredom. While the majority, perhaps, succeed in "living their emotions," regulating their living so imaginatively and constructively that their relations with their world are vital and sthenic, and their emotions a natural expression of that living, others are "lived by their emotions," feel pressured, caught off guard, depressed. In their need some try to use emotions as one would use a cup of coffee, to tide them over their low spots. They play at love, seek excitement, need chemical boosters (many of which only help momentarily by dipping into biological reserves and leaving the person eventually depleted). The millions of whom we are speaking make this an "addicted society." They complicate their lives by unhappy liaisons, by alcoholism (from four to six million, conservatively estimated, are chronic alcoholics), and by the use of drugs. This is the soil in which many psychoneurotic adjustments to life flourish. Emotions, which are capable of being sthenic in character, of supporting good designs for living, are allowed to serve as diversions, distractions, biochemical fillips, or they become overwhelming and depressing. On the asthenic side we call emotions exhausting, arresting, fixating, disorganizing. They possess the individual rather than express his own vital engagement with life.

Is it only the fortunate ones, well-endowed, the tough and healthy, the quick-witted and imaginative, who can escape these low spots of neurasthenic malfeasance? Is it only those who were fortunate in having been disciplined to endure and persist until they work through to satisfactions who can now bear up under stresses and penetrate the frustrating barriers, without turning aside to play the illness game? Are the nonneurotic simply so well-placed among the objective conditions and the supporting circumstances (including family and friends) that a healthy adjustment and a subjectively wide area of psychological freedom is easy to acquire? Whatever the answers to these questions are, the fortunate ones will not need to seek the forced reverberations or the "pep pill" type of solution. Their emotions, arising under a natural pressure in conjunction with their own healthy response to challenges, become a tonic and natural part of living. In a special sense, such a person can regard his emotions as his own. His attitude toward his emotions is neither one of blind trust nor one of fearful mistrust; he neither depends on them nor strives to eliminate them. He certainly would not dream of "cooking up" an emotion by the deliberate use of another human being. He would be too busy living.

On Freedom for the Neurasthenic

Living his life day by day, the neurasthenic will not see all the relevant relationships that an experienced counselor might consider. Indeed, this gift of seeing ourselves as others see us is not only rare, but often painful; a certain toughness is required of each of us if we are not to allow "the look" of the stranger to weigh too heavily. If bodily complaints have become a focus of attention for the neurasthenic, the counselor who would divert his attention and disrupt every form of excuse-making will require all of the tact he can summon, for he is suggesting that another "living gestalt" would be better. To explain the pattern by reference to causes of which the patient is unconscious, to things that have been done to him (by parents or other nuturant authority figures), is often accurate, but it is also good strategy, as a point of attack.

How can a "design for living" be converted into such bodily symptoms? What justification is there for that notion so central to the thinking of many counselors: Think right, live right, shift your accent to the positive, act more wisely, and your body will take care of itself? It sounds, at first, like a brand of Christian Science. It is also very optimistic, and it places the final responsibility, in the end, back upon the person himself.

The psychologist or psychiatrist who works with the Pepitas, or any other type of addict, is confronted with a particular version of the problem of human freedom. As a scientist, studying the behavior of these patients, he seems to be seeking the laws that underlie their emotions and actions. For this purpose, he assumes a determinism that makes these precise outcomes the inevitable consummation of a constitution, a press, a history. Behavior is caused! But as counselor, therapist, or spiritual advisor, he sometimes seems bent upon breaking up those very laws. He is full of the conviction that, even with these constitutions, in spite of these histories, and even under these precise circumstances, *there are other and more productive designs for living that these very same individuals can manage.* Otherwise psychotherapy would descend to mere compassionate support, custodial care, and a diagnostic naming of the categories of malfeasance.

As the young clinician grows "case-hardened," he may lose some of his optimism. He may begin to say to himself privately, even when he is overtly encouraging his patient and guiding him through a reeducation process, "This man is no millionaire of the spirit. I ought not to encourage him to aim too high. He simply lacks integrative power." Or he will remind himself that a recent survey of alcoholics treated in one of the best-staffed clinics showed many relapses among the cures and a minimum of improvement in three-quarters of the cases accepted for treatment. His optimism undergoes attrition as he tests his own powers as therapist, and the powers of his own patients. His own level of aspiration is gradually lowered to "what is possible."

Nonetheless, as surely as he remains a therapist, he clings to the belief that there is a better life-style than the one his patients have found, a way of functioning that—if it is not optimal well-being—is more tolerable. It can be designed! Sometimes it seems to the therapist that there is some inner barrier, some lack of imagination, some paper-thin wall of inhibition that, with a little conditioning, could be penetrated. He designs a reeducation that can more than undo experiences which, if one merely counts the repetitions of errors, one would believe to be a basis for an insuperable fixation, firmly believing that insight, a new enthusiasm, fresh motivation, can overlay the past with a new level of performance. As expert, as therapist, he will believe that he can see possibilities that his patient cannot, that he knows the precise steps that the patient cannot find by himself, that his patient can become free in a sense that he is not now.

That such a therapist should have difficulties within his own family some-times shocks the layman. ("Psychiatrists' children!" the schoolteachers say, as they once spoke about ministers' children.) Is the divorce rate for these "specialists in living" lower than that among other professionals of a similar economic status? The facts give little ground for optimism. Sister Kelley (1961) reports that the rates of depressive mental illness among nuns are as high as the rates among other women of similar ages in similar social strata: another embarrassing fact. Is this freedom which the specialist hopes to bring about only a freedom for patients, for others?

When we begin thinking about therapy for the therapists, we are reminded of the difference between a purely intellectual and technical knowhow, which can be taught as one would teach a skill, and the capacity to live out that same knowledge productively in a world we did not design and with shipmates not always of our choosing. There is a difference between a therapy for Pepita, the ability to so change her life that she will never again fall into that trap of boredom and romantic fantasies, and the ability to make one's own marriage work *if one's partner happens to be a Pepita.* There are limitations inherent in any dependent therapeutic relationship in which a patient must borrow strength from his counselor. Such "gifts" or "borrowings" from a therapist are quite different from the wholly autonomous effort to achieve self-regulation through personal hygiene that does not need pep pills, human or otherwise.

CLINICAL PROBLEMS OF NEURASTHENIA

The clinician who deals with the problem of neurasthenia is plagued by certain "mixtures" of symptoms in which organic and psychological causes are both at work. He can commit the error of treating an essentially psychological problem as though it were medical, physiological, organic. He can be equally wide of the mark, overlooking physiological and organic bases for the symptoms, treating the patient's problems as though they sprang from a "state of mind," acting with all of the certitude of a faith-healer. The succeeding pages discuss some of these mixtures of organic and psychological causes, and point to the need for broad training of clinicians in both medicine and psychology, or for a type of staff structure that permits men of widely differing viewpoints to collaborate with and learn from each other.

SIMPLE PHYSICAL EXHAUSTION

Consider the simplest case, where overwork, genuine exhaustion, under-nourishment produce a subjective state of fatigue and a depression of mental functioning, an inability to concentrate that closely resembles the symptoms of neurasthenia. In their most severe form, these symptoms approach that sense of utter hopelessness and worthlessness that we find in the depressive phase of manic-depressive insanity. Samuel Kraines (1941, p. 155) reported a case that illustrates the clinician's problem.

A 37-year-old woman presented the symptoms of an overwhelming fatigue. Her bodily pains reminded her physician of the complaints of a neurasthenic, but her recent loss of weight inclined him to consider Addison's disease, since the adrenal deficiency in this disorder is also accompanied by marked feelings of fatigue. Failing to find confirmation for this hypothesis, he altered the diagnosis to neuras-thenia. When her history was taken, there was some evidence of an unhappy childhood, of a home that lacked parental harmony. An analyst might have focused on the early mothering, building a case for rejection as the cause of her feeling unloved, unworthy of love, helpless.

It was not long before her physician learned that this woman, the sole support of her four children, was unable to stretch her meager relief allowance to feed the family; rather than eat it herself, she had been giving the food to the children. Iron-ing, washing, caring for the children and the home, making the clothes and keeping up the morale of her flock, although her own was sagging under the bleak and hopeless outlook, she developed these symptoms of fatigue and bodily pains.

A social worker saw that an increase in food allowance was given which de-creased her anxiety. A few days of rest in hospital with a high-caloric diet removed the rest of the "neurotic symptoms." No residual neurasthenic symptoms remained. Like the four out of five cases of combat fatigue that improve with rest, proper food, and security in wartime, this case of "civilian combat fatigue" needed a very simple therapy.

SYMPTOMS TREATED AS BAD HABITS

The application of Pavlov's classical conditioning and other learning principles to psychotherapy has been noted in Chapter 1. Behavioristic (or "action") therapists concentrate on behaviors which other therapists regard as symptoms, treating them as bad habits, with little consideration of their causes. For instance, Wolpe (1961) has developed a technique he calls "systematic desensitization." This starts with a list, composed by patient and therapist, of stimuli that arouse anxiety in the patient, ranked from weakest to strongest. Therapy consists of training the patient to relax, sometimes by means of hypnosis, while imagining the anxiety-arousing stimuli. The patient is "desensitized" to the stimuli progressively until the strongest imagined stimulus fails to disturb his state of relaxation.

Operant conditioning, which is associated with the work of B. F. Skinner, is a form of learning in which desired behavior is successively reinforced with rewards. Bachrach *et al.* (1965, p. 157) report a clinical experiment involving a woman suffering from anorexia nervosa who had been hospitalized weighing 47 pounds. Before the experiment the patient was placed in a hospital room lacking the forms of electronic entertainment which she found rewarding.

At first, any portion of the meal that was consumed would be a basis for a postprandial reinforcement (a radio, TV set, or phonograph would be brought in by the nurse at a signal from the experimenter); if she did not touch any of the food before her, nothing would be done by way of reinforcement and she would be left until the next meal. More and more of the meal had to be consumed in order to be reinforced until she was eventually required to eat everything on the plate.

This subject was discharged after two months of treatment weighing 64 pounds. A year and a half later she weighed 85 pounds, was employed, and had an active social life.

A SOMATOPSYCHIC MIXTURE

Harold Harris (1944) has given us a description of a patient that illustrates both the problem of diagnosis and the fact that neurasthenia commonly presents two faces. The fatigue of the neurasthenic may represent a lack of integrative power that rests on a solid physical basis, but it may be complicated by a kind of "learned withdrawal from action," a psychological form of fatigue that emerges in a not quite adequate personality. His ways of coping with his tasks, less than adequate, can be combined with a feeling of worthlessness, unlovableness, rejection. A clinician can be puzzled about whether he should concentrate primarily on the problem of building up physical strength, or on improving the morale (or social skills) of the patient, or on reducing the press of circumstances that have proved too much for this system of limited strength. He may toy with ideas of a rest cure, a simplification of life, some type of support and encouragement, or an endeavor to lower a too high level of aspiration.

Dr. Harris's case represents an interesting mixture of the two facets of this disorder, and reminds us that life does not obey our neatly ordered categories.

A 47-year-old naval officer, seen in Naval Hospital, complained of fatigue, weight loss, headaches, and general nervousness. The condition had persisted over 15 years, and the symptoms had, in this period, shifted from one complaint to another. His nervousness, gas pressure, palpitation, high blood pressure suggested a chronic emotional tension, and the complaints sounded like that "windy melancholia" that was once believed to center in the hypochondrium.

In his discussion of his complaints, the patient revealed feelings of inferiority; he expressed the fear that his symptoms might be of neurotic origin (his anxiety anticipating a corresponding evaluation from his physician). The case was diagnosed as "psychoneurotic anxiety with neurasthenic symptoms," and a routine course of psychotherapy was planned.

Tests undertaken in the course of treatment revealed a Brucella infection.[45] The brucellosis was treated and the patient returned to full duty with his parting observation: "I've always known that I had various evidences of neurosis, but I knew it wasn't all neurosis. I can live comfortably with my neurotic manifestations now that I feel so much better physically."

A PSYCHOSOMATIC MIXTURE

A clinician is called on to assess the personality that bears the symptoms of fatigue. If he deals with an adolescent, he may have to treat both phases of the disorder, acting *in loco parentis* while struggling to eliminate physiological symptoms by a biologically oriented medicine. Wendell Muncie (1941) has presented the case of a man in his early thirties who was less mature than his years would lead one to anticipate.

"The patient had been bedridden for three years before coming to our clinic last year. He was known to have a low basal metabolic rate and had been treated with thyroid extract by thoroughly competent physicians with only transient and indifferent success. He had taken to bed through the conviction that rest was his only salvation, and this had reached the point where he was resting in anticipation of the effort which he never was quite able to get himself to make. He lived on his inheritance and so managed to get along without actually calling on the charity of strangers. Repeated examination at our clinic confirmed the hypothyroid status, and he again was placed on thyroid extract. At the same time an attack on his attitude to life was made by means of a personality study and the encouragement to socialized effort with definite goals within his immediate reach, to increase his self-confidence. After about four months this patient was leading an active life, and was doing volunteer work several hours daily in the medical school library. He left the hospital and continued to do well."

Here a defeatist attitude had developed over a long period. The readiness to take to bed, the passive acceptance of guidance, the lack of any very lively life-plan, all made the hypothyroidism and the chronic fatigue seem a small segment of a much larger problem. If the symptoms of this rather weak and immature personality function as a roundabout and substitute method for direct coping with life, for enlisting aid, acquiring pity and a certain minor form of affection, and for rationalizing his nonfeasance, whoever undertakes to eradicate them opens up the problem of encouraging a normal maturing to a proper adult status. The fact that, with support, this 34-year-old man achieved the status of a volunteer part-time library worker is not the kind of victory that would make us extremely confident about the future; it implies a "need for guidance" of a type that is in short supply. His very weakness tempts a counselor to become his spiritual advisor, to use the energetic forms of therapy that leave little for the patient to do.

---

[45]Milk is a common source of this infection, which produces undulant fever, weakness, loss of weight, and anemia.

Hypoglycaemic Fatigue: Somatopsychic or Psychosomatic?

Alexander and Portis (1944) have called attention to a type of fatigue that is associated with lowered blood sugar. This condition may involve faulty action of the pancreas, an overactive vagus nerve, a hypothalamic parasympathicotonia. Pushing their description of nine cases that they report still further, these clinicians suggest that behind the faulty autonomic responses there are also failures in living, a more global failure affecting the patients participation in social life and producing a poor centering of any life plans. Each of their nine patients studied presented three features:

1. *The asthenic syndrome.* The symptoms reported included boredom, ennui, a general loss of the zest for living, a let-down feeling, a feeling of emptiness, and a general sense of drift and aimlessness. For these patients, household duties, social obligations, office work, vocations, and avocations had all become dull and distasteful. The doctors identified a characteristic daily cycle: the patients awakened, tired. Their fatigue mounted as the forenoon advanced. After lunch it lifted slightly; and then, once more, the spirits sagged to a low point in the late afternoon. The cocktail hour, a hearty dinner, would bring relief. At the lowest points of the day the patients complained of headache, sweating, vertigo; on a few occasions there would approach a feeling of incipient bodily collapse, a fear of loss of control. As in many aging persons, there was a "fear of action" and of those demands for effort that role responsibilities bring.

2. *Low-grade stress; a chronic, unrelieved sense of "ungratified living"; and an expectation of failure, rebuffs, and rejection.* The behavior of these patients suggests that their action systems are never fully tuned up, tensed for the fray: they meet life with something less than full emotional participation. They do not "feel things," they say, as they did formerly.

3. *A flat sugar-tolerance curve.* The curve in Figure 4 suggests that there is something unusual about the patient's conversion and use of sugar, that too much insulin rapidly sweeps the blood stream clean of that energy-supplying glycogen. This suggestion, in turn, raises questions about the pancreas function, about the vagus nerve that innervates the pancreas, about the parasympathetic center regulating vagus action from the hypothalamus, and about the whole psychodynamic and emotional pattern that involves the hypothalamus. If the physiologist is content to stop at the hypothalamus and to speak of a "vegetative retreat" (see Gellhorn 1963, p. 302), the more holistically minded psychologist will want to know what underlies the "failure of nerve," the retreat of the *person*. These patients show a parasympathetic dominance, where the normal "fighter" has a healthy adrenal-sympathetic action that compensates for the challenges and puts a physiological floor under effort.[46]

---

[46]The hypertonic parasympathetic nerve also produces activity in the acid-secreting gastric glands; it lowers heart rate and blood pressure. The organism is on a "rest footing," prepared to digest a meal, to relax, to withdraw from action, even while the situation makes the person tense, anxious, tired.

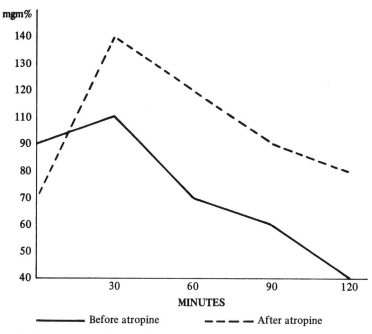

FIGURE 4. THE FASTING BLOOD-SUGAR LEVEL OF HYPOGLYCAEMICS.

For the therapist this description poses a problem. Can he reverse the cycle by proper analysis and treatment of the patient's problems in living, so that, with new insights and encouragement, a new design for living can remove the *psychological* causes of this "vegetative retreat"? Or is his proper port of entry the chemical one, as when he uses atropine to check the overactive vagus or gives some type of "hypothalamic booster" that will set respiration, heart, thyroid, adrenals into a pattern of sympathetic dominance? Rennie and Howard (1942) had reported a series of patients treated by the first method: they had employed psychotherapy to restore a normal level of activity, and, as a result, found that the glucose-tolerance curves of these treated patients returned to the normal form. They concluded (p. 282), "The hypoglycaemia seems secondary to the psychiatric disorder since it has been shown that it disappears with the management of the psychiatric condition.... Treatment of hypoglycaemic symptomatology in a certain group of such patients might better be focused on the personality disturbance." In short, they suggest that the "physiological parts obey the whole."

According to the Alexander and Portis analysis, which favors the psychogenic interpretation, an ideal condition for producing this ennui, fatigue and vegetative symptoms is a chronic low-grade stress, an anxiety that is not sharply focused on any object and, especially, whose causes are unknown, repressed, forgotten, vaguely grasped if at all. The homeostatic failure (with the overactive branch of the parasympathetic supply) becomes a critical link in a vicious cycle, secondary to the psychodynamic failure but, in turn, an essential cause of the fatigue. High insulin, low blood sugar, failure in energy are then seen to emerge in personal action as an intensification of aboulia, incapacity for effort, and withdrawal from action and "failure in living." "Body" and "mind," which we have so long separated, here are seen as inextricably interwoven. The practical question is "Where shall we first intervene in the cycle?" It is not "Which is the cause?"

The therapy pursued by Alexander and Portis was a "buckshot mixture" of atropine, altered diet, and psychotherapy; a proper evaluation of the therapies is therefore difficult. Five of their nine cases responded to medical management alone; four were treated by varying mixtures of medication and psychotherapy. The possibilities may include: (1) a type of physiological failure that is the primary factor, with secondary, psychological "neurasthenic features" a consequence; (2) a type that closely resembles other types of neurasthenia, but in which there is an additional and secondary parasympathicotonia that helps to fixate a vicious cycle that originated in psychological causes.

An Evaluation of the Therapies

Genuine fatigue that has been "earned" by hard work, real dangers, and short rations—including combat fatigue—responds quickly to rest, food, liquids. We saw this in the case reported by Kraines. A disabling bad habit—refusal to eat, for instance—may be removed by means of operant conditioning, as in the experiment reported by Bachrach *et al.* (though we cannot be certain whether this patient would have resumed eating without the rewards she was given). Successful treatment of a debilitating organic ailment can help a patient to cope with "chronic feelings of inferiority," as in the case reported by Harris. On the other hand, in a case of hypothyroidism reported by Muncie, the patient only left the hospital after getting strong "encouragement to socialized goals within his immediate reach." In nine cases of hypoglycaemia reported by Alexander and Portis, five patients responded to medical management alone, whereas four seemed to require varying mixtures of medication and psychotherapy. But large questions remain. To what extent was the procedure emphasized by the therapist reporting the specific cause of improvement? To what extent will the reported symptoms, or other symptoms recur? Finally, to what extent have the patients become dependent on their therapists, and can a dependent patient be considered cured?

When a "need for guidance" is great, and when some very directive method of therapy can give such a patient the feeling that he is understood and accepted, that he has the support of a strong personality who will make him feel good and capable again, something akin to an addiction to guidance can develop, and more quickly than any true consolidation of autonomy. Janet, who used hypnosis in many of these cases, speaks of a "trance need" (1898, I, 423 ff). This restful, sleeplike trance state asks so little from the patient, and gives in return for an easy submission a lifting of the burden of fatigue, pain, and general sense of incompleteness. Cured of an "attack," these patients tend to react to any return of their fatigue, or of their gnawing sense of incompleteness, with a clear sense of their need to return to the clinic to "get their battery charged." With this type of weakness and this type of treatment, physician and patient may rest content with a recurrent dependency as a modest type of therapeutic goal. A more radical therapy would have to find some way to increase that integrative force, that tolerance of stress, which seems so lacking in these psychasthenics.[47] Wherever the constitutional view prevails, so that such patients are regarded as basically and biologically weak, the clinician is apt to settle for half a loaf, using any ameliorative devices that can render the patient symptom-free for a short time. Such a view also tends to make him urge the patient to keep his level of aspiration within attainable limits, and to choose some relatively secure and simple niche in life, there to regulate his energy output in the light of those symptoms that regularly warn him when he has transgressed the boundaries of safety. This is certainly a course more easily followed than any that attempts to bring about a full maturing of the personality and an optimal development of integrative powers.

This constitutional view is completely rejected by some theorists. Consider the position of Angyal (1965, p. 87):

"If one considers the person's total course and conduct of life, what is it ultimately that makes neurotic living different from healthy living? The basic human tendencies are the same in normal people and in neurotics, and all the potentialities are the same. There are as many gifted, finely organized people among neurotics as among healthy people, if not more. I think it would be very difficult to defend the thesis that neurotics are basically inferior because of constitutional factors; such theories exist, but they do not have much empirical support. Neurosis is nothing but an attitude acquired by the child in the process of re-relating himself to the world after his original separation from it. On the basis of the experiences he has had at the time, one or another kind of attitude may develop. In either case the person pursues the same general goals, but in a different spirit, with different kinds of expectations about the outcome of his efforts."

Such a view is to be contrasted with that of Janet who said, in effect, "these are not millionaires of the spirit! There is such a thing as *misère psychologique*." Even Freud, whom Angyal follows in many things, did not deny all constitutional differences.

The data revealed by the laboratory studies, where experimental neuroses are produced and treated by conditioning principles, show that the symptoms are apt to recur. Enthusiasm for a particular type of cure tends to wane as recurrent attacks point either to some more fundamental weakness untouched or to the need for a more radical therapy. The Freudian view of this illness did not prevail for long; as psychoanalysis developed, clinicians who followed his emphasis on a sexual factor showed an increasing concern about the structure

---

[47]The trance need closely resembles the kind of addiction developed so easily by these patients when they discover any chemical which "boosts their ego." Amphetamine, mind-expanding drugs, alcohol, mescaline, marihuana, heroin, all have a fatal attraction to those who live on this fringe of life.

of the personality, the importance of reeducation, of insight and a deepened self-understanding.

When one is certain that there is a large constitutional factor in neurasthenia, one can understand how the fact of recurrent attacks is bound to present a challenge to every theory and therapy. Sometimes, when a case is finally reported as treated in late life, the history of the previous attempts at cures makes the case a veritable museum exhibit of types of psychotherapy. The evidence that Eysenck (1966) has gathered points to the conclusion that all types of therapy can succeed, that none has any demonstrated superiority over others, and that spontaneous remission is about as frequent as the cures by any or all methods now in use.

Muncie (1939, 1941) has some pertinent suggestions as to how neurotic fatigue can develop:

1. It may be simply a prolongation of that infantile dependence on a supportive and indulgent family frame, a form of parasitism and an inability or unwillingness to tolerate the stresses involved in moving out from this first protective haven. Instead of persisting *through* difficulty and discouragement, such a neurasthenic learns an easy fatigability, a quick withdrawal from stress, the utilization (and exaggeration) of attendant symptoms.

2. It can arise where goals are vague, far off, unrealistic. Such goals do not generate effective striving or provide the kind of proximate reinforcements that strengthen integrations. Such a person may settle into a rather monotonous and "unpunctuated" sort of living, without risk-taking and without triumphs, particularly when efforts at involvement have led to frustration and disappointment. Not only does the weary round of "forenoon, afternoon, and night" repeat itself, but perception is dulled, and bodily sensations creep into the foreground of attention, where lively interests and proximate goals should be.

3. It can arise out of imitation of those nearby models (parents, relatives) who also live by a neurasthenic plan, and who, therefore, instead of setting the pattern for vital interests and active efforts, create a model of nonfeasance, using their complaints where others put forth effort.

4. The status of an impaired person, since it offers justifiable excuses for nonfeasance, may become a goal in itself.

Once the pattern develops, the soil is prepared for chronic anxieties, limited risk-taking, a defensive, ultraprudent, rigid, and easily exhausted pattern of living. The person sometimes assumes a "hard-done-by" attitude, complaining of the very great pressures he is under, the multiple duties, his enforced role, and shows that he feels that he is somehow an outsider, not quite up to the demands of living.

Muncie points out that the difficulties in treatment arise from the very task of getting the patient to face up to his weaknesses and immaturities, and to the need for some rather painful and unpleasant self-discipline. Some of the clinician's difficulties arise from his uncertainty about the relative weight to be assigned to physical, interpersonal, and historical (rooted in infancy) causes.

The patient, having long used the defenses of a set of physical symptoms and bodily complaints, is loth to have these deemphasized. The therapist who does not accept the patient's self-diagnosis may easily be counted as lacking in understanding. The counselor is faced with the difficult task of preserving a patient's self-esteem while encouraging him to face a view of his symptoms that undermines it. When the much stronger ties to parents and relatives have not been able to produce a normal development, the counselor's slender claim upon him is severely tested. (The counselor is, let us face, it, a "paid companion," a "hired supporter," unless, perchance, he happens to be one of those volunteers who work out of a fund of good will or some deep religious conviction.)

One of the difficult phases of the therapist-patient relationship arises out of the actual personality weaknesses of the neurasthenic. When this type of patient responds quickly to the preferred dependent role and to that authority figure who supplies guidance (and the decisions the patient cannot make himself), and when the patient seems either unwilling or unable to move toward autonomy on his own, it is all too easy to settle for a compromise in which a therapist's strength and skill are in uneasy balance with the patient's craving for dependency. A busy clinician is tempted to assume too great a role in such lives, and, in supporting such a patient, fail to free him.

EPILOG: QUESTIONS THAT STILL PLAGUE US

The summons to action, the challenges that normally arouse the autonomic nervous system to produce a good underpinning for effective effort, seem to produce a kind of vegetative retreat in the neurasthenic.

1. Is it a bad life situation, a monotonous and exhausting type of work, the "trap of a poor marriage," or some other combination of circumstances that leads to this retreat, this sense of failure; is it basically an unpunctuated living with a vegetative retreat as a secondary feature?

2. Is this a vital failure, a constitutional weakness, some basic organic condition that transforms the stresses others find enjoyable and challenging into overwhelming, deadly, exhausting routines?

3. Is it even possible, as some behaviorists assert (see London, 1964, p. 76), "that symptoms may not be meaningful expressions of their motive states, but may be nonsense learned by chance association with some unhappy event" and therefore subject to "unlearning" through conditioning techniques?

4. Is it some indefinable lack of "emotional participation," a lack that originated in some earlier trauma, which has produced this loss of zest, the boredom, that (secondarily) leads into the abnormal vagus action and high insulin output?

5. Does such readiness to retreat indicate a delayed maturity, a prolonged dependence, a weakness in decision-making and positive action, that have gradually produced a cumulative incapacity, not revealed earlier simply because life had sheltered the individual?

6. Are there some more specific developmental causes, such as that improperly liquidated Oedipus attachment that the Freudian looks for?

7. Is it a simple expression of a life failure, a weakness in integrative power, that can spring from a thousand small causes and end in a failure to find a satisfying centering of life on goals that are exciting and worth effort, and that can be faced with confidence?

8. Is this type of organization (psychosomatic) an example of a poor use of the person's psychological capital, a matter of hygiene and the organization of effort?

9. Are the neurasthenic symptoms, the self-doubt, the aboulia, the sense of guilt, "symbolic" of deeper meanings which must be sought by special methods of analysis, and is the patient's haste in departing from his analyst (once medical management has reduced the symptoms) evidence of a distaste for exploring these deeper meanings and facing an evaluation of his life style?

Each of these questions implies a type of theory, and each finds a group of clinicians who prefer a particular line of approach. For example, there must be various types of hypoglycaemic fatigue, and many therapeutic "ports of entry."

When (in 1869) Beard grouped the symptoms of an exaggerated tense fatigue with an accompanying indecision and incapacity for action under the rubric "neurasthenia," the disorder was not new. Chaucer described one form of the pattern in his *Canterbury Tales* (pp. 296-99), when his Parson described *accidie*. St. Theresa, in *The History of Her Foundations,* warned her Mothers Superior who watched over her Carmelite nuns to be on guard against its dangers, along with those of other forms of depression. If and when the term is finally discarded, as some of our contemporaries urge that it should be, for not discriminating among its many forms, and for implying a specific cause (nerve weakness) that has never proved to be a source of useful hypotheses, the pattern of symptoms will still continue to exist.

Since the symptoms sometimes originate in a local organic process, and sometimes represent a more holistic failure in energies and in motivation, the therapist must not only discriminate among several types, but also be prepared to deal with a faulty constitution, a set of psychogenic causes that date from infancy, breakdowns traceable to faulty types of conditioning, an infection in the tissues (e.g., brucellosis), a faulty hygiene of living and poor regulation, or a "dependency addiction," and to use widely ranging hypotheses and many different therapeutic approaches, ranging from atropine and diet to a new design for living, from a very direct and energetic reconditioning to a nondirective or psychoanalytic exploration of a fringe consciousness. The clinician must not only be equipped with the diagnostic skills to discriminate the particular type or mixture that he is dealing with, but also be able to work flexibly and at all levels, biochemical to social and interpersonal.

In contrast with such a flexible and eclectic approach, there have been attempts like those of S. Weir Mitchell or Freud to lump all types into one and to assign a single cause and a single type of therapy. Every new discovery (experimental neurosis, low blood sugar, adrenal deficiency) has a way of being applied to these morose inactives, as explanation and as indication for therapy. Even LSD-25 and the newest of the psychotomimetic drugs have had their takers, and sensory deprivation, the newest form of the oldest rest cure, and other forms of prolonged narcosis have been tried.

Neurasthenia is a peculiar kind of fatigue that does not respond to the simple treatment of rest. Though it is often described as the mildest of neuroses, it can arrive early and persist throughout adult years, incapacitating the sufferer and making him a chronic invalid confined to the sickroom. Because of the vague, elusive, and therapy-resistant quality in some cases, many clinicians dislike this type of patient, suspecting him of malingering and of playing the illness game. Successful treatment can sometimes require an investment of concern and an amount of effort that few therapists are ready to make. Although four out of five patients recover from their "attacks," recurrence of the symptom cluster is common. The moping apathy, the morose inaction, can progress to a serious depression, or it can disappear overnight as the patient is caught up in some new exciting adventure.

Like an "unknown" that tests the skills of the young chemist, the tense fatigue and morose inaction of the neurasthenic test the diagnostic skills of a clinician. The symptoms can alternate with obsessions and compulsions, with the somatic complaints often diagnosed as anxiety attacks or gastric neurosis. The pattern can be left as a kind of residue of weakness as a depression is lifting; it can herald the onset of schizophrenia, or be replaced by hysterical symptoms. Until we have examined other syndromes, we shall not realize the degree to which neurasthenia is related to all of them, even to the organic changes that come with senility.

Chapter 6 • Hysteria

To the older clinician who observes, "Hysteria today is not what it used to be," one might answer, "It never was." In the long span of its recorded history (on which see Veith 1965), from records on papyri dated 1900 B.C. to the current case studies appearing in our journals, its meandering course has involved so many changes in the concepts of the disease, in the observed facts grouped under the term, in popular beliefs and in the attitudes of physicians (or witch doctors or priests), that one is tempted to say that the disease itself has changed. New concepts, new methods of observation, and new attitudes toward the phenomena actually generate new facts. The older categories of mental illness placed epilepsy, Parkinson's disease, catatonia, and many symptoms of the chronic and deteriorated forms of senility under hysteria. The new categories permit the clinician to exclude every disorder with a clear organic basis from the diagnosis of hysteria, which thus takes on quite different properties.

The Egyptians and the Greeks confined the concept to a group of "female complaints," for in their thinking the symptoms were produced by a wandering of the uterus. Displacements of this organ were blamed for such remote effects as a loss of ability to speak, convulsive attacks, and amnesia, and elaborate ad hoc explanations were developed to account for the relation of cause and effect. At other times (as Plato indicated in his *Timaeus*), the uterus was conceived of as a kind of animal within, whose passions and appetites had to be gratified, and whose lusts were responsible for disease-producing excesses (a view which vaguely foreshadows Freud's concept of libido, and the ego's problem of control). Treatment consisted of driving the uterus back to its proper position by tastes and odors that would repel it from above, or of applying to the genitals perfumes and "inviting" substances that would summon it back from below. This emphasis made physicians completely overlook the possibility of hysteria in a male. As late as 1885 Charcot was still taking time out in his lectures to correct this oversight.

We have already commented on the likelihood that many of those punished for witchcraft were hystericals; we might also note that during all this period the medical approach to hysteria virtually went underground. These "patients" were freed from the demons who tortured them sometimes by the flames which devoured their bodies, sometimes by a priest who had learned how to exorcise evil spirits. Meanwhile, in China and Japan, it was the fox spirit that disturbed the susceptible. Neither in Europe nor in the East did the healers discriminate between neuroses and psychoses or between organic and functional disorders. Thus the phenomena we now call hysterical were buried in a mishmash of poorly discriminated illnesses, while here and there relics of the superstitions about the uterus remained.

The category has expanded, at times, to embrace almost half the chronically ill,[1] but in our own time it is undergoing sharp delimitation. The American Psychiatric Association no longer uses the term in its standard nomenclature, except in the special form of "conversion hysteria," a term which implies that bodily malfunctions have been produced by the conversion of impounded libidinal energy into contractures, anesthesias, and inhibitions of functioning. In this particular usage we can read the triumph of Freud's ideas in current medical politics.

Whether the phenomena which until recently have been studied under the rubric hysteria are to be so named in the future, or be referred to as the hysterical component of some other disease, or be completely integrated and explained in new concepts of some other (and possibly organic) disease, or be overlooked altogether (as a social-ethical matter not within the province of psychiatry), it is still instructive to witness what this concept has generated in the most recent past, for without a clear grasp of this past, we shall be in danger of repeating some of its errors.

A young resident-in-training who was privileged to hear the brilliant lectures of Charcot at the Salpêtrière in the 1880's, as Freud, Janet, and Babinski were, might easily have concluded that at last the disorder had been given its definitive form, so authoritative were the pronouncements, so complete the demonstrations before the eyes of the audience. Yet before Charcot was ten years dead, each of this famous trio had published a version of what he had heard that differed as much from the others' versions as it did from that of this charismatic teacher. Charcot gathered together the best of the medical and neurological understandings of hysteria of his time, used what he believed to be the most objective of methods, and added some new features that were then possible as a result of a hundred years of study of hypnotic phenomena. This latter addition took considerable courage, for, since the scandal of Mesmer in the early 1800's, hypnosis had led a clandestine existence, driven underground with other forms of quackery and "fake healing." Only a few had been willing to risk their reputations by openly studying and using the hypnotic state. In Charcot's hands it became, for a time, respectable. As others took it up, it was made to reveal the existence of an unconscious set of mental processes, beneath the level that had been traditionally studied. Without this beginning, Freud and Breuer would have lacked a certain foundation for their

---

[1] Ey, Bernard, and Brisset (1963, p. 394) date this inclusive usage as 1682, and name as their authority Thomas Willis, English physician and anatomist.

new system of thinking, and the *dynamic unconscious* would have had to wait for some other, later formulation.

We shall therefore begin our account of hysteria with a discussion of Mesmer and Charcot, and with a brief survey of the changing concept of hypnosis. Then we shall pay our respects to Babinski and Janet, especially to the latter, whose extended laboratory and clinical studies offer the most complete and objective account of the range of hysterical behavior we have. Next in importance is the development that led Freud and his followers in a radically different direction in search of the causes and cure for hysterical symptoms, a development which today dominates the psychiatric field. Lastly we must pay our respects to the followers of Pavlov, who have used conditioning procedures as a method of eliminating symptoms, content to bypass all considerations of the structure of consciousness, the meaning of symptoms, and the possible involvement of the personality as a whole.

Unsatisfactory as our present state of knowledge is, we can use the discussion of hysteria as a way to understand current scientific theories (and their limitations), even as we use these theories to illuminate the symptoms of patients who suffer from this disorder.

HYSTERIA AND HYPNOTIZABILITY— FROM MESMER TO JANET

The modern conceptions of hysteria can scarcely be understood without a brief backward glance at Mesmer, and without paying a special tribute to Charcot, who had the courage to revive the practice of hypnotism after it had been twice condemned by the highest medical authorities of France. Some of Charcot's friends believed that Charcot was positively foolhardy; as it turned out, he was led by the nose for a while by compliant hysterical subjects who produced for him what they believed they should, an unhappy consequence that has followed many efforts to make a science of hypnotism. It is indeed surprising to find Charcot, a neurologist with strong interests in anatomical findings and in new advances in chemical medicine, risking his scientific reputation in such a fringe area.[2]

MESMER AND MAGNETISM

It was while men were still talking about animal spirits, and before the concept of reflex circuits in the nervous system had developed, that Mesmer developed his speculations about animal magnetism. He was 33 when he published his thesis (1766), which attempted to explain what many had believed since the ancient astrologers had affirmed it: the planets have an in-

---

[2]Perhaps it is our stereotype of the "objective scientist" that is in error. Certainly Freud was not afraid to come out for telepathy, notwithstanding the low repute enjoyed by works on "psychical research," nor did he hesitate to speculate about the inheritance of acquired characteristics (and a racial unconscious) when neo-Darwinism and the works of Thomas Hunt Morgan were making the notion seem foolish to most biologists. Only today, in some of the wilder speculations of those who are interested in the DNA substance, is there a shred of conceptual foundation for his notions.

fluence on man. Is not *lunacy* a word that transparently reveals this ancient intuition? The moon pulls the tides; why not the anima within us? Does not the action of the magnet, at a distance, show that one body may influence another at a distance? But a thesis is only a thesis, and it was more than ten years before Mesmer got around to applying his rather vague notion to human illness. Suppose that a magnet, which can make a compass needle spin or rearrange a group of iron filings, could also act on the fluids which circulate within a human body. Suppose further that Galen was right, that the difference between health and illness is a difference in the animal spirits, the doubly distilled fluids that rise to the brain. Suppose in addition that, instead of being disturbed in their *composition,* as Galen taught, they are disturbed in their "inner" *arrangement.* An ordinary bar of iron that is not *polarized* need only be placed near the strong magnet; its diffusely arranged particles assume an alignment and it now has a *force* that will make a compass needle spin.

These speculations were not wholly new. For hundreds of years the magnet had impressed physicians, but no one since Paracelsus (1493-1541) had seemingly known how to work a cure or develop the theory, until Mesmer. He asked an astronomer friend to prepare a magnet for the treatment of one of his patients. It worked! And all Viennese society heard of it. Mesmer's biographers picture a man who had been something of a socialite and medical dilettante, whose home had been one of the more popular salons of the city. His beautiful home and garden suddenly became a crowded clinic, overflowing with all sorts of patients. He could not begin to treat each one individually and it occurred to him—as he saw the crowd around one of his fountains—that there should be some way to "magnetize" the water so that its good influence could automatically spread to all those who needed it.

Intent on healing, making no discriminations among the disorders he treated as to whether they were "polarization illnesses" or some other type of organic, cellular, or chemical illness, and confining his thinking to the idea of transmitted "magnetic" influences, he must have met with many failures. The medical council and finally the state authority acted to oust him, and in 1778 he fled from Vienna, his departure hurried by a scandal that had developed around one of his failures (and a consequent court action).

But Mesmer was not discouraged. He had even made a great leap forward, for in the course of his work he had discovered that it was not the magnet his friend had prepared for him that did the work. His own hands, *his magnetic passes,* could produce cures. Indeed, he could "magnetize" a tree, a rope, a bottle of water, a fountain; and those who came in contact with any of these objects would "feel the influence." He continued to believe that by this process of "magnetizing," now transformed into a "personal" magnetizing, he could cure illness, and so, driven from Vienna, he went to Paris. There he became "the last word," the newest fashion, and as though a vast reservoir of human need had been tapped, all Paris came to take the cure. Society, both high and low, flocked to his clinic, the Knights of Malta endorsed his treatments. Societies of Harmony sprang up, and large sums of money were raised by popular subscription to support his research. Mesmer walked among the crowd at his clinic in a lilac-tinted silk coat, pausing to touch the body of a patient with a long wand that he carried, to fixate the eyes of one, or to make passes over the body of another. Sometimes he would seat himself opposite a patient, knee to knee, and place his hand on the patient's abdomen, or, making a pyramid of the fingers of his hands, sweep downward from the head and shoulders to the feet, repeating the sweeps until the patient felt that he was saturated with the fluid, for Mesmer was still trying to rearrange the animal spirits, to repolarize what had become disarranged within. Outside the clinic, in the street, the poor were permitted to cling to a rope attached to a "magnetized" tree. (What therapeutic gains followed this diluted influence we are not told.)

From the time of his hasty departure from Vienna to his similar departure from Paris, in 1784, there were only six short years, during which Mesmer rose to the pinnacle of fame; then followed an investigation by the Academy of Medicine, charges of quackery, and disgrace. Even while the friends of one of his famous patients were testifying to the remarkable quality of the cure, the newspapers carried the death notice of this same patient, the Count de Gobelin. Nevertheless, the tide that his promises had released is impressive, and it testifies to the existence of something that therapy had not touched.

For a long time any study of the phenomena he had produced was difficult. Animal magnetism was taboo, and its study ran underground. There the concepts were radically changed, as well as the procedures; when they reemerged as hypnosis, the changed conceptions produced new facts. As Mesmer had practiced his art, he had become interested in a certain "state of crisis" that seemed to overtake many of his patients: some of them would break out in a sweat, become agitated, and finally enter into convulsions, rolling their eyes, crying out, weeping. Others, less agitated, seemed to fall into a deep sleep. There were some who felt nothing at all (the skeptical members of the investigating committee sent to pass final judgment on Mesmer fell into this group). Since the impervious ones were not helped and the agitated ones were so obviously affected, Mesmer worked to produce these crises, in the belief that it was in the seizure that the animal spirits were being rearranged and repolarized.

CHARCOT'S APPLICATION OF HYPNOSIS

The successors of Mesmer who took up his work, usually motivated by the same desire to heal the sick, continued to work for a special state. But in their hands it grew less and less dramatic, less and less like an epileptic seizure, and more and more like a quiet sleep. By the 1880's the "trance state" had become a second level of mental functioning, with increased suggestibility and hypermnesia. Most of the operators were producing a sleep-like state, and the concept of suggestion had replaced the magnetic influence. Only in Charcot's clinic were there major convulsive seizures; so great was his authority that for many years hypnosis became linked with hysteria.

He expected hystericals to be easily hypnotized, and patients who were susceptible to hypnosis became, *ipso facto,* potential hystericals. He demonstrated hypnosis in his Tuesday lectures, showing three clearly defined stages: lethargy, catalepsy, and somnambulism. With the precision of a classifier, he demonstrated five phases to the full-blown attacks of hysteria:

1. A prodromal condition (comparable to the aura of the epileptic), marked by palpitation, a lump in the throat, visual disturbances, and ovarian pain, and ending in a loss of consciousness and fainting.

2. An epileptoid state, with (1) a phase of tonic contraction, arrest of breathing, and a stiffening of the whole body; (2) clonic convulsions, beginning with minor spasms and grimacing, and ending in generalized contractions of the whole body; and (3) complete calm, with stertorous breathing.

3. A period of contortions varying from mimicry and clowning to a struggle (with cries) against some imaginary being.

4. The period in which the patient seems to act out scenes of violence or erotic passion (a single patient following the same recurrent pattern on repetitions of the attack) and with some fixed idea at the center of the action.

5. A terminal period in which the patient returns to consciousness, repeating phrases inspired by what he has just acted out and with residues of visual hallucinations and postural contractions still in operation.[3]

Years later, Pierre Marie offered an explanation (see Guillain 1959) of what most of Charcot's colleagues had come to look on as a curious lapse in the clinical work of this great neurologist, to whose clinic the brilliant young neurologists of Europe were flocking. Three factors were involved. (1) A building housing a mixture of insane, chronically ill aged, epileptics, and assorted neurotics had to be abandoned; Charcot used this opportunity to house the two episodic illnesses (hystericals and epileptics) together in a single ward, as the patients were reallocated. (2) Charcot relied on his assistants to prepare all cases for demonstration, and to do all of the hypnotizing, while he busied himself with the preparation of his famous lecture demonstrations. (3) The principal subjects on which he based his first outline of the disorder were three young women, whose hysteria, in the hands of the zealous assistants, compliantly demonstrated all the facts that were taking shape in his mind. To what extent they simply imitated the epileptics whose attacks they witnessed on the ward, and to what extent Charcot's assistants were the responsible agents, is not clear, but the contrast between the findings at the Salpêtrière and the work that was unfolding at Nancy became, finally, a medical scandal.[4] It was the great Charcot who lost in this round.

[3]Ey, Bernard, and Brisset (1963) still offer this historical core of "fact" as the starting point for their description of the many variations and minor forms of the "classic disorder."

[4]Axel Munthe (1937, Chap. 19) makes a melodramatic tale of his efforts to rescue one of the three hysterical patients, who he insists were kept prisoners on the Saltpêtrière wards so that Charcot might have material for his demonstration lectures. Munthe's tendency to exaggerate for the sake of telling a good tale, as well as other internal evidence in his writings, does not make this a very trustworthy source of information.

JANET AND THE NANCY SCHOOL IN MODERN PERSPECTIVE

Three of Charcot's pupils were to develop and extend his use of hypnosis, but with changing and divergent emphases in theory and practice. The Polish neurologist Babinski developed the notion of a *pithiatic constitution* that is especially susceptible to suggestion and that must be handled with special care by the examining physician, lest he produce the very signs of illness he must treat. In Babinski's hands hysteria became a disorder that develops out of suggestion and can be cured by persuasion (or hypnosis) in these most susceptible constitutions. Freud, whose use of hypnosis was soon abandoned, learned from Charcot that ideas could indeed cause symptoms, but the existence of trance states that permitted all manner of actions promptly forgotten on waking led Freud to speculate about this possible "unconscious" source of symptoms, to ask how systems of ideas were segregated in such a split-off portion of the mind in the first place. In the course of answering this last question, he developed his sexual theory of the neuroses, which we shall later have to consider in greater detail.

In the hands of Janet, whom Charcot appointed as chief of the psychological clinic and laboratory at the Salpêtrière in 1899, three years prior to his death, hypnosis became a second sleep. Janet used methods similar to the one described by Bernheim of the Nancy school. In this technique the hypnotist merely asked his subject to be seated comfortably, to lean back and relax, to think of nothing but sleep while paying close attention to the operator's words: "Sleep. Think of nothing but sleep. Your arms are tired, your legs are tired, your eyes are tired. You cannot hold them open. Closing, slowly closing, think of nothing but sleep. Rest." Some physicians used fixation on a bright object, taking their cue from a Doctor Braid, who believed that a kind of optic-cerebral fatigue facilitated this unusual "second state." A few continue to make passes, as though in concession to the still extant folk beliefs that Mesmer originated.

More noteworthy than the mere outward changes in technique was the change in the concept of the second state that the new rituals produced. What the operators expected of it, and how they explained the phenomena and the facts which were recorded, seemed to change together. (No wonder that R. W. White [1941] has defined the hypnotic state as a form of "meaningful, goal-directed striving, its most general goal being to behave like a hypnotized person as this is continuously defined by the operator and understood by the subject.") The new facts that emerged seemed to require a new theory of the mind, or of the structure of consciousness and its relationship to objectively recorded behavior.[5] Four main changes are to be noted:

1. In the first place, the minds of the hystericals and of the subjects placed in the deeper levels of somnambulism by hypnosis seem to become dissociated into two functional organizations. The facts which required this formulation

---

[5]The reason for this qualifying phrase is that later experimental studies showed that a subject who denied all awareness of pain when pricked with a needle nevertheless showed the effect of the stimulus by changes in heart rates, galvanic skin reflexes, and respiration. See Hull 1933.

emerged as observers watched a subject speak, carry out commands, and discuss memories before a group of witnesses, but, when wakened, seem to be astonished to hear what had taken place, and even deny it. To this extent we may speak of the events as *forgotten,* yet, when rehypnotized, the subject will be able to recall what took place in the first seance, work out a second chapter in this strange underground, and again, on wakening, forget the whole matter. Perhaps we should not use the word *forget,* for the memories are still there. They are simply not available to that smaller, vigilant waking consciousness.

2. The special state known as the hypnotic trance, seems also to be the one in which remote memories, forgotten bits of experience, are more available than in the waking state. This *hypermnesia* proved invaluable to Charcot and Janet in their treatment of hystericals, for they discovered that many of their patients were literally suffering from memories they could not recall. A mad dog, a train wreck, a fall from a horse, a sexual assault, the widest range of traumatic events, had left their *scars* as an anesthesia or paralysis, but no conscious process of recall could summon a memory of these occasions when the subjects were fully awake. If we refer to these scars as *traces* in the neural tisses, we have to add that in these patients the traces were functionally dissociated from the normal waking consciousness, were not available to the recalling ego.

3. The third fact that made this concept of a divided mind, a separated pair of memory chains, necessary emerged as soon as the hypnotist tried to use the second state as a lever for influencing the normal state of functioning. A command could be given under hypnosis to carry out some action, say, winding a clock, when awake. When the subject wakened, experimenter and subject carried on a weird dialogue. "Why did you just do that?" "I thought it was in need of winding; it sounded as though it were running down." (And the experimenter wondered: Is he a malingerer? Is he fooling me? Does he *really* think this is the reason for his action?)

Or let the action in the subsequent waking state arise spontaneously, but refer to something that has occurred under hypnosis, something forgotten by the subject but remembered by the experimenter. Clark Hull (1933, pp. 28-31) reports an instance in which a subject was given a toothpick. Told under hypnosis that it was a match, he was instructed to light it. He made the gesture. Then he was told to hold it as long as possible, and then to reverse the ends so that it would burn up completely. Wetting his thumb and forefinger he carried out the instructions and watched the match burn down. But at the last the operator told him: "Watch out, it is burning your fingers! Oh, I am sorry, that must be painful," and the subject protested, and shook his hand as though in pain. Wakened, this subject said that he could not remember anything that had occurred, yet he kept rubbing thumb and forefinger together. Questioned, he said: "It's odd. My thumb feels so smooth. It is almost as though the surface had been burned."

This third type of fact led Charcot and Janet to the assumption that, certainly *in these subjects,* the lower half of this two-layered mind continued to function, after the hypnotic session was over and beneath the conscious level. Things could evidently be put into the mind, be retained, and continue to produce changes in behavior, *even though not available to conscious recall*. Further, the surface layer of the mind, called on to give an account of what it was doing, trying to integrate and make sense of what was actually moving within the person, might develop plausible and reasonable, but wholly false, explanations, thus *rationalizing* what it did not understand, and assigning both goal and cause to what would otherwise have seemed wholly spontaneous, automatic, and without explanation.

4. The school of Charcot and Janet developed an additional set of concepts by means of which they hoped to explain this splitting process.

a. In the first place, the conscious ego, the system of processes that summoned and integrated the memories from the past and acted as a kind of *organizer of the mind,* is only a small part of the total system of active neuromuscular processes. Figuratively, it is like a central lighted portion of a field, a limited area under the spotlight, with the whole darkened auditorium forming a huge penumbra around about. (Bats could be flying around, or darkly seen shadows moving just outside the well-lighted portion, but there would be no clear awareness of these.)

b. This lighted area, the conscious organizer, the summoning ego, is sometimes fairly large, sometimes smaller. It narrows as we fall into reverie, and doze, or become very tired. It expands as we are startled into "vigilance." In the half-waking stage just prior to getting up in the morning, it may still be almost obliterated—little more than a vague or anxious ache that fills our poorly structured consciousness. When we are fatigued or exhausted, the upper level shrinks; this restriction of the conscious field seems to release some of the more automatic and poorly structured processes from control. The more it shrinks, the less it can recall the past and order new actions in the light of present needs. Like the man who "knows" a name but cannot recall it, the ego cannot summon memories. Sometimes the mechanisms not only romp about: they *possess* their bearer, completing themselves in actions, movements, cramps, paralyses; the poor ego can only observe, puzzled. The Salpêtrière group believed the cure required an expansion and strengthening of this restricted consciousness, a conversion of automatisms to disciplined recall and directed planning that is subordinate to an organizing group of processes.

Although preoccupation with the role of these buried memories tends to make us think that if we could just "get them back and hold them" the battle would be won, it seems to be a fact that:

1. The descent of a particular system into the lower regions may be due to a *general* weakening of the system. Thus fatigue, illness, loss of blood, overwork, the exhaustion that comes with failure, loss of love, loss of support, or death in the family can alter the shape of the total system, the *proportionate strength* of ego and subconscious automatism, and produce the splitting.

2. The descent of the particular system may be attributed to the unpleasant or morally disagreeable quality of the memory. A disgraceful failure, a

shameful debauch, an episode in which one made a fool of oneself, can be quickly swept out of mind, for to dwell on it is painful, and whatever announces its emergence into awareness may signal alarm, set in motion distracting actions (*reaction formations* we call them, now). To the degree that the energies of the ego are tied up in keeping down what never should have occurred, the balance of free energy, which is required both to appraise the present field and to look ahead, is limited. The field is restricted.

3. The sensitivity of some persons' systems is so great that minor events possess a traumatic quality. They reverberate long after these occasions should have been forgotten. If such a person digests his experiences poorly, keeps an unreasonable portion of his energies bound up in reverberating circuits, these circuits will also tend to sink below the level of recall. We could call him *frangible,* meaning that he is "easily split." What would be no trauma to the tough-minded is fracturing to him, producing a restriction of the field of awareness. In the most extreme form, narcolepsy occurs: the person meeting a challenge simply sleeps. (Pavlov was later to find a type of dog that reacted to a difficult discrimination by going into a state of stupor.) The thought of the Charcot-Janet school is that in the trance state of the easily hypnotized subject, this narrowing of the field is not complete, but partial: he meets the command of the experimenter with a prompt narrowing of awareness until the hypnotist and his words are all that remains within his narrow focus. There is nothing to oppose the command: and it is acted out.

Accounts of hystericals give evidence of easy access from the trance state to dreaming. We could diagram the relationship as in Figure 5, which gives a visual form to what many have believed: that these two "second states" are in better communication with each other than with waking consciousness; and that dreams have a better access to the waking state and so can bridge from the trance to ordinary levels of awareness. To measure the communication among these three states would require an experimental program of testing that has not been carried out.

From this changed conception of mental functioning, a number of changes in the treatment of hystericals have developed. One of the first orders of business may be the unearthing of the hidden fixed idea that underlies the hysterical patient's symptoms, but it will be apparent from the above analysis that such unearthing may not be sufficient. Therapy may also have to involve a general strengthening of the system, excitation, support, arousal, consolation, exhortation, scolding, or even, as appears in the case of Achille, a change in the buried memory itself, until it is no longer dangerous and disorganizing.

Janet's Achille

Where superstition abounds, hysteria often takes the form of a "possession," as it did in the days of witchcraft. Achille's possession was an acting out of some folk beliefs common to the people of the Midi, where the world of modern science has been slow to penetrate (see Janet 1898, pp. 373-406).

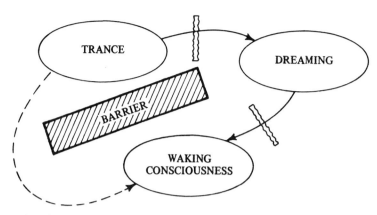

FIGURE 5. HYPOTHETICAL CHANNELS OF ACCESSIBILITY BETWEEN TRANCE STATES, DREAMS, AND WAKING CONSCIOUSNESS. The barrier drawn between the trance state and waking consciousness indicates the fact that, on waking from the deeper levels of somnambulism, the subject usually forgets all that has transpired. The dotted line around the barrier symbolizes the fact that, without instruction, occasional bits of the trance state do irrupt into waking consciousness. There are two additional facts symbolized by this line: (1) Instructed under hypnosis that he will later recall what takes place, the subject can break this barrier. (2) Repeated questioning can lead to recall of the hypnotically induced events.

When his "acting out" began, Achille had just wakened from sleep, eyes bathed with tears. He called his wife and child to his bedside, embraced them as though in the last stage of despair, and stretched out on the bed, motionless. He stayed motionless, terrifying his family, who waited, almost certain that he would die.

Then all at once, after two days of this "dying," Achille sat up and, with eyes wide open, broke out in a terrifying laughter, jumped out of bed, and called for champagne: "It's the end of the world; they are going to burn me, cut me to bits." After a night of agitated sleep, he told the family about a host of little, menacing, horned devils that had tormented him. He would break out in blasphemous shouts, expressing all the obscenities about religion he could summon up. His arms and legs contracted convulsively, as though violently acted on by some force not his own. He ran from the house when he was not observed, hiding in the woods or the cemetery, where he would fall asleep. He took laudanum and other mildly poisonous medicines. Once he foolishly bound his own feet and then threw himself into the lake, but he came to the surface and made his way to the bank. When the family could no longer manage him, he was brought to the Salpêtrière. There he demonstrated his possession, carried on a struggle with his demon, described his voice. "The head of the devil," he assured his physician, "is the clearest of all, black, frightful, with horns, and, most satanic of all, his head does not hide the objects behind it completely. It is half-transparent."

Achille's symptoms had begun after he had returned from a business trip, depressed, full of ruminations which he kept to himself. The first physician who examined him found symptoms of diabetes, and a second one convinced him that he had angina. Before a month was out, he took to his bed, and the "acting out" began.

Achille resisted Janet's questioning and refused, at first, to allow himself to be hypnotized. Through a roundabout stratagem, automatic handwriting was induced; a pencil placed in Achille's hand began to write messages from his demon while Achille was distracted, questions being whispered in his ear. A three-cornered conversation between Janet, "the demons," and Achille began, one result of which was the induction of hypnosis and the unearthing of the idea that had been tormenting this patient. In the somnambulistic state he told Janet about an episode of infidelity on that last business trip, just prior to his rumination, guilt, and certainty that he would be punished. His illness, the demons, his suicidal gestures, and his refusal to talk to anyone lest he blurt out the truth, now became understandable, at least to some degree.

Characteristically, in addition to the use of hypnosis for exploratory purposes, Janet gave his patient suggestions, guidance, physiotherapy, support, and encouragement. Using hypnosis, he made a direct attack on the memory of the critical event that had started the trouble. He tried to help Achille digest the experience, to bring him to forgive himself for his lapse. He also made certain modifications in the remembered event while Achille was in the somnambulist state, until, in his unconscious, Achille had so altered his "fixed idea" that a kind of scientific absolution had been accomplished. All of this was forgotten when he awoke. His delirium subsided, his nightmares and pains ceased, and the anesthesia that had involved both arms when they were contorted in convulsive movements was gone.

Only the vague memory of his devil remained, and it now seemed to amuse him. As he recovered, his susceptibility to hypnosis declined, as did his ability to carry out automatic handwriting. Occasionally, at first, his "devils" would torment his sleep, but these nightmares disappeared, too, and Achille went back to the Midi. He corresponded with Janet, and when the latter finally published his report of the case, Achille had been free from symptoms for eight years.

Now that we have the benefit of 75 more years of research on hypnosis, we have some reason to question what Janet's "exorcism" seems to imply, namely, that once an idea is implanted in the state of somnambulism, it will stay implanted until removed by the operator. Experimental measures of the persistence of habits set up by verbal directions given under hypnosis indicate that they are as fragile as conditioned reflexes and as subject to extinction. Enduring for a few weeks and growing weaker as unreinforced trials accumulate, their existence in that subconscious or dissociated stratum of the mind does not preserve them from the usual forces of attrition. However, when a vicious cycle or an exaggerated generalization of some traumatic experience can be broken in this fashion, the shift to more realistic patterns of behavior, together with the support brought by more adaptive behavior and its reinforcing effects, may be made permanent. This gives hypnosis, in addition to its value in exploration and in heightened suggestion, a special use in "emergencies" where a stubborn vicious cycle has to be broken.

A Question That Has Persisted

The revival of hypnosis by Charcot and his pupil Janet helped restore the dignity of the procedure as a diagnostic and therapeutic tool, and provided us with an experimental procedure for the study of subconscious phenomena. But like the hystericals, whose compliant behavior has validated such a variety of theories and therapies, hypnotic subjects have produced such varying and contradictory phenomena that we still lack the firm foundation of experimental evidence we need. The rapport between operator and subject may fluctuate widely from day to day, or be completely disrupted by events occurring outside the laboratory or clinic.[6] Although one operator has claimed success in 90 per cent of his attempts, the modest claims of experimenters who have attempted to measure "hypnotizability" have shown that operators with considerable experience may succeed in producing a full-fledged state of somnambulism in less than 25 per cent of their cases.[7]

One generalization that has persisted in some quarters since the days of Charcot is still a matter of dispute. Although most observers agree that hystericals as a group are easily hypnotized, we would hesitate to reverse the relationship and state, as Charcot did, that all who are good hypnotic subjects are, *ipso facto,* hystericals or potential hystericals. Even the general consensus is challenged by Brenman and Gill (1947), who state that hystericals as a group are the most difficult patients to hypnotize. In his last summary of the question, Janet (1919, I, 247 ff) showed that, toward the end of his career, he was still laboring under the influence of Charcot. He gives the following reasons for suspecting the person who easily slips into the full somnambulistic state with consequent amnesia to be of the hysterical constitution.

1. Such a trance cannot be distinguished from those which occur in the hysterical spontaneously.

2. A full and impartial examination will show that these subjects also have other forms of dissociated reactions that occur spontaneously.

3. Epileptics, scrupulous doubters, obsessive-compulsive personalities are not hypnotizable in this fashion. The susceptibility is related to hysteria, among the neuroses.

4. Artificially induced somnambulism will gradually wear off naturally, and, like the hysterical who gets well and who then ceases to be hypnotizable, the susceptibility varies from time to time.

5. Spontaneous somnambulists make the best subjects for hypnosis, and their sleepwalking, or states of possession and of awayness, can be easily transformed into hypnotic states.

---

[6]A young resident-in-training (Spiegel 1967) reported the successful use of hypnosis to block the pain his patient was experiencing following laparotomy. A drug which had been in use could be discontinued. When he told these facts to his analyst, who was supervising his training, he was forbidden to use such a technique. His supervisor agreed, however, that he might continue the hypnosis until another physician (who had taught him the technique) could take over. But on the following day, he found that the same procedure that he had previously used now failed, and his patient had to be placed on meperidine HCl again. When his successor took over, the hypnoanaesthesia was easily reestablished, and the narcotic could again be withdrawn.

[7]Davis and Husband (1931), who studied 55 patients in all, tried to establish a scale of hypnotizability, and identified 30 gradations of this trait. Slight changes in procedure, the substitution of different operators, a change within the subject can produce changes in such indices. And new population samples will in all probability give a new distribution of the trait.

6. Somnambules, subsequently hypnotized, can recapture memories of what transpired in this dissociated state, when properly guided. The reverse is also true: what transpires in artificially induced trances may emerge in spontaneous somnambulist states.

7. In 120 cases from the file at the Salpêtrière who showed the greatest ability to pass into the deepest states of somnambulism with subsequent amnesia, each was suffering from hysteria at the time.

8. The recovery of health in the hysterical is usually followed by a period in which he is no longer susceptible to hypnosis.

From these observations it appears that statements about "hypnotizability in general," without qualification as to groups studied, the competence of the operators, the methods employed, or the criteria used to define the effects, have limited validity. Chertok (1961, p. 34) describes a practice in use at the Vienna Psychiatric Clinic at one time, in which "professionals" were employed so that, out of their experience with these "easy" subjects, young psychiatrists-in-training might gain confidence in their use of a method. At the other end of the continuum, there will be a few subjects who cannot be touched even by the most skilled operators.

Although most observers suspect that there is a certain "prestigeful personality" that has the greatest success in inducing the state, the components which make up this outward impression of prestige have not been easy to identify, and since there are two persons involved, we have to ask, "Prestige for whom?" Common experience would suggest that a long experience of success would contribute to both skill and confidence, but others (Chertok, Ferenczi) have insisted that they were completely successful at the start; they suggest that the young practitioner does not yet realize the limitations in his powers and in his methods. One American practitioner insisted that he had lost his skill as a result of a psychoanalysis, during which he discovered that some of his motives were open to question.[8]

As for the "good subjects" who are easily hypnotizable, some have described them as hysterical, others have found them most normal. Chertok and Cahen (1955) report that those whom they could not hypnotize were also markedly maladjusted socially, and often full of somatic complaints. Their good subjects (who were also patients) had a good contact with reality, and, while troubled by some conflicts, were coping successfully with most problems of adjustment. Like Janet, they find that obsessionals are not good subjects. Their hystericals are divided by these authors into two groups: the severely ill are poor subjects, the milder cases are the best of all. (Others have suggested that hypnotizability is a favorable prognostic sign.)

The subjects of Eysenck (1947, pp. 173 ff), measured by an independent test for suggestibility, showed a fair degree of correlation between suggestibility

---

[8]Schilder (1921) argues that the hypnotizer has an unconscious desire for magical power and domination over his patient; he points out that many subjects fear just such libidinal domination by the operator.

and hypnotizability. When a group of neurotic soldiers were separated into suggestible and nonsuggestible groups, he found that the more severely ill patients tended to fall into the suggestible group.[9]

Instead of being a simple trait that is easy to measure (like height or weight), hypnotizability turns out to be a relationship between subject and operator. A subject resistant to one operator will trust and obey the next one, although the latter has no better record of inducing trances. Mutual expectations based on social roles seem important (see Sarbin, 1954). Some subjects who resist hypnosis on the first trial, succumb to a second attempt or to a 300th. Even for a single pair, operator and subject, hypnotizability varies from day to day, and a subject's need can develop into a positive "addiction." With the variety of opinions now extant, each supported by extensive experience, it will require a very extended and well-controlled study to provide the "final word."

JANET'S VIEW

Through more than half a century of active study and teaching, on the wards and clinics of the Salpêtrière and in his classes at the Collège de France, Janet's notions about hysteria had crystallized around two ideas. Somewhat against his better judgment, for he had seen dozens of such "definitions" come and go in his own time, he once tried to compress his understanding into a definition: "Hysteria is a form of mental depression characterized by the constriction of the field of personal consciousness and by the tendency to dissociation, with emancipation of those systems of ideas and functions whose synthesis constitutes the personality" (Janet 1908, p. 345).

Like all such summarizing statements, Janet's definition needs to be understood in the light of those facts which underlie his two major concepts, as well as in the light of his general theoretical viewpoint and his metapsychology. Read by a student unfamiliar with his writings, it is both unclear and misleading. Hystericals are not depressed, as a rule. In fact, what usually strikes the clinician is their calm indifference to their disabilities, their lability of mood, and their tendency to excesses of expressive gesture and speech and to a certain theatrical manner. They are outgoing, as a rule, and easy to relate to. (It was early noted how easily they establish rapport, and this ease was made a point of contrast between hysterical and obsessive-compulsive personalities. But when this rapport often turned out to be superficial and a sign of excessive dependency, and many cures transitory, many physicians began to think the line between hysteria and malingering to be very fine.) Why, then, does Janet speak of a *mental depression?*

---

[9]Eysenck also relates hysteria to extroversion. When we have boxed the compass so as to include the healthy and the ill, extroverts and introverts, hystericals and nonhystericals, suggestibles and nonsuggestibles, the intercorrelations leave us as confused as the bettor who is trying to predict the outcome of the game from comparative scores accumulated in the season. Furthermore, one subtest counted as a good test of suggestibility does not correlate highly with the next subtest.

Conceiving of human development as a progressive integration of functions, in which simple reflexes are grouped into habits, and habits, in turn, subordinated to a system of conscious regulation, Janet looked on any dissociation of functions, any splitting into subsystems, any escape of the parts from the central controls, as a depression, a lowering of the integrative force in the system. Searching for a name for this latter synthesizing power, he called it *psychological tension.* So interpreted, the definition becomes a restatement of the clinical facts, a regrouping of his observations around a single central idea. The crucial questions raised by his definition then become: What causes this descent in integrative power? Is there any therapeutic procedure that can raise this power to its former state?

FOUR CLASSES OF SYMPTOMS

Four groups of facts formed the empirical basis for Janet's concept of hysteria. All four of them, or only one of them, may be found in any one case. Their frequent association and their *equivalence* (sometimes the cure of one of them, say, an anesthesia, is followed by an appearance of a new sensory deficit or an amnesia or an attack of somnambulism) suggested to Janet a common underlying weakness, a deficit in integrative powers.

Anesthesias

Losses of tactile sensibility on a portion of the skin's surface had long been regarded as one of the diagnostic signs of abnormality (since the days of the witch hunts). The hysterical's loss of sensitivity is of a special sort:

1. The area varies in extent from day to day, expanding as the patient's general condition worsens, constricting or disappearing as he improves.

2. The areas do not correspond to any distribution of nerve trunks. Occasionally they appear to conform to an idea (as when a glove anesthesia corresponds to the surface that would be covered by a glove).

3. Unlike the anesthesias that depend on severed nerves or central lesions, the hysterical form is reversible, as when the patient responds abruptly to persuasion or to suggestion under hypnosis, or when sensitivity returns under the impact of a sudden access of interest or of a fright.

4. Therapeutic efforts concentrated on one area may restore sensation to that area, only to be followed by an appearance of new anesthetic areas in some other place, as though the perceptive-regulative consciousness were like a blanket, too small to cover the entire body surface. (Pull it up, the toes are exposed; pull it down, the shoulders are bared.) The new area is thus viewed as an equivalent, insofar as it expresses the same basic weakness in integrative powers. (This concept is to be distinguished from the Freudian concept of equivalence in symptoms, in which the equivalence is in meaning, in a similarity of function. The function of the anesthesia, in Freud's eyes, is to both express and conceal that which has been repressed from awareness.)

5. Sensory deficits appear in all the sense fields. Vision may be lost in one eye and not the other. The visual field may be constricted so that objects

falling outside a small central area which occupies less than a third of the normally visible field are not seen. There is also a form of hysterical deafness. In hysterical anorexia there is a loss of all awareness of hunger pangs. A hysterical form of frigidity or impotence is accompanied by a complete insensitivity of the genital region.

6. Under hypnosis these anesthetic areas can be restored to function, and with proper preparation for posthypnotic tests, it can be demonstrated that a signal falling on the insensitive zones can cue some planned response. Even when the hysterical anesthesia persists in the waking period, the subject's response to the prearranged cue reveals that the area still functions at a subconscious level. The paradoxical quality of these anesthesias is beautifully illustrated by the subject who complains that he can see no colors with his right eye. Nonetheless, when he is invited to peer into a box so devised that the color seen by the right eye appears to be located on the left side (by reflecting mirrors) he will name that color. His notion that his right eye is not functioning properly seems to be the controlling factor.

7. Two facts militate against the notion that the symptoms have been produced by suggestion alone. Babinski's notion, that since all hysterical symptoms can be duplicated by procedures employing suggestion, we should look on those which we observe clinically as also caused in the same way, does not appear to apply in all cases. In exploring the visual field, for example, some hystericals and their physicians discover for the first time that there is a nonfunctional fringe at the periphery of the field. Large areas of tactual anesthesia turn up in the course of an examination, areas that had not been noted, that had in no way interfered with action, that had not produced any "secondary gains" such as concern and sympathy from those who surround the patient, or proof of an impairment that would provide an excuse from work or validate a compensation claim. These special instances of anesthesia of which the subject has not been aware argue against many of the teleological interpretations currently offered in explanation of the hysterical's symptoms. They point, Janet thought, to factors outside the awareness system itself; instead of being explained by unconscious motives, they should be accepted as evidence of something that restricts the area of perceptive-regulative control, a "something" that reduces normal vigilance, and that could be as impersonal as a microorganism, a metabolic failure, or a fever. The facts do point, undoubtedly, to the existence of a lower order of automatic functioning; the hysterically blind subject does not see, consciously, but he uses unconscious visual cues in the course of action. For example, such patients can avoid obstacles and participate in sports in a way that would be impossible if their impairment were based on lesions in the visual-motor paths.

8. This unseeing form of seeing, these anesthesias that still permit sensory cues to function (through some lower network that does not elaborate conscious responses), tempt the clinician to diagnose his case as malingering, to accuse his patient of having unconscious reasons for not responding, to

think of hysteria as a willful and deceptive sort of illness, based on intentions of the patient (even when these intentions are unconscious, denied). Janet discounted both the truth of this interpretation and its value as a clinical strategy. The dissociation, or break in the response circuits, was studied with the same impersonal attitude that Pavlov was to use in his approach to experimental animals that developed conditioned inhibitions in the experimental-neurosis training. Like an engineer trying to locate the "fatigue" of the materials used in the construction of a bridge that has collapsed, Janet looked both at the strength of his human materials and at the stresses that had produced the collapse, and not at "intentions" or "secondary rewards." What had shunted the reactions into the lower circuits, the memories into a lower form of recall? Why did the perceptions not elaborate themselves into the conscious form?

Amnesias and Fugue

The second group of facts, about amnesias, presents us with a similar set of puzzles. Just as the anesthesias represent an incomplete registration of the stimuli (but with full elaboration of perception possible under hypnosis), so both forgetting and recall are incomplete: the person who had forgotten some "island" of his past could recall it under hypnosis; the one who could not even remember his identity when awake (as in fugue states) could cleverly skirt those persons who would identify him. Defective function of memories, not memory loss, was the rule. This defect is reversible and can disappear spontaneously. Again, it is distinguishable from irreversible losses, such as those based on frontal-lobe or temporal-lobe lesions.

The hysterical memory loss may take the form of a *fugue*. Here the patient may appear in clinic pleading for help in establishing his identity. He has no memory of his family, his profession, his place of residence, although other memories and habits, such as his language skills, are unimpaired. Under hypnosis such a patient will reveal how he traveled, where his family is located, what his previous work had been, and so on. Such "flights" may endure for months, even years, the patient taking up a new life and constructing a new history within whose bounds his memory functions fairly well.

Amnesia may occur in the form of an attack of somnambulism. These episodes of trancelike "awayness," in which a patient sometimes reenacts some scene from his past (a scene that is often heavily charged with emotions), can occur in broad daylight. The patient appears to have all but completely lost contact with his surroundings; when he once more resumes this contact, he will have completely forgotten all that took place (much in the fashion of a good hypnotic subject who can scarcely accept the account of his performance others give him). The block of activities, forgotten as he recovers consciousness, is not actually lost. It is simply not open to voluntary recall. There is a functional dissociation between this block of experiences and normal perceptive-integrative awareness. Such somnambulistic episodes, occurring spontaneously in the hysterical, not only plummet into the unconscious themselves, but may also take with them memories of the events just preceding the attack, so that the memories for a considerable period in which the subject appeared to be functioning normally are also lost (retrograde amnesia).

In rare instances, such as those reported by Prince (1905), Thigpen and Cleckley (1957), and Franz (1933), the self-system seems so divided that rather large blocks of perceptions, memories, and actions function independently, each out of contact with and not controlled by the other selves. Like the controlling sets involved in speaking a language, each of which can function without interference from the other language sets the person possesses, these partial self-systems alternate in a strange Dr. Jekyll and Mr. Hyde fashion, producing alternating personalities. In Prince's account of Sarah Beauchamp, one of the personalities seemed to have full knowledge of another one; the former plotted mischievously to create predicaments that would disturb the latter, and spoke with some contempt (to Prince) of this other, "stupid" portion of the self-system.

The evidence which emerges from the studies of these divided selves shows that subsystems out of touch with the waking consciousness (sometimes rather large subsystems) can operate autonomously, and carry on an independent existence. When, as in Morton Prince's case, an impish Sally steals and destroys money from Sarah's pocketbook, or puts angleworms in her jewelcase where she will find them, we can see dramatic examples of conflict between selves. We can also see that a dissociated system not available to conscious recall, and existing outside the field where habits can be partially regulated, can irrupt, disorganizing the course of thought and action. Paradoxically, in these hystericals, what drops into oblivion is not forgotten: it continues to exist and even to enjoy a certain exaggerated power in its isolated form.

In Janet's view, the descent of any system of ideas into an unconscious existence was not so much the result of repression (an active "holding back" of something fearful or disagreeable) as of weakness in the integrative powers that normally contain and organize our experiences into a communicable form, a history of our actions. In order to restore normal functioning, a clinician would naturally assume that some kind of psychological dragnet should be used to fish up these submerged systems that have put too much strain on the integrative powers. Their *liquidation* would involve their reassimilation into the system that had digested them so poorly. No mere *abreaction* (expressing or reliving them) would be enough. Their owner would have to come to terms with them, and reintegrate them with the rest of a personal history, until they could be recalled normally, placed in their proper setting, and used in present actions and future planning.

Janet's logic would lead us to suspect, however, that unless the more basic integrative powers were somehow improved, any mere restoration of particular memories would be followed by other (equivalent) losses. The constricted blanket of consciousness (and regulative powers) has to be restored to its normal size and power. The fishing expedition that would restore some particular forgotten (but subconsciously existing) past would be fruitless if, as fast as the new catches entered the boat, other old ones dropped back into the dark waters, unless (and Freud was to press this alternate hypothesis) there is some particular quality about that which is forgotten, something unusual in its relation to the censoring-regulative self that controls habit systems.

Disorders of Movement

Persistent paralyses and contractures affecting whole systems of movement rather than the simplest reflexes suggest a failure of one of the higher brain circuits through which our more complex learned integrations are routed. But again, Janet discovered that movements which cannot be carried out voluntarily can be executed if the subject is distracted, hypnotized, caught off guard, commanded. Hysterical mutism and the inability to write or walk yield to hypnosis and suggestion.

Janet's No. (1919, I, 356-58) suffered for 21 years from recurring abdominal contractions that made her feel forced to assume an exaggerated and absurd posture. Appearing initially after surgical removal of one of her ovaries, her posture was first interpreted as a protection against real pain. When Janet hypnotized No. and suggested that she could and must straighten herself up, she would do so and remain free from the contractions for a period of months. Then, upset by quarrels in the family, she would again experience the symptoms and return to Janet. This routine was repeated at varying intervals, usually twice a year.

Thus the hysterical presents us with a paralysis that is no paralysis, an anesthesia in which sense organs still function, an amnesia that is not a complete forgetting, and a set of complex trancelike states (fugues and somnambulisms) with autonomous control existing outside normal awareness and creating a separate subsystem of memories. Again, the dissociation of these memory subsystems is sometimes incomplete, since the subsystems clash at times, irrupting and penetrating whatever other system is dominant at the time.

Disorders of Character: The Psychology of Hysteria

There are three traits that recur throughout the foregoing groups of hysterical symptoms; their ubiquitous presence points to an underlying common nature in these symptoms.

First, consider the hysterical's suggestibility. This fact is so obvious that Babinski wanted to make it the key to all phenomena (see Babinski and Froment 1917). These patients are easily hypnotized. They are quick to pick up a suggestion. Moreover, they realize the implanted ideas, even in their tissues. Some observers have even claimed to be able to raise blisters or to remove warts in these patients by suggestion alone. Babinski was of the opinion that many of the symptoms commonly reported in case histories of hystericals were physician-caused. He believed that the anesthesias, pains, paralyses, and contractures were produced by a clumsy and inexpert examination procedure that had suggested the very phenomena "discovered."

This notion of Babinski's is supported by those who point out that the old "major attacks" which so closely resembled epilepsy (with tonic contractions, arched back, involuntary cries, loss of consciousness) are now rarely seen. Were such attacks created by Charcot's housing his hystericals on wards with epileptics, who provided the model for the hystericals to imitate? Is the rarity of split personalities of the type described by Prince, Thigpen and Cleckley, and Franz—where as many as five separate subsystems of the personality are reported—due to the simple fact that they were artifacts produced by clinicians who, in using hypnotic procedures, inadvertently permitted their own theoretical interests to be communicated to very compliant and suggestible subjects?[10]

Without entering these controversies or pretending to possess more data than are in fact available, we can at least note this fact: the word and the idea possess a power in the hysterical that they do not have in the normal. In them, we could say, "The word is made flesh." The operator who repeats the formula, "Your eyes are heavy, your legs are tired, your whole body cries out for sleep," will find that his hysterical subject passes into the deep somnambulistic state, before his eyes, in minutes. Others who watch the operator and his subject with an amused and skeptical smile, and who ask (or rather challenge) him to repeat the process may hear the same words without experiencing any such effect. Some of these difficult subjects may actually be curious to find out what it is like to be hypnotized, and are so busy watching instead of obeying that nothing happens. A few are busy raising counter-suggestions, repeating to themselves, "I am *not* tired. My eyes are not a bit heavy. This operator seems to be carried away by his enthusiasm."

The hysterical is different: he is less critical, more submissive, or perhaps more prone to permit one idea to develop and expand to the exclusion of any contrary notions that might inhibit, limit, and deny the validity of the controlling idea. "What," we have to ask, "is the condition or state that permits such a dominance of a single impression?" Like a crystal dropped into some supersaturated solution, the idea given to the suggestible hysterical or-

---

[10]A similar discordance in reported facts has haunted the students of hypnotism. Mesmer's patients who entered the trance state had "seizures" that sometimes resembled epileptic attacks, but the subjects of Bernheim, Liébault, Janet, and De Puységur seemed always to pass easily into a gentle sleep. In similar contrast to the hystericals demonstrated by Charcot, the modern patient diagnosed as "conversion hysteria" is a tame successor to the "classic" form. The sexual meanings that Freud was to revive were more apparent to the physicians of Plato's time, when the cause of hysteria was traced to a misbehaving uterus, than they were at many subsequent periods, or in Janet's clinic. Does the physician select symptoms to report? Are the symptoms produced out of Janet's beliefs a collaboration between a physician with a theory and a compliant patient who responds to his suggestions? Does a set of folk beliefs send the hysterical to an exorciser of demons in one period, and to a specialist in psychosomatic medicine in a later period? Is the diagnosis of hysteria reserved for a "residue" of patients that physicians find so hard to treat and so irritating that the physicians *know,* by their own reactions, what class the patients belong in?

ganizes congenial and congruent crystalline forms around it, as though such congruent ideas were the only ones the person possessed. Or, like a person eager to please, who brings supporting evidence to each statement of his interlocutor, the hysterical actualizes the proffered word in the flesh, when a normal regulative consciousness would test it, and then assimilate it or reject it in terms of a larger body of experience. The radical, critical empiricism that John Dewey wanted to develop in opposition to some of the more dogmatic or revealed philosophies is the very antithesis of *pithiatism,* as Babinski called the suggestibility of the hysterical.

Second, consider the hysterical's distractibility. In one sense the hysterical concentrates too well: he is completely attentive to the single idea that occupies his consciousness. But the other side of the process is equally striking: his unawareness of that normal penumbra of attention, the outlying fringe, the wider field, is also complete, or at least much more complete than in the normal.

Directing the attention of a patient with a constricted visual field to a set of numbers placed in the center of the field, and instructing him to carry out certain simple mathematical operations, Janet found that the borders of the visible field had been pulled in.

Such a patient acts as though a field-making and -encoding process, normally always at work constructing a life-space around us, operates as a power that is present in limited supply. The hysterical seems able to hold a very limited range of experiences in a lively state of organization at any one time. He is, therefore, both distractible and suggestible. The good "field-maker" establishes a wider-ranging cognitive map. He assimilates and owns, in a personal sense, the events that move into his field. The hysterical's field seems weaker and narrower, and his ownership less vital; as a result the more restricted systems are under limited controls. The idea of the moment, the proffered suggestion, assumes more importance. In its structure such a system is more like that of a child; in a sense the hysterical has regressed, since his regulative awareness-structures are simpler, more limited, even as those of a child are limited to the here and now and to a very limited range of cues.

There is a second sense in which the hysterical patient tends to regress. To the degree that old, automatic organizations occupy the field, or that old conditioned responses tend to irrupt, uncorrected by intervening experience, the hysterical is past-ridden. We could translate Janet's notion of psychological tension, and its companion idea of the making of a present field, into the statement: "Lacking normal integrative (or field-making) powers, the hysterical's depressed level of functioning results in distractibility, suggestibility, and a proliferation of automatisms, all of which permits him to become 'entrapped' in his own past." We should now begin to see the full implications of Janet's definition, in which the facts have forced us to include: (1) a depressed level of functioning; (2) a constriction of the field of awareness; (3) a weakness in the response-regulating power of a personal consciousness; and (4) the tendency to dissociation, in which subsystems within the personality dominate action instead of remaining consistently subordinated to a more highly integrated and complex system that ordinarily "owns" them.[11]

Third, consider the *equivalence* of the hysterical's symptoms. The facts about this equivalence are consistent with Janet's belief that the basic weakness is in the integrative powers, not in some peculiarity in specific organs or in some unusual quality in the lost functions. He found that if he concentrated his therapy on getting his anorexic patient to eat, he would discover that she had developed an anesthesia. Exhorting his subject to carry out a movement in a paralyzed member, he would discover that the functional loss emerged elsewhere. When he had restored sensibility to the right side of the body (in a case of hemianesthesia), he would sometimes find that a new insensibility had emerged on the left side.[12]

Even where the therapeutic work is more successful and the hysterical appears to be cured, a thorough follow-up over several years will typically reveal a recurrence of symptoms. The protean character of the behavior changes brought back into the clinic indicates that something about the patient remains untouched by the therapy. Janet assumed that this something was a constitutional weakness.

FEELING AND EMOTION IN THE HYSTERICAL

Janet used another approach to the symptoms of the hysterical, one that was suggested by the psychology of his time. He examined, one by one, each of the major facets of action which were then called emotion, intellect, and will: faculties that the phrenologists once wanted to locate in specific brain areas (as their modern successors still try to locate emotions in the hypothalamus). In every one of these traditional "aspects" of mental functioning, he found that the hysterical was operating at something less than a normal level.

Consider feeling and emotion, first, since so many of our contemporary theories of mental illness tend to speak of emotional tensions as the *cause* of mental changes. For Janet, feeling was the great stimulator and regulator of action. When a person aims at some target and then watches his arrow of effort fall short, he promptly adds a fresh charge of effort to his next try, especially if he carries an inner standard. Köhler, watching his apes reach for the banana that lay outside their cage, just out of reach, imagined their reaction to be a kind of unverbalized animal equivalent of our "arm too short."

---

[11]These facts should remind us that the "holism" of a Goldstein or Angyal may very well represent a kind of ideal functioning. Below the state in which such maximal integration exists, there are in fact states in which all degrees of partial functioning of subsystems exist. Do we not forget the parting instructions and good intentions with which we left home, and return in the evening having completely forgotten to bring home the shoes that had been left at the repair shop? The hysterical seems to forget even more easily and more completely.

[12]These shifts in area of insensibility emerged in Charcot's clinic in a curious form. Charcot demonstrated his ability to force such shifts by the use of magnets applied to the insensitive surface. This curious bit of evidence seems to hark back to Mesmer's belief in the healing power of the magnet. The idea that metal plaques of gold or copper could also cure an anesthesia represents a similar "throwback," and reveals how suggestible and how compliant these patients are.

Objectively, they did look about; as their eyes fell on the stick lying on the floor of the cage, the stick was transformed by this "feeling" into a means-to-an-end. This stress of the felt want, this reaction to our actions, moves us to raise our sights, correct our effort, and try again. "Once more, with feeling," the director says, for an empty action, a mere movement, is not the way we *act*. If one is competing with or threatened by others, acting under difficulty, the sympathetic nervous system will participate in this charge of effort, accelerating the pulse rate, stimulating the liver to pour out its blood sugar, increasing the tonus of our muscles, putting a floor under the striving.

Such a conception of feeling fuses the perception of relations (arm too short) and the disturbance down among the cells (including an increase in the oxygen-carrying corpuscles) into a single process; the regulative awareness is united with a compensatory striving. Such a view makes an observer say, "Feeling and emotion are good things, sthenic in their influence, sustaining and regulating in their effects."

But let the complexities and difficulties mount to the point where an individual's limited coping powers begin to fail consistently: feelings of anxiety and fatigue will become prominent; a progressive disorganization will enter into what had hitherto been controlled movements; the feelings will begin to initiate rest behavior, giving up, and withdrawal of effort; and a *vegetative retreat* will set in. In the autonomic nervous system, the parasympathetic branch will be in ascendance; separate segments will begin to function in an excessive and autonomous fashion. Although there will be feelings and emotions in good measure, they will not operate on the sthenic side. The person will begin to cast about for an escape, to look for help, to anticipate a catastrophic defeat or a complete collapse, or to break out in wild expressions of angry frustration. Pushed far enough and long enough, he can feel despair and apathy; when this latter feeling is chronic, and his characteristic response is "What's the use?" we begin to speak of *aboulia* (a failure of will). Both output and effort decline. His aim is disorganized, and his actions and feelings may even turn against himself.

In such an end state, at the end of a curve of output that rose with the first joyful efforts, passed through anxiety, and descended into progressive disorganization and apathy, should we think of the end-state emotions as the *cause* of the collapse, or as one expression of a state of disorganization? Shall we think of those feelings and emotions at the beginning of the curve, as we seemed to be doing just a moment ago, as the *causes* of a steady improvement in performance, or as one facet of good psychological functioning?

Janet's theory of emotions makes them play a series of roles.

1. They can be sthenic influences. Janet makes use of them when he tries to rouse, threaten, cajole, bestir, encourage his hystericals to achieve a better integration. His patients realize what they have lost, and some of them beg him, "Emotionize me." They have experienced, before, the tonic effects of these supporting forces which make them come alive to their very fingertips. Janet suspects that some of his patients, like Pepita, have a kind of "addiction" to these states, as though an emotion were something that could be made to

function by itself, abstracted from its normal setting in the midst of action, used as a tonic, manipulated by itself.

2. They can also be energy-depleting. Janet records a recurrence of hysterical symptoms in some of his hystericals after they have gone through a period of intense emotions (e.g., those centering around grief, disappointment in love, failure in examination, breakup of a marriage, exhausting effort ending in a general disorganization of behavior). In these instances, the emotions are not sthenic, for they are followed by a lowering of psychological tension and an increase in "emotionality," that is, by a readiness for exaggerated responses to small blows, responses that also disorganize and incapacitate.

3. Emotions can also be described as *effects* of lowered psychological tension. Whatever decreases our power to cope with life, whatever depresses our power to gather our forces and to attack problems in an integrated way, also frees emotions. The little things that we would ordinarily take in our stride or use as cues in our coping efforts are now reacted to as though they were major disturbances: they flick us on the raw, revive old unpleasant memories of insults, catastrophic failures, or disasters. In the hysterical they are enough to produce a new round of symptoms: anesthesia, or amnesia, or a contracture returns.

We can thus use the single term "emotion" to describe qualitatively different dynamic fields. Emotions at the beginning of successful action have a different functional significance from those at the end of a series of exhausting efforts. We should bear this fact in mind as we consider those classes of occasions that precipitate neurotic symptoms. For example, in his *Psychological Healing,* Janet mentions the following classes of occasions that keep cropping up in the histories of hystericals, just prior to the onset of symptoms: the first communion, the entry into life (leaving home), social functions, rest (holidays), occupational responsibilities, changes in environment, quarrels (or dangers), death of a near kin, betrothal (marriage), education of children, and old age. Reading the titles of these categories is not wholly convincing, but when we have followed Janet through his analysis, we can see that each of the categories he has named is interpreted as an occasion for new and difficult adjustments. Consider, for example, the extended period of rest, the holiday or vacation, and ask, "How could this be the occasion for an outbreak of symptoms?" Janet invites us to consider the man who has been leaning on a work routine as a protective organizer that crowds out fearful thoughts and provides a pattern for his days; for him a long rest is like an enforced retirement. He is at a loss to occupy himself, having lost the one basis of worth that he had, and is instead faced with endless decisions as to how to spend this free time, and with quarrels with the rest of the family. The man who is boss at the office is now forced to "fetch and carry," lug the picnic basket, start the camp fire, kill the spiders and bees, and so on. We can begin to see how Janet is going to find in each of his categories the types of occasion that lead to exhaustion and disorganization, and that call for more integrative power than the person can supply. He could have added others: the birth of a child, occasions that reinforce a sense of inferiority, demonstrations of impotence—there are as many classes of such occasions as the wit of a classifier can construct.

We can expect clients to enter clinics with an immediate past history of one of these "precipitating causes." We have to remember, however, that every developmental task, every occasion for new learning, can be an occasion for two radically different outcomes, depending on the balance of forces. These occasions challenge us and test us; they can make us stronger when we discover a way to master them, or can defeat us, depress us, and reduce us to apathy and despair. (Martin Luther facing the occasion of his first mass, André Gide entering a public-school classroom after having been tutored at home, a nervous young teacher facing his first class can be so disturbed at these first encounters that their task seems impossible; a little support and encouragement, or an added bit of difficulty, can throw the balance from positive to negative learning.) Should the clinician be moved to identify these occasions as the cause of hysteria, he should not overlook the fact that he is also identifying the most banal transition points in life, the common occasions which each of us must learn to live through. In meeting them the strong will discover improved strength through mastery, whereas the weak will emerge with fixations, false generalizations, and neurotic symptoms as end-products.[13]

What kinds of generalizing statements can we make, then, about the feelings and emotions of the hysterical? They tend, Janet felt, to be shallow and weak, instead of being the sthenic supports for integration that fill the "happy warrior" with energy. They tend toward extremes that break out of containment. (Or is it simply that the forces of containment are weaker?) Since they function, in the hysterical, within a constricted behavioral field, where the brakes of reason and the more remote concerns do not operate as effectively, the extreme expressions, which are also shallow, are more easily triggered by slight blows and local frustrations. Easily triggered, they have less sthenic value, and offer poor support for sustained effort. Where they are "cooked-up," as in the "emotion-addict" who uses them to arouse a sluggish system, they are apt to wear out rapidly. Depending on the degree to which the integrative forces are depleted, the feelings of the hysterical patient thus tend to drift toward states of emptiness, apathy, and boredom.[14]

Histrionics

Perhaps we should remember both that not all hystericals have "a typical hysterical character," and that, in accusing the hysterical of *histrionics,* we are repeating the kinds of evaluations that ran through earlier discussions of

---

[13]The clinician who finds that his adolescent patient has been sent into a depression on the occasion of his first communion may grow angry at the priest or look upon his patient's conflicts as "implicit in the religion on which he had been reared": cf. Roland Bainton's (1950, p. 42) comment on Luther's mighty wrestling with evil. Yet the plain fact seems to be that the same religion accommodates all manner of men, easily. Was it not their very laxity that Luther fought against?

[14]Some of the plays of Chekhov and novels of Dostoevsky give us the impression that a whole social class in Czarist Russia had arrived at a group malaise of this type.

malingering. Nevertheless, it has become something of a tradition, since Janet's day, to point to the hysterical as an "actor," as a bit of a "phony." While his expressions may be stormy, like a summer thundershower they may be expected to pass rapidly. If, as Ey suggests, he would feel at home in theatrical circles, it is because he can live out simulated emotions in this milieu, where they are the stock in trade of everyone.

Still another way of describing this type of person is to suggest that he is more mask, more *persona,* than authentic self. Such a person is forever taking up some new role, putting on a new face and manner, as though he were not a deeply committed and solidly integrated person who knows who he is and means what he says. Those who like to trace such matters back to early infancy tend to suspect one or both of the parents of originally refusing to accept the child's deeply felt emotions, authentic wishes, and real desires, in which case, they argue, the child in his insecurity must pretend to have feelings that he does not feel, to seem to desire goals that are not really his own. Such a "shell of pretense" becomes a way of getting on with parents, a way of achieving peace in the family. It expresses a need for affection and approval that, under the circumstances, is warping the course of development.

This kind of displacement of the person from his natural center means that what he undertakes under such outer-directed and enforced conditions is a shallow shell of role-playing. It also means that the person is constantly in danger of being exposed, that he has to overdo the expressions of his feelings to cover the inner emptiness or lack of conviction behind his actions. In his moments of truthfulness such a person might turn on the one who began this split between persona and real self, as André Gide turned upon his mother in his autobiographical novel, *Si le grain ne meurt* (1928, p. 363): "You never loved me for what I really was, but for what you thought I ought to become."

From such a "displaced person's" unhappy feelings comes a resentment against being put upon, a rebellion against requirements to conform, and a special commitment to the ideal of liberty. The liberty of a truly tough and autonomous agent is both the last thing such a person could manage and his deepest desire. Of all the authorities, the judges, the evaluators, who are continually giving him trouble, he could say, as Housman does in "The Laws of God, the Laws of Man":

> "Their deeds I judge and much condemn,
> Yet when did I make laws for them?
> Please yourselves, say I, and they
> Need only look the other way."

But *they* never do, nor does he let them, any more than André Gide could allow his mother to preserve her illusions. "Look at me," he seems to say, "See what I really am," for deep within him remains the need to be valued as he really is.

Thus one conflict of the hysterical (some would urge it is the basic one) is caused by a displacement of action from the authentic center of motivation, and by the development of a persona, a false front, an outer shell of conformity. The expressive movements of this superficial self may be dramatic, outwardly visible, but they are also shallow; secretly the true self may watch this phony self, as though from over his shoulder, and say, "Oh, come now. You're putting it on." He sees his own tears as "crocodile tears," and accuses himself, "You are not even sure that you feel anything. All of this is for them, for effect!"

PERCEPTUAL DEFECTS OF THE HYSTERICAL

The hysterical's perceptions can be so severely defective that the skin surface, eyes, ears, do not seem to function at all, yet when he is distracted, or is in hypnotic trance, he can respond with normal sensory thresholds. In the less severely depressed functioning of some hystericals, objects can be identified and named, persons recognized, but everything has an aura of unfamiliarity, of unreality. Like the student who, studying late, can still read the words but fails to sense either the poetry or the meaning of what he is reading, these neurotics perceive incompletely; their reactions are not fully developed or elaborated. The parts do not jell into a solid synthesis or make a complete figure. A pseudoneurological description would be easy to construct: somehow the impulses that reach the cortex do not set in motion the normal range of reverberations and elaborations that enrich, identify, and qualify a particular figure, and that place it in a broader context of meaning. When the hysterical confesses to a vague feeling and asks, "Haven't I been here before?" or when he reports a weird sense of unreality that he can neither explain nor shake off, we are inclined, again, to put down these experiences to the incompleteness of his perceptual responses. These are low-grade perceptions, incompletely developed, poorly related to past and future, and capable of arousing only a vague feeling of familiarity (that is sometimes false). Such patients are also known to say (when it is patently false), "I have never been here before." One of Janet's patients insisted, "That is not my sister!" when, in fact, it was. Pressed to note her features, down to the little details of the fillings in her teeth, the patient could be forced to admit a remarkable resemblance, but one thing still remained lacking: the *feeling* that this was really his own sister. Something vital about the relationship had been lost, and with it the readiness to act on his identification.

Jamais vu and *déjà vu* are thus two phases of a more general defect in perceptive regulation. In an analogous way, the paralyses and contractures of the hysterical patient are aspects of a single inability to control and coordinate action. Possibly both his wild rages and his complete apathy are also signs of his incapacity to will, to keep his emotions within bounds, to produce effective coordinations that cope with reality, to relate his acts to an authentic core of motivation.

Continuing with the intellectual facet of behavior, we can note the two sorts of memories that Janet, along with Bergson, described. A good memory of an event places that event in its proper niche in time and space. Such a memory can be used to fill out and strengthen a stance in the present field that, in turn, serves as the launching platform of actions directed into the future. A poor memory, on the contrary, is a mere rehearsal, even if it has some of the qualities of total recall. It can be kicked off by some external conditioned stimulus, or can represent a diversionary routine (like a pun) that splits off from what was, initially, an organized train of thought. Once a part of some other setting, this poor memory merely rehearses the old sequence of thought and action, lives over the scene. Inappropriate to the present context (or rather, not made appropriate), it is an intruder. Such memories can live us (i.e., possess us, interrupt us, arrest our actions), rather than enrich our lives and make our purposes more efficient. They preoccupy us and devour us, like the beggar's lice. In the obsessive they defy his efforts to control them (like the lascivious thoughts that bother the maiden who is trying to compose her thoughts in preparation for taking communion). Such memories are neither summoned by the whole, active person nor regulated by him. In their simplest and lowest form, such memories are not even an awareness, but function outside the perceptive-regulative field, with all the automatic quality of a pulsebeat or the intestines' peristaltic movements. They may be partially conscious, merely the exposed tip of that buried iceberg of an old memory.

Janet described a patient who entered the clinic complaining of acute abdominal pains. Careful study revealed that the patient had suffered burns and lacerations in a railway accident years before, when, as engineer, he had piloted a train into a head-on crash. A long and painful recovery, following surgery, had finally been complete, and he had gradually forgotten the accident. At times, when he was very drunk, the memory came back to haunt him, and it assumed such painful proportions when he became intoxicated that he was obliged to give up drinking. When he entered hospital he did not associate his abdominal pains with the old accident at all, but looked on them as some new digestive difficulty. The pains were conscious enough, but the rest of the scene, of which they were once a part, failed to emerge. He could not identify his pains, place them appropriately in a past. He had recently experienced the death of a daughter and of his wife; in the ensuing depression the old pattern was partially revived. In this same fashion, an old phantom limb, long forgotten but originally very painful, will return to haunt a patient going through a time of troubles (see Kolb 1954; Ewalt, Randall, and Morris 1947). When the current organization of action is weakened, the old traumatic memories can irrupt, but they do not always return in a form complete enough for them to be placed in their proper context.

VOLITIONAL DEFECTS OF THE HYSTERICAL

Looking at the third great facet of mental life, the volitional, we can almost anticipate Janet's emphasis, for the defects in the patient's "will" will match those in the two facets just described: the will is incomplete; it exists in the form of unregulated impulses and in an inability to plan. Janet's view centers on the patient's power to act effectively in the real world, to construct a future, to create new combinations, to deal with a practical and novel reality. Janet noted that the whole class of behavior changes which he classified as psychasthenic was somehow less vital, less real, less capable of being transformed; he considered hysteria a subtype of psychasthenia in which amnesias, somnambulisms, anesthesias, and contractures were found. Bound by his past, fantasying an unrealistic future, playing the role, the hysterical was less vitally engaged with his milieu.

Just as there are restrictions of the field of awareness, of remembering, and of perceiving, as well as restrictions in feeling and emotion, so there are *restrictions in action.* Purposive movements always occur within a field, require a vigilance that will correct and redirect them as they unfold. They must be constantly reshaped in view of their goal. If the field is enlarged, the number of factors that have to be synthesized in such corrections increases, and the process grows complex and difficult. The leader of a discussion group who would like to involve all participants and draw out every divergent viewpoint faces such an increase in difficulty as his group grows larger and the membership more varied.

Who cannot walk a two-by-eight-inch plank, when it is stretched between two blocks that raise it a few inches from the floor? The act of balancing seems easy, even if the plank sways a little as we walk. Place the plank on two window ledges, across a narrow areaway between two buildings at the first story; the fall would not be more than twelve feet, but walking becomes something of a challenge. Place it at the top of the buildings, at the seventh floor, and the action will become impossible for most of us. Neither the width of the board, nor the distance we must walk, nor the amount of bending and swaying under our weight, if we move properly, has changed but the *action* of balancing has changed. To synthesize such an action under the pressure of inhibiting fears, and to regulate our motion (and our visual fixations) against the new and distant background, is a much more difficult action. Likewise, to perform in public (where the "fall" is a shameful failure before an audience) or to discuss a serious matter before an audience of persons with strong and distinct personalities will involve us in conflict, fill our minds with inhibiting thoughts of the multiple consequences occurring in each of our hearers; such a situation is too difficult for some of us, particularly when we are required to "take a position" and to act in authentic and responsible fashion. It is such a difficulty in a particular performance that makes it a candidate for hysterical nonfeasance, Janet believes, rather than its special content, its peculiar relationship to a basic instinct or urge, or its social or ethical value.

Even the mere number of items that have to be synthesized in a single action may make that action too difficult. Janet notes that his hystericals can attend to only a few things at a time. The patient at the Salpêtrière ball who complained to Janet that she could not see the costumes because she had to attend to the dancing showed this difficulty in synthesizing. Eating and talking before others were too difficult for another patient, who had to eat alone. For some sensitive persons, talking to a stranger can be like walking a plank suspended between the roofs of two buildings; it is so disorganizing that they "draw a blank," to use their own words.

New actions, multiple actions that require fusion and synthesis, actions in which conflicting impulses have to be harmonized and inhibitions over-ridden, voluntary actions, responsible actions with multiple consequences, actions that are related to a wide field of personal involvement are all difficult and costly, and these are the ones that the abouliac cannot perform. If such an aboulia (which Janet identified as a part of a hysterical attack) were a consistent personality trait, we might use it as one of the indices of the more or less enduring hysterical character. Since it is also a dynamic property of an action system, may appear for a short while and then disappear, we might also expect to find that persons who at one time have flagrant signs of hysteria may have succeeded in noteworthy accomplishments at others. St. Theresa, with her stigmata and ecstasies and depressions, was also the founder of the Carmelite order, and an able administrator and negotiator with civil and ecclesiastical authorities.

The Nature of Aboulia

Aboulia is associated with suggestibility. Having a will of one's own, having a place to go and a goal to win, makes one think twice before acceding to some idea or request that comes from without. The will-less are the soft and compliant. They may even fear the effect of being with others, complaining of the horsecollar of the bureau, of the pressures toward conformity, of the impossibility of inserting their will in that organized life we call society.

It could be circular to define aboulia as a state and then say it has *caused* the suggestibility. The two are merely facets of a single trend in personality structure. The same might be said of the beliefs of the hysterical. These patients do not achieve rational convictions *on their own,* yet, strangely, they are, of all men, believers, arriving all too quickly at an automatic and unreflective form of belief, and with a special craving for certitude.

They are also poor beginners and poor stoppers; that is, they are poor at self-regulation. They dislike change, yet they are quick to grow bored with difficult actions, quick to rebel against a discipline that requires hard work of them, quick to imagine that the grass must be greener elsewhere. Although they are in fact healthier and happier under routine, they make liberty their highest value. Some of them are ready to escape into mystical experiences, into states where they can be completely spontaneous. Some of them begin as conscious dreamers, seeking the solitude in which revery is easy, planning their "meditations," executing adroit introversive maneuvers. Executed intentionally, these maneuvers sometimes end in the hysterical being "dreamed" by his automatisms, possessed by mechanisms which run themselves. As mystics or mediums, some hystericals have learned how to put themselves into the relaxed state in which their visions come; but they warn others against "trying too hard." They instruct the novice to approach the experience with the attitude of surrender, to drop all concerns, even the concern about entering this special kind of consciousness.

Hypnagogic Images

There is a variety of image that appears before the closed eyelids of a person who is drifting between waking and sleep. It seems to be present in richer supply in those who sleep lightly and who have difficulty in falling asleep. *Going to sleep* is one of the actions the neurotic often finds difficult. That the hysterical should be a good customer for the pharmacist who sells hypnotics is an interesting datum we owe to Janet. Like eidetic images, the hypnagogic images have an objective quality: they are as definite as an afterimage, and as completely "out there." They can be studied, like a foreign object, although those who have observed them warn against allowing interest to grow too keen; for they evaporate the moment the observer is aroused from his drowsy, half-waking state. As though one were watching these "pictures" through closed lids, they can be observed as they come and go (see Leroy 1926; Ey 1948, pp. 189 ff).

These images arise in the transition between waking and sleep, in a twilight zone in which our thoughts are freed from the constraint of immediately pressing practical concerns. They represent a kind of automatic functioning of part of the central visual apparatus; they have a quality that reminds us of the aboulia of the hysterical, an independence or autonomy; they cannot be directed at will but must function automatically; and they possess the observer in a way that is analogous to some of the symptoms of the hysterical and the obsessive. Yet this possessed observer knows they are images; they do not take over completely in the way the trance state possesses the somnambulist. The two systems exist side by side, in an uneasy coexistence: the placid observer, who can take them or leave them and who can snuff them out by the effort to waken; and the automatisms, which have a kind of life of their own and do not obey the observer's wishes. Henri Ey believes that they are most abundant when one is exhausted and less completely in control of one's mental functions, when one is troubled with insomnia, or when one is suffering from a neurosis. The normal "tired feeling" that comes at the end of a good day's work will prompt us to fall asleep as soon as we go to bed. The exhaustion that goes with aboulia is of a different sort: hypnagogic images multiply, sleep is shallow and less restful; and the inferior type of sleep is matched by inferior planning and action the next day.

In a discussion of the acute psychoses, Ey (1954, pp. 691 ff) develops the notion of a "destructuring threshold." Since the making of a figure of action offers special difficulty for the hysterical, his suggestions may have a bearing here, as well. Objectively, this "threshold of destructuring" is revealed by the dosage that is required when tranquilizers are used: the less firmly structured are susceptible to smaller doses of drugs. In these susceptible ones there is a wide band of borderline states that are not fully conscious, not fully integrated, not "managed," and in which subordinate parts escape from the control of the normally regulative awareness system. Within a part of this band, the person can act as both voyeur-observer and dreamer; although he is conscious of the march of imagery, he cannot control its course. In this twilight state he can watch the images and know them for what they are, a product of his own imagination, yet he watches their independent unfolding with a fascinated interest.

Under this view "the unconscious" tends to be a series of levels of functioning, the deeper layers of which are submerged and out of range of waking consciousness altogether, the upper levels being within view yet possessing a certain autonomy. In the prophet and seer, these processes have sometimes escaped from normal controls and are then reacted to as though they were from a divine source; a Mohammed will carry on a conversation with the angel Gabriel, or a Moses will listen to a voice from a burning bush. The homicidal schizophrenic becomes a menace when he acts under the guidance of the voices. The obsessive remains fully oriented but is troubled by the thoughts which he cannot banish from his mind and which irrupt into his normal concerns. The little spiritualist who entered the Geneva circle studied by Flournoy did not know what to think, at first, when his automatic handwriting, first tried skeptically, began to intrude into his daily life. Depending on their anchorage in a general system of beliefs, those who discover that they possess eidetic imagery, and that these images, projected upon a neutral surface before them, sometimes move independently and change before their eyes (instead of remaining fixed, like an afterimage), may be tempted to assign them more significance than they have. The hysterical who is aware only of a moving system of images, and not of the context to which they should be referred, may misidentify them as signs of an organic ailment, only to be invited by his psychiatrist to refer them to his unconscious.

Less bound within a system of intentional actions, these half-conscious and unconscious automatisms unroll in a mechanical and haphazard way. A conditioned response can operate in a similarly independent fashion, as it does in the alcoholic who unwillingly submitted to conditioned-reflex therapy and who knows that it was merely an association between the sight of his favorite cocktail and the emetine that now makes him nauseated. However, the "cured alcoholic" has the means to correct matters: knowing the origin of his slight nausea, and familiar with the process of extinction, he can repeat the conditioned stimulus without reinforcement and thus restore his capacity to drink without nausea. His automatisms will once more be "under control."

If this kind of automatism can run underneath the surface awareness, it can irrupt to form the "bright idea" that is transformed and reshaped to fit a current need, or it can take over control of action, especially when there is any weakening or abdication of normal vigilant control. The student of the abnormal witnesses a kind of seesaw struggle between these automatisms and the rational, reflective, vigilant powers of the individual. Whatever weakens the latter, loosens the individual's hold upon reality, gives greater scope to the automatisms.

Jean Lhermitte (1951, pp. 52-55) has some interesting personal observations which show that these automatisms can, under special conditions, pass into full-blown hallucinations. Here the "waking dreamer" loses his critical awareness and accepts the dreams, with whatever powers of belief remain, as reality itself. On the morrow, he may vouch for their authenticity *as experience,* while injecting doubt now supplied by his fully functioning critical faculties. It was at the end of a long, three-day march when, too long without sleep and almost drugged with fatigue, Lhermitte began to have hallucinations of extreme vividness. He saw the dappled flanks of horses, caught in the moonlight that penetrated the trees, as he nodded, exhausted, riding a caisson on a long retreat. Others in the troop saw a village on a distant mountainside, a village that was not on any map. Neither horses nor village could be verified as the kind of fact that exists when our attention turns away.

Similarly, the extreme lassitude and boredom that come to the prisoner under prolonged solitary confinement (or the condition that is produced in some subjects in the sensory-deprivation experiment, where the normal support of external cues is cut off) permit a weakening of that normal stance that keeps the automatisms in their place.[15]

As a neurosis or psychosis develops, this in-between band of half-conscious processes grows wider, and the person who watches it encroach on that area normally under his control may feel he is losing his mind precisely because it operates with its own powers. The weakening of the organizing and integrating process (as in aboulia) and the invasion by the automatisms are two phases of a single process.

Janet's Marcelle

Marcelle (on whom see Janet 1893, pp. 103 ff) showed in extreme form what a less severe instance of aboulia would reveal only obscurely:

Extending her hand was too much for Marcelle. She had to be urged, cajoled, even threatened, and then when she made a feeble attempt she quickly withdrew it, saying, "But I can't." She would sit, crocheting automatically, scarcely moving otherwise, and resisted all invitation to other activities. Urged, she began to show emotion, pouted, grew stubborn. She could not dress and undress herself without assistance. Left to her own devices, every action was interminable. She kept begin-

---

[15]See Solomon *et al.* 1961. In the light of Janet's logic, we can understand why there should be a great deal of individual variation in such destructuring, even when there is an effort to standardize the external conditions, for the toughness in the integrative process that is put under stress varies from subject to subject. Some can keep alive that life-space to which they know they will return, and make every effort to keep up morale under captivity. Compare the efforts of Nehru (1941), described in his autobiography, of Edith Bone (1957), or of Jean Cazeneuve (1945). three imprisoned ones who felt there was a "work" they could perform to preserve their integrity.

ning over, again and again, what she started out to do, or she sat, in suspended animation, as though she could not move into the next phase of action. If we could think of each action as a schema that has to be set in motion, corrected in course, and then discharged and replaced by the next schema, Marcelle lacked the power to charge the schemata and to start and stop them. Those that ran at all seemed to require an external instigation and guidance. Janet found her, one day, sitting empty-handed. "I am so bored," she said, "without my crocheting. Will you hand it to me?" (for it had been there, all the time, on the table). Marcelle was not paralyzed, unless we can speak of a paralysis of will. The tougher normal regards such a person with a certain contempt: "Such people would sit on a burr rather than get up."

Fully charged schemata are similarly lacking in the young student who cannot fully visualize and feel the consequences of nonfeasance, as he mopes, doing little or nothing, or, if he weakly feels them and can verbalize them, he cannot act in accordance with what he anticipates. The victim of aboulia is often left with routine habits fairly intact; he may be able to obey, or act under urging. It is when he needs to "make up his mind," to act as a responsible and authentic person with a plan, particularly when he has to act in the midst of novel reality, that the deficit appears.

Marcelle wanted to go out in the sun, but she was sitting, and it seemed too much effort. She wanted to speak to the physician when he was there, but she was too slow to respond, and before she could form the phrases he had gone. The wishes were there, in feeble form, but she could not execute them. Such a patient may sit during an interview while the counselor probes, questions, tries to put words in the patient's mouth; although the patient betrays little interest, he returns, a week later, for another bout with the "helpful" therapist. There is no paralysis of the speech apparatus. Sometimes an answer forms, but the sentence is half-expressed, left hanging, incomplete. The frustrated counselor begins to wonder if the patient is playing a game with him, for his own attention is quickened. It is almost as though a part of her fell asleep in the middle of a sentence. With her eyes wide open, she is "too tired" to function, to communicate anything.

The Inability to Charge the Schemata

Commonly this motor aboulia does not affect simple movements. But since many simple actions involve decisions, or function within a developing plan, even such simple actions as eating, dressing, or writing a letter may fail. In general, it is the purposive action, rather than the part-movements, that is weak. For these patients every decision seems to be painful. For every argument "pro," they can find a matching "con"; some of them delight in playing the game of getting up both sets of arguments. Janet's Claire wanted to be an actress, or to go into a convent, but she couldn't make up her mind which. She wondered whether she should become a saint or a completely abandoned woman. In a not too obscure way these two extremes are alike, as burning hot and icy cold are; both are easier than the life of compromises in which "nothing too much" is the rule. Such people cannot choose a dress or a box of writing paper, any more than they can choose a career or a husband. "Tell me," they say, "which should I do?" They are constantly trying to entrap their friends into declarations, and then promptly present the *opposite* side. If their friends are too insistent, they are accused of trying to run the lives of these doubters.

Decisive action seems to require a kind of force that these patients lack; it is the occasion that will require such action that they will avoid in advance, as they try to regulate their lives in psychasthenic style. It is not the touch of the doorknob that Marcelle fears, for if one is placed passively in her hands by someone else she does not recoil. It is making the decision to open and enter a door, and face what lies beyond it, that is too much for her.

Such indecisive ones complain that the examination is too long, the questions too ambiguous, instead of selecting those questions that can be answered in the allotted time. They complain, "If there were only more time," and tend to come too late to a meeting. Their actions unfold slowly. Their efforts fall just short of what is needed for full achievement. They tire easily and leave work at loose ends. They cling to the habitual and shun the new. Janet felt that they also shun the social forms of action, and found in these patients unusually great timidity and searching for isolation, for some means of putting and keeping a distance between themselves and others. "When I want to play some little piece on the piano before someone," Janet was informed by Nadia, "even before you, whom I know so well, it seems that the actions become difficult, something inhibits me, and if I try to overcome it, I have to put forth an extraordinary effort. My face flushes and I feel lost. I wish that the earth would open and swallow me up" (Janet 1903, p. 355).

There are two forms to every action, Janet reminds us, one when we perform the act in solitude and the other when we do it in front of or in collaboration with others. "I can talk freely with a single person," says one patient, "but when two or three are present, I grow confused. I seem to want to please everyone, to include everyone in my action, and it is all too difficult." "I would be perfect, I could do everything, if I could be altogether alone, like a savage on a desert island; society is made to prevent people from acting. I have the will for everything, but I do not have it except when I am alone" (*ibid*).

If these abouliacs have trouble in the "affection department," it will not be surprising, for their impulse to withdraw is easily interpreted as coldness. They, like the rest of us, are in need of affection, collaboration, and support, perhaps unusually so, for their need for guidance, direction, even unconditional consideration, is excessive; yet to find this affection and consideration requires a certain tougher, more active, more potent type of social participation. If we call theirs a passive love, it is also a wish for an unconditional love, and, of course, for a very unrealistic form of love.

The aboulia that Janet describes is not so much a fear-ridden inhibition, a disgust, or a lack of desire as it is a weakness in "stance-making," a lack of the power to affirm and persist, a failure in becoming an autonomous center of forceful action. Autistic activities are less inhibited; daydreaming, imagining, thinking about action, automatic actions are present in good supply. But the collaborative ones that involve a person in social actions, in a persistent struggle with novel realities, are in short supply.

Janet accuses his abouliacs of breaking up their actions into little loads, of acting piecemeal, of going through interminable series of preparatory approaches, in contrast to persons who have a more rugged capacity to plan and execute a whole action in one continuous trajectory. The abouliac has to be sure of himself, and sure that he is sure, and sure of the setting in which the action is to function. He therefore has to preplan, preorganize, rehearse in advance, cross all the bridges, prepare for all contingencies. He writes out his speech in advance, plans the interview down to the smallest details, goes over the agenda to be followed in the conference, for he can afford to leave nothing to chance. He even writes down his symptoms on bits of paper lest he forget to tell his doctor all. His writing is full of digressions, and he finds that he has to "get up" a number of subtopics before he can approach the goal he had intended. As a matter of fact, he had not been able to *intend* it fully, sharply, clearly, as we can see from his distractibiliy and from the ease with which novelty inhibits him. It would seem that this insecure person is present in Everyman, and will emerge whenever the going gets rough or the integrative forces are in short supply.

Intellectual Aboulia

There is a semantic agnosia that corresponds to these defects in action. The lack of the integrative force which would hold an action on target also emerges as a defect in the perceiving process such that parts can be seen, but not the whole. Never was the slogan of the gestaltists more true, "The whole is something more and other than the sum of its parts." Some researchers have reported similar perceptual deficits in frontal-lobe patients, who are unable to build up a whole out of parts that are exposed and reacted to correctly enough, as parts. Or consider the student who is struggling to master a difficult presentation, forcing himself to underline passages, to make marginal notes, still emphasizing the parts, while the larger whole still fails to take shape easily and spontaneously.

This unseeing form of seeing, this uncomprehending form of looking, has been called *aprosexia*. The example of the uncomprehending student should show us how general this limitation on perceiving is. Janet quotes St. Theresa as observing, one day, that as she read the life of one of the saints she found herself reading passages sometimes four and five times before she could comprehend them, though the words were those of a familiar language, and she threw the work aside in disgust. Janet also notes that St. Theresa was subject to attacks of spiritual dryness when she could not read from the book of life in any better fashion. In these special periods she found that she could go through the motions of familiar rituals; but they did nothing for her. She felt that her prayers did not ascend, that her heart was not in her work, and that the life of devotion that had begun like a proper spiritual marriage seemed suddenly empty and without meaning. She feared these attacks, for in them her faith faltered and her doubts seemed to put her immortal soul in jeopardy. The hysterical, it seems, shares something with the obsessive, the bored neurasthenic, and the depressed. "The hystericals of today," Janet wryly remarked some time ago, "seem to continue to follow the pattern of one who might be called their patron saint."[16]

Janet asked his patient Marcelle to read a certain short passage for him. She did so, but complained while complying. "Now," he continued, "tell me in your own words what you have read." But Marcelle could not manage this; she complained that, although she had read the passage, it had not "entered her head." "Read it again, this time aloud!" she was ordered. Janet noted that she read her native tongue as if it were a foreign language: the words came forth, but in a wooden, uncomprehending manner. When she had completed the second reading, the result was the same. To read the words, to perform the parts, is not to make a whole. In aboulia, the patient's actions and perceptions fall short of this last stage of synthesis. It was as though she had forgotten the beginning before she had reached the middle of the paragraph. Should we explain her difficulty by referring to her poor memory? Not if it is a question of repeating something old, something long remembered, something learned on an earlier day. Yes, if it is a question of imprinting and organizing a new passage with understanding. In the extreme form, this deficit does include a continuous amnesia, in which a patient who is aware of what he is doing at any instant seems to forget it as soon as it has passed; although an observer might imagine that he must be aware of his surroundings, the patient does not in fact "make a history" of his doings in hospital. The parts glide in and out of awareness, but they are neither organized into a meaningful whole nor left as useful memories.

This semantic agnosia can be studied in the laboratory. Looking through a tube that permits only a very small portion of a figure to be seen at one time, a subject can learn to trace its outline. He can learn which movement follows what preceding movement. He can even make a recital of the process. Curiously, he may form no conception of the shape or meaning of the figure that the lines bound, yet when the figure (say, a shoe) is exposed as a whole in a tachistoscope, for as little as a tenth of a second, he can name it and discriminate it from others (a trunk, a mirror, or a table). Like this subject who has the penumbra of the field screened away from his vision, the hysterical suffering from an intellectual aboulia can move through the parts of an action without generating the forward thrust into the future or developing a sense of the whole. Normally there is a tension to complete a figure. But if the patient forms the whole poorly, if at all, this tension must be at a very low ebb. This low degree of tautness in psychological systems is here

---

[16]See Quercy (1930, I, 173-348) for an interesting discussion of her health, from a Catholic point of view.

described as an intellectual deficit, but other observations of the hysterical indicate that there is also an affective aboulia (an emptiness, an inability to feel) and a volitional aboulia, which Janet describes as a constriction of action.

More striking is the demonstration with Marcelle that there is no defect in her rote memory. After reading a short passage several times and failing to discover its meaning, Marcelle was asked to repeat the words in the two lines, and did so correctly. Still she did not comprehend them. What teacher has not discovered students with such a capacity to repeat words or phrases without comprehension? This incomprehension of a large figure is not limited to reading or to speech, but also appears in this patient's grasp of the real events in her life. Often a person, distracted by his own thoughts, is unable to pay attention to what is before him, showing a temporary "absent-mindedness." Such a momentary lowering of the perceptual powers disappears as the distracting thought is dissipated and the person returns to full vigilance. The hysterical's deficit in figure-making also disappears when the attack of the illness is over. How tempting to imagine some inner and possibly sub-conscious source of distraction! Yet, if we follow Janet's logic, we must consider the destructuring or splitting off of such a subsystem as itself a part of the changes we call hysterical, and to be explained by that same complex set of causes that underlie the lowering of psychological tension.

This inability to give the kind of complete attention that grasps and orders the field of action can be of all degrees of severity. If it is very severe, we could speak of a state of emptiness, in which the patient is so empty of feeling, and so apathetic, that he is indifferent about his incapacity. Less severe, the deficit is felt as such, and it is painful. The patient complains of his lack of integrative power, of his lack of interest in anything, of his boredom, of his restlessness, of his inability to do completely what he can do in parts. Thus, on a curve which shows the rise and fall in the structure of action, we can conceive of a graded series: first, exaggerations of effort and fatigue, a feeling of pressure that does not quite produce the complete action desired; next, as the integrative force declines, the feeling of effort is replaced by anxiety, then by a tense and morose feeling of incapacity, inaction, and rest-lessness, and then by the *feeling* of emptiness; finally, there is the calm and indifferent *state* of emptiness.

Janet pointed out a relationship between this failure in the attention process and some of the other symptoms of hysteria. Aside from the slowness of attention, there is a certain frangibility in the process; when the patient is urged, cajoled, forced to attend, then the twisting and turning, the anguish and anxiety, the sweating and other autonomic symptoms break out, and the clinician may witness an outbreak of side-effects such as anesthesias, tics, contractures, paralyses. The latter, which Janet called *derivations,* could also be called conversions, transformations, equivalents. The hard currency of organized and purposive action is cashed in for the cheaper and inflated currency of symptoms. The forces or energies assembled for a "high-level" or difficult action that fails can be converted into the simpler forms: the fretful, automatic, emotional, visceral, reflexive, or random forms of action, which express a low order of tension and accomplish little. "Pull yourself together," we admonish such a person, when we see the disintegration begin; sometimes he can, briefly, as though with a force we have summoned, but the added pressure may also intensify the outburst of automatisms and visceral symptoms. What we might call an "effort syndrome" could be described as a substitution of low-level and disorganized activity in glands and muscles for the highly coordinated and directed patterns that seem to require a type of integrative power which is absent in these patients. The collapse of willing is the occasion for the emergence of symptoms.

JANET'S THERAPY

Janet's Irene (1893, pp. 506-44), 23 years old when he first saw her, had been suffering for more than two years from recurring somnambulistic attacks, which irrupted spontaneously into the rather dull and apathetic condition she had fallen into after the death of her mother. In her seizures she lived through the scene of her mother's death with hallucinatory vividness, dramatically portraying in actions and comments what she had been unable to recall during the months that had elapsed. Interviewed at the clinic, she insisted that she could remember nothing of her mother's death. She also could not recall certain incidents before that event, especially if they related to her father's drunkenness and her mother's neuroticism, or immediately afterward.

Another peculiarity in her remembering emerged when Janet questioned her about her life since she had entered the hospital. She could give no sensible account of what she had been doing or of what had occurred about her. Later, when hypnotized, she could recall this hospital life. If she had been constructing memories, making a figure of her days (as a gestaltist might say), it was at some lower level of her mental functioning that represented a less than fully vigilant form of response.[17]

Irene had been told that her mother was dead. Her relatives forced her to put on mourning. She could name the date of the event, since she had been reminded so often. Finally, with Janet's help and the use of hypnosis, she was learning to speak about the details of the event. But even with this educated form of posthypnotic recall, her mother's death remained unreal:

---

[17]Referred to, in the literature of hypnosis, as the *hypermnesia* of the trance state, this superior recall gives the impression that both the hysterical's subconscious and the hypnotic trance state extend farther than our ordinary waking recall. The hypnotized army officer can remember the number of the form he used in issuing passes to the members of his company ten years ago, whereas, awake, he refuses even to try to recapture such a detail. Perhaps it is a similar resurgence of old and long-forgotten memories that makes some clinicians refer to LSD-25 and other psychotomimetic drugs as "mind-expanding." The cult of hypnosis (or mesmerism, as it was then called) that led the leader of the Knights of Malta to advise all members to take the cure has been replaced in our time by the "psychedelic churches" that today promise so much to their parishioners. In terms of the subject's grasp of a present outer reality while these states are in effect, neither hypnosis nor the psychedelic drugs expand awareness.

she did not feel it, believe it. A memorized newspaper account of a stranger's death could not have seemed more artificial or remote from her own experience. She did not *own* the memories, nor refer them to her own past life. She "knew" that her mother had died. She could no longer remember what her mother looked like. Yet she also said that her mother had gone away on a trip and would return soon.[18] She would jump up when someone knocked, thinking that her mother was about to enter. She showed no sorrow. Indeed, she advanced her incapacity to feel anything as evidence that her own private belief was correct: "Would I behave this way if she were really dead?" In her constricted conscious field, there was room only for an abstract skeleton of an idea of that death, whereas in her expanded trance consciousness it was too real, vividly present in all details.

Janet set to work to restore the integrity of this system of memories, seeking to bind it with the rest of her conscious system of recall. He found that the trancelike dramatizations could be duplicated by the use of hypnosis, and, placing her back in that scene, by his suggestions he sought to transport the details she produced into the subsequent waking period by giving the appropriate posthypnotic suggestions. He turned to this type of reintegrative task, this "liquidation of traumatic memories," since the other therapies in standard use for hystericals at the Salpêtrière had failed.

Janet soon discovered that, both in the posthypnotic state and in the trance recall, Irene's capacity to absorb these memories had distinct limits. For example, the group of memories that centered around the death scene itself proved beyond her capacity to handle, at first. Either she dropped into them, or she found that she could not properly talk about them or represent them. Janet confronted the problem of retraining her memory even under hypnosis. She was urged to recall the events, to talk about them, to represent every detail in words, and to work inward from the events preceding her mother's death to those painful and critical last moments. Encouraging her, prompting her, which he could do since she had dramatized it all in the deeper somnambulistic state, Janet succeeded: the final traumatic scene was finally rehearsed until she *owned* it.

Finally, after this education of recall under hypnosis, the process had to be repeated in waking recall. There were momentary successes followed by relapses, as though, with the ebb and flow of some integrative power, she could tolerate now more, now less, of this traumatic past. He noted that when some emotional crisis in her waking life upset her, the carefully restored memories would plummet out of sight again, and she would drift back into her former divided state. Years after her recovery, when she was 28, she found that these slumps were still recurring, and she sometimes behaved like an obsessive-compulsive, with scruples, hesitations, indecision, anxieties, and

---

[18]Both the wakened somnambulist and the amnestic whose loss of the recent past is caused by brain lesions show this tendency to *confabulate*. They bridge the gaps in recall by "stories" which they seem to expect their hearers to find plausible.

feelings of inferiority, instead of with this island of amnesia or any return of hysterical attacks.[19]

Irene had lived in a special kind of time: her orientation to her past was poorly structured, and she lacked a lively future, when she was in her abnormal states. When she had recovered and assimilated her memories, she felt the change with keen appreciation: "I am no longer the same, I am taking up a new life, my head feels new. It seems to me that I am seeing things for the first time. Before I saw the same things but they were in a fog, as though in some faraway dream. Now for the first time I can truly recognize you."

As Irene improved in hospital, she became more sociable, and she talked to the patients on the ward without her terrible attacks of shyness and anger. She began to plan her life. Although battered and troubled by the memories she had regained, and full of anguish, she also felt a profound joy at the restoration of integrity.[20]

Irene's therapy could be described as a "lifting of the level of psychological tension," which not only lifted her spirits, restored her motivation, and brought back memories, but also banished the amnesia, aboulia, dissociation, and lack of vital contact with surroundings.

A VIEW OF MEMORY

Remembering, Janet repeatedly reminds us, is an action. The behaviorists will hasten to agree: a behavior sequence that unfolds in time under appropriate stimulation tends to be reproduced in a similar order on a later occasion when the earlier members of the sequence are aroused. Such a sequence has even been named a *redintegration*. But such a definition applies to a lower form of memory. The higher form that occurs in a talking social animal such as man, the form that must function in voluntary and vigilant action and in good communication, involves the power to represent and speak about past actions. It is an essential part of our social responsibility. We are often required to give a recital of what we have done, and to prepare for doing so we have learned to transform the events we live through into an ordered history to whose events we can point when required. Effective action into the future also requires that we make a stance founded on this recalled past, evaluating what has happened as we anticipate fresh consequences.

Otto Jespersen (1922) gave a hypothetical story of how language might have begun. Imagine a war party, he suggested, falling on a group of enemy

---

[19]This point is worth emphasizing, since Janet had worked hard to set up a distinction between the hysterical and other psychasthenics, between the "hysterical character" and the corresponding life style of the psychasthenic "obsessive-compulsive." What he here records points to the facts that these are dynamic conditions, that one can replace the other, that the effort to find a special constitutional weakness or a special period of development in which each type of trauma originates is misguided. Neither Janet nor his successors have fully understood this idea.

[20]That Irene felt such deep joy presents a problem to those who use the pleasure principle to account for repression. It also answers, at least in one way, those who suggest that it might be better for a patient with Irene's symptoms to be allowed to continue to forget her past. Perhaps we fail to distinguish pleasure and joy.

tribesmen, and suppose that a terrific battle develops, ending in a victory for the attackers. Imagine, further, that in their jubilation the victors express their feelings in a dance, and that as they dance they fall to shouting some rhythmic chant, so that a recurrent pattern of vocalization develops, like "Ta-ra-ra-boom-de-ay." When the whole affair has subsided and been forgotten, for a while, should one of the participants cry "Ta-ra-ra-boom-de-ay," the others would laugh, or shake their heads, or nod, or wince. Now the differences between the responses of his hearers might arise from the fact that one heard the meaning, "Come, let us form a war party and go forth to conquer some more enemies"; another heard him mean "Do you remember the day when we met the enemy from across the river and vanquished them?"; while another heard "We ought to be prepared, for we may find ourselves in that kind of fight any day." By gestures, by facial expressions, by his excited and anxious manner, the speaker might try to reduce the ambiguity, and of course the context in which this signal for recall is given would also add some power to discriminate. The agglutination of possible meanings would force the tribesman into many refinements of syntax, into the use of modifiers to sharpen this "pointing back," in order to increase the efficiency of such cries.

As language has developed, man has learned how to transform his actions so that they will prove effective bases for analysis, reporting, planning. As he pays attention to what he is doing, he also transforms his actions into another form, so that he can later stand questioning. Like a sentry who has been well-trained, and who not only knows how to take cover when he hears an enemy patrol but can also note the uniform, the insignia, the number of soldiers, and the kinds of weapons, we who must be ready to collaborate, or obey, or explain our commands, have to *perceive in terms of possible later uses of what we see.* Later, like the sentry relieved from his post and brought before his commanding officer to give a full report, we will not have to repeat the movements of peering, ducking, trembling, reliving what we did in pantomime; instead, we summarize, refer to what occurred, speak about the events, represent what we saw, and as we speak we are figuratively pointing back to that other time in the past, placing our memories in a precise context in time and space, referring to contexts others have shared in, utilizing a social type of life-space. "You remember," we insist, "it was on that camping trip into the Sierra."

A child begins to perform this type of action when he first watches his mother disappear through the door into the kitchen; as he waits expectantly for her return, he hears her movements in the next room. Since he has learned to expect her to reappear in that same doorway (as she has done on so many occasions) he knows, now, that she is there, out of sight, behind the wall, an absent but active "presence." He represents her, carrying her in his set of reactions, and in his posture. He continues to develop this representational skill as he trudges home, late from school, building an account of himself and preparing a story that will explain why it has taken him so long to appear before his mother, for he knows that in her thought she is following him, and he has learned to anticipate questioning. He may even learn to shade the account he will give her, since he has had to learn that certain types of answers create an unfavorable reaction. He finds himself caught between that superior power of adults to represent what a schoolboy could possibly do between his dismissal from class and his appearance on the doorstep and the limitations in that same omniscience which can be mollified by certain types of answers. The family life, with its shared concerns, its rituals of eating and sleeping and outings together, teaches each member to "carry" the other ones as he learns to anticipate the nodal points where paths cross. Each member is trained to be ready to meet these nodal points and to give an account of himself.

As our behavioral field enlarges, even though mutual concerns may be less intense, and confined to specific areas of responsibility, this type of representational activity and capacity for a recital continues to develop. As our observation is whetted by every intense and significant relationship, it tends to grow selective. Sometimes a father can grow so preoccupied with what is happening at the factory that he is all but unaware of what is going on before his eyes in his home; or, absorbed and distracted by family conflicts, a schoolboy cannot hear what is going on in the classroom.

As this development of the power to represent, to make a history as we go, to presentify, to attend to, to structure, and to grasp a present scene progresses, it is both sharpened and distorted. We learn to see with the shared prejudices of our group, to select those aspects that will make a good tale, to overlook what is before our eyes and to become old fogeys bound by our past. We even try out various recitals, subvocally, rejecting some as inappropriate. The schoolboy formulating stories to tell his mother, the consultant shaping his report for a government agency, the matron planning a version of her experiences for the bridge club—all construct a history that is selective, and sometimes very loosely bound to the realities lived through. Shared experiences and folk beliefs can so absorb and distort the events that, as in the Chinese village, one neighbor can report to another that he saw a person seized by the fox spirit. Between the shared beliefs and the warping of stories into forms suitable for private purposes, there develops what we might call *inconsistent language.* Sometimes a conscious liar has to develop a double-entry system of representation, in which what he did has to be retained and kept separate from what he is prepared to tell an audience. In the "unconscious liar" there is a subtle contamination of the very sources of recall, even at the perceptual origins.

In an exhausted and dulled state of consciousness, such as must have existed in Irene at the time of her mother's death, things were happening to her, but they were being encoded poorly. She did not grasp them in their full significance, convert them into a history, or formulate them into plans. Though she lived through these events, the pieces of action did not form into higher units that could function in recall. They passed through her mind and dropped out of it. They were not first fully grasped, *then* repressed. They never developed into that higher recallable form, and so were poorly imprinted, poorly assimilated, and not properly acted on. For example, Irene did not make the funeral arrangements, or care for the body of her mother, or put her house, or for that matter, her memories, in order. In the course of her therapy, Irene had to be brought to the point where the process could be completed, assimilated, and liquidated.

When, months after her mother's death, Irene experienced her hysterical attacks, she was descending into a hallucinated form of reliving those events. They were not representations but repetitions, a lower form of memory, a mere redintegration of action, a repetition of what is not properly recognized as something to be placed in the past, and without that backward pointing that is properly contained in a correct stance in the present field. In a trance-like state, unaware of where she is and of the inappropriateness of her actions, her physician and the hospital have dropped from her cognitive map (that set of postural expectations that gear us into a present field). The fifth time she repeated her little drama it was like the first time and the second. Janet's therapy was consistent with his theory of recall: he worked to restore the memory to its higher level of functioning. He tried to transform mere traces of old experience into the more highly structured form that could be assimilated and used in future planning.

By the time Janet published the English translation of his *Les Médications Psychologiques,* he had realized the gulf which existed between Freud's interpretations of hysteria and his own. He had come to reject the psycho-analytic view of repression and its central emphasis on the role of sexual development, and he felt called on to use the case of Irene as evidence against the Viennese theories.

"Throughout that period [of ten years following her mother's death] I watched her closely; I am familiar with all her thoughts and all her mental states; and I can asseverate that she has never had any sexual disturbances in the strict sense of the term, or any sexual adventures or mishaps which have produced a strong impression on her mind. Brought up in an easygoing proletarian environment, she made an early acquaintance with all kinds of sexual phenomena without attaching much importance to them; she is capable of experiencing normal sexual sensations, without going out of her way in search of them, and without trying to avoid them; it is difficult to conceive of a more normal sexual life than hers—and yet I do not know a more typical case of major hysteria."[21]

---

[21]Before Freud and Janet had finished arguing about the causes of the disorder, Freud had accused Janet of basing his judgment on Parisian morals, while Janet accused Freud of being as corrupt in his theorizing as the life in Viennese society. As for Freud's "anti-Puritan" complex, which was as violent as that expressed in England in the days of the Restoration, it seems to have been aimed at something which deserves another name, something which has always existed in a few individuals in every clime. It is amusing to read Perry Miller's descriptions (1939, p. 472) of the thunderous denunciations of their congregation which were made each Sunday by the Puritan divines in New England. By implication they suggest that what went on in the daily lives of their parishioners was something far removed from our stereotype of Puritan behavior. In their totality these sermons make a staggering index: "criminality, worldliness, fornication, uncleanness, drunkenness, hypocrisy, formality, oppressing of debtors by creditors, usury and profiteering,...and rudeness and incivility among the young." If these evils were rampant, even in Cotton Mather's parish, then the repressive atmosphere of Puritanism did not succeed in choking all expression of that instinctive mainspring within us.

The Hysterical Character

One of the less satisfactory chapters in Janet's discussion of hysteria is that devoted to his analysis of the *hysterical character*. While describing the suggestibility and distractibility of these patients suffering from a mild depression, a lowering of psychological tension, and a constriction of the field of consciousness, he inserts a class portrait of them that is a physician's stereotype long associated with this disorder. Compounded of medical folklore that dates back to the Egyptians, of masculine dislike for feminine "vapours," and of a clinician's tendency to group together obscure complaints that seem to have no organic basis and to be coupled with an almost perverse tendency to outwit the physician, to remain ill in spite of therapeutic efforts, and to achieve the secondary gains that go with an impaired status, there is an attitude which develops among those who deal with this category of patients. To be sure, Janet phrases it not so much as a moral judgment as an estimation of a lack of integrative power:

"Their flitting enthusiasms, their exaggerated despairs so rapidly evaporating, their unreasoned convictions, their impulsions, their caprices, in brief, this unstable and volatile combination of extremes, seems to us to depend upon this fundamental fact: that they give themselves wholly to the present idea without any nuance or reserve, without mental reservations of the kind that give to thought its equilibrium, and its transitions."

This is no "man for all seasons," no Portia, not even a person one would like to see on a jury. When such a sketch is advanced as the typical hysterical character, we tend to think of it not as a passing dynamic state, or an episode of depression, but as something that is permanent in the makeup of the person.

This view of the hysterical is repeated by Ey, Bernard, and Brisset (1963), with a slightly different emphasis; they emphasize three facets of this "fundamental hysterical character": suggestibility, mythomania, and sexual disorganization.

The first facet refers to the fact emphasized by Charcot, Janet, and Babinski: these patients are easy to hypnotize, are open to all forms of suggestion and autosuggestion. Easily influenced by their last contact, identifying themselves with their most recent "crush," they are so plastic as to be fickle and inconsistent. They lack an authentic identity.

The second facet refers to their little comedies, their constant role-playing, their pretending, and, in fact, their downright lying. Instead of taking a firm grasp of reality, with a firm stance in a real field, they are forever playing out some role, seeing the world through some fiction, such as playing a Don Quixote, whose constant effort was to imitate the great Amadis of Gaul. Never settling down to be themselves, they overreach themselves as they form these shallow and changing identifications that lift them momentarily to heights of grandeur from which they fall, crashing, to their troughs of depression. Furthermore, both the peak experience and the mild depression have a certain phony ring.

The third facet has cropped up in every generation since 1900 B.C., when the Egyptians first identified a group of "female complaints" as the outgrowth of uterine displacements. Sometimes the afflictions have been attributed to excessive abstinence and unsatisfied longings, and sometimes to excesses of sexual indulgence, but the aura of erotic involvement and disorganization has influenced the physician's judgment and his evaluation of the symptoms. Ey and his associates do not imply that hystericals are nymphomaniacs or hypersexed; they hint, instead, at a general disturbance of sexuality that may take the forms of impotence, frigidity, Don Juanism, or Messalinism. In short, hystericals do not find "the middle way."

From these three basic traits flow the tendency to falsify existence, to see the world as it is not, and to assume an identity that does not fit the facts of their existence. In a proper dosage this tendency is the work of a stimulating imagination, such as that of the creative artist or the scientist who transcends ruts of habit, or of the great technologist or politician who actually changes the shape of the world into a new order. What is most precious and noble in man, when overdone and limited to its fantasy form, becomes hysterical, misleading, and disorganizing. "The hysterical way of life," Ey suggests, finds its natural milieu in the backstage corridors and dressing rooms of the theater. The world of starlets and movies, the salons or studios haunted by esthetes, and the world of high fashion, artificial as they are, become the preferred world of the hystericals who gather in these artificial milieux to share their secondary gains and enjoy a mutually supported feeling of superiority.

It is from these same roots that these authors derive the hysterical's tendency to repress memories, to overlook a reality that is before his eyes, to produce false memories (or feelings of *déjà vu*), and to confabulate. His forgetting and his "screen memories," like his anesthesias and his attacks of delirium, produce symptoms which express his misdirected desires.

It follows that the persona (the outer and conscious self that the hysterical assumes) hides what is real and authentic, concealing from the bearer himself his own true nature. This makes the work of the therapist one of revealing the real or authentic self to this "displaced person." Thus the hysterical character that Janet described is transformed into a neo-Freudian schema that requires a psychoanalytic therapy to penetrate the surface disguise, the shallow hysterical consciousness.

FREUD'S ALTERNATE PATH

In the very year that Charcot was writing a brief foreword to Pierre Janet's study of hysteria, recommending it to the medical public as the work of one of his pupils, another pupil was finishing the page proof of an article that was to appear in the *Neurologische Zentralblatt* for 1893 with the title "Concerning the psychic mechanism of hysterical phenomena." This article, a collaboration of Joseph Breuer and Sigmund Freud, was to open up a development in psychiatry that has finally come to dominate the practice and teaching of this discipline. The Salpêtrière school, the center of the world's attention in the decade 1880-1890, attracting the most promising young neurologists from all Europe, offering the famous Tuesday lectures to which all Paris flocked to see hypnosis demonstrated and hysterical paralyses cured, has dropped into the background today. On the wall of the amphitheater where Charcot once held forth is a bronze plaque announcing the fact that at one time Sigmund Freud spent several months studying under him.

Charcot impressed everyone who heard him. Soon after he had arrived in Paris, Freud had written to his fiancée: "Charcot engrosses me; when I go away from him...my brain is sated as after an evening at the theatre. Whether the seed will ever bring forth fruit I do not know, but what I certainly know is that no other human being has ever affected me in such a way." The seed did indeed bring forth fruit, but how strange a fruit Janet himself did not realize at first. As he wrote a review of the new Breuer-Freud view, he described it as a development and extension of the concept of the role of subconscious ideas that he had learned from Charcot and had himself been developing. He understood it to be an independent confirmation of his own work. In fact, neither Janet nor Freud followed the lines laid down by Charcot, and each differed from that third pupil, the brilliant Polish neurologist, Babinski.

Janet began to realize just how greatly Freud was going to diverge from his path as, one after another, Freud's brilliant studies appeared, and his new methods, his total revision in the theory of mental illness, were advocated by a tightly knit coterie that grew dogmatic and aggressive, and which finally succeeded in convincing the bulk of the psychiatric profession. Reviled, laughed at, discouraged at first by an almost complete rejection, Freud has since been enshrined by his followers as one of the three great thinkers on the nature of man in the industrial age, along with Charles Darwin and Karl Marx. By 1925 the cleft had so deepened that Janet's reviews and criticisms characterized the new Viennese school in caustic terms, as something bizarre and puerile, as a method that twisted facts and treated patients in an unprofessional manner. Freud never forgave Janet these critical shafts, nor those of Janet's pupils, who tried to establish the priority of the Salpêtrière teachings and to show that Freud's ideas were both borrowed from Janet and distorted. When the son-in-law of Janet tried to arrange a meeting between the two, in the period after Freud had been driven to London by the Nazi invasion of Vienna, Freud refused to unbend:

"No, I will not see Janet. I could not refrain from reproaching him with having behaved unfairly to psychoanalysis and also to me personally, and having never corrected it. He was stupid enough to say that the idea of a sexual etiology for the neuroses could only arise in the atmosphere of a town like Vienna. Then when the libel was spread by French writers that I had listened to his lectures and stolen his ideas he could with a word have put an end to such talk, since actually I never saw him or heard his name in the Charcot time: he has never spoken a word. You can get an idea of his scientific level from his utterance that the unconscious is *une façon de parler*. No, I will not see him. I thought at first of sparing him the impoliteness by the excuse that I am not well or that I can no longer talk French and he certainly can't understand a word of German. But I have decided against that. There is no reason for making any sacrifice for him. Honesty the only possible thing; rudeness quite in order."[22]

If Janet was slow to realize that their thinking was diverging, Freud was not. In 1898 he wrote: "I picked up a recent book of Janet's on hysteria and *idées fixes* with beating heart, and laid it down again with my pulse returned to normal. *He has no suspicion of the clue.*" (Bonaparte, Freud, and Kris 1954, p. 247; my italics.)

A part of the great secret, which Freud was afraid would be discovered by someone else, before he could fully establish his priority, was not at all new. The Egyptian-Graeco-Roman conception of a disorder that originated in a "wandering of the uterus" had been repeated in dozens of versions, all of which considered some sexual factor at the root of this disease of women. This notion of a sexual etiology of hysteria had passed into folk beliefs, until even the most uneducated peasant could say of such a woman, "What she needs is a man."

The rest of his secret had to do with a method of exploring the unconscious without the use of hypnosis, and a theory of repression which was designed to account for the presence of the hidden *idée fixe* in the first place. Refinements in procedure, and intensive analyses of the patient-physician relationship that developed with the application of Freud's new concepts, have produced a literature of enormous extent. Freud's metapsychology has spread, penetrating all the life sciences, and has so influenced the arts that, whether he accepts these views or not, the knowledgable person has to take them into account.

THE CASE OF BERTHA PAPPENHEIM

We might begin with the case of Bertha Pappenheim. It is first reported in the original Breuer-Freud study (1895) as "The case of Anna O." Ernest Jones suggests that her actual name deserves to be commemorated in some fitting fashion, since it was she who taught Breuer, and through him Freud, the value of a special technique for casting out morbid thoughts which lurk in the unconscious (or at the fringe of consciousness).

The patient had come to Doctor Breuer late in 1880. Her symptoms had been incubating since July, Breuer thought, when her father had developed an abscess of the lung which did not yield to treatment. Breuer thought that he could link Bertha's paralysis, anesthesias, and contractures, which had reached a peak of intensity at the year's end, with this illness of the father; this linkage was what he had to explain. She had a distressing nervous cough and disturbances of sight and speech, and could not eat properly. She was paralyzed in the right arm and in both legs, and the right extremities and the muscles of the neck were contracted. In addition, she seemed to function, at different periods, on two distinct levels of awareness: in one of these she

---

[22]Quoted by Jones (1957, p. 213) from a letter from Freud to Marie Bonaparte, April 9, 1937. The hostility that had developed between these two leaders of different schools is visible in Freud's "History of the Psychoanalytic Movement" (Brill 1938a, pp. 952, 956).

seemed "absent," confused, and she could not speak or understand her mother tongue, although she could converse freely in English, or read aloud in French and Italian.[23] Jones, reviewing the case in the course of writing Freud's biography, sees the alternations in personality as somewhat like those in Morton Prince's famous case of Sarah Beauchamp, for in one state, like Sarah, she was sad and anxious (but relatively normal), whereas in the other she hallucinated, was "naughty," scolded, threw pillows, ripped the buttons from her clothing, and complained that she was going crazy. She also offered evidence of hallucinations of black snakes, mistaking her hair or shoelaces for the reptiles, yet chiding herself for being so stupid as not to recognize them for what they really were.

It is very difficult to discover which functions are preserved in each of the states, for Breuer's original account contains none of the meticulous measurement and careful description we find in Janet's studies. Breuer was struck by another fact: he found her troubled and tormented by some ideas at the fringe of her awareness, when he came to make his professional call in the evening. The two of them got into the habit of talking out these fringe thoughts, all of the disagreeable events of the day, along with each of her hallucinations, and it seemed to bring relief. The talks went back to the beginning of a symptom and the mere "talking out" seemed to bring relief. Soon so much material was pouring forth that Breuer added a morning and evening hypnotic session, devoting hours every day for more than a year to this hysterical patient.

"I came in the evening when I knew that she was in a state of hypnosis, and I took away from her the whole supply of fantasms which she had collected since my last visit. In order to obtain good results this had to be accomplished very thoroughly. Following this, she was quite tranquil, and the next day she was very pleasant, docile, industrious, and cheerful. The following day she was always more moody, peevish, and unpleasant, all of which became more marked on the third day. In this state of mind it was not always easy even in hypnosis to induce her to express herself, for which procedure she invented the good and serious name of 'talking cure,' and humorously referred to it as 'chimney sweeping.' She knew that after expressing herself, she would lose all her peevishness and 'energy,' yet whenever (after a long pause) she was in an angry mood and refused to talk, I had to resort to extorting it from her through urging and begging, as we'l as through some tricks, such as reciting to her a stereotyped introductory formula of her stories. But she never spoke until after she had carefully touched my hands and had become convinced of my identity."

(Breuer is here describing a procedure that he used when Bertha had been taken to the country and he was able to see her only at intervals.)

It is apparent that objectively the treatment had a resemblance to that which Janet was to use later, in his treatment of Irene, as he developed a different theory. Breuer was working toward a conception of catharsis, of

---

[23]Had Bertha Pappenheim's losses of function followed the lines that are usual in cases of exhaustion, brain injury, or simple forgetting, it would have been the least stable, the newly acquired language habits that would have been the first to suffer.

abreaction, a symbolic method of reactivating old traumas, of working through them, and by this means purging the system of its tensions. Like the old tribal conception of the scapegoat, who carried on his body leaves and twigs that symbolized the sins of the tribe, the words that were pouring out of Bertha were thought of as carrying pent-up emotional tensions out of her system. Like the Salpêtrière conception of "trance need" that developed when hypnotic sessions were too widely spaced, Breuer found that Bertha's "need" developed to the point where, to appease her resentment at his absence, he had to employ special stratagems.

When, soon after this, Freud took up the Breuer method and extended it, he began with hypnosis and the talking cure, working for an abreaction that would unveil the traumatic core and at the same time release the subconscious causes of the symptoms. He found hypnosis distasteful and soon abandoned it, offering a number of reasons: (1) it is not necessary; (2) it is not always easy to achieve the proper depth of hypnosis; (3) it is very embarrassing to the physician and harmful to the rapport with the patient; (4) its effects are, in any case, brief, and less valuable than when the recall can be made with full attentive awareness; (5) it tends to encourage too great dependence and passivity on the part of the patient; and (6) with most patients, the barrier to these unconscious processes the physician is dealing with can be penetrated by patient and persistent questioning without hypnosis.[24] In his Clark University lectures he reported an additional reason, with complete candor: "One time a patient whom I had repeatedly helped through nervous conditions by hypnosis, during treatment of an especially stubborn attack, suddenly threw her arms around my neck. This made it necessary to consider the question, whether one wanted to or not, of the nature and source of the suggestive authority."

Freud, already suspecting that there was a sexual factor at work in hysteria, was modest enough not to attribute his "attraction" to any personal qualities. He began to see that the physician who worked with hystericals had at his command a powerful instinctual force. It was this force that he assumed was at the basis of a "transference relationship" that inevitably developed between physician and patient. At times it was charged with resentment and hate, as the relationship between a son and father might be, and sometimes with a misplaced love and submission. He said, in 1914,

"The fact that a gross sexual, tender or inimical, transference occurs in every treatment of a neurosis, although this is neither desired nor induced by either party, has always seemed to me the most unshakable proof that the forces of the neuroses originate in the sexual life. This argument has by no means received the serious consideration it deserved, for if it had, there would have been no arguments. For my own conviction, it has remained the decisive factor beside and above the special results of the analytic work." (Brill 1938a, pp. 936-37.)

---

[24]Bernheim had taught him this fact when he visited the Nancy clinic during his studies in France. The posthypnotic amnesia, after the somnambulistic trance, can be made to yield, if the operator insists.

Before Freud had finished his reflections on Breuer's handling of Bertha Pappenheim, he was to conclude: "Poor Breuer was an innocent." The two had discussed Bertha's fear of snakes. When she had been sitting by the sick-bed of her father, with her right arm falling asleep as it hung over the back of her chair, she had fallen to dreaming. Bertha was an imaginative girl, anyway, often spending hours at what she called her "private theater," and she could plunge into reverie at will, becoming lost in a waking dream. This time she saw a black snake come out of the wall toward her, fangs bared, ready to strike. Breuer tried to lead her to common-sense interpretations: undoubtedly there were snakes in the lawn near the house. Had one of them frightened her?

As Freud reviewed the case, thirty years later before an American audience, he was ready to add an interpretation. Now, with the *Interpretation of Dreams* worked out, he knew what the symbols meant. "Whoever will reread the history of Breuer's patient in the light of the experience we have gained since then, will have no difficulty in understanding the symbolism of the snakes and her rigidity, and the paralysis of the arm." (Breuer's note had read: she wanted to drive away the snake but felt that she could not, that her arm was paralyzed.) Freud went further: this was the sick-bed of her beloved father. One "can easily guess the actual meaning of that symptom-formation. His opinion as to the part sexuality played in the psychic life of that girl will then differ greatly from that of her physician.... Now I have strong reasons," Freud wrote, "for thinking that after the removal of the symptoms, Breuer must have discovered the sexual motivations of this transference [that was growing between them], but that the general nature of this unexpected phenomenon escaped him, so that he stopped his investigation right there" as though hit by "an untoward event." Freud hints that Breuer had never come straight out with it, merely hinting enough to give Freud the basis for his deductions.[25]

Breuer had written, in the case summary: "The sexual element in her makeup was astonishingly undeveloped. The patient, whose life became as transparent to me as seldom happens in the case of one person to another,

---

[25]These are reflections of the mature Freud, 49 years old when he wrote this reevaluation of Breuer's work. If we note how, on a slender basis of fact, he wove a plausible story that provided a meaning for the patient's symptoms, with two pages of interpretation for every page of data, we can sympathize with his problem: he had assumed an explanation of the illness that had puzzled generations of physicians, and he needed a bridge of rationalizations to make the theory work. We must remember that much of what we read in Freud's narration of the case took place in Freud's mind, and that some portion of the reported facts may very well have been produced as so many hysterical phenomena have been, by the suggestibility of these compliant patients as they collaborate with physicians who have theories.

The alliance between father and daughter, who jointly denigrated the mother and her role, could have influenced the daughter's struggle to establish her own identity at puberty, a theme Freud's successors were to develop and expand. Why, they were to ask, should a daughter identify herself with such a woman, accept and incorporate her as one to be copied, attempt to take up a feminine role? Better to be like a male, superior, some of these daughters were to conclude. (See Erikson 1956, 1964; Angyal 1955; Horney 1950.)

never experienced any love, and in the whole mass of hallucinations, which characterized her disease, this element of the psychic life never appeared."

The story of Bertha Pappenheim erupts, once again, in the Jones biography of Freud. Mrs. Breuer did not make any open charges, but she became obviously bored with her husband's talk about Bertha day after day. Perhaps Breuer's imaginings helped him to divine the source of his wife's uneasiness. He broke off treatment. Although Breuer believed that Bertha had improved to the point where she could accept this, she began to act out the throes of a false pregnancy and childbirth that she had been secretly nurturing (one of the cobwebs in her mind that she had not discussed with her physician). Freud was later to ask: Why do adults behave like a fantasying infant, unless such an infant still exists within their unconscious? Breuer was shocked. He hypnotized Bertha and fled the house in a cold sweat. The next day he and his wife left on a second honeymoon, which resulted in the conception of a daughter, repairing the rift that a hysterical girl had threatened to create —in the wife's imagination.

After Breuer's departure Bertha had to be hospitalized; and when Breuer returned to check up on the case, he found her quite unhinged. This does not seem to be quite in keeping with the ending that Breuer gave to the story, when he wrote, "In this way the whole hysteria came to an end. She has since then enjoyed perfect health" (1895, p. 27).

It is true, however, as Jones reports, that ten years later Bertha was sufficiently recovered to serve as one of the first social workers, to become an ardent feminist, and to assist in the rescue of Polish, Roumanian, and Russian children whose parents had died in pogroms. A lay nun, she never married, believing that her life was devoted to God; yet she ended by committing suicide in New York City.

FREUDIAN PSYCHOANALYSIS

Two generations of post-Freudian novelists have sensitized the general public to the interpersonal relations within the family; it is therefore somewhat difficult for us to recapture the impact of Freud's analysis on his contemporaries. If the disorder is constitutional at base, as they believed, and if it represents a state in which integrative forces are at low ebb, or if it is the expression of a pithiatic personality, as Babinski and his followers were asserting, the description of personal relationships in the patient's family or the attempt to build up a personal history with emphases on infantile experience would seem shockingly irrelevant. Freud stressed the patient's emotional life and tried to place the symptoms within a unique family constellation; this was something distinctly new. Moreover, he attempted to give the symptom a meaning and to look on it as the language that expressed an unconscious process.

We begin to see what a psychoanalytic case study requires, as a symptom is finally placed against a life in a family setting. The organicist and the laboratory worker may shrink from such an abandonment to subjectivity and interpretation, from the ambiguities of multiple determination, from the risk of self-revelation, of exposure of the clinician himself, by his own interpretations, and from the need on the clinician's part to keep analyzing his own mental processes. As Freud trained his own disciples, he insisted that anyone analyzing the mind of another must first be analyzed. Few could be expected to do for themselves what Freud had accomplished for himself. Worse, each analyst must continue the process as he meets each new and challenging case: it is a never-ending form of self-discipline. If the process requires an exploration of fantasies, dreams, gossip, and fringe consciousness, by means of interpretations that are full of ambiguity, then so much the more difficult it will be to achieve clarity, but if this is the route required because of the very way the human mind works, clouded as it always is by this same ambiguity and disturbed by that underpinning of subconscious processes, then it is also the *one* way to get at the psychological truth. If to get to the goal one has to become deeply involved in the life of another, with rather intense affectivity (both affection and hate), and if this affectivity makes objectivity increasingly difficult, this, too, is still the only road which can penetrate that chilling barrier of defenses which each person constructs for his own safety. Interpreting the symptoms in this fashion gives more than understanding: the process shows how the symptom both expresses and conceals the truth. As the patient achieves insight and the kind of emotional reeducation that enables him to abandon his symptoms, no longer useful or necessary, the analyst can say: "You see! These were not merely hunches, or guesses, or mere fantasies. These are the forces that produce the illness, the psychological tensions that were converted into breathing difficulties, convulsive attacks, and other symptoms."[26] The patient who leaves the physician's office, ruminating over what has been said in the analytic hour, feels the presence of this counselor accompanying him. This continuing rumination will be there as he falls asleep until finally, in the dream, it will touch off those deeper

---

[26]In Freud's time that borderline between epilepsy and the hysterical attack was still obscure, as it had been in the days of Mesmer and of Charcot. Penfield and Jaspers (1954, pp. 661-62) note that today the diagnosis of epilepsy would be withheld when the seizures have not become habitual. *Usually* the nonepileptic seizures have normal electroencephalograms even during their seizures. A normal electroencephalogram does not rule out epilepsy. Freud's practice dates long before the use of this diagnostic tool, and, like Charcot, he entertained the possibility of a band of disorders in that area between hysteria and epilepsy that he called *hysteroepilepsy.* In 1945 (p. 267) Fenichel was still writing: "There is a gradual transition between genuine epilepsy and conversion hysterias, in which epileptiform seizures express a definite idea and show all the characteristics of hysterical motor symptoms."

At one end of this continuum the psychoanalyst looks upon the hysterical convulsion as a kind of body language, as a kind of symbolic orgasm; at the other end of it the organicist believes that he is dealing with an impersonal "brain storm," a discharge in a specific group of cells that is as impersonal an event as one could conceive. Recently investigators have reported cases in which true epileptic seizures are set off by specific stimuli (lights, music, noises). By reducing the intensities of these triggering stimuli, investigators have succeeded in gradually developing a conditioned inhibition so that the attacks no longer follow the stimuli (reported at the Fourth World Congress of Psychiatry, Madrid 1966, by Dr. Francis M. Forster of the Wisconsin School of Medicine). This fact is of some interest to those who have tried to condition the audiogenic seizures of experimental animals without success.

layers of memory not yet openly discussed. Even if the dream forms are vague, they will be related to this ruminating process which aroused them. The task is to properly decode and interpret them.

In addition to this relationship to what has gone on in the analytic hour, there is the fact that dreaming, less bound by conventions and by the rules of logical communication, has greater access to all manner of half-formed processes that lie at the deeper levels of the mind. As Freud carried on his work with his patients, it was as if he assumed that somewhere, on the other side of the patient's defensive consciousness, there was another force (or person) striving to speak to him. Distorted as the language of the dream was, vague and concealing what was behind it, it was also a communication.

That dreams mean something, or are trying to say something, and that they can be decoded, interpreted, and used as guiding lines for conduct, is a very ancient belief, as old as Daniel's efforts to interpret the dream that Nebuchadnezzar could not quite remember, as old as the belief in the messages given out by an oracle, or the whispering wind, or the burning bush. Both the dreamer and the inspired prophet have had to drop the logico-deductive stance of a practical everyday consciousness, to listen with a third ear, to let a fringe consciousness speak. Some have even resorted to drugs in order to open up their minds to this other kind of process.[27]

Hysteria presents a puzzle. In Freud's hands the problem was attacked by a method that assumes the cause to be unconscious and that postulates early repression of sexual energies. By using and interpreting the patient's free associations, especially to the reported dream fragments, Freud found evidence of unconscious incestuous attachments, parental seductions and rejections, early fantasies about impregnation, and unconscious linkages between sexuality and aggression, between sexuality and eating, and between sexuality and a death instinct. Out of the mouths of his patients he was able to draw the evidence to validate his theories, as fast as these developed, even as Charcot was able to demonstrate the classic stages of *grande hystérie,* which began to disappear at the Salpêtrière shortly after Charcot's death.

Today it is difficult to find the classic forms of hysteria described by Charcot. It is also difficult to recapture the violence of the rejection that first greeted the papers of Freud and his pupils when they were read before scientific meetings: vitriolic criticism, red-faced denunciations, followed these expositions. His accusers insisted that Freud had soiled the relationship between infant and mother, and had besmirched everything with sex. Today such papers

---

[27]In World War II, psychiatrists confronting the problem of combat fatigue and hysterical symptoms, unable to spend the time needed for prolonged interviews and free associations, made use of the artificial sleeplike state produced by sodium pentathol. There they could achieve something similar to the state of hypnosis, with its hypermnesia, and accomplish in a very short period what the long hours of free association on the analytic couch managed to do. Freud was trying to do something similar without drugs, without hypnosis. Since the patient's communications in the form of dreams were so obscure, ambiguous, and fantastic, Freud assumed that the dream action was symbolic; but he also assumed that by giving the patient time and a free rein, his associations to these reported actions would lead inevitably to the root process that had been causing symptoms.

are accepted with little comment, save an occasional defense by the more orthodox of Freud's followers against attempts at revisionism, or occasional criticism by some skeptic who senses the absence of statistics, the lack of controls, the failure to consider alternate hypotheses. The work of Freud's successors has been done so thoroughly that there is even hesitation to revise the work of the master.

In particular, psychoanalysis is aimed at reviving the memories of the earliest relationships between an infant and its parents. The Freudian hopes that the "transference relationship" between analyst and patient will reactivate these oldest conflicts. Although the dream language is symbolic and terribly vague, he seeks to interpret it and to project its meanings into these forgotten primal scenes. What was preverbal when it first occurred left its traces nonetheless, and what was verbalized and experienced as fantasies and then repressed still exists beneath the crust of conventional attitudes. Each of these processes has to be disinterred, put into understandable discourse, ventilated in a process of emotional reeducation, and allowed to complete itself until it can be discharged. The mixtures of love and hate that have crippled the power to act, in their frustated and entangled forms, can now be expressed effectively; expressed, his needs can find fulfillment. The reliving with feeling, the discovery of insights, now enables him to act, and in these final transformations of the world about him, the cure finally completes itself. The restoration of the patient's power to speak and act effectively often produces some surprising results. The analyst sometimes warns the parents of a young patient, or the husband of a neurotic wife: "She will seem to get worse before she gets better." Those who live within the family circle have to be prepared for the impact of impulses long repressed, for the expression of feelings that remained in an unconscious and unverbalized form.

A VIEW OF MEMORY

Freud's great discovery that every neurosis has a sexual root set him to looking for sexual traumata in the life-history of his hystericals. Searching for assaults, seductions, adolescent adventures, and failing to find them, he was led to examine earlier periods and to speculate about the process of forgetting which had screened away what he assumed was there. He finally settled upon the period before six as the place where the basic character structure was formed; for the gravest mental afflictions (such as schizophrenia), he turned to the early oral period of the nursling for the root causes of the disorder. The more his explorations led him into this preverbal past, the more he had to depend on interpretations and reconstructions; for the early infancy of each of us is screened away by a complete amnesia.

When Freud's daughter addressed Vienna schoolteachers, she used the phrase "infantile amnesia" to describe this process of forgetting which makes us all into men and women without a past. Ask your six-year-olds to tell you about the past: "They willingly talk about the events of the last few days or weeks, about holidays which they have spent in strange surroundings, about a former birthday or saint's day, perhaps even about the Christmas festivities of last year. But then their recollections come to a standstill, or at any rate they lack the power to impart them to others." She reminded her audience that, as adults, none of us can go much farther back in memory than the age of three (see A. Freud 1947, p. 20). Somehow a curtain is drawn over these earliest memories so that we cannot recall them. What blocks them?

Perhaps the simplest thing to say is that they never were verbalized, that what was never formulated in recallable form cannot strictly be said to have been forgotten. The infant of three weeks can be conditioned; but these changes in his reflex responses have no accompanying verbal patterns. He lives through the sequences, but makes no history of them. Yet he makes traces, so that objectively we can show the influence of the past, the existence of the "aftereffects," at a time when his psychological time-space field is not yet structured and verbalized. He is laying a foundation, forming a life-style (placid or restless, irritable or smiling), and his approach to people has a recognizable shape. We are forced into saying: (1) foundation of the personality is being laid down; and (2) it exists in an unverbalized form that, later, he will be unable to recall. The more importance we attribute to this foundation, the greater will be our dependence on the reports of outside observers, unless, that is, we can hit on some method of interpreting what an adult says (or dreams about) in such a way that, like the work of the archaeologist which recreates the entire vessel from a potsherd or two, we can reconstruct this shrouded past for him.

Anna Freud was sure the first-grade teachers would agree with her. The six-year-olds are already formed into personalities, highly differentiated from one another. The preschool teacher also finds that some are aggressive, some timid, some affectionate, as though the parents had shaped them in the very early months. Either the basic lines of development are laid down genetically, or the foundation traces have been laid down in an unverbalized and unre-callable form before the child enters kindergarten. Freud's successors have chosen the latter tack: they find the disciplines that shape the basic personality trends in feeding and toilet-training, in the training to inhibit and restrain expressions of sexual curiosity and aggression. Though it makes a lasting imprint on the mind of the developing child, it cannot be recalled even in the hypermnesia of hypnosis. Perhaps we ought to say merely that the body remembers it.

To choose a single possible event, such as a separation from the mother at nine months of age, the six-year-old would not be able to recall it in words, but it could be reactivated when his mother leaves him at the door of the schoolroom. His rages when his mother spanked him for wetting the bed may be forgotten, but his teacher can reactivate them when she tries to discipline him for his messy homework. Unlike Janet's engineer, who does not consciously recall the train wreck but who can get it all back under hypnosis, the child, who is affected by these very early traces laid down before speech developed and before that habit of converting experience into a recital was established, cannot make any understandable communication at all, save, perhaps, in that body language which only the skilled interpreter can convert into understandable form.

Let us examine some of the options open to us, as we try to understand the facts:

1. We could say, simply, that since the earliest events occur before speech is well-established, and before the child has learned that he will be called on to make a recital of his experiences, these events are laid down in the nervous system in a nonverbal form. Feelings, attitudes, readinesses to act are there, but in a form that is unattached to any moment of history, any specific objects or settings; as a result, they are highly generalized. They spread to all manner of inappropriate settings. Without a temporospatial structure, without words, they have a kind of timeless and universal quality. Underneath and outside of our well-structured actions, they provide, nonetheless, a foundation for those actions, and may even change the direction and quality of those actions we do verbalize quite accurately. Our reason is thus corrupted by something that lies outside of reason! The histories we make are affected by a prehistory of which we are unaware.

2. Since adults also have experiences that they do not, or cannot at the moment, translate into words (fringe experiences, ineffables), but which they can revive and at least partially translate into communicable form when it becomes important to use them, the nonverbal existence of the foundation underlying our conscious mental life does not wholly explain the elusiveness of these earliest memories. I may not be able to verbalize a description of the criminal, but I can pick him out of the lineup. My Sylvia, whose charms leave me dumb, affects me like no other; I can visualize her, and I will accept no substitute.

It is quite possible, therefore, that early experiences are in their nature so different from later ones (even those which we do not stop to verbalize) that they cannot be summoned. They do not fit our present structured stance, they do not respond to our summons, and they would not be recognized if they were now active. Their effects slowly summated, leaving residues which altered our behavior, but it was a dumb erosion-accumulation process, in which "deposits of affects" make a difference in spite of the fact that discrete patterns are not available to any ordinary summons. The adult is therefore affected by this mass without knowing precisely what affects him.

3. Before we arrive at the verbalizing, experience-structuring, time-and-space-ordering stage of development, a mass of traces has accumulated. The inarticulate mass of attitudes and expectations formed a necessary base for the later structured forms of memory. But even while the articulate memories were taking shape, another process was at work, so that some memories, potentially recallable, were laid away, repressed, forbidden as too dangerous to use. They were as much outside the acceptable territory as incest, were as ugly as murderous hate, were entirely outside that character which, we

hoped, would make us well-liked. The more highly charged with emotions these "laid-away" memories are, the more closely tied to needs which persist, the more their effects will be noticeable, and the more effort will be required to keep them out of sight.

It is this third form of amnesia that Anna Freud chose to emphasize. It is this which shrouds our past in darkness, creates an unconscious that can cause symptoms, produces highly charged memories that are unavailable, and makes the work of the analyst so difficult, for the patient will deny, resist, evade all effort to penetrate this territory, and for the very reasons that made him hide these memories away in the first place. We might call this the psychoanalytic article of faith. Working on this basis, the analyst makes it true as he fits the facts he discovers into this prepared framework.

This third view is not without its difficulties. Since all of us have this form of infantile amnesia, why does the unconscious that it creates in the neurotic produce symptoms, while in the normal it does not? Since all adults have many private thoughts, many of them so shameful and intimately personal that one does not share them with anyone, so insistent that one wishes, indeed, that he could repress them, why does the hysterical convert them into symptoms while the normal does not? Our amnesia for infancy extends to innocuous events as well as to all others, and some of our most disturbing adult memories do not drop into the unconcious.

The great empty space created by this universal infantile amnesia has created a field which the analyst can fill with hypothesized causal relationships. It may contain events which are imputed and not observed. The forgetting which screens away incestuous thoughts and murderous fantasies, which are inferred, also screens away innocuous events. Is it possible that the intensity of the repression has to match, in theory at least, the improbability of the events imputed?

The hypothesis of the sexual origin of neuroses, of a process of repression that created a dynamic unconscious, or of "affects" that charge symptoms with instinctual energies, could both be in error and still serve to structure events in the life of a disturbed patient. Another type of unconscious process, other detached and generalized emotional reactions, other unverbalized components in behavior, might conceivably be favorably affected by the analyst's efforts to give a structure to the lives of his patients, by his supportive interest, by his common sense outside the area dedicated to his theory. Priests have succeeded with an entirely different approach; as we shall see later, the neo-Pavlovians succeed in eliminating anesthesias without making use of this framework of theory or the prolonged rituals involved in the daily sessions on the analytic couch. We shall have to have much better measures of the success of therapies before we have a pragmatic test of the value of these speculations and therapeutic rituals.

There is another factor that has persuaded many to adopt the analyst's views. It is a fact that the infant is very dependent: for his very life he has to be sensitive to every mood and command of those persons responsible for his nurture. He is safe and comfortable when his relations with these nurturant ones are good, anguished when they are bad; it is quite possible that some of his solutions which bring safety and peace of mind at this dependent stage will cause him difficulty later. Worse, his demands and appetites grow as they are gratified, asking finally for the impossible. He may not possess his mother; the outer world intrudes again and again to force him into an autonomy. "Now," it insists, "is the time to put away childish things." At every stage there are developmental tasks which force him out of his comfortable infantile ways: too quickly, too slowly, too roughly, too permissively, until as an adult he has to face responsibilities, citizenship, war, love, demands of a vocation, and so on, sometimes poorly prepared.

In the life of every individual, and in every culture, this process of achieving an autonomy that is adjusted to others goes on. In one tribe the infant will be nursed until he is five, in another for a bare five months. One will be bedwetting until six, his brother toilet-trained at six months. One will be overprotected until he is 25, the next forced to fend for himself as he sells papers at a busy street corner in downtown traffic when he is scarcely ten. In all cultures the majority manage to come through the most diverse training schedules to the typical adult patterns. We try to read back into their history some subtle differences that explain the ones who falter. When the specialist centers his interpretations on a period that is shrouded by this universal infantile amnesia and protected by the energies that first generated repression, he is free to project and to interpret to his heart's content. The Freudian, exploring this shrouded area, explains the amnesia and the later neurosis by the following implications:

1. The infant wanted his mother to himself, even sexually.
2. He was jealous of all with whom he had to share her (siblings, father).
3. He experienced hatred and death wishes directed against anyone who interfered.
4. He experienced the same hatred and death wishes toward the mother when she corrected him, disciplined him, refused some of his demands, readied him for autonomy; and in like manner he experienced a similar ambivalence toward the father.
5. He is doubly hurt when he is forced to act out love when he is really filled with hate.
6. He has to cope with a family that is far from that ideal one we imagine to be filled with affection and concerned with the infant's security.
7. He has to forget, deny, and act falsely about what in his dependency he dares not express openly.

One factor, in the Freudian theory that has developed in our own time, has plagued the theorist and experimentalist who would like firm data to validate the analyst's procedures. Almost from the beginning Freud discovered that he had to interpret both facts and fantasies. The patient imagined a mother who was an ogre; the objective data did not fit the fantasy. Imagined seductions proved to be more frequent than the real event. Firm correlations between precisely described parental behaviors and developing neurotic symptoms were not postulated or discovered. Evidence based on a retrospective construction of an individual's life-history took the place of objective and statistical studies. They were demonstrations, of the type Freud made in his patient Dora, not proofs (1905a).

When Anna Freud told the teachers of Vienna that the children they dealt with differed from each other because of experiences of early infancy, fantasied interpretations of real events, sibling rivalries, death wishes that had to be repressed, she expressed her beliefs in the form of a scientific proposition that lacked supporting data. It was the precise, but deviant, behavior of the parents that had produced the products.

"The children whom you designate as quarrelsome, asocial, and never contented with anything, are putting their school companions in the place of their brothers and sisters, and there, at school, are fighting out with them the conflicts which they were not able to finish in their own homes. And the older ones who react so violently if you endeavor to exercise the slightest show of authority, or those who are so cowed that they do not even venture to look you in the face or to raise their voices in class, are in truth the same little children, but they have transferred to you the longing for the father's death and the difficult suppression of such wishes, with the resultant anguish and surrender." (A. Freud 1947, p. 35.)

The Freudian tale is rendered believable, finally, by an appeal to our common sense. If even the well-born child, in comfortable socioeconomic circumstances, living in what appears to be a "good" home, sometimes develops neuroses, how much more vulnerable will be the child who has been passed from one nurse to another, and has had no single mother to identify as his own; who comes from a broken home; who has a father who is a drunkard; or who has neither father nor mother? She pictures the reasoning of the waif whose father and mother are about to separate: "If my father does not love my mother, then my mother does not love my father, and they can't like me. Then I don't want them. And then the whole family is no good." She adds: "He is like an employee in a bankrupt firm who has lost all confidence in his principals and no longer therefore feels any pleasure in his work, or reason to anticipate and obey the wishes of his superiors."

The credibility of the hypothesis which asserts that a neurosis is related to the many pressures that are working to make integration difficult, in adults as well as in children (but especially in children), tends to spread to validate an imputed psychosexual theory of neurosis, to support the procedures of dream interpretation, and to permit a fanciful reconstruction of that infantile past shrouded in amnesia. Unchallenged, the psychoanalytic reconstruction passes for something factual, and a therapeutic ritual is allowed to continue in the absence of a better one.

THE NEO-FREUDIAN CONCEPT OF HYSTERIA

The historian of the future may very well note that, by the second half of the twentieth century, the psychoanalysts had come to dominate the American Psychiatric Association. The word "hysteria" was eliminated from the association's *Mental Disorders Diagnostic Manual* in 1952, and replaced by "conversion symptom," that is, by Freud's concept of the process whereby psychic conflict is transformed into bodily symptoms. Had Babinski's view triumphed, the manual would have listed the classification "pithiatism"; and had Janet's successors been more numerous, they might have insisted on a listing of "dissociation symptoms." The names change, and both theory and therapy that deal with the categories change. Even the symptoms seem to have changed, since our contemporaries report so few instances of those major convulsions that Charcot demonstrated at the Salpêtrière.

In spite of all this, W. M. Millar (1958) informed his colleagues, in a Maudsley Bequest lecture in 1956, that "the situation of the hysterical patient today is very much as it was when his grandparents and great-grandparents submitted themselves to the awesome scrutiny of a full neuro-psychiatric investigation." Millar seems to imply that "the more hysteria changes, the more it remains the same." What remains the same, he is persuaded, is "the situation of the patient" before his puzzled physician, who, in spite of the most recent high-powered concepts, cannot reduce the phenomena to a conceptual schema that permits him to handle the illness with precision and dispatch.

The anesthesias, amnesias, contractures, paralyses, delirious attacks, and fugues persist, but in our time they require the use of such concepts as identification, incorporation, and somatic compliance. They are treated as though they were a body language, a primitive type of communication, as though a man were forced to keep his mouth in a perpetual open-jawed cramp and could not simply announce that he was hungry. The convulsive *arc en ciel,* which Charcot's patients demonstrated, with body thrust upward and its weight resting on neck and shoulders at one end and feet at the other, could be viewed as a symbolic orgasm expressing a sexual need. The therapist, confronted with this curious language, is required to discover what the symptom means, what the patient is trying to say, even as Jesus appeared to do when, commanding the paralytic to get up and walk, He said, "Thy sins are forgiven." Thus the "situation of the patient" has not changed inasmuch as his improvement still awaits the clairvoyant healer who can penetrate his symptom disguise. At any rate, the psychoanalyst belongs in this tradition, but with this difference: he now offers us a method which, with the collaboration of the patient, can penetrate to the core of the hidden meaning.

The Symptom as a Statement

Conversion hysteria is a concept that raises questions. Why does the patient have to resort to bodily language? Does the symptom communicate a single meaning, express a single thwarted impulse, or does it convey so many meanings that we could call overdetermined, literally choked with meanings? (Religious symbols carry such a heavy freight, and, like metaphoric language, stir up ambiguities.) Why is it so stubborn, so resistant to therapy? Because it somehow "binds anxiety" and serves as a kind of bodily scapegoat to carry away guilt? Because it justifies nonfeasance, and enlists sympathy and pity from those who surround the patient? Because it bars a course of action demanded by impulses that are taboo (aggressions, cowardice, lust)? Because it is a way of getting even, of expressing hatred and of settling old scores, of defeating a stubborn mother who has insisted upon a hateful course of action? Because it is a roundabout way of preserving a dependent status, of finding security, of being excused from military service, of avoiding marriage or a career?

The very fact that we continue to raise such questions suggests that the old concept of the hysterical as a malingerer is still very much in our minds. Even the behaviorist, who uses the concept of "secondary reinforcement," will join with the irritated analyst who makes the symptoms of his patients unpleasant, for he uses "negative reinforcement" when the symptom appears and introduces "positive reinforcement" whenever it decreases in its intensity.

The work of tracing out the gains, both primary and secondary, which the patient enjoys as a result of his symptoms, serves to rationalize them. The functional values that the analyst calls primary and that arise because he is kept in ignorance of what remains unconscious consist in a reduction of anxiety and guilt. The secondary gains arise from the consequences of the symptom in the patient's life-situation, from the reactions of others, from the reduction of pressures for performance. Paradoxically we seem to find it easy to explain the persistence of the symptoms by a kind of learning theory which stresses gratification and reinforcement, in spite of the fact that the symptoms arrest growth, and have a maladaptive quality with serious consequences. (The writer's cramp threatens the bank cashier with the loss of his job, with debts, with the loss of his home, with loss of status for all members of his family who depend on him.)

What this type of functional explanation does not clarify is the fact that the normal person, who also has similar motives (e.g., to get out of the service, to avoid making the speech), does not react to his crises, accidents, or difficulties in this way. In spite of all of the secondary gains that would be open to him, he will retain his skin sensibility after the accident, preserve his control over his vocal cords and leg muscles. He scorns to merely evade his responsibilities as a soldier or citizen, to regress to childlike dependence, or to plead an impaired status. He stands on the side of his commander and his medical officer in trying to maintain his own morale, or, as a conscientious objector, does alternative work or takes his case to court. Even more puzzling is the fact that, after we have succeeded in imagining multiple sources of gains and have reinforced our interpretations by the words produced by the patient in his free associations, sometimes his "compensation neurosis" suddenly ceases, so that he can resume his work and throw aside all of these secondary and primary gains. (See Cameron 1963, pp. 305-37, and Denker 1946.)

To add to the confusion that arises from this attribution of a function to the symptoms is the fact that the prognosis for a *particular* attack is usually good. The interpretation of the symptom's "language" works. Then the symptom, or another like it but different (an anesthesia in an area of the body that has quite a different symbolic value), returns, and the process has to be repeated. The symptoms improve as the person as a whole improves, as his situation improves, as his depression and confusion and aboulia lift, only to return as his general psychological economy worsens. When one has read a long series of interpretations made by psychoanalysts, one discovers a terrible monotony in the imputed meanings: in the midst of a wide variety of bodily signs and symbols, the meanings seem to be curiously similar. No matter what words are used, they seem to refer to a limited set of schematized meanings.

This functional view (which is also a purposive-expressive-symbolic concept of the illness) does not fit those cases that have entered the clinic with functional losses of which they were totally unaware until a thorough neuropsychiatric examination revealed their presence, losses which had not come to their notice because they neither impaired their adjustment nor provided them with any secondary gain. Peripheral vision can be restricted in the hysterical; until his range of vision is tested in the perimeter, he is quite unaware of the fact (as unaware as the patient with an injury to his occipital lobe and a small lacuna in his visual field). Binding no guilt and anxiety, yielding no secondary gain, such symptoms do not fit the ordinarily compliant analytic brand of teleology. The beautiful indifference of the hysterical that has been identified in many descriptions of the illness is here a "beautiful ignorance." Where psychoanalysis prevails to the point where neuropsychiatric examinations are deemed unnecessary, this "beautiful ignorance" is shared by the physician, whose therapy, when successful, improves functions without his knowledge.

According to this functional-analytic view, psychotherapy will strip the patient of his pretenses: the hidden motives of which he is unconscious will become conscious problems, and they will create fresh responsibilities the moment they are revealed. A "clarification therapy," such as psychoanalysis, will thus necessarily intensify guilt and anxiety, destroy the secondary gains of his neurosis, reveal the precise meanings (however horrible) that the body symbol so obscurely implied and concealed. Such a treatment must rob the patient of many forms of psychic income, force him to live up to some of the mature responsibilities he has been avoiding, release inner anxieties and conflicts that the illness had "bound" but which he must now face. Though he does not use the crude and painful electric shock of those German psychiatrists in World War I, who tried to make "shell shock" unpalatable to the malingering soldier, the analyst's methods may involve an equally unpleasant, even if more "refined," form of cruelty. If he is to be successful in the long run, such an analyst-counselor would have to become an educator and spiritual guide, assisting his patient to mature, serving as a diplomatic buffer against those persons in his environment who—with the best of intentions—still work to keep him prisoner. If we believe that there must be corresponding "gains" to compensate for the losses he has incurred, this therapist must help the patient find those other, more mature satisfactions which more than compensate him. If the analyst merely substitutes a dependence on himself for the dependence on a parent that his analysis has revealed, or if his own tendency to seek the cause of the neurosis in parental mismanagement merely ends in a kind of "scapegoating" that leaves the patient at the same arrested stage of development, the method would fail except as a temporary safety valve.

Thus one is driven to conclude that, although there may very well be a certain amount of truth in this neo-Freudian "functional" view of the hysterical's symptoms, and although the view also helps explain a certain resistance on the part of the patient and a certain fixity in the symptoms, we are required to make certain discriminations:

1. Most of the hysterical's symptoms can be produced in nonhysterical normals by means of hypnosis. There is no independent evidence that unconscious motivations of the type imputed to the hysterical are here responsible.

2. There are cases of hysteria that do not fit the type of analysis supplied for conversion hysteria.

3. Many of the hysterical's personal conflicts are entirely within his powers of conscious recall. The killer-soldier whose paralyzed and anesthetic hand can no longer hold a gun knows what he has done and is fully aware of his desire never to shoot again. And if instead of developing a neurosis, he were to choose to shoot himself in the hand, as many soldiers did in World Wars I and II, would we here speak of the "conversion of a conscious conflict" into bodily symptoms? Where the psychoanalyst makes use of old infantile conflicts, long repressed, we could wish that there were independent validation of their existence.

4. Some forms of hysterical symptoms, amnesias and anesthesias, are "silent." The patient does not even know about them, nor do others until examination reveals them. Like a sudden loss of spirit, they seem to represent a descent in integrative powers.

5. Appearing spontaneously and disappearing without therapy, the symptoms of some hystericals have to be described as behavioral changes of unknown origin. When conditioning techniques can restore sensibility to an anesthetic area without the use of interpretations, and without any effort to understand hidden motives behind the symptom, the analytic procedure appears superfluous. Sometimes the descent in integrative force can be traced to such causes as loss of blood, the toxins of fever, a dramatic failure in a course of action pursued with maximum effort and an exhausting expenditure of energy, loss of love, or excessive outer stress. Since, as in the case of combat fatigue, others who stand beside the hysterical under similar stresses do not succumb, one is tempted to postulate a constitutional weakness of some sort.

6. The temptation to use learning theory is great: the secondary gains provide the reinforcement to account for fixations. The "multiple causation" revealed as analysis unearths a plethora of motivation gives a multiple rationalization for the symptom. All this becomes excess baggage the moment spontaneous recovery sets in. The fact of recovery, by whatever means, calls for

new concepts of reinforcement. Insight has to bring other values if it is to be expressed in action and reinforced by the new consequences, in which self-realization and a joy in truth (though it be painful) triumph over all the other neurotic gains that once accounted for the persistence of symptoms. We have to be alert, as theorists, if we are not to become tagalongs who rationalize the course of events after the fact.

7. Finally, we have to remain alert to that two-fold nature of psychotherapy. In part the therapist is a technician. He brings about a new awareness by his use of hypnosis, free association, dream analysis, interpretations, or management of the patient's hygiene. But he also assumes the burden of further guidance and education, and functional interpretations of the symbolic body language do not help him here. His own personal force, his philosophy of life, and his grasp of life make him either a successful artist, here, or a miserable failure. His training as a physician seldom imparts such a skill, although his teachers, as persons, may sometimes supply good models.

Symbols and Symptoms

The neo-Freudian attempt to look at the symptom as a "statement" couched in body language is expressed succinctly by Cameron (1963, p. 327):

"Eyes and ears help us to build our worlds of internal and external reality from the earliest phases of infancy. They come to participate in human interaction to a degree rivalled only by hand and tongue. Eating, swallowing, regurgitation and elimination, the comforts of body contact and body warmth, the multiple meanings of movement and posture—all these have influences upon personality development and personal functioning that leave their anatomy and physiology as irrelevant to what they symbolize as is the chemistry of a painting. The anatomy and physiology must be understood, taken into account and allowed for; but they cannot be made central to an understanding of the final product, the meaning conveyed."

This is well said, yet its truth obscures other truths. The anatomy of the hand of Michelangelo may have been, in truth, much like that of the hand of an Italian farmer, stonecutter, quarry worker, or sailor, or of any other person whose hand is strong and skilled. But the moving beauty and strength revealed in the sculptor's *Moses* is something more and other than anything we could discover by any anatomical analysis of the hand that carved it. No more could any anatomist discover the secret of Einstein's genius by postmortem microscopic study of his cortical cells. The whole man in action is, as the gestaltists never tire of emphasizing, more and other than an aggregate of parts and can never be grasped through an analysis of parts as parts.

Eye, hand, and tongue movements, digestion, elimination, contractions of the muscles of leg and foot, a cramp in the muscles of the shoulder girdle, can each be taken up into a "higher organization" that we describe as the person in action. They are absorbed into a dynamic process that imagines a future, speaks to friends, reasons with enemies, fights, deceives, seduces. So well-organized are these "higher units" that, in the main, they can communicate a meaning from one person to another, a meaning that symbolizes some shared event in the past, or points to some desired goal in the future so clearly that what does not yet exist can form within the mind of a hearer, so that he, too, can focus on the relations between ends and means that will be significant in an act of collaboration. Occasionally, as in the cramp of the shoulder-girdle muscles of the student with "piano arm," the parts get out of hand to the point where they block the practice that the student is intent upon. His teacher may have to reevaluate his instruction methods, if too many of his pupils develop this cramp, or give some attention to his pupils' hours of practice or to their posture before the instrument. The teacher's superior may want to review the relationships which obtain between this teacher and his pupils.

It is true that in such a shoulder-girdle cramp, which can be felt by palpation of the muscles, there would be changes in the electrical record of the shortening of the fibrils, but the muscular changes thus recorded would not point clearly to the cause of the cramp (practice schedule, anger at teacher, poor posture). If used as a "communication," this language is ambiguous in that it does not point to the cause.

It is also true that meanings can be transmitted without intent. The restless movements of his class tell the lecturer something. The limp hand that withdraws from the palm of a guest too quickly tells more to the latter than the hostess intended. Our gestures and our posture express *us* to a perceptive viewer (even when we wish to remain hidden). Harry Stack Sullivan insisted that his residents should pay more attention to the voice quality of those they were interviewing, use changes in quality to read what was transpiring behind the remarks of the patient, to read meanings that may have been hidden even from the speaker. But all such readings have to be made with a dash of skepticism and some self-criticism; and those who are very sure of themselves can be in error here. The rest of us realize that the viewer and hearer can read what is not there, utilizing their own shaky hypotheses and projecting their own private feelings about the interlocutor. (A weakness caused by a slight case of polio in childhood may lie behind that fishy handclasp that is interpreted as "coolness.")

To that limited portion of the integrative network that communicates clear and unequivocal meanings (as when we use speech and gesture intentionally and effectively) there must be added a fairly wide fringe of partially integrated expressive movements, and some residues of *schizokinesis* that "speak" of other not yet extinguished traces from the past. Schizokinesis, a splitting of movement systems, emerges as a learner is put through conditioning and extinction procedures. Records taken from heart, intercostals, adrenals, pupils, and the like, show that the segments do not arrive at an in-phase state at the same time; and as the responses are extinguished, some lag behind the others. In the talking human subject who can predict whether or not he is going to get the shock following a signal, the man as a whole may be fully aware of what is to come, but his breathing rate, pupillary response, and heart may lag behind. Where "shock" and "no-shock" members of a series follow a pattern that can be named, we might say that the man has insight but that parts of his response system have not yet received the message. In a rapidly changing field the laggard systems produce a schizokinesis that disappears as an experimental sequence is stabilized and an outer steady state permits the parts of a response system to fall in line. Too rapidly changing, too closely crowded, conflicting signals may make demands that the organism cannot parse out so that all segments of response are appropriate. (Gantt, in Miner 1953.)

This fringe of reactions, this schizokinesis, offers something that is more than anatomy and physiology but also less than clear speech. These surplus patterns, organized by conditioning in some other scene, or grouped by the very configuration of the autonomic nervous system that overflows with impulses when some strong emotion moves us, are frightfully ambiguous: they carry surplus meanings, contradictory meanings, not quite shaped meanings. They are hard to read. They were not intended as communication. They are not completely planned voluntary acts. A frown can mean eyestrain, astigmatism, too intense illumination, indigestion, extra effort, "nerves," or vexation.

Such patterns can be irrelevant, inappropriate, and outside the actor's field of awareness at times. They may be transferred from some setting that is remote in time and only vaguely similar in structure and meaning to the one that preoccupies the person, or they may be so rooted in anatomy and physiology that they are present but without meaning (such as the breathing changes in emphysema). Such "transferred" expressions, whose sources are unknown to the actor and to the person who is watching him, may be as inappropriate as any pun that arises in the midst of serious discourse simply because a sound touches off a klang association, and may express the fact that the subject's attention (and his integrative forces) is simply not strong enough nor well-structured enough to exclude them.

Some of this fringe of partial integrations is appropriately called automatic, since, like the shoulder-muscle cramp that invades the pianist's performance, it operates without his conscious intention and against his repeatedly affirmed wishes. But there is also a class of actions that is neither wholly voluntary nor wholly automatic. The unwilling partygoer who suffers from a slight indisposition (a mild headache, a lead-cap dullness, a barely perceptible nausea) has a choice. He can dwell on it, expand it, recall previous migraine headaches, speak as though his pain is actually greater than it is. With the cooperation of a solicitous spouse, he can avoid the dinner party, escape from an occasion that is a bore. If the hysterical happens to be a wife, she can irritate and frustrate an ambitious husband, express her contempt for her hostess, win pity and sympathy from her family, or avoid sexual relations that have grown burdensome. Should she, in fact, be a genuine hysterical (with marked suggestibility, with a restricted life-space, with a slight depression of integrative powers), the autosuggestions are realized and the pains become "real." Barred from going out, she can now ask, plaintively, "Why am I punished so, when I so wished to attend the dinner?" Her not quite conscious performance permits her to spoil the party, irritate her husband, play the martyr, claim that she really wanted to go; yet these secondary effects which partially reinforce the pattern may not be the primary reason for the headache, for that original malaise that started the cycle.[28]

In this in-between zone, the symptom has an ambiguous role. It can be taken up, amplified, used as language, made to serve as a tool for manipulating others. Or it can be recognized for what it is, kept in its place, and laid aside while effort is turned to more direct attacks upon problems.[29] As we approach the borders of more serious illness, however, the symptoms begin to possess the person. The headache is painful and overwhelming. The "identity crisis" shatters the last vestige of self-regulative powers. The writer's cramp and the pianist's painful shoulder girdle make work impossible. If we still insist that the symptom is a kind of body language, we have to realize how far this kind of "communication" has departed from the ordinary use of symbols. The process is strongly supported; its support lies outside of our awareness; and if there is a "will" involved, it is not that of the conscious patient.

The average person has difficulty in appreciating the range and complexity of this borderline zone of automatisms. They produce problems for others outside the medical profession. Consider the case of Madame Guyon, the seventeenth-century mystic who was condemned and imprisoned for her heresies by the Catholic authorities (see Knox 1950, Leuba 1925, Malebranche 1922).

Madame Guyon believed that she was operating under divine inspiration, possessed by the Holy Spirit, and when her hand raced over the pages at furious speed, taking down the "dictations" that became her commentaries on the Bible, she asserted that she was a mere onlooker. Amazed at what her own hand wrote, she denied that she possessed any such theological wisdom, or that she could have composed the lines at such a speed that four copyists were kept busy writing out a legible manuscript, transcribing her frenetic scribble. It *must* have come from without; she was *sure* of it. "Not my will but God's," said Madame Guyon. ("Not the patient's conscious will, but the will of an unconscious mental process," add the neo-Freudians of our time.) Exalted in her mood, yet passive, Madame Guyon was

---

[28]The seminary student may begin with small doubts, such as many other pastors in training go through. Added to these are the upcoming examinations, his own rather poor record as a student, and the family expectations which originally helped him set his goal, expectations which he never more than half-shared. The impasse that he works himself into is a real one. If we wish to give it a fancy name, we can call it an "identity crisis," as Erik H. Erikson does. The question is, "How will he use the crisis?" And, "How will those around him contribute to his solution of the problem?"

[29]The normal person, bent on his goals, is sometimes suspicious of his own complaints, hesitant to report them lest they be dubbed "psychosomatic." Among a series of hysterical patients (see Ziegler, Imboden, and Meyer 1960), there will be a large proportion who insist that their disability is organic. At the other extreme of the continuum, the psychotic will insist that the voices he hears are real. There is also the effect of a supporting milieu: in spiritualist circles, automatic handwriting is accepted as a "communication." The analyst who trains his patient to believe that his dreams are valuable communications from his unconscious belongs somewhere in this series, encouraging a certain passivity in the face of automatisms and utilizing these for their persuasive power. They become evidence of the patient's disability.

happy to let God work his will. Indeed, the purity of her revelations and their free flow depended upon her keeping out of it all. "Keeping out of it" became a new and conscious maneuver (just as the proper free associations now require the patient on the analytic couch to keep out of it, to let his thoughts flow freely so that they can express what underlies consciousness, and the symptom; he must not talk to the analyst or try to impress him, nor should he criticize his own ramblings).[30]

Madame Guyon also made use of bodily symptoms. Feeling her body distended and aware that her corset was too tight, on one occasion, she asked an attending duchess to assist her in unlacing it. She interpreted her feeling of fullness as due to an "engagement with the Holy Spirit, for it had interrupted a seance in which, sitting opposite the duchess (as Mesmer was to sit opposite his patients in trance, a hundred years later, to allow the magnetic fluid to flow into them), she was acting as a kind of lightning rod for the Holy Spirit, allowing divine grace to flow through her and out to her interlocuter.

This was a much more dramatic kind of framework of belief than that which the modern hysterical uses to interpret his symptoms: today the patient plays an "illness game"; then it was a "holiness game." Madame Guyon was sure that she was God's special deputy. If she had a special misfortune (e.g., if her carriage overturned on a mountain pass), the event was immediately interpreted as a "sign," or utilized as a special opportunity for her to receive (or transmit) God's grace, or as a Heaven-sent suffering to prove (and improve) her own moral state.

In usages of this sort (which convert a bodily symptom, an accident, malicious gossip, or a victory over the Irish into "signs and portents"), the hysterical typically becomes the center of things. Even when he is punished, he is the great suffering hero. In Madame Guyon this egocentrism was fused with and concealed by a theocentrism: the latter disguised the former so that she appeared to be pointing toward God even while calling attention to herself as His agent. The modern hysterical is given a much less important role, yet he is able to draw on a superficial medical knowledge and a smattering of psychoanalysis while his "interesting colitis" enables him to become the center of the concern of family and physician. By making his paralysis a symbol of very dramatic events in his history, his analyst helps him to suffer in the grand manner. It is not quite the grand role of the principal actor in a miracle play that would be reenacted were he to undergo "treatment" at Lourdes, yet to receive the undivided attention of a skilled psychiatrist for an hour a day, for weeks, is something.

If our sense of the matter is correct, the *cause* of the hysterical's symptom does not lie in its symbolic value. God is not to be blamed for Madame Guyon's tight corset, or for overturning her carriage. Before we have explained this sort of usage we would have to run down the origins of her delusional

---

[30]The Church, of course, did not accept her "inspirations" as coming from any divine source, and it warned against the passivity of Quietism, which seemed to imply that a Christian could relax, become one with God, without strenuous voluntary effort to save his immortal soul. In the analytic procedures the "Quietism" of the patient is corrected by the analyst who interprets what is fished up from the unconscious.

beliefs, the roots of her egocentricity and her immaturity, her poor capacity to structure thought and action, her hysteria. To insist on the central significance of the symbolic value of the symptom, and to make the communication value into a cause, is somewhat comparable to making dreams the cause of sleep. Hysteria (and the sum of those conditions which produce it) must be viewed as the explanation of this use of body language, and not the reverse.

The two become intertwined, however. The feverish patient with his restricted powers of thought and action, the immature patient who has never developed a realistic and vital contact with reality, may begin to experience bodily complaints, which may have a simple and natural origin (flatulence, tight lacing, too tight a hat band, a bit of schizokinesis from some remote and irrelevant scene). Such "symptoms" may serve the person's needs or cause endless anxiety and effort. (When Mary Baker Eddy felt the baleful influence of "malicious animal magnetism," she had to choose a new house as headquarters and move all her belongings.) Some of them may serve purposes which the person has but is reluctant to own. Once the process of interpretation, misuse, misidentification begins, the symptom can be absorbed into an interpersonal network and into a plan of action. The comedy of errors that ensues may involve a pyramiding of misinterpretations, as in the adventures of Don Quixote or the wanderings of "the chosen people."

In all of this discussion, we need to remember one quality of symbols. The flag is a symbol, and so is the cross, and thumbs up, and the V-for-Victory, and the Presidium and the Pope, and the thumb to the nose, and God. Into these symbols we crowd more meanings than we can, or care to, make explicit. "Thumbs up" means "Let the beggar go," Live well," "Keep up your courage," and is also a slightly obscene gesture. Some symbols are like worn banknotes; their frayed meanings prompt redefinitions and the invention of new terms. What is that "Republicanism" that means Lincoln, Barry Goldwater, freeing the slaves, living within the national income, and so on? To some it has a vague and hollow ring, to others a warm, rich coloring; the quality of the user's voice gives it more meaning than the dictionary. We communicate both more and less than we intend; the symbol can be used to conceal what ought to be made explicit by a better language.

The analyst who sets himself the task of unraveling all the significant meanings of the symbols follows a course that is full of risks. His own favorite meanings intrude, as when Erik H. Erikson keeps finding "identity crisis" behind both symptoms and dreams of his patient, whereas his mentor, Freud, found more specifically sexual wishes. The whole process has a way of overleaping many possible causes to center on ideas, thoughts, or psychic processes, much as the Christian Scientist does, much as the ancient exorcist did in searching for mortal sins. A special risk is created whenever the analyst forgets that the id, the source of our instinctual energies, is also a part of a biochemical network that can be analyzed according to another kind of impersonal logic. The Freudian, sticking to his own method as he tries to free these id energies that were once impounded and distorted in the early training of an infant, can overlook another type of causal relationship. With his notion of repression, which thrusts these forces into unconscious channels, and through his technique of derepressing, he arrived at a method of searching out particular kinds of buried meanings, at an interpretation of symptoms as symbols of these same buried meanings. Looked at from a great distance, his method consists in a retraining of reason, an education of perception and willing, by the use of a method that is so loosely structured it can entrap both patient and analyst into "explanations" that are as fanciful as those Madame Guyon gave for her sense of fullness. The theory, it would seem, mistakes effects for causes, and provides an analyst with an opportunity to insert whatever favorite moral counsel he wishes.

August Strindberg

Symptoms as symbols call for an analysis. The biographer who is *au courant* with modern clinical findings can make the life of his subject transparently clear as he reduces the conflicting and chaotic facts to order by the use of analytic theory, particularly when his subject is also full of a sense of his own destiny, and in the habit of seeing "signs" everywhere. August Strindberg used all manner of "happenings" in this hysterical fashion. It was not limited to bodily complaints; the events of his childhood, the scribbles on a wall, the movement of a weathercock, the flight of ladybirds, the shapes he saw in the cinders, all had a meaning for his destiny. His encoding was, of course, highly selective; he was the center of the unfolding drama; and his struggle with these "forces" that were trying to work his destruction was that of a Titan against the devil himself. One of his dominant nightmares had to do with Woman. "He could no more break free from his mother than from his father. Early jealous for her love, early bereft of her, all his life he went on seeking her, and could never grow up to become a normal lover. And from life's harshness he had acquired a sadistic desire to trample, a masochistic desire to be trampled."

"Always," Lucas (1962, p. 19) says, "he longed to kneel before his beloved, to lay his head upon her knees, to set her on a pedestal, to become her child. But the instant he suspected his mistress of assuming the mastery, he changed in a flash from a docile child to a raging rebel, who leapt up and ground the poor woman underfoot. Further, his sense of sin regarded guiltily the healthy physical side of human love. A difficult lover."

Because the hysterical has not won through to a normal "identity" and is still rehearsing those childhood years when his mother was the Queen of Heaven and an Ogress, when his father was both a God of Sweetness and Light and a wrathful Jahweh, when his siblings were good companions and "lice," the "history" that he helps the clinician write is full of seducers, castrators, rejectors, tyrannical parents, and grand and dramatic struggles. It is this blown-up brush heap of his own unresolved past that now interprets the immense overhead of schizokinesis that spoils his relations with sweetheart, boss, colleagues, who undermine his authority, throttle him, dominate him, seduce him, in this same grand manner. He, too, is a poet: the wilted primrose by the river's brim is *also* beset by too great difficulties; the world resounds with his own inner struggle; he can feel the telepathic and spiritual forces zeroing in upon him. These histrionics, his compulsive exhibitionism, his grand roles, give a cosmic significance to unimportant things; even his bodily symptoms have an exaggerated significance. And the psychoanalyst is playing along with him, as he utilizes dreams and free associations to reveal a rich structure of meanings behind the symptoms. "You are indeed an interesting and dramatic case, the very center of the plot." Yet he has to lead his patient to the realization that he is merely human, that his parents are neither tigresses nor Visigoths, that the vast unconcern of the world can also be a blessing that yields great freedom.

The Symbolic Process

One of Freud's favorite spots in Rome was where he could look on Michelangelo's statue of Moses, which stands in the Church of St. Pietro in Vincoli. He puzzled over what meaning the artist was trying to convey. He focused on the position of the hand and the way the hair of the beard fell over it. What had Moses just done? What was he about to say? Suddenly, he became absorbed in the meaning of the whole Moses tradition for the Jews and for the rest of the world, a meaning that he tried to write down in *Moses and Monotheism*. The statue was the first to serve as a kind of three-dimensional projection test; subsequently the mythical personage who, some have insisted, was an Egyptian and not a Jew, came to preoccupy him. Both symbols are ambigous enough; we do not have the sculptor or the Egyptian archives to set us right, so our free associations can run wild, or rather, as in Freud's case, they can tell us the meaning of fantasied patricide, of the killing of a tribal leader, and of the subsequent incorporation and identification that made his "laws" a part of the Jewish character.

A symbol does not have to be grounded on precise historical data in order to be an effective point of reference for the tribe which adopts it. The hand of the father who believes in the symbol gives it a fresh charge of energy as he beats its meaning into the flesh of a punished child. It remains doubtful, perhaps, for the archaeologist (who finds the tale of the child lodged in the bullrushes all over the world, not just in Egypt), but it has a lively quality for the child whose bottom still stings. For the childhood of the race, the patriarchal figures of Abraham and Moses may have provided just the kind of "father figure" needed to make an authentic religious experience work.

The statue of Moses is a symbol, one art historian suggests, of action in repose, of awesome force, of a man capable of wise and realistic leadership as well as of towering rages that called down the wrath of God; he is well within the legendary subject matter with which the sculptor was also familiar. Others, searching for the artist's intention, believe they can see angry scorn on the face of the statue, sensing the feeling of a man who may have been turning his eyes on men and women who caroused and worshiped the golden calf in utter disregard of the laws engraved on the tablets brought down from

Sinai. With varying emphases, the viewers have insisted: he is agitated, angry, contemptuous, about to denounce; he is proud, relaxed, calm in his possession of the ultimate truths; he is saying farewell to his people; his animal-like head (with horns) symbolizes a brutal fanaticism; his poise is the calm before the storm; he is about to hurl the tablets down; he is profoundly shaken; his nostrils are distended; the lips are about to speak; a blazing scorn is on his face; he quivers with horror and pain and has already let the tablets slip; he has just released his beard after having grasped it in some tense moment. And why should a Freudian not add: the animal-like id that protrudes in the horns symbolizes both the half of man that his better nature has to repress (even as the teachings of Moses saved the Jews from the fate of Sodom and Gomorrah) and the wrathful and sometimes violent half of Moses that, no doubt, was foremost in the minds of that tribe of shepherd folk when they killed him.

The free associations of generations of critics have packed this Moses symbol with meanings. Perhaps every meaning read into it is correct, as an expression of what the viewers have seen there. It is this kind of *truth* that the collaborating analyst and his patient find when they treat the bodily symptom as a communication. The symptom, too, becomes a projection test.

Incorporation, Identification, Incarnation, and Deification

There is a psychoanalytic concept, still widely used by the neo-Freudians, that has caused generations of students much difficulty. We have to turn to anthropology and to the history of religions to appreciate the concepts of incorporation and identification to their fullest: it was in our past that we actualized them in flagrant fashion. In their most vivid form the concepts appear in the stigmata that were reported on the body of St. Francis, who had so internalized an image of Christ that the wounds of the crucifixion were reproduced in the saint whose ecstasy had climaxed long contemplation. In their most trivial form, they appear in the posture of the youth who swaggers out of the movie, Marlon Brando in the flesh, and with tone of voice and gestures that imitate his hero, this tough, good guy.

When cannibalism prevailed, the meaning of incorporation was clear: the believers ate the flesh of the brave warrior in order to take on his qualities. In Freud's myth of the slaying of the old man of the tribe (*Totem and Taboo*, 1912), the leader's qualities were internalized, along with the guilt that arose with his murder; they, too, are pictured as eating his flesh. They acquired at the same time, in fact, other powers that he had possessed, such as free access to the women of the horde. This symbolic tale became, in Freud's mind, a kind of reference symbol that portrayed what every son must do, psychologically, as he cuts the bonds of his dependence and submission in the course of his maturing. Guilty, a murderer in fantasy, the son also internalizes the traits and values of that father, in spite of himself, and is most like him when he has completely finished with him. Awesome fear, resentment and hate, worship and submission are the extremes that he has to throw away as he discovers that his idol has feet of clay and as he learns what it is to be a man such as his father was.

In our own tribal past, just a few centuries ago, these processes of identification and incorporation included a kind of deification. Some saints experienced what they believed to be a oneness with God, a spiritual union during which they were no longer separate from Him. Long fasts, lonely vigils, and horrible acts of penance, not wholly different from those of the Indian who awaited the visit from his spirit guide, sometimes preceded these ecstatic moments of union, and were enough—the reader cannot help feeling—to get them into a state wherein the ordinary reflective powers are in abeyance. Madame Guyon knelt with bare knees on venomous snakes, stood passively before a dangerous bull, bit the flesh from her own arm in order to relieve the pain of a disciple and to take it upon herself, licked up spittle from the street, sucked suppurating sores, had her sound teeth extracted, all in the effort to court divine compassion and to prove herself before God. When she felt that God's spirit had indeed descended upon her, as when she wrote with furious speed in order to get down all of her inspired revelations, she *was* God; she felt a complete identity; her old private self had been crowded out, burnt away in the flame of her passion.

Now the person who has adopted a more matter-of-fact language that expresses the skills suitable to running tractors or computers, and who tries to keep the objects of his material surroundings in their place (even when he turns his vision away from them), has difficulty understanding the words of the seer and saint possessed of his God. He has difficulty finding the words to break up this process into its components, difficulty in making any analysis that would do justice to what is occurring and still preserve what he calls "the necessary rationality" to remain properly oriented in the real world. What the possessed tells us surpasses our belief, as it surpassed the belief of Madame Guyon's contemporaries and of the ecclesiastical court which tried and sentenced her. She was not God. Her much-touted love of God was a very impure affair. They regarded her as foolish much in the same way we consider Father Divine foolish. Only yesterday he was telling his followers, who repeated, "Father Divine is God."

The concept of incorporation has entered our vocabulary for want of any better name for such a process. We come very near to repeating the ancient cannibalism, in a virtual and symbolic ritual, when we repeat in the communion service the phrases supposedly spoken long ago, "This is my body, broken for you." The devout who rehearse this service seem to be striving to accomplish some magical thing, to perform a miracle. The prudent onlooker who keeps his skepticism sees either a mystery or foolishness. How can words be incorporated and gestures "made flesh"?

We approach an experimental demonstration of this process when we tell a hypnotized subject that he is some well-known figure and then instruct him to act true to form in some setting that we structure for him. He seems to become the character as he acts out this role, or as he gives his version of what he thinks he is expected to do. The Madame Guyons have needed no operator to produce the action; if there was suggestion, it came from the tradition, from the books, finally assuming the form of autosuggestion. Some who enter ecstasy or a state of transport are indeed possessed, and far away from normal contact with their surroundings.

It is from such roots that the terms now current in psychoanalytic usage have grown. They are of course grossly altered as they become a part of the analyst's schemata. It is in the family setting that a child's identity (and identification-incorporation) is worked out. Confusions in identification (such as those of the "Nice Nellie" who is a male dress designer and who walks, gestures, and talks like his mother) can occur, since the "incorporation process" begins so early and has so many interpersonal tensions to throw roadblocks across the normal course of development. New as its present locale seems, new as the surrounding beliefs of current healing cults are, it is again a kind of automatic transfer of traits from one person (or image) to another. Neither the transmitter nor the receiver may intend what transpires. It can be a wordless process, as in early infancy it must be. It can exist beside and in contradiction to both intention and verbal communications. One can see a later form of this same identification process in the old married couple who have spent half a century together; bits of one spouse have entered the spiritual marrow of the constant companion until each unconsciously identifies with the other. A wordless glance communicates. The resonance defies attempts to deceive.

This kind of automatic transfer can also occur between a hero (now gone to join that host of unseen witnesses) and his biographer. Long days of reading and meditating on the life of Lincoln must have opened up channels to create similarities in a Sandburg who unwittingly internalized some of the turns of thought of his subject. The young novice who starts on his course that he describes as an imitation of Christ can succeed in incorporating bits of his model. Normally, such an identification remains quite incomplete. "He is there; I am here," and history retains its structure, as it should, but a Madame Guyon falls into a lower form of misidentification. "I am God," she says, "at such moments. He is in me. I write his thoughts. There is no scrap of my former worldly ego left."

There are also wordless and unintentional incorporations. A child shows such a process in the flesh when his way of cocking his head on one side is a clear imitation of his father's gesture. Even the acting out of headaches, stomach complaints, and a fear of cancer can arouse our suspicions of some incorporation process at work.

The hysterical whom we suspect of incorporating some model is not usually as wildly histrionic as was Madame Guyon, but his suggestibility makes him sensitive to every model in his orbit. So much of this transfer operates below the vigilant-reflective level that, even in the days of Charcot, physicians were beginning to urge isolation as the first step in therapy. The recurring tale of epilepsy being portrayed by hystericals who had lived in the presence of these organically rooted seizures gives some substance to the possibility of incorporation and acting out of patterns first portrayed by another.

This process of identification-incorporation-incarnation of patterns seen and heard has remained too complex a problem for the laboratory. Depending on a process we call suggestion, it has remained an interesting idea rather than a mechanism easily reduced to laws; we use it after the fact rather than as a precise method of predicting. Even when we approach an experimental use, as in the laboratory study of hypnosis, we discover gross limits to the process: the subject's performance represents his version of Paderewski, and is no more skilled than his own waking performance on the piano. Some "models" that are suggested to a hypnotized subject are flatly rejected, as when a modest young woman refuses to play the role of a striptease artist even under hypnosis.

This process can also generate conflict within the individual, especially when the pattern he sees himself taking on almost automatically is one that he has come to hate. A young woman who had "attacks" of overeating would purchase a dozen doughnuts, eat them at one sitting, and then make herself vomit, and a period of fasting would follow. "I have no more control of appetite than my father," she confessed. Her father, who had lately become an alcoholic, was the family problem, with his weekly alcoholic binges. Here the daughter was irritated with her own weakness, afraid that something had been inherited, and in conflict with and determined to suppress whatever she had identified and incorporated. Her identification was conscious; she was quite aware of the mixture of affection, shame, and resentment involved. But in her case the identification is only a vague analogy, a way of speaking; it does not solve the problem of how this girl arrived at a state where she could no longer regulate her appetite, nor does it indicate a clear line of attack on the task of establishing an improved self-discipline.

Identification in the Clinic

Cameron (1963, p. 319) describes the case of a young resident on a neurological service who watched his chief demonstrate a case of torticollis and listened to a careful description of the organic changes underlying the disorder. Soon thereafter he developed a similar tic and assumed that it must have a similar organic basis. We could say that he identified himself with the patient; the half-teasing attitude of his chief toward the patient was one that he had also shown to the resident. We could even speculate about passive desires, unconsciously at work, that were striving to perpetuate and extend themselves by means of this "incorporated" torticollis. He, too, could become an interesting case and receive attention from his chief. "Look at me," we imagine him saying as he used the symptom as a way of communicating.

After the resident had been carefully studied by the staff of neurologists and psychiatrists, who could find no supporting evidence of organic involvement, a psychiatrist took up the problem and with the help of the patient worked out a history. There had been conflicts between the mother and father, the mother being somewhat contemptuous of her husband. The close bond between this son and his mother and his turning away from the father were later succeeded by a strong aversion against his mother, a resentment which set in when he was bullied by his playmates and thereupon projected all blame on the mother who had made him, he was convinced, so soft. This double aversion continued to weaken his sense of identity as a male, and was a factor (his psychiatrist was interpreting now) in his insecurity as a young and inexperienced resident. Consciously he idealized his chief, but he was also disturbed by the latter's teasing. This background and present condition facilitated his new and surprising identification with the patient. The process of psychotherapy carried him back through old conflicts, and permitted him to relive them in the presence of a wise and tolerant guide. It helped him to formulate a realistic role for himself, to restructure his present goals, to discard his pathological identification with a patient, and to slough off the remnants of fixations and aversions that had never been properly worked through, closed off, and replaced by more mature attitudes.

This case could be used to illustrate the fact that a fairly sophisticated adult can betray hysterical symptoms and suggestibility. In fact, it was the young resident's neurological sophistication that provided a precise channel for his attitude and beliefs. The case also suggests that secondary gains are often designed to gratify an immature portion of the self that remains in spite of a superficial maturing. The gains that would accrue to a "mature resident in neurology" were discarded under the cloak of, perhaps, a vague hope that he would get by as a passive patient. Or did he want the attention of his chief and invite, in fact, the kind of discipline and help in maturing that neither his mother nor his father had provided?

It is the psychiatrist's speculation that makes the aversive tic (in addition to imitating the patient) express unconscious conflicts. It is the psychiatrist who makes it into a body language that only a clinician with his training can interpret after long hours of discussion. In this process of interpretation a pun served as the link between a head-averting movement and an aversion from mother and father. It is also this psychiatrist-interpreter who makes the symptom into a punishment for the resident's hostility to his parents, into a response that binds anxiety and guilt, and expresses a contempt that he feels toward himself and that his chief's teasing had reactivated.

The hypnotized subject will sometimes take on assignments, act out suggestions, that in his waking period he will reject out of hand. As though his stance in the world had somehow been weakened by the operator's procedures, he submits, actualizes, consents. The state is one of markedly increased suggestibility. Now these "states" recur in the life of the hysterical. They come and go. When he is in one of these troughs of mild depression of his integrative powers, such a demonstration as that of the chief before the young resident can produce dramatic aftereffects. Just as a hysterical girl can take on the politics, opinions about dress and manners, and religious beliefs of her new "flame," this resident seemed to take on the role enacted before his eyes, to put himself in the place of the patient.

Although the hysterical patient is not usually as wildly incorporative as Madame Guyon, he seems to be operating at something less than a fully vigilant and reflective level. He is so vulnerable that what he does becomes cluttered up with automatisms of whose origin he is unaware and whose relevance to his present aims and purposes is not critically examined. Before we place him in a class apart, in this respect, we need to recall how widespread this suggestibility is. Before we know it, we have incorporated the role our family designed for us, or some successful lawyer friend of the family portrayed for us, and then some ten years later discover that this is not a profession for us at all. If the conflict between the persona and some deeper-lying protest within us comes to a head as late as in the forties, it will take a very skillful clinician to interpret all the bodily tensions and somatic expressions that we bring into the clinic in terms of hasty identifications, conflict between role and capacities. If this clinician is fully aware of how many ways there are for a lawyer to live out his profession, how many roles and what diverse satisfactions are available to a man with this training, he will also have to explain the inability of his client to find satisfactions within the role that he has pursued for so long.

Identification and incorporation are concepts of very uncertain value. Wherever they are used, they present as many problems as they give solutions (or rationalizations). Guillaume Monod acted out his delusion that he was Jesus Christ returned for more than sixty years. The moviegoer who comes out of the theatre with an internalized image of an actor has abandoned it by the next morning. A young lawyer may strive to outdo his uncle for ten years before he wakens to the fact that he is living out a role that is really not for him. There are states (such as hypnosis and the mild depression that some hystericals show) that make their bearers unusually susceptible to presented copy, but these states pass, and with them the "incorporations" disappear. (Posthypnotic suggestions are dissipated in the course of a few weeks, usually.) Since the clinical usage of these concepts is "after the fact," the identification hypothesis can at best present a problem, not an explanation.

THE PSYCHOANALYTIC SCHEMA

The neo-Freudians have a certain advantage over the other clinicians, somewhat like that of all true believers who know precisely the origins of all things, and who have a clear conception of that destiny toward which life moves. They possess an over-all schema of development, with the stages at which "arrests and fixations" occur. Once these oral, anal, and genital stages are posted, they can be used as reference points for the later pathological behavioral changes. To the developmental tasks that must be accomplished at each level, if there is to be a normal progression to maturity, there will correspond special pathologies. If a symptom proves to be so complex an affair that it can not be adequately explained by reference to a developmental failure at one of these levels, the rather loose schema will permit whatever flexibility is needed. Thus an anorexic girl who refuses to eat may be struggling with her oral cravings (especially with those not properly worked through when she was a nursling); she may be holding back an unconscious desire to bite the breast. Fused with it may be the desire not to get too fat (i.e., to grow up, to look like a pregnant woman, to have fully developed breasts). Or she may be resisting an unconscious wish to be impregnated orally (acting out a long-forgotten fantasy about childbirth). Or it may express a resistance against an unconscious desire to eat the male genital. Or she may be pitting her will against that of her mother, as she did in her toilet-training days. The pegs on this developmental model are like convenient hooks on which to hang speculations (as these are prompted by interview material). As the analyst traces out a pattern of hypothetical motivations, these spots on a developmental schema become linked in a kind of dynamic map, useful in exposition and serving to symbolize an interlocking set of unconscious forces that determine symptoms.

Freud once compared human development to a march into the desert. He used the figure of a foreign legion sent to occupy a colony that had been overrun by indigenous hostile bands. During the march the leader must establish outposts as they penetrate this territory; at each point supplies and men must be left behind. Finally, as his marching column is depleted by this long string of posts that dot the land, the commander has to meet and overcome one more band of tribesmen that sweeps down from the hills. He may have to turn back to one of the posts previously established, if more men and supplies are needed. If the natives are too many, this regressive movement will have to be greater; sometimes the retreat may carry the troops all the way back to the coastal border. So it is, Freud argued, with the adult overcome by pressures from without and conflicts from within that exceed his power to master them; he, too, falls back to once-secure positions. Suddenly he begins to feel and act as though he were a motherless child, filled with oral cravings, overcome by a blind rage, acting as though he had just been punished for resisting his mother. Or he is nauseated (as he was when his mother stuffed food into his already resistant mouth, as she insisted on following the doctor's orders to the letter). Or, suddenly, he is moved to give up, as though he expected supporting arms to sustain him, and his paralysis of the legs reenacts the earlier time when he balked at walking further and forced his mother to carry him.

Such a parable for the neurotic's tendency to regress invites another parable for the normal, whose development is like the winning of the West. The pioneers set up outposts, planted crops, developed their herds, and only occasionally sent back for iron, special seeds, ammunition, and other supplies they could not yet manufacture for themselves. Ultimately the outposts became autonomous communities and the natives were subdued (not without residues of guilt, to be sure). There was no neurotic weakness in the series of "rootings in life" in this latter saga, no flight back to security, no arrest in growth, no crises in identity that left the pioneers confused.

If one were to adopt Freud's figure, the balance in forces that determines forward movement or regression would be both variable and unstable. As he might have put it, it is an "economic matter" (i.e., dependent on the relative quantities of supportive and nocuous influences). One might want to anticipate that the points of arrest, and of regressive movement, could lie at any point along the march, and the extent of the recoil could carry the column back to any level, depending on the severity of the opposition. What we might call "affective resonance" could conceivably direct the regressive changes toward any one of a number of earlier points of reference. For example, if he feels abandoned, or if he is blind with rage, or if he cowers in fear, these moods may point to old positions, old solutions. If the hysterical is, in fact, a person of extremes, these incubating and expanding emotions in the present can summon old resonant traces, stir the most remote memories, and penetrate those barriers that, in the normal, seem to remind the person: "You can't go home again. You need not go way back there. There is strength here, and power enough to go ahead. You are not a child." Thus, the backward reverberation, the dominance of the past, and the weakness of the ties to the present would produce most variable forms of regression.

These parables, which some find helpful frames for thinking, set certain problems. What weakens the hysterical's integrative strength to the point where he has such a poor grasp of the present field? Why do his old crisis points have such an exaggerated and magnetic power? Why are his old affective memories so easily set into vibration that he begins to act, now, like a motherless child, or like a willful three-year-old who is still rebelling against a mother bent on toilet training, or like an adolescent girl afraid of womanhood? After all, every man has traveled this way. Why does he not keep his emotions within bounds and make the proper references to his history and his present life-space, expressing them in ways of coping with the reality that is producing them? Why must he regress from the adult level to find some old pattern to bind them?

In short, the grand schema raises a great number of questions. The reasons for the particular form of the symptom, for the regression to a particular level, for the use of old defenses, for the turning to secondary gains that only help to arrest growth remain to be determined. The neo-Freudian has a way of explaining the particular symptom by viewing it as a displacement, a condensation of motives from many sources, and as an identification with some significant figure. Each of these principles represents one of many possible ploys that can be used to fit the symptoms into a life-history and give it meaning. None of the principles has predictive value, nor does any combination of them explain why this particular patient took this particular path of regression.

Since the growth and development of an individual are not precisely like that column of troops marching into the desert, and since there are many hysterogenic factors that lie outside such a schema, the latter can serve as a screen to block fruitful hypotheses (just as it would have led clinicians to overlook brucellosis or hypoglycaemia as causes of neurasthenia). Those forms of hysteria that are somatopsychic require us to take a wholly different orientation from this figurative schema. Where the symptoms arise out of a poor hygiene of living in the present, or where special constitutional disabilities require the invention of a special design for living, this constant reference of a single schema of development will make effective diagnosis and treatment of the disorder harder, not easier.

THE PAVLOVIAN APPROACH

A neurosis can be viewed as a learned response, the outgrowth of conditioning. In the case of hysteria, a particular constitutional makeup, combined with special schedules of reinforcement or with conflicts between opposed response tendencies under high-level motivation, can produce, in experimental animals, analogs of the anesthesia, paralysis, and nonresponsiveness that human patients bring to the clinic. In the case of the human patients, the conflicting motivations and the schedules of reinforcement or frustration are often unknown; to unravel the threads of causation would require patient study and in all probability would produce more speculative questioning than firm answers.

Fortunately, the Pavlovian argues, in "behavioral therapy" no historical review is necessary. This is not a talking cure. There is no need to view the symptom as an expression of the personality as a whole, or as revealing unconscious motives, or as the product of erroneous ideas. The Pavlovian is not interested in the patient's philosophy of existence, or in locating and diagnosing some obscure ego-weakness that has permitted sensory or motor functions to "escape from control." He does not feel called on to offer a new hygiene of living, although specific work schedules may sometimes be identified as the source of a cramp or an anesthesia. He is not interested in some obscure relationship between the man and his mechanisms, nor in providing a "will discipline" that will improve a patient's consciousness or ego-strength. What other therapists would regard as a weakness in clinical technique is offered by the Pavlovian as its essential source of strength, its great economy.

The Pavlovian view of stimulus-response relationships would imply that the patient is a bundle (and a loosely integrated bundle, at that) of specific S-R bonds, and that his symptom is merely one local set of connections that needs to be set right by a specifically designed series of "forcing stimuli" aimed at a specific malfunctioning of reflexes. The local inhibition that has developed to block the pathways rising from an anesthetic hand requires carefully aimed excitations that will break through a particular inhibitory barrier. Advice, encouragement, suggestion, psychotherapeutic probing of dream material, free associations are all beside the point. Not only are these person-to-person methods fruitless, they are relics of a psychology of another day when, after dismissing a mind that acted on the body's levers, psychologists developed a conception of psychophysical parallelism in which mental events were envisioned as somehow reflecting or running in tandem beside bodily changes. At long last, the Pavlovian says, it is time to abandon concern about these images and subvocal "comments" on action, since they do not move the body's levers.

An example will make the Pavlovian's emphasis clearer. A patient with a hysterical anesthesia of the left hand (which is insensitive to touch and to pain) could not recognize objects placed in her palm, out of sight, nor respond when the hand was brushed with a wisp of cotton. From other studies (such as

Janet's), we know that there is not a complete loss of sensitivity in such cases. Under hypnosis the patient can react to touch. Conditioning procedures offer an additional proof that there is no lesion.

Applying the wisp of cotton as a signal that is followed one second later by a strong electric shock applied to the surface of the normal right hand, and giving fifty paired stimulations, failed to produce in the patient a conditioned response. Reversing the relationship (applying the wisp of cotton to the normal right hand and the strong shock to the left) produced a conditioned response after two trials. Then, returning once more to the first sequence of stimulation, and substituting deep pressure (which was normally perceived) for the light touch (in the form of a tap of the knuckles of the left hand), produced a conditioned response after one trial. By the twelfth trial the wisp of cotton was substituted, at first without success, but then, after alternating the touch with the rap of the knuckles (followed by the usual reinforcement by the electric shock), the cotton wool began to evoke conditioned responses in the right hand. Through succeeding days, with many trials at each experimental period, the sensitivity of the surface of the anesthetic hand gradually returned. There was, at first, a period in which the light touch which evoked CRs was not felt, then gradually the normal perceptions returned.

By this method of attaching a reaction to the stimulus, and thus forcing a discharge of impulses through the barrier of inhibition, the experimenters (Sears and Cohen 1933) brought a return of that normal process of elaboration of sensory impulses that enables the adult to name, classify, and identify the source of the stimulation.

Hilgard and Marquis (1956) repeated similar procedures in a case with a paralyzed and anesthetic area of such long standing (six years) that considerable atrophy had occurred. The forcing procedures restored sensitivity, forced the return of responses in the paralyzed muscle, and finally enabled the patient to resume active control of movements.

Hysterical deafness, blindness, phobias, and aphonia have been treated by various modifications of conditioning techniques, operant conditioning, avoidance training, and exhaustion methods (repetition of conditioned stimuli without reinforcement). Combinations of reward and punishment have been applied to control the ebb and flow of recovery. When these forms of training are combined with "desensitization procedures" (which may involve considerable verbal persuasion), relaxation techniques, hypnosis, and direct suggestion, it becomes difficult to evaluate the weight which should be given to the Pavlovian elements in the therapy.

The fact that behavior therapy is founded on "a rigorous process of deduction from certain general laws or principles, independently established," is offered as one of the great selling points of this new school of "scientific therapy." But no rigor can save the theory if the basic assumptions of Pavlovian psychology are not adequate to cover the phenomena to which they are applied. Whoever uses the holistic approach will find the assumptions wanting,

and to such theorists as Janet or Freud, who focused on the relationships between the man and his mechanisms as the central problem in psychotherapy, the
Pavlovian's assumptions are too simple. The person is not a mere bundle
of reflexes, casually formed into a loose aggregate. This system as a whole
undergoes changes of a global sort; when the hysterical is afflicted with
aboulia, or when a dissociation process splits a half of the system from
another half (as in a fugue), one is at a loss to imagine how a local conditioning process can accomplish the change in the system as a whole. It may
be that, in evaluating the work of the behavior therapists, we are unwittingly
taking a very limited sample of those cases that have been judged as "good
bets" for the more particularist approaches. Simple addictions, phobias, anesthesias, paralyses, can be fitted into the procedure with greater ease. Even
here we find Malmo strongly suggesting to his patient that the machine
which will deliver the electric shock will cure her deafness (Malmo, Davis,
and Barza 1960). We may be witnessing one more occasion on which the
man in the white coat (and a theory) is taken in by his compliant hysterical
subject. A room full of apparatus is as full of persuasive power as was the
great Charcot on the podium, and he was taken in.

An additional aspect of the theory ought to be brought into question.
Although one of its advantages lies in the fact that the therapist does not
have to make any inquiry about the patient's past, the behavior therapists
have felt forced to construct a "just-so" story as to how neurosis must come
about. Some special account is doubly necessary since they are fully aware
that conditioned responses (and a neurosis is a conditioned response, they
claim) tend to be extinguished when not reinforced. How is it that a maladaptive phobia should become *fixed,* then? A three-stage process is postulated:
(1) a traumatic event with all of its autonomic overflow and disorganization
of behavior; (2) its spread through generalization and second-order conditioning so that the response is cued by a wide range of stimuli; and (3)
the human animal (not strapped in a harness), free to escape, avoids the
very setting where relearning would be possible and secures the tertiary
reinforcement of anxiety reduction that comes with the avoidance of the
original danger.

There are two things wrong with this picture. In the first place, the
unreinforced avoidance should itself die out. Cat phobia or not, the person
would grow careless and inevitably discover that "nothing happens" when a
cat is present. In the second place, and this is reported by the behavior therapists
themselves, when the hysterical deafness, which was supposed to serve the
patient's need to escape, was removed by conditioning, *no anxiety was uncovered.* Or to speak more accurately, anxiety was imputed by the theorist who
invented the "just-so" story. Others have failed to find it.

Perhaps weakest of all is the essential mechanism, the conditioned reflex.
When we have adjusted our vocabulary to the requirements of Pavlovian
theory and have come to look on the strength of a habit as the natural outgrowth of hundreds of thousands of repetitions and reinforcements, the thought

of the long struggle with painful extinction, repeated errors, and slow build-up of contradictory habits is enough to make one put off buying an electric typewriter. And what does the purchaser discover? That in two weeks he has adjusted to the new keyboard: he no longer "fans the air" to hit the lever that returned the carriage on the old machine; he has given up punching the keys to make an impression; he lets the mechanism and key advance the machine to the new position for the next line. The same could be said of the person who has been conditioned to light a cigarette with his coffee, at the office door, at dozens of other occasions as he consumes a pack a day for thirty years. Surely the conditioned responses will have set like plaster, as James once said of habits. The man may have set, but not his conditioned responses. If, as we so vaguely put it, *he makes up his mind,* the clamor for a cigarette that arises in his tissues when he first cuts off this response, and that is most annoying, will have subsided at the end of the second week. At least, that is the story, according to surveys, for nineteen million older Americans who "got the message" from the Surgeon General. (To be sure, more than nineteen million younger Americans have responded to the call of the advertisers, so that total consumption has not decreased markedly.)

These examples suggest that the behavior therapists have misplaced their emphasis on something peripheral, and have forgotten the one who makes up his mind, the relationship between the ego and its mechanisms, the quality in the system as a whole that enables a man to decide and act appropriately. "Here is my body," the patient might be pictured as saying to the behavior therapist. "You condition it, since I can do nothing with it." Little does he realize that of all the mechanisms psychologists have turned up, the conditioned response is the most ephemeral.

When we learn that this new therapy conditions patients so that they stay conditioned, that it eliminates symptoms without recurrence or displacement, that it does not need to delve into a patient's past or know the circumstances which first gave rise to symptoms, that it does not need to treat "the individual" or to deal with consciousness or to use the slipshod verbal techniques of the more conventional psychotherapies, we can afford to reserve our final appraisal until more evidence is in.

It has many praiseworthy features. It invites the therapists to look for conditions in which near-normal functioning is possible and to start retraining from there. The person with a writer's cramp, it has been found, can write without a cramp if the arm is fully extended to the right (in the right-handed), so that extensors are tensed in opposition to the offending flexors. Beginning here, and proceeding slowly back to the normal posture, a reeducation is possible, without going into the relationship between the bank teller and his father-in-law who is president of the bank. Perhaps going into that relationship would be more important than retraining the muscles of the forearm, but the therapist has a starting point from which to make visible changes. On the other hand, consider the puffy hands of the sophomore who cannot play in recital, or the piano student with a shoulder-girdle cramp.

The first might need to reconsider her capacities, her vocational choice, and her relationship with the mother who chose music as her career; the teacher of the second pianist might need to be studied as well as his "driven" pupil. It is one thing to identify immediate conditions which can be changed with good effects, and it is another to overlook the major aspects of a person's life setting. In the latter case, should the causes lie in the larger setting, the removal of a partial symptom, a single expression, leaves person and milieu in an unchanged condition. The "soil" in which symptoms grow has not been improved.

In one respect, behavior therapy is modest. It leaves "the mind" and "the person" alone, limiting itself to the work of a technician. We do not want personal advice from dentists; why should we seek it from a behavior therapist? It deals with the peripheral mechanisms and leaves the imperious self untouched. It charges flaccid muscles and does not bother about "me." It is a great economizer of therapeutic effort. But it also misses much.

TESTING THE THEORIES AND THERAPIES

EMPIRICAL STUDIES OF THE "HYSTERICAL CHARACTER"

Neither the generalized portrait of Janet nor the neo-Freudian modification of the concept stands up too well when a number of cases diagnosed as hysteria are studied intensively with this clinical stereotype made the center of concern. In an extended survey of 381 cases diagnosed as hysteria, Ljungberg (1957) could find no noteworthy and consistent personality deviation common to the group. Of those "unusual" personalities that he found in 39 per cent of the case records, only 21 per cent possessed a "hysterical character" that even loosely approximated the pattern identified by Janet or Ey and his associates. In this fraction of the total population, he did find suggestibility, distractibility, rapid learning and easy forgetting, and easily aroused enthusiasms which fail to persist. These patients were also described as being bored very easily, and as needing to be the center of attention.

Ljungberg found a second pattern, in 10 per cent of the case records and not altogether remote from the above, that he called *psycho-infantile;* he described this group as childish, credulous, easily led, fixated on relatives, and deeply in need of their affection, guidance, and support. Immature, not quite autonomous, this type of person reacted to external pressures with a collapse (attacks, anesthesias, restriction of field, paralyses, and so on).

Another 8 per cent showed the easy fatigability of the neurasthenic and an exaggerated anxiety; they were described as working to reduce their energy expenditures by maneuvers that seemed to conform to Zipf's "law of least effort" (Zipf 1949). They avoided fatigue, sought to prevent all surprises, and tried to escape from all situations requiring firm decisions; as a group these persons were described as shy, withdrawn, "routineers," meticulous, and dutiful, but also as irresolute and vacillating.

The majority of Ljungberg's cases did not show any marked personality deviation. We can only speculate whether 39 per cent represents a saturation that would be extremely high for any random sample of the population which could be studied by the same close clinical scrutiny as that given to these patients.

A second study that throws some light on the hysterical character is reported by Slater (1961). He was able to find 24 pairs of twins of which one member had been diagnosed as hysterical. Twelve of the pairs were dizygotic, twelve monozygotic; these relationships held out the possibility of identifying a genetically caused concordance in the identicals if "the hysterical character" is, indeed, an inherited disposition. Such evidence to support the genetic interpretation was not found, although in both sets of twins there was evidence of nervous ailments in the ancestors as well as in other relatives of the patients, with a frequency that Slater judged to be higher than one might expect to find in a random sample of the population. The patients diagnosed as hysterical had one common element: he described them as complicated cases, resistant, histrionic, hard to diagnose. But the more closely Slater studied their records, the more he became convinced that he was dealing with a complex relationship between patient and physician rather than some clear-cut disease entity:

"In some sense it is true to say that 'hysterical' is a label assigned to a particular relationship between observer and observed; it appears on the case sheet most readily if the doctor has found himself at a loss, if the case is obscure, and if treatment has been unsuccessful. *Of all diagnoses it is that which is least likely to be made in a spirit of detachment.*"

It is interesting to note that Slater's comparison twins (none of whom had been diagnosed as hysterical) were described as less anxious, less tense, less inclined to worry, but the traits of excitability, suggestibility, and shallow affects were present in both the patients and their twins in about the same frequencies (and in about the proportion noted by Ljungberg). The patients were judged to show more of the "histrionic" trait than their normal twins, and greater difficulty in achieving a normal sexual adjustment, but these differences were differences in degree rather than absolute differences. For example, there were ten of the twins in the nonhysterical group whose sex interest was judged to be late, feeble, or too weak to prompt marriage, and two of the marriages of normal twins had ended in divorce.

When he turned to study possible pathogenic pressures, he found that the items identified in the case histories of the hystericals were banal, varied, and often present in the twin. The cluster of traits that Ljungberg had identified as "hysterical characters" (suggestibility, distractibility, easily aroused enthusiasms) were present in about one-fourth of the cases, and with only slightly higher frequency in the probands than in their twins.

One factor is worth emphasis, in evaluating the data of studies of the type here under consideration. Both studies begin with cases that had been diagnosed as hysteria. Although the textbooks strive to present a clear-cut conception of a disorder that can be discriminated from other mental illnesses, the cases so diagnosed on actual hospital wards may include brain lesions, epilepsy, schizophrenia, endogenous depressions, simple anxiety states, and neurasthenia.

Among the cases reviewed by Slater, a few improved without therapy; others proved to be chronic. All manner of therapies were used in those cases given treatment, including leucotomy, electroshock, drugs, psychotherapy. The differences between those who recovered and those who did not were not easily accounted for.

If the concept of hysteria is to be rescued from the dustbin where some would place it, much will have to be done before it is rehabilitated. The subjective factors must be removed from diagnosis, and therapy will have to be superior to that slogan "make it unpleasant and destroy the secondary gains" that some evidently feel is germane. Such a descriptive term as "histrionic" (which often reveals merely that the patient is a poor actor and deceives no one) needs to be replaced by more objective descriptions of behavior.

EVIDENCE REGARDING BEHAVIOR THERAPY

Eysenck makes a strong case for the Pavlovian approach to therapy. It is relatively brief, requiring perhaps ten to fifteen hours (in the place of the 300 hours of an average orthodox analytic procedure). It requires no exploration of personal history and no interference with the life of the person as a whole. In many of the reports of "cures," there is no report of recurrence, or of the substitution of other hysterical symptoms (as though some general weakness had remained untouched). As a technique it makes less demands on the therapist, either for high-quality interpersonal skills or for a great quantity of concerned effort. Since the procedures have arisen out of an extensive body of experimental work and rather precise theoretical formulations, they promise a future in which greater precision in treatment can be expected (with objective measurement of success as attainable as in any other conditioning study).

In his summary and evaluation of evidence that has accumulated in recent decades, in which more than a thousand patients have been treated, Eysenck is quick to point out, however, that adequate follow-up studies are rare, that controls are often lacking, and that comparisons with other therapies (and with spontaneous recovery without any therapy at all) are still something for the future. The reports of recovery vary widely (as with other methods of therapy). Perhaps best are the results of Lazarus (1963), who reported results for 126 cases of "severe neurosis": 62 per cent were apparently cured or much improved, and in his follow-up two years later, only one of the patients had relapsed. Of the 126, 27 patients were diagnosed as hysteria; within this group 71 per cent had recovered. There were "only the most tenuous suggestions" of symptom substitution.

In the special form of aversion therapy used by Voegtlin and with longer follow-up study, the evidence does not support the notion that once conditioned a patient stays conditioned. At intervals of two, five, ten, and thirteen

TABLE 7. *Prognosis in the Psychoneuroses.* (From Hinsie 1937, p. 167.)

Institution	Number Treated	Average Duration	Per Cent Recovered	Per Cent Improved	Per Cent Recovered or Improved
All New York State mental hospitals, 1917-1934	5,700	—	32	40	72
Maudsley Hospital, 1931 and 1935	1,531	6	15	52	67
Cassel Hospital (Kent, England), 1921-1933	1,186	4.1	45	25	70
New York Psychiatric Institute, 1930-1935	119	6.1	40	47	87
Berlin Psychoanalytic Institute, 1920-1930					
Total cases treated	312	—	22	36	58
Total cases completed	200	17.1	35	56	91

years after therapy, follow-up data on 4,000 patients treated showed that the percentages of alcoholics remaining abstinent dropped from 60 per cent through 51, 38, and 23 per cent. From the earliest studies of Pavlov, one of the outstanding characteristics of the conditioned response has been its fragility and the speed with which it is extinguished. And the extinguished conditioned reflex fluctuates, with flurries of spontaneous recovery, and stability seems to depend on a stable matrix of supporting reinforcements.

Eysenck's stress, elsewhere, on the high percentage of neuroses that recover spontaneously is in sharp contrast to his enthusiasm for the new behavior therapy.

STUDIES OF CHRONICITY: COURSE, OUTCOME, AND CURE

From the Biblical account of the healing of the paralytic, through Savonarola's exorcism of demons, to the latest effort to apply Pavlovian extinction procedures or direct conditioning techniques to an anesthetic area, there have been reports of the sudden and almost miraculous cure of hysterical symptoms. In Table 7, which summarizes the experience of some hospitals, both public and private, with all psychoneuroses and without distinction between subclasses, Hinsie points out that at least two out of three patients treated are discharged as recovered or improved. (The estimates for the Berlin Psychoanalytic Institute are somewhat confusing, since a large proportion of the cases did not complete a course of therapy, and we are not told why.) Combining the figures given by Hinsie with those summarized by

Eysenck in Table 8, we can see that for the general class of psychoneuroses—disregarding any differences between neurasthenia, anxiety neuroses, obsessions, psychosomatic illnesses, and neurotic character disorders, and any between the severity of the disorders—somewhere between 40 and 80 per cent of all cases treated respond to psychotherapy. The measures are crude. The therapy ranges from mere custodial care (in public hospitals where the physician-patient ratio is approximately 1 to 300) to the intensive, hour-long, daily sessions between one therapist and one patient. Reports from psychoanalytic institutes in London, Chicago, and Berlin published in the 1930's and reported in Hendrik's study (1941, pp. 256-57) of this form of psychotherapy range from London's 99 per cent (satisfactory or improved) to Chicago's 19 per cent (cured or much improved), with Berlin reporting 40 per cent (cured or much improved). These three figures deal with all cases treated and with hysteria rather than with psychoneuroses as a general class.

A study (Denker 1946) of disability cases who were receiving insurance compensation for incapacities of neurotic origin and were treated by general practitioners, most of whom had slight acquaintance with the illness and many of whom merely diagnosed and certified the extent and nature of the disability, showed that in the records of 500 consecutive cases 45 per cent had recovered after one year, an additional 27 per cent after two years. By the fifth year, 90 per cent had been removed from the disability roll as recovered.[31] In general, treatment was relatively superficial, and consisted of reassurance, suggestion, and sedatives; when one considers the "secondary gain" of disability payments, these patients might be said to have improved in spite of receiving reinforcement for continuing to show symptoms.

A Study of 25 Hystericals

The cases of No. and Irene reported by Janet warn us that, although the prognosis for a single attack is good, the likelihood of a recurrence is strong. Guze and Perley (1963) followed their cases after their discharge for periods ranging from six to eight years. The average age at the time of first diagnosis was 40, and their illnesses had existed for some time before they found their way to this clinic, nine reporting illnesses that had begun before age 20. Two of the 25 seemed improved at the time of the final study, but were not symptom-free. Only one of the 25 regarded herself as well, finally, but the clinician who studied this case discovered that she was anxiously trying to conceal her former illnesses from a third husband, so this single "recovery" was listed as doubtful. The two improved cases had not been hospitalized in the follow-up period. The rest of the group had been in and out of hospital with a total of 53 hospitalizations for the 23

---

[31]In this study the criterion for recovery involved a return to work for at least a five-year period, no further serious complaints, and a successful social adjustment. This, too, was an undifferentiated group of neurotic disorders, and was not classified in any way according to severity, except that in each case the physician certified that disability payments were warranted.

TABLE 8. *Summary of Reports of the Results of Psychotherapy.* (From Eysenck 1952.)

Cases Reported by	Number of Cases	Cured or Much Improved	Improved	Slightly Improved	Not Improved; Died; Left Treatment	Per Cent Cured, Much Improved, or Improved
Psychoanalytic therapists:						
Fenichel	484	104	84	99	197	39%
Kessel and Hyman	34	16	5	4	9	62
Jones	59	20	8	28	3	47
Alexander	141	28	42	23	48	50
Knight	42	8	20	7	7	67
All cases	760	335			425	44
Other therapists:						
Huddleson	200	19	74	80	27	46
Matz	775	10	310	310	145	41
Maudsley Hospital Report (1931)	1,721	288	900	533		69
Maudsley Hospital Report (1935)	1,711	371	765	575		64
Neustatter	46	9	14	8	15	50
Luff and Garrod	500	140	135	26	199	55
Luff and Garrod	210	38	84	54	34	68
Ross	1,089	547	306	236		77
Yaskin	100	29	29	42		58
Curran	83	51		32		61
Masserman and Carmichael	50	7	20	5	18	54
Carmichael and Masserman	77	16	25	14	22	53
Schilder	35	11	11	6	7	63
Hamilton and Wall	100	32	34	17	32	66
Hamilton *et al.*	100	48	5	17	32	51
Landis	119	40	47	32		73
Institute Med. Psychol.	270	58	132	55	25	70
Wilder	54	3	24	16	11	50
Miles *et al.*	53	13	18	13	9	58
All cases	7,293	4,661		2,632		64%

women.[32] They had received electroshock, surgery, psychotherapy, osteopathy, and chiropractic treatment for their disabilities during this period, but had been, in general, resistant to psychotherapy as they had met it; the physicians report that their experiences had made them doubtful of its value. Only five had actually been seen for extended psychotherapeutic interviews, and of these, four had been in psychotherapy for several months. The symptoms this group had brought to their physicians included headache and other pains, vomiting, menstrual disorders, and sexual and marital difficulties. Ten of the 25 had been divorced by the time of the follow-up.

The sample of cases selected by Guze and Perley had satisfied several severe criteria, which eliminated single-symptom cases, such as aphonia, paralysis, anesthesia, trance states, amnesia, unexplained blindness, diplopia, and urinary retention; such cases are more responsive to treatment, although they, too, may have a persisting and underlying disease process or may reveal, later, latent schizophrenia, drug addiction, alcoholism, or sociopathic personality. By their criteria, which selected long-standing cases, multiple symptoms, repeated hospitalization, and disturbed functioning of several bodily systems, they selected, in all probability, a severe form of the disorder.[33]

A Study at Johns Hopkins Hospital

In a recent summary of cases seen at Johns Hopkins Hospital, Ziegler, Imboden, and Meyer (1960) have studied the records of 134 cases diagnosed as hysteria during a four-year period. The patients were classified into four categories: (1) those showing the classical losses of function (amnesias, anesthesias, paralysis, aboulia) described by Charcot and Janet before the turn of the century, when they constituted about 8 per cent of the patients seen on the Salpêtrière neuropsychiatric service; (2) a form of *grande hystérie* in which attacks are somewhat similar to those seen in epileptics, a form that has grown increasingly rare; (3) a third form that simulates *myasthenia gravis;*[34] and (4) forms of hysterical pain (found in 75 of the 134 cases). In a case in the first group, a 34-year-old woman showed

---

[32]It is noteworthy that all cases followed were women. Guze and Perley, in drawing up their criteria for diagnosis, quote Purtell, Robins, and Cohen (1953) as believing that the syndrome occurs primarily, if not exclusively, in women. In spite of the long series of clinicians who have struggled to correct the notion of the Egyptians and the Greeks, and who have identified male hystericals, there seems to be a stubborn conviction that haunts the corridors of clinics, the stereotype of "the hysterical woman."

[33]Their comments on the meager results of psychotherapy in these cases find an echo from the other side of the Atlantic. Ey, Bernard, and Brisset (1963, p. 411) note that "the hysterical patient is a poor candidate for psychoanalysis," but add, "analysis is the only therapy capable of bringing about a cure." The best candidates, they point out, are the young, the intelligent, and those strongly motivated to correct their personality difficulties. The others, stubbornly fixated in the hysterical pattern, not very interested in getting rid of their symptoms, or reluctant to give up secondary gains, are not promising material for any form of psychotherapy.

[34]Myasthenia gravis, described as a "bulbar palsy without visible anatomical changes" and as a disease of unknown origin, is more frequent in females than in males, and is obscure enough to make a good candidate for "hysterical simulation." The fatigability of the skeletal muscles and the weakness in voluntary movements makes the aboulia of hysteria a "functional twin."

paralysis in all four extremities and anesthesia from the neck down. She deceived her physician so well that he—fearing an ascending paralysis that might involve the respiratory center at any moment—performed a tracheotomy in the accident room without anesthetic. All of this patient's symptoms had disappeared by the end of the next day.

The myasthenia gravis group, restudied after first being diagnosed as having some "organic" disease, were placed on a new drug dosage and reclassified as psychoneurotic; the symptoms raised the question of a possible collaboration between physician and patient that had unwittingly created symptoms and the incorrect diagnosis. One of these patients, closely studied, found that her new diagnosis was not especially helpful: she could not afford psychotherapy; she admitted that she was "too bitchy and impossible at home"; and her history showed that she had been counted an unstable child who had learned to avoid doing whatever was difficult or unpleasant by the use of a combination of "cuteness and histrionics."

Reviewing the results of such therapy as could be applied, Ziegler and his associates were unable to report any impressive therapeutic success. Most of the cases had been discovered on the medical wards, convinced that they had bona fide organic illnesses and preferring it that way. One bright farm wife chided her physician, "My back pain is immotional, not emotional," when he tried to formulate a psychodynamic explanation for her conversion hysteria. The psychological symptoms which they experienced (such as anxiety or depression) were readily interpreted by the patient as a reaction to their *real* illness. In general they were reluctant to look on their symptoms as being psychological in nature; nor did they wish to be referred to psychiatrists or transferred to that wing of the hospital. A few exceptions who did accept treatment by a psychotherapist responded fairly well. Perhaps, these physicians argue, these patients might be placed on the convalescent wards of a hospital, where surgical patients are recovering from severe operations. On such wards there is typically a good morale and an eager interest in returning to active life. With a minimum of psychotherapy for the hystericals, perhaps some of this high morale of the other patients might rub off; and modest improvements might open the way for more intensive psychotherapy.

In the list as a whole there were 82 per cent females and 18 per cent males, a ratio that has recurred in clinical reports over the last hundred years. There are still a few who repeat the ancient dictum of the Greeks that it is impossible for a male to have hysteria; and these feel a certain surprise at finding males afflicted with the disorder. Such a prejudice makes these clinicians look for a special cause at work in the males.[35]

---

[35]For example, Robins, Purtell, and Cohen (1952) concluded from their studies that hysteria is not found in the male except in a compensation setting, where the secondary gains are obvious. However, Margaret Gildea, who led the discussion of the Ziegler paper and who expressed a particular interest in the males in the series, added that, from her experience, the motivation in such cases is quite similar to that found in female patients: conflicts in the home, difficulties with a wife, business worries, and so on.

Ziegler and his associates repeat the common judgment that the cruder forms of simulated illness are found in patients from comparatively backward rural areas, but they note that their cases include two physicians, two nurses, and two secretaries employed by neurologists. Although most of the simulations were described as crude, and easily detected by the experienced physician, their own records include cases that do not fit this description. Aside from the paralysis which led the physician to perform a tracheotomy (a "sophisticated error" on his part), one neurologist's secretary produced symptoms normally associated with a cyst of the third ventricle, and the other secretary "imitated" multiple sclerosis. Since there is a fairly widespread, even if superficial, medical sophistication (what with reports of medical discoveries appearing in the illustrated weeklies), the number who possess the kind of half-knowledge that can deceive both themselves and some physicians would seem to have increased. Should the unwary physician use diagnostic procedures which would help these suggestible patients become good collaborators, there may be many more cases than are reported: the hysterical patient who is put to bed for two years would be "out of sight and out of mind" as far as the records of contemporary hysteria are concerned. The 134 cases turned up on the wards of Johns Hopkins Hospital may testify to a greater sophistication and diagnostic acumen in that center of psychiatric pioneering.

One new emphasis appears in the Ziegler report. The 75 cases of the series who reported pain as a prominent symptom represent a trend different from the older Salpêtrière series, where there were few cases with severe hysterical pain. Pain proves that "something is wrong," and both in popular understanding and in the minds of many physicians it is likely to suggest something organic (as when a pain in the right shoulder is diagnosed as a "referred pain" of visceral origin). The bulk of these 75 cases chose to believe this. The pain marks such a patient as an impaired person; it provides a real (i.e., organic) excuse for nonfeasance; and it is an effectively disguised appeal for help that is likely to produce the desired effect, perhaps more so than some mute anesthesia.

EPILOG

Hysteria, as a concept, may be on the way out. The problems once covered by the rubric will remain, nonetheless, to plague the newer theorists who handle those constellations of symptoms into which the old symptoms have been placed. There are enough contradictions in the facts already discovered, enough divergence in therapies and claims of ability to modify the symptoms, to occupy us for decades to come.

One interesting possibility is suggested by Hollingshead and Redlich (1958), who have studied the relationship between diagnostic trends and social class. Their findings suggest that a case of hysteria arising in a member of the lower fifth of our stratified society would more likely be diagnosed as psychotic (perhaps as borderline schizophrenia) than a case originating in our highest stratum, where the patient will be treated by a private physician, will likely be called a severely disturbed personality with a severe neurosis, and will be given the extended psychoanalytic therapy that Freud and Breuer first developed with Bertha Pappenheim. Janet's Achille with his demons, coming from a backward rural area, would likely be given some form of chemotherapy or (two decades ago) a prefrontal lobotomy. The "culturally deprived" patient is likely to get such "rough and ready" treatment if his therapist is convinced that the "classic" form of hysteria is a "peasant illness" or a pattern confined to the hinterland, where "hexing" and other superstitions prevail.

Angyal, Fromm, and Horney, among the neo-Freudians, have stressed alienation from the self. When the person's actions indicate a consistent policy that could be phrased as "I will be as you desire me," the center of his striving may be too remote from his own needs. True, among his needs is the need for affection, for approval, but in striving to fill this need, he becomes alienated from other important ones, which are left frustrated, unexpressed, unfulfilled. For the sensitive, the insecure, those who have felt inadequate and rebuffed from the start, the need for affection and approval forces the creation of a protective outer shell. At the same time, not only is this outer shell robbed of the support of the inhibited needs, but the latter offer a continuing threat to the security and peace of mind of the person. Such a formulation, it must be noted, creates a very extensive conceptual net, since civilization itself is "against nature," at least cruder forms of nature. Both civilized man and the neurotic have fantasies about the perfect past that "might have been," when self-acceptance, acceptance by others, and full and free expression of all impulses were simultaneously possible.

This compulsion to "be one's true self," rather than to accept the perfection (or corruption) others desire, is an experience that can occur in any culture. Frequently the individual (whether neurotic or normal) takes the position that it is society, or those in authority, or, as in the case of Luther, the ecclesiastical authorities, that are corrupt and unjust. The "gap" need not be always between a good nature and a bad society, although from the days of Rousseau the *good natural man* has been set in opposition to the *bad artificial demands for conformity* from a society. Unshaped human nature (if we could find any of it) would be just so much raw material, as the reflexes of an infant are so much "stuff" to be socialized and shaped into a personality (with appropriate defenses against the shapers). It is neither good nor bad, as the raw clay, which is to be shaped first into bricks and then into buildings, is neither good nor bad architecture. The civilization which shapes these raw materials may defeat itself, if it produces creatures so seriously in conflict with themselves as to be self-destructive and destructive of the stability of civilization itself. In this instance, the shapers would be against nature. But only the foolish believe that "what comes naturally" is bound to be both good and fit to live with.

The neo-Freudians are correct at least to this extent: striving for any form of perfection, if extreme, is bound to generate its own set of lagging impulses and organic protests. The quarter-miler, or a Schumann at the practice keyboard, can damage heart or hand irreparably, driving the very tissues until they break. Each attempt at "perfection" creates its own protests, its own "unconscious," and the yearning for its opposite, its own form of regression. Thus, whatever breaks up a particular pattern of perfection may very well reveal what has remained hidden during its dominance, its success.

Neo-Pavlovian studies have been useful in demonstrating the extent to which symptoms can be manipulated (established and extinguished) even without the participation of the man as a whole, and without or in spite of the conscious intent of the individual. This type of simplification should make us reexamine some of our concepts, such as unconscious motivation, repression, early infantile fantasies, that plague psychoanalytic formulations, as well as other types of ad hoc hypotheses never tested operationally (lowered psychological tension, suggestion, nervous fatigue).

Some of the findings have had a serious impact on our concept of the rational man. Just as Freud showed the neurotic to be helpless in managing his instinctual (and repressed infantile) impulses, Pavlov's followers have shown that human subjects can be conditioned in spite of their intention to the contrary and can persist in fixations in spite of insight. More radical in some respects than the Freudian emphasis, these Pavlovian studies show that even the subject who knows better, who understands the procedures, who can verbalize his brief laboratory history, cannot suddenly command his heart to slow down, his postural tensions to relax, his sleeping-waking rhythms to resume their normal cycle. But the studies have also shown that such a man can accomplish these ends indirectly, by following through on the appropriate reinforcement routines, and by performing appropriate actions in a free field. When no amount of verbal explanation or exhortation or compassionate support or helpful chemotherapy will do the task, the correct actions can still accomplish the objectives.

Because of these studies we have been forced to take another look at our still somewhat naive faith in the power of the word, not to discard it, but to use it in a way that will do the most good. The conscious man has a role, and words are still our most precious tools. The limitations that its organic embeddedness impose on the ego and the new type of usage of these tools still call for patient and persistent study. Properly extended and controlled, these studies will lead us back to a fresh look at both the man as a whole and at his mechanisms. We shall discover a fresh "insight into insight" and a new respect for those humbler mechanisms that the ego has to learn to manage.

After describing the persistent controversy between the behavioristic, or "Action," and the analytic, or "Insight," schools of psychotherapy, Perry London (1964, p. 173) concludes with this comment on psychotherapists in general: "As their ability to control and manipulate behavior improves, the moral character of their enterprise will become more visible, and more embarrassing. But at the same time, their knowledge of man should also improve, and their moral stand thus become more defensible."

Chapter 7 • Psychosomatic Disorders

The idea of psychosomatic illness is not new. Its roots can be found in Hippocrates, Aristotle, and Galen. During the history of psychotherapy it had often been noticed that many bodily conditions could be influenced by suggestion. Many a general practitioner had come to say "The trouble with *this* patient is in his head." For generations, however, the emphasis had been on the other side: medical progress had come from the application of anatomical and physiological knowledge, and biochemistry had made so many advances that medical answers were increasingly sought in terms of the functioning of cells and part-processes. So many part-processes had been farmed out to those who pursue laboratory studies on animals that the specialists had come to look for part-answers, forgetting the questions that have to do with the man as a whole. Holistic medicine was in poor repute; consideration of "mental states" smacked of Christian Science or "medical moralization," and scientifically trained physicians wanted tests, measures, X-rays, laboratory reports. They seemed to feel that if they could keep the processes running smoothly down among the cells, the self-regulator up in the cranium could be left to choose what he wished, or to seek a spiritual advisor if his choices got him into trouble. The man as a whole was not a medical problem.

The group that founded the *Journal of Psychosomatic Medicine* in 1939 felt that this process had gone too far, even to the point where it was defeating medicine itself. A second group, centering in the Washington School of Psychiatry and the William Alanson White Psychiatric Foundation, which published a journal of interpersonal relations directed toward psychiatrists, joined in this medical reformation. Not only the whole man, but the man among his fellows, the man in society, were to be considered when physicians studied the sources of anxieties and frustrations, and study them they must, for these emotions penetrate the tissues and disorganize the vital functions.

Before the decade was out, these innovators were joined by the existentialists, who suggested that "what happens down among the cells" ought to be related to "crises in identity" and to cosmic questions of being and nonbeing. The

Journal of Existential Psychiatry, founded in 1960, invited practitioners to become philosophers, and made some wish that holistic teachings could be included in the medical curriculum. John Hunter, concerned about his heart, had resignedly pointed out, in 1790, "My life is at the mercy of any damned rascal who chooses to annoy me" (Wolff 1953, p. 92). Now bits of common sense that medical practitioners had always understood were about to be systematized, and even organized into a philosophy of mind-body relationships. Weiss and English (1943) announced that, in their opinion, a third of the patients who consult general practitioners or specialists in internal medicine belong in the "psychosomatic group" whose disordered functions are either caused or aggravated by emotional conflicts that arise as the whole man struggles to adjust to his society.[1]

When fully developed, the programs of these groups threatened an invasion of the general medical wards of our hospitals by men trained in taking a psychological history, in assessing interpersonal relations, in assisting a patient to solve his economic problems or some crisis in identity. It began to look as though medical schools would have to train young physicians in psychological, psychoanalytic, sociological, and even philosophical matters which had previously been considered outside the province of *scientific* medicine, for, should the new view prevail, the new role of the man at the bedside would include the task of serving as a spiritual guide, or at least a guide who could help the patient understand problems of adjustment about which he had been confused or imperfectly conscious, and which he could not correct without expert assistance. He needed something more and other than medication or surgery. Many of the founders of this medical reformation were psychoanalytically oriented, and believed that nothing short of analytic procedures could provide the "microscope of the mind" that would lay bare the psychodynamics and emotional conflicts that were expressed in the physiological disarray that constituted these functional diseases.

The founders of this reform movement found it necessary to take time out to give their new emphasis an acceptable underpinning, a kind of philosophical rationalization, for they were raising, in new form to be sure, a very old problem. The mind-body problem is an ancient stumbling block for all of us, and for psychologists in particular; its "solution" usually stirs up more academic dust than it succeeds in settling. At one time, when religious interests were involved and the problem of the detachable soul (with immortal life) seemed threatened by materialistic science, the issue was hotly debated. The question also troubled meticulous persons who did not want any nonmaterial process to invade or disrupt a series of physical events. How could it, when matter cannot be created or destroyed, nor physical laws abrogated by some spiritual force? A simple example and a practical problem can suggest the gist of what this new school was working toward, better than some series of extended

---

[1] A few enthusiasts put the figure higher, asserting that two out of three who enter the doctor's office have problems that are basically psychological.

quotations from these physicians, who, after all, are not trained philosophers.

A 26-year-old male complaining of vomiting and epigastric pain that had recurred during a four-year period and had increased in severity during recent months, with daily nausea and vomiting, was studied in a San Francisco clinic by W. B. Faulkner (1940), who reported:

"I encountered the most marked esophageal spasm I have ever seen. None of the lumen was open and the spasm involved the entire esophagus. No portion of the esophagus escaped, but the region of the inferior constrictor of the pharynx and the cardiac end showed the most extreme degree of constriction.

"Ordinarily the instrument can be slid either up or down the esophagus with great ease but, in this instance, at each point throughout its entire length, the esophagus clamped down so hard upon the esophagoscope that the procedure was a slow, difficult process, requiring considerable force to pass from the cervical to the cardiac end. Attempts at withdrawal were even more difficult than the introduction of the instrument. The esophageal muscles clasped the instrument tightly and would not let go. The withdrawal of the esophagoscope even as little as one cm. demanded considerable strength.

"I had known in advance that this patient was extremely nervous and apprehensive, and that his home and economic environment had caused a tremendous emotional strain; but I did not see how this knowledge could in any way facilitate the esophagoscopic examination and treatment.

"As the operative difficulties increased it occurred to me that here was an opportunity to determine whether the degree of esophageal spasm could be altered in any respect by the patient's mental outlook. Accordingly, while still looking down the esophagoscope, I suggested to the patient that it was very probable that we could arrange work for him which would bring social and economic security. To my utter amazement the spasm relaxed immediately and the esophagus opened to normal size.

"It was very hard to believe that the suggestion of a pleasant environment alone could bring about this prompt favorable change. Was it not more likely that the relaxation was a mere coincidence?

"To test this point, I then asked how he would like to think of a future with even greater poverty and insecurity than that in which he was now living. And promptly therewith, the spasm returned. I repeated this experiment several times and noted alternating spasm and relaxation, depending upon the emotional and functional response to the environment pictured."

Simply stated, a man's life-situation can tense the muscles of his esophagus. Equally simply, even the mere discussion of a changed way of life can release the pathological tension.

The mind-body relationship is a two-way street: the changes down among the cells, which in turn are traceable to bad dietary habits, smoking, or addiction to drugs, can alter a man's view of himself, his life-plans, his way of coping with difficulties. The pure psychophysical parallelism of the psychology laboratory at the turn of the century has to be broken in practice, as a series of mind-body problems is tackled either through the manipulation of the tissues or through the treatment of the man as a whole; if we call the latter type of manipulation mental, and the other physical (or bodily), then mind influences body and the body's conditions alter mental states, whatever metaphysical statements are contructed to make this comprehensible.[2]

The persistent belief dominating most of these new studies assumed that psychological causes underlie much physical disease, and that pathological bodily processes can be altered by changing the mental state of a patient, or by restructuring his personality, or by altering his relationship with his human milieu. Playing a central role in their writing and research was a group of changes that physiologists, following Cannon, had been describing as "the bodily changes in emotion." While one group set out to identify the groups of cells in the rhinencephalon that made up the "center" for rage, a second sought to give precision to the peripheral physiological changes in smooth and striped muscles and in the endocrine glands, and a third listened to the free associations of patients who experienced such rage or hostility, and guided the patients through interviews in search of a psychological understanding of the phenomena. By "stress interviews" these research workers sought to identify "hot topics" capable of sending up the blood pressure, altering blood sugar, constricting the small blood vessels in the hands, making the stomach wall flush (or blanch), opening the bronchioles of the asthmatic patient, and so on.

In one patient, a man with a gastric fistula, one observer was able to watch the development of an ulcer, inspect the gastric mucosa during an hour when the subject was filled with resentment, measure the concentration of HCl in his gastric secretions, and take introspective reports and assess the patient's life-situation at the same time (Wolf and Wolff 1943). Other research workers (Mahl and Karpe 1953) have run parallel series of observations, so that the same interview could produce assessments of anxiety (or psychological status) made by a psychiatrist and observations by a psychologist with physiological interests who used a system of recording physical and physiological measurements.

In an earlier day, when philosophers were debating whether the soul was located in the brain or in the heart, Hippocrates chose the hollow ventricles of the former, while Aristotle held out stoutly for the latter. Its motion could be felt, he noted, in pleasure, fear, and pain. He thought, further, that its central position, with ducts leading in and out of the organ, marked it as a suitably located controlling center. Time and tradition have worked against Aristotle: the *psyche* has been promoted to the brain, and, barring the few who still follow James, it is the brain that is thought to be the "seat of the emotions," a center where emotions are first felt and from which the autonomic outflow is regulated. The final motions in the tissues and glands are now identified in psychosomatic research that has examined every bodily part: from the electroencephalogram of the cortex, down to pancreas, kidneys, heart, bronchioles, skin capillaries, stomach, and colon.

Our language still retains the imprint of an older dualism. Wolf and Wolff

---

[2]A *monism* in which the single mind-body entity can be approached from two sides, and "manipulated" from either, is one way of getting around the problem. In this view, the divergent methods of study have fractionated the unity into seemingly separate kinds of phenomena.

look on the bodily changes as *expressions* of their subject's resentment (when he was falsely accused of shirking his responsibilities in the laboratory of the Cornell Medical School, where he was employed), and his anger, his red face, and his "blushing" stomach mucosa were the final terms in a chain of responses initiated in the first place by a change in his life-situation. When such stresses become chronic, the steady stream of autonomic innervation that spreads down from the hypothalamus to the tissues can disrupt normal digestive sequences, increase acidity, and finally produce a literal "digestion" of a portion of the stomach wall. The pitting of the mucosa can be seen on the X-ray photograph: the chronic emotional tension has finally etched its signature in the tissues.

THE AUTONOMIC NERVOUS SYSTEM AND THE EMOTIONS

The tubes and pouches of the alimentary canal, the smooth-muscle walls of the blood vessels and the heart, and the secretory cells of the duct and ductless glands are all innervated by a system of nerve fibers originating in the two chains of ganglia that lie in front of the spinal cord (see Fig. 6). Preganglionic fibers, in turn activated from head ganglia that lie in the rhinencephalon, supply these ganglion relays. Two divisions of this last relay system, the parasympathetic and sympathetic, distribute impulses to smooth muscles and glands. The parasympathetic is composed, in turn, of two divisions: a cranial outflow that supplies the middle and upper segments of trunk and head; and a sacral outflow that supplies colon, bladder, rectum, and genitals. Terminating in a single organ such as the heart, the two branches of autonomic fibers can control its action, one set of fibers (sympathetic, in this case) accelerating the rate of its beat and the force of its contractions, and the other slowing its rate and cutting down the force of its stroke. The excitation of the vagus nerve (one of the subdivisions of the cranial system) can increase gastric secretions, slow the heart, and stimulate the secretory cells of the pancreas to pour forth more insulin. The branch of the sympathetic that reaches these same organs has opposite effects. Sometimes a gland's activity is controlled indirectly, by the contraction of smooth muscles in the walls of the blood vessels that supply the secretory cells. Thus, either directly or indirectly, the smooth muscles and glands are under dual control, regulated from the rhinencephalon, and are excited or inhibited, accelerated or retarded, according to the "calls" that are made on this center. In turn, the rhinencephalon sends impulses upward to the cerebral cortex and receives impulses in return, so that this "automatic regulation system" becomes both "driver" and "driven": the viscera poke up the projicient system to care for bodily needs, and the system as a whole calls on the viscera to support its projects.

These autonomic distribution systems tend to react en masse. The crack of the twig just outside the circle of light cast by our campfire sets the autonomic overflow to work, from the smooth muscles at the roots of our hair follicles in our scalp to the arterioles in our feet. There are glandular, respiratory, and circulatory changes that are set in motion; and we could not produce them

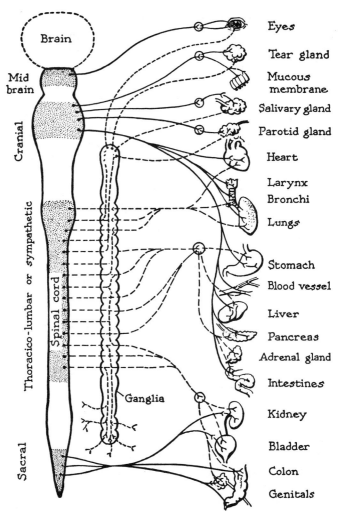

FIGURE 6. SCHEMATIC DIAGRAM OF THE AUTONOMIC NERVOUS SYSTEM. From the spinal cord (at left) two sets of fibers carry impulses to the organs: the *sympathetic fibers* (dotted lines) which inhibit salivation, accelerate the heart, and so on; and the *parasympathetic* system (solid lines) which constricts the pupil, stimulates gastric activity, slows the heart, and so on. (Reprinted by permission of Appleton-Century-Crofts, publishers of Walter B. Cannon, *Bodily Changes in Pain, Hunger, Fear, and Rage* [1920], in which the original figure appeared, p. 25; and of Harcourt, Brace & World, Inc., publishers of L. E. Cole, *Human Behavior* [1953], in which this adaptation appeared, p. 249.)

voluntarily if we tried. Digestive secretions and the churning movements of the intestinal walls are checked; respiration and heart rates are increased. From head to toe the alerting signal puts us on a war footing. It all occurs reflexly. The heart pounds. We do not voluntarily accelerate it, nor could we slow it by saying, "Be still, my heart." The only control open to us is to get up, investigate, and take care of whatever is prowling about the camp. There are other changes, such as those appropriate to postprandial relaxation, which favor digestion, assimilation, and repair; here the parasympathetic system is in ascendance. Cannon (1929) once described the sympathetic (commonly active in pain, fear, rage, and lust) and parasympathetic systems as like the loud and soft pedals of the piano, the former modulating the whole keyboard at once, while the cranial and sacral systems act as separate banks of keys. Although its range is limited, the vagus will alter the state of affairs in heart, pancreas, pupil, and bronchi.

These autonomic changes are so perceptibly present in our emotional states that many psychologists have been tempted to measure them, as a way of calibrating the intensity of these otherwise elusive mental states. The galvanic skin reflex, for example, can detect changes in the action of the sweat glands that cannot be reported introspectively. Small or large, with or without awareness of an emotional quality to the experience, these indicators can betray what might be called a "subthreshold" (or an unconscious) emotion. A list of stimulus words can be read to a subject, one at a time; as a galvanometer records the slight changes in electrical resistance of the skin surface, the words that produce the reverberations in the autonomic system can be identified. Some of the recorded disturbances may puzzle the subject as much as they do the experimenter, for if the stimuli trigger an "emotional" reverberation, it is via the trace of some remote experience that he cannot identify, evoked through some ramifying train of associations that he has not consciously elaborated. Sometimes an operator may be convinced that the subject knows full well what the sources of the changes are, but does not choose to tell.[3]

We need to be wary of identifying the bodily reverberation with an emotion, or of making the varieties of autonomic reaction the basis of classifying human affective *experiences* or emotional *behavior*. This was the error of James, who wanted to describe human emotions as the way we feel these bodily reverberations when some blow sets the tissue changes in motion. He argued that the purring cat, the setting hen, the moorhen frightened into diving by a barking terrier are set into characteristic patterns of reverberation as they react "instinctively" in appropriate fashion. If the hen looks on the clutch of eggs as a "never to be too much sat upon object," is she not a kin, even if a remote one, to the mother who looks upon her newborn son with overflowing love; is not the conscious state the way the body feels when it reverberates to significant cues or blows? James seemed to be thinking of an upward reflection from the peripheral changes reflexly induced and then relayed to the "little

---

[3]In the case of the suspected criminal, when the GSR is used as a part of a "lie-detecting" technique, the emotion is clear enough to the subject, but suppressed. In the medical student (Syz 1926) who *reported* an emotion in response to the word "mother" (while the galvanometer recorded a very small change) and who *denied* any emotion in response to the word "prostitute" (which evoked large GSRs), the verbal reports seem to be more related to a convention than to the affective state itself. The myth of motherhood, on the one hand, and the notion of how a young man who has "been around" should bear himself, on the other, may alter communication and conscious attitudes more than they affect the actual autonomic reverberation. The guest who insists that he is having a wonderful time may fool his hostess, and sometimes himself. The autonomic system has a stubborn quality, and blurts out what the conscious man conceals.

man upstairs," the perceiver. Perhaps James's all too vivid memory of a day in the room upstairs, when depression struck him and he felt the bodily changes occur as though he had been struck a blow, led him to want to put the peripheral tissue changes first, the feelings and emotions last.[4]

Cannon attempted to correct James by showing that experimental animals whose "bodily reverberation" had been grossly altered by the excision of the chain of sympathetic ganglia, continued to claw, bite, hiss, and otherwise act out their "emotions," even when changes in gastric secretion, erection of tail hairs, and other sympathetically innervated actions no longer occurred in their customary fashion. In effect, this argument puts the emotions, so central to psychosomatic theory, back in the class of reactions of the organism as a whole: they were as much an affair of striped muscles, attitudes, movements in the making, verbal retorts (or pleas), and gestures, as they were of gastric secretions, pounding heart, adrenal hormones. Perhaps Cannon's studies did little to determine just where in the cycle of changes consciousness should be placed (before, after, or in parallel with bodily actions, or as another "aspect" of these same changes), but at least they remind us that it is the man who *lives his emotions,* the whole man in action that we must consider. No study of the peripheral structures alone, as organs, nor of an observer upstairs (who, like a helpless prisoner, can only receive reports of what is happening in the effectors) will be an adequate method of investigating emotional behavior. Certainly Cannon showed that an emotion is not an autonomic "it" that operates mechanically, apart from the rest of the system.

Sympathicotonia and Vagotonia

This first rough draft of autonomic functioning needs to be revised and complicated. For example, although a "standard man" in resting condition would show a steady state in which sympathetic and parasympathetic branches are in balance, there are in fact some 8 per cent (according to Losse *et al.* 1956) who show a chronic sympathetic dominance. These *sympathicotonics* (with dry mouth, cold extremities, accelerated heart, low acid content of the stomach) are easily aroused to those glandular-visceral expressions of sympathetic activity, as though they carried a smoldering hostility or a latent anxiety that had readied the organs for minimal triggering stimuli, tuning the sympathetic system in advance. There is another 8 per cent who are *vagotonics.* These subjects are slow to respond with a sympathetic pattern; when the sympathetic is briefly aroused by stress, they tend to swing back toward the chronic state of parasympathetic dominance, as though a weak sympathetic component was easily fatigued, or as though some neurohumoral or homeostatic imbalance tended to restore the chronic condition. In such persons the very stress that first checked pancreas and gastric secretions and accelerated the heart now ends in producing high acidity, hypoglycaemia, excessive fatigue,

---

[4]"My theory," James (1890, II, 449) wrote, "is that *the bodily changes follow directly the perception of the exciting fact, and that our feeling of the same changes as they occur is the emotion.*"

and hyperinsulinism. Alexander, who frequently used the term "vegetative retreat" to describe his exhausted patient with an ulcer, fatigue, and low blood sugar, could have used this concept of Losse and his associates, at least to name the constitutional predisposition. (See also Richter 1957.)

The physiologist (Gellhorn 1963, pp. 244-53) tends to look on these two extremes of the distribution curve as genetically different from those standard types composing the middle 84 per cent of the sample. He notes that when one of a pair of identical twins is a sympathicotonic, his twin tends to be one also, whereas fraternal twins are more likely to show dissimilarities. Sheldon, Stevens, and Tucker (1940) believe vagotonia tends to appear in ectomorphs (who are more prone to develop ulcers), whereas the short, heavy endomorphs are more likely to be sympathicotonics.

Gellhorn also shows that the autonomic can be tuned (either by stimuli or by drugs that affect one branch of the autonomic more than another), and that such tuning will create a sensitivity to new stimuli, even if its existence is not revealed by any presently measurable elevation or lowering of activity in the peripheral organs that the autonomic system supplies. With sufficient tuning, the autonomic response to standard stimuli can be reversed, so that stressful stimuli produce parasympathetic reactions instead of the usual sympathetic ones. In addition, after prolonged sympathetic action a "homeostatic balancing" follows: the parasympathetic will then be hyperexcitable and hyperactive in the resting intervals. (It is possible that the high acid secretion in ulcer patients during their sleep may represent such a compensatory swing.)

In addition to such physiological tuning, there is such a thing as "emotional tuning." The depressed patient who has hitherto reacted to stress interviews, in which there was a discussion of an intolerable life-situation, by an angry outburst ("I would like to strike him with the frying pan. There are times when I could cheerfully kill him"), will, on another day, verbalize her helpless and hopeless feeling. Defeated, lonely, feeling there is nothing she can do about her situation, she expresses her emotions by tears, and she betrays her defeat at her fingertips. A loss of tone in the minute blood-vessel walls permits a dilation of the small blood vessels, and the formerly blanched skin grows cyanotic, gorged with blood (see Graham 1955).

Duncan, Stevenson, and Wolff (1951) found that when their cardiac patients were experiencing despair and discouragement and were given a standard exercise test, the effort produced a cardiac *hypoactivity*, with heart rate and blood-volume flow below normal instead of the increases found in other moods. Such a "loading" of the autonomic system by a chronic emotional condition was found to exist *without measurable changes* in the cardiovascular levels in the resting states, whereas the effects appeared as an "exercise in-tolerance" the moment effort was required. These patients added complaints of dyspnea, palpitation, weakness, and discomfort to the atypical measured changes in heart rate and output. Security, relaxation, resentment, despair could be revealed as states of autonomic tuning, even when their existence could not be revealed by current recording techniques.

These still somewhat pervasive and general tunings of the autonomic system must be complicated still further. There are, it seems, "nose reactors," "stomach reactors," "pulse reactors," as though the conditions within a particular organ make it momentarily resonant to the stress-induced autonomic outflow, or as though because of some genetically determined vulnerability it is regularly the first to "speak," the organ most likely to show pathology under extreme and chronic stress.

One is reminded of the French typologists of World War I who divided their officers' training candidates into abdominal, respiratory, muscular, and nervous types, distributing the men they examined to those branches of the service where their particular capacities would be most useful. The muscular, for example, would not be as phlegmatic as the abdominal types, nor as excitable as the respiratory, and were believed to be better adapted to tasks which called for stamina and patient persistence. The "nervous type" would contain the intellectuals, the versatile and adaptable ones who could quickly summon reserve powers in emergencies. Now we seem about to identify organ systems and physiological functions as "types."

The Attitude Theory

It is when we come to explain the differences between the "nose reactors" and the "stomach reactors" that we run into differences of opinion. It is a matter of *attitude,* suggest Grace and Graham (1952), an attitude that is moreover near the surface and capable of being verbalized. An attitude, for these investigators, involves a feeling about what is being done to the patient, about the patient's position in a field, about what action he must take. The patient with urticaria (hives), these investigators report, sees himself as being mistreated; he is the target of things said and done; he is preoccupied with what is happening to him, not with retaliation or with finding a solution. Such statements as: "They did a lot of things to me and I couldn't do anything about it. I was taking a beating. My mother was hammering on me. The boss cracked the whip on me. My fiancée knocked me down and walked all over me. But what could I do?" were reported spontaneously. There was no attempt to utilize dreams or to probe deeply (through free-association techniques) into underlying affective positions.

In the case of urticaria, the clinicians seem to be utilizing a form of "psycho-analogy" to explain the relationship between attitude and symptom, for they point out that an abrupt blow to the skin surface of the urticaria patient will raise a welt and produce changes in the tonus of blood-vessel walls. These changes are direct, reflexive. They also appear in corresponding areas on the opposite side that has not been struck, rather like the flushing of the skin in the left hand when the right hand is plunged into warm water. Because reactions of this type can be conditioned (see Menzies 1937, 1941), it is not too difficult to extend the simple reflex to "psychological blows" (my mother was hammering on me): what a physical punishment did originally, the "conditioned stimuli" now do.

Grace and Graham have identified characteristic attitudes shown by patients who suffer from psychosomatic disorders, with each disorder characterized by a specific attitude (see Table 9).

The Complexity of Emotional Patterns

Later investigations have raised questions that throw doubt on any simple form of the attitude theory. Attitudes, freely verbalized and resembling those found in the patients Grace and Graham studied, may exist without any corresponding autonomic changes (Graham *et al.* 1962). We could dismiss these exceptions as due to the subthreshold intensity of the attitudes or to high constitutional stress tolerances, if it were not for other experimental findings still more puzzling. Gottlieb, Gleser, and Gottschalk (1967), for example, induced the "Raynaud's attitude" and the "hives attitude" in subjects who were under hypnosis; although they found measurable changes in skin temperature, blood pressure, and heart rate, the changes did not conform to the predicted patterns. Curiously, these effects became measurable and reasonably consistent when directed toward an assistant, but not when directed toward the hypnotist himself. (As in other studies of hypnosis, this evidence points to the fact that the hypnotic subject "sleeps with one eye open" and that, in spite of his heightened suggestibility, he still manages to participate as a regulator of his responses.)

As we face up to the problem of correlating attitudes with symptoms, we begin to see that:

1. Many patients express attitudes that are typical of those listed by Grace and Graham, without showing the autonomic changes these experimenters found to be correlated with psychosomatic illness.

2. These patients with "subthreshold" attitudes are matched by others who show the somatic patterns without the predicted accompanying attitudes.

3. The theory may have to be extended to cover instances where (a) the attitudes exist but are unconscious, (b) the patient has reason to suppress his true feelings.

4. Real situational tensions and special organic susceptibilities may escape the examiner who concentrates upon attitudes, and either of these variables may be the significant causal factor.

5. Schizokinesis, produced in earlier exchanges with the environment, can register its effects long after attitudes have covered these traces of former interchanges with new surface postures and expectancies.

If man were a simple machine capable of expressing only six types of affective response, as Allport (1924) once suggested, with each prepotent system capable of a rather precise differential description, we might be able to move rapidly to a description of psychosomatic problems. We could sketch the way in which each of the six facets is completed on the afferent side by a conditioning which adds wider and wider ranges of signals, and on the efferent side by differentiated expressions in words, gestures, and precise striped-muscle movements that are on target. Hopefully, we would then emerge with awareness,

TABLE 9. *Relationships between Psychosomatic Symptoms, Attitudes, and Verbal Statements.* (Adapted from Grace and Graham 1952.)

Disorder (Number of Patients)	Attitudes and Feelings	Verbal Statements
Urticaria (31) (skin eruption, also called hives)	Mistreated, but preoccupied with what was being done to him. No thought of retaliation.	They did a lot of things to me and I couldn't do anything about it. I was taking a beating. My mother was hammering on me.
Eczema (27)	Interfered with, frustrated, and with no way to deal with frustration. Preoccupied with frustration.	I want to make my mother understand, but I can't. I couldn't do what I wanted but there wasn't anything I could do about it.
Raynaud's syndrome (4) (spasm of the capillaries, especially those of the fingers and toes during exposure to cold)	Hostility, with intent to carry out hostile action.	I wanted to hit him. I wanted to strangle him. I wanted to put a knife through him.
Vasomotor rhinitis (12) (allergic inflammation of mucous membrane of the nose)	Facing a situation that he didn't have to do anything about, that would go away, that he did not want to have anything to do with.	I wanted them to go away. I didn't want to have anything to do with it. I wanted to blot it all out. I wanted to go to bed and pull the sheets over my head, to hole up for the winter.
Asthma (7)	Same as rhinitis.	I wanted them to go away. I just couldn't face it.
Diarrhea (27)	Patient wished to be done with a situation, to have it over with, to get rid of something or somebody.	If I could only get rid of it! (a defective auto). I want to dispose of it. If the war was only over with. I wanted to get it finished with.
Constipation (17)	Grimly determined to carry on with an insoluble problem.	I have to keep on with this, but I know I'm not going to like it. It's a lousy job but it's the best I can do. This marriage is never going to be any better, but I won't quit.
Nausea and vomiting (11)	Thinking of something he wished had never happened. Feels responsible.	I wish it hadn't happened. I was sorry I did it. I wish things were the way they were before.
Duodenal ulcer (9)	Wished to injure the person or thing that had injured him.	I wanted to get back at him. I wanted revenge. He hurt me so I wanted to hurt him. I did it for spite.

TABLE 9. *Relationships between Psychosomatic Symptoms, Attitudes, and Verbal Statements.* (Adapted from Grace and Graham 1952.) (Continued)

Disorder (Number of Patients)	Attitudes and Feelings	Verbal Statements
Migraine headache (14)	Intense effort to achieve, having ceased, no matter whether followed by success or failure.	I had to get it done. I had a million things to do before lunch.
Arterial hypertension (7)	Feels that he must be constantly prepared to meet all possible threats.	I had to be ready for anything. It was up to me to take care of all the worries.
Low back pain (11)	Wanted to carry out action involving the whole body (running away, walking out).	I just wanted to walk out of the house. I wanted to run away. I felt like taking a flying leap off that island.

expressive movements, viscera, and verbalizations all functioning in parallel, each affective type accompanied by its typical cognitive and volitional counterpart. But man turns out to be a much more complex affair: the emotional *patterns,* in both visceral and striped muscles (including vocal and subvocal components), become so varied and intermingled that neither six nor sixty categories can do them justice. Even the "original" patterns that Watson, the Shermans, and Bridges set out to describe show great variability under standard stresses. As conditioning attaches these patterns to contexts with complex mixtures of cues and "forcers," and as varied methods of coping with the environmental press are developed, differentiating attitudes, expectancies, and purposes break up the original autonomic patterns, fuse them with precise superimposed striped-muscle contractions, and add culturally defined identifying names and values to socially defined situations that have cultural consequences. The relationships between awareness, naming, movements, attitudes, and this visceral underpinning make the effort to categorize difficult; any category constructed on any one of the facets (social situation, visceral pattern, attitude, striped-muscle postures and movements, verbal naming) will include a great variety of members in the other facets. No wonder the puzzled adolescent wonders, "Am I really in love?" or his older brother asks, "Is this really the vocation I want?" or another asks, "Should I laugh or cry?"

As a result of our learning, the verbalized attitudes and visceral changes need not be expected to have very precise relationships; neither attitude nor action nor visceral changes can be expected to show close correlations with specific stresses. (Two weeks in the operating room alters the young nurse's reactions to the sight of the cutting scalpel and blood.) Not even in Sparta, where the weak were quickly eliminated, would such selection eliminate those whose "vegetative retreat" might leave a willing soldier stranded, without good autonomic support for his role in the phalanx, and certainly not in a permissive democracy (or a tenderizing home) that tolerates and accepts individuals with widely varying styles of life. In between those who curse their weaknesses and those who learn to exploit them, we can expect the widest variation in attitude-response relationships. Indeed, it is precisely because of this "split" between the various measures of response that so many have been driven to postulate unverbalized and unconscious attitudes where the unusual relations recorded violate a clinician's suspicions.

We might overlook the exceptions that appear in the neonate (one infant whom an experimenter tried to condition to a pistol shot remained calm but curious), and posit that the gross relationship between certain crudely defined stresses and the bass chords struck out in autonomic reflexes will be closer than the relationships between these same stresses and our definition of the setting, our associated gestures and actions. The experiments of Carney Landis touched on both of these points, as he dealt in one study (Hunt and Landis 1936) with the startle reflex and in another (Landis 1924) with the relations between the five classes of variables just named. (See also Oken *et al.* 1962; Lipton, Steinschneider, and Richmond 1961; Bridger, Birns, and Blank 1965; Wenger and Ellington 1943; Sontag 1944; Jost and Sontag 1944.)

In fact, the whole range of phenomena which we are describing as psychosomatic illnesses indicates how these six "measures" can be thrown out of phase in the course of development and to a pathological degree. Whether his physician sits at the patient's bedside giving expression to a kind of medical moralization, as Dr. Dubois did at the turn of the century, or tries to recondition him by an active process of desensitization, as the behavior therapists do, or tries to put him into a new life-setting that will permit normal relationships to be restored, or tries to lead him by a long process of analysis to identify and express things about himself and his personal history that he has never done before, the therapist is trying to bring the part-processes back together once more, so that, in phase, the patients' reaction systems can show the standard visceral responses, while the other levels fall within that plausible-rational design for coping with stress permitted in his society. We are in danger of overlooking the obvious, the gross lack of correspondences *which exists* in these illnesses. Genetic constitutions, personal histories in a family and with peers, histories with stresses and challenges that follow no predesigned pattern, learning situations that deflect and separate the levels until an inevitable schizokinesis is produced. The lack of standard correlations should be seen as natural, even if it leads sometimes to an unwanted outcome, a pathological relationship.

CRISES CREATING MEDICAL PROBLEMS

A child may experience his first asthma attack when he is separated from his mother at her death; a mother bearing "smother love" may precipitate an attack when she visits her daughter, now escaped from the sheltering, repressive household and living a free existence away from home. A father may experience a coronary attack when, at the sound of a car crash in the street, he rushes to his bedroom window to see that his son and the family car have been hit by a racing motorist. A student, finding that his medical training is growing increasingly difficult and that he cannot both "take it easy" and live up to what his wife (mother) expects him to do, may experience examination black-outs and gastric ulcers. A hostess, preparing to serve a dinner for a group of critical guests whose approval is important to her ambitious husband, may be overwhelmed with a paroxystic auricular tachycardia (a racing heart, suffo-cation, fear of imminent death) and a full-blown anxiety attack, until the cancelation of the dinner brings complete relief. The psychosomatic literature records such onsets of medical problems by the thousands.

The list could be extended until every organ and every tissue reveal how these crises produce bodily changes. Flanders Dunbar (1938) constructed a veritable encyclopedia of such changes. From graying hair to constricted arterioles in the foot, from a sudden attack of glaucoma to an increase in white blood corpuscles, from the adrenals to ovarian hormones affected by sexual conflicts, there seems to be no group of cells immune to the impact of these stresses created by crises in our lives.

Sometimes the stress reveals a weakness in the individual's carrying capacity (whether it is the carrying of physical loads by an aging dockworker or the capacity to carry and cope with interpersonal adjustments). Sometimes the crisis point reveals a long-latent and slowly developing constitutional weak-ness. An epileptic's constitution may be revealed, for the first time, in a crisis-precipitated attack. A condition in the coronary artery of the heart that has been thirty years in the making, through heavy smoking and poor dietary and work habits, will suddenly appear in an emergency. Sometimes the weakness seems so little linked with an obvious behavioral cause that the observer is inclined to say, "Small matter who is involved, no matter what his personal and interpersonal history may have been, no matter what type of stress initiates the collapse." The clinician is tempted to generalize:

1. If each of these subjects were more mature, more competent in handling personal problems, the tensions could then be more efficiently liquidated, and no persistent overflow of autonomic innervation into the tissues would produce pathological changes. At most the emotional tensions would alert him, provide the autonomic "fillip," the "alarm reaction" that energizes action systems and puts a supporting floor under the striving that is called for, by increased muscular tonus, increased endocrine supplies, heightened metabolism, increased blood flow, and increased oxygen and glycogen. A little anxiety is a good thing, a little more begins to lower efficiency, and too much can etch its chronic presence in irreversible tissue changes. Instead of searching for a "psychosomatic personality" as some have done,[5] attention should be turned to the particular

---

[5]Halliday 1948, Ey, Bernard, and Brisset 1963, p. 854. Abstracted from the traits common to the group of illnesses most thoroughly studied by the physicians interested in psychosomatic medicine, the *psychosomatic personality,* with its fragility and its proneness to these biological accidents that threaten life, becomes a kind of *basic weakness* in the structure of action. Aside from its obvious tautology, there is the question why this general weakness pitches on the respir-atory system (asthma) in one, the circulatory system (coronary attack, high blood pressure) in another, and so on.

stresses, to plans for an improved method of coping with them, and to that ratio between press and carrying capacity that has a critical point at which the tissues begin to act as indicators.

Stated most simply, and in the most general terms, we are dealing with a balance between the person's powers and that mixture of visceral demands and the circumpress: a little less pressure or a little more power to integrate and cope with conflicting demands, and the pathological residue would disappear. Perhaps those patients who were so promptly operated upon (and who had a background of successful adjustment) would never have suffered a recurrence of ulcers with or without vagotomy.

2. The rest cure, so popular at the turn of the century in the treatment of neurasthenia, reminds us that sometimes psychosomatic problems can be resolved by the simple reduction of pressures. The therapist is moved to urge changes in the environment, a simplification of life, an easing up of the pressures on the medical student, a foster mother for the asthmatic child separated from his mother. Whether a clinician is dealing with a young child or an older person who is childlike in his dependency cravings, this reduction of pressures may have to be so marked that his counselor will judge the person as neurotic, as having excessive dependency needs. Noyes and Kolb (1963, p. 389), commenting on therapy for ulcer patients, suggest that:

"There are on record some excellent therapeutic results from prolonged psychoanalysis, but whether these outcomes exceed the frequency in patient groups treated by medical measures alone has not been demonstrated. It may be recommended that the repressed dependency needs of the patient be gratified directly or indirectly without inducing shame, guilt, or resistance. This can be done by environmental manipulation, including vacation, enlisting the support of key figures in the patient's environment, or by strengthening the patient-physician contact through regularity and frequency of visits. In those individuals with an infantile personality, the facing of the conflict by psychiatric treatment may well lead to serious depression, and a more disturbing personality reaction than that accompanying the primary ulcer symptomatology.[6]

3. Some of the pressures that the clinician sees appear to be self-generated. Some of them are retaliations by others who are irritated by a patient's excessive demands on them; others express excessive ambition and are the outcome of undertakings that tax capacities beyond safe limits. When Thomas Carlyle was working on his *Sartor Resartus,* and suffering from a chronic dyspepsia which the most elaborate dietary precautions could not correct, his friends could see an easy solution for all his difficulties. If he could only compromise with the tastes of his public, come to terms with the suggestions of his editors, and forget for a moment that he was a Messiah to set the world aright. But no! He had something to say, something that would make their ears tingle! Like Freud

---

[6]To this we can add the judgment of Ey, Bernard, and Brisset (1963, p. 864), who note that in general a classic psychoanalysis is not to be recommended. Describing this group of patients as having less ability to tolerate the analytic experience, and as having a greater vulnerability to all emotional traumata, they recommend a briefer form of psychotherapy, more active, less permissive, and less time-consuming than psychoanalysis.

(also troubled by heart symptoms and other somatic ailments), who also knew that he was destined to trouble the sleep of the world, this lonely Scotsman, holed up at Craigenputtock, had assigned himself a difficult task which, if he was to keep his self-respect, had to be done in a certain way.

Here a clinician may hesitate to rush in where fools tread so fearlessly. He has to observe caution in recommending changes in a patient's design for living, in his ambitions, in his way of coping with the world, lest he recommend measures that violate conscience, destroy an inner coherence, and threaten "sacred" values. Changing the world, changing his objectives, changing his situation, adapting himself to the world or forcing the latter to adjust to him: to choose among the alternatives is the patient's task. Lacking the coping power, he may tempt the clinician to play God.

Considering the alternatives, a generalization forms in the clinician's mind: psychosomatic illnesses call for "improved adjustment." Simple in principle, difficult in execution, this principle seems to imply that *there is a way* of coping with the combined pressures of tensions from within and demands and threats from without, in order to produce a sound and healthy life.

Because some of his clients are immature (in spite of their age) and neurotic (with exaggerated responses to pressures that others carry without an emotional overhead and without symptoms), this professional "adjustor" may leap to such conclusions as the following. "Psychic factors play a decisive role in regard to the blood pressure level in all stages of the disorder [essential hypertension] and therefore ... in all hypertensive patients the major emphasis should be on the treatment of the psychic element" (Fahrenkamp 1931, in Dunbar 1938, p. 227).

It is the "allness" of these generalizations that is currently being challenged. Swept into hasty conclusions by the first enthusiasm for this new extension of medical skills, students of peptic ulcer were ready to say, "In all of the patients with peptic lesions ... [there was] an emotional frame within which they occurred [and that] had important effects on the patients" (Mittelmann and Wolff 1942). Groen (1947) asserted that "every onset or recurrence ... was preceded by an emotional trauma." Of patients with neurocirculatory asthenia, Dunn (1942) asserted that "the majority ... show a psychological disturbance."

Weiss (1939), on the contrary, suggests that the emotional and mental strains found in the history of hypertensives play a purely accessory role in the genesis of the disorder. Rival hypotheses that relate coronary occlusion to atherosclerosis, overweight, faulty diet, or excessive use of tobacco tend to turn attention away from the emotional and psychological factors, save as these, in turn, help explain the excesses that lead to poor cardiovascular functioning. Whether the difference in the rate of incidence of cardiovascular accidents that has been found to exist between Westerners and Orientals is due to genetic differences in temperament and physical makeup, or to some as yet undefined differences in child-rearing techniques, in life-style, or in cultural pressures, or, more simply, to differences in diet, is still being debated (see Arlow 1945).

The truth seems to lie in between these two "enthusiasms" and two types of therapy. Proper diagnosis and treatment will require clinicians to separate

those suffering from psychosomatic diseases into those that have a large psychological factor associated with the complaints, those that are principally organic
cases, and those (probably the majority) that involve both factors. The emphasis on psychological factors in the immature patient has to be balanced by
a concern about his somatic condition (even though, on the face of it, he is
so obviously a psychological problem). The same dual approach must hold
for the aging patient whose signs of advanced arteriosclerosis make his predicament so obviously organic. The optimism of the clinician who is sure that
there is a way of adjusting the person to his milieu (and to his visceral needs)
has to be matched by a caution that recognizes organic limitations and constitutional predispositions. Both the person and his aspirations, as well as interpersonal and cultural demands, have to respect these organisms. This field is
not one in which sweeping generalizations should be made, either by medically
trained clinicians or by Christian Scientists.

"DREAM WORK" AND METABOLIC PROCESSES

There never has been any lack of speculation about the function of dreaming, as was noted in Chapter 3. Some have wanted to make it a process of
assimilation and digestion of the conflicts of the previous waking period, or a
preparation for the morrow. Actions begun during the day and left incomplete
may be liquidated in the dream; thus viewed, the dream is a recuperative
reorganization. Others have seen the dream as a period of ventilation or expression, in which repressions and frustrations could be at least symbolically vented,
like some head of steam in need of release. Others, sure that dreams are symbolic, saw the symbols as concealing a deeper meaning and thus shielding
repressed materials undergoing repression from a dreamer who would have
been alarmed, otherwise, if his conflicts were frankly exposed.

Those who gave the dream a forward reference, and who looked for symbols
relating to the subject's future, viewed its function as that of planning, organizing, preparing for the work to come. A few, following a cue suggested by
Jung, looked on the dream as a symbol of archetypal forces, a kind of tribal
unconscious that persists within us and that we forget at our peril; these
theorists, who thought of the dream work as a "getting in touch with the
deepest layers of the self," saw it as a work of harmonizing the surface life of
the individual with his deepest nature. There were skeptics who saw the dream
as merely a low-grade, poorly structured form of thought, prompted by current
endogenous or external stimuli, a process which does little or nothing for the
individual that a sound and dreamless sleep could not do better.

We can see these speculations about the dream function emerging in the
interpretations of experimental findings. Fisher (1965) noted that on the days
following interrupted dreaming his subjects were irritable, tense, and anxious,
and complained of difficulties in concentrating, fatigue, and lack of muscular
coordination. These reactions were not as intense as in subjects deprived of
sleep altogether, yet the disorganization of behavior was similar. Fisher and
Dement speculated about an accumulative "pressure," as though the inter-

ruption of dreaming dammed up an important liquidating work. Mandell and Mandell (1965) suggest that dreams may accompany a periodic neuroendocrine discharge triggered by metabolites accumulating during sleep; certain threshold levels of such accumulations may call for periods of dreaming to purge the blood stream. On such a theory "dream work" and dream content might have no important psychological significance. If such metabolic ebb and flow occurs, dreams might be counted as similar to the whistle on the steam engine, as Thomas Huxley once suggested, a kind of irrelevant pipsqueak occurring whenever the biochemical pressure rises to a certain level. But, as James once reminded us, the stream of conscious events serves whatever value and function it serves no matter what biochemical events may form its source.

THE EXPERIMENTAL ANIMAL AND THE HUMAN SUBJECT

A physiologist whose studies usually center on organs, biochemical changes, and responses to measurable physical and chemical agents, and who can surgically sever a vagus or sympathetic nerve, implant electrodes to stimulate or record cellular changes, collect gastric juices, measure blood sugar or excreted substances that show excess of hormones or enzymes, usually operates "below decks," in the body's engine room, one might say. He can produce ulcers by giving his experimental animals histamine-saturated beeswax pellets which increase gastric secretion (unless the action is blocked by vagotomy). The ego upstairs may be having an identity crisis, in the human subject, but it will still be the rise in HCl (or the inhibition of growth in new cells in the gastric mucosa) that is the focus of the physiologist's interest. He is trying to identify the ultimate stages in which emotional tensions become tissue changes, the symptoms that patients present to the clinician.

Sometimes in his experimental work, he eliminates or bypasses the so-called psychic factor by placing electrodes in the anterior portion of the hypothalamus, so that he can give direct stimulation to this center, from which fibers radiate to activate the autonomic nervous system; in an experimental animal such direct stimulation will produce ulcers. Instead of gathering his subject's free associations, if he studies human subjects, he will take nighttime samples of gastric secretion from ulcer patients, discovering that the HCl content is from four to twenty times that of controls (Dragstedt 1958). This excessive acidity (either in animals whose hypothalamus is stimulated or in the sleeping ulcer patients) is reduced after vagotomy, or when his subjects are given atropine to inhibit vagus action. Thus he narrows attention to that final common path which involves the anterior hypothalamus, the vagus outflow, and the acid-secreting cells of the stomach wall, *whatever the cause of the excessive hypothalamic stimulation may be in the living human subject,* whatever the crisis the "man upstairs" may be living through.

Occasionally, an experimenter has attempted to induce these same changes by manipulating the behavior of the organism as a whole. He may train his animals so that, confined to a harness for hours on end, they "earn" their food by pressing levers which also enable them to avoid electric shocks. Anticipations of reward and anticipations of punishment can be pitted against each other, and the mastery of the problems can be made increasingly difficult by delays, partial reinforcement, conflicting programs of stimulation, warning cues that are difficult to discriminate, and such constricting confinement that very little freedom of movement is possible. Under stresses of this type, Porter *et al.* (1958) were able to produce gastric and duodenal ulcers, mucous colitis, and enteric intussception, in their monkey subjects, 11 out of 19 showing measurable changes in their alimentary canal. In a few of the animals who seemed about to master the problems, lethal changes suddenly terminated the experiment: they died of their success.

In the Porter study the combinations of training procedures, effective in producing bodily malfunction in more than half their subjects, were so varied that the authors were not prepared to identify the precise nature of the stress factor. Their method of selecting and testing their subjects did not permit any evaluation of the nature of stress tolerance in the eight animals who came through the same training schedules unscathed.

In a limited study of four animals, two used as experimentals and two as controls, the experimental animals could avoid electric shock, but at the price of constant vigilance. The control pair were given the same warning signals, but had no way of cutting off the shock. The latter pair actually received more shocks, suffered the same confinement, received the same schedules of stimulation, but had no "exit" save a gradual negative adaptation.[7]

Both of the vigilant animals, who had a way of mastering the task, developed ulcers. "The experiment was terminated in each case by the death of the experimental animal." In one there was little indication of the impending fatal outcome of the successful avoidance training. The day before his death, this monkey failed to eat but continued to respond effectively. The animal was found dead on the morning of the twenty-third day, during one of the six-hour "avoidance periods." The ultimate question as to what was involved in this transition from "mastery" to ulcers to death remains unanswered. The authors note: "Although the pathogenesis of such gastrointestinal pathology is far from being well understood, it has been presumed to develop as a consequence of physiological exhaustion of the organism's somatic defense mechanisms in the face of overwhelming stressful stimuli."

Porter and his associates point out some of the possibilities that need to be tested before the essential factors in such stress induction of ulcers can be identified. Some will want to identify the nature of a constitutional susceptibility; others will search for earlier experiences (either interpersonal or

---

[7]Anyone who studies the distribution of pain endings on his own skin surface discovers just how large an "anticipatory suffering" is commonly added to the reflex component. As he explores a forearm surface, not only does he find anesthetic spots where pressure alone is felt, but the residual pain in other spots is steadily reduced until "the bodily reverberation" is minimal. The "subjective pain" (suffering) decreases as exploration proceeds.

impersonal) that make one animal stress-resistant and another stress-susceptible; still others will try to identify more precisely the elements in the procedure itself.

There have been many studies of this type, far too many to review here. All in all, they warn us against excessive interest in a concrete and highly personal account of a unique conflict, and against too heavy a weighting of biographical details (analogs of which occur in most lives). In the physiological-behavioral studies, there are quantitative factors (rate and intensity of stimuli, dosage with histamine), programs and patterns of stress, degrees of confinement or freedom, which will have to be measured. One is tempted to generalize: the ulcer-producing mechanism is as impersonal as the telephone cable that is ready to conduct any sort of message; the conflicts and stresses may vary from a Luther's identity crisis to a schoolboy's struggle with algebra. As long as they are heavily charged, producing an autonomic overflow, as long as they are of sufficient duration, as long as they require a chronic vigilance from which there is no exit, the "breaking point" of the tissues can be surpassed.

Laboratory Animals Contrasted with "Free" Human Beings

This impersonal formulation gives the clinician who deals with human beings only a brief respite, however, for two principal reasons.

1. The "confinement" that is so uniform a factor in the animal laboratory as to almost escape notice, is of a different type where "free" human beings are concerned. The boy struggling with algebra may be confined by an *inner* barrier created by the medical career he has elected: a career studded with requirements but leading nonetheless to something he has admired in his father, or to becoming the kind of man his mother wished she had married and was determined that her son should become. The prosecutor at the Moscow trials, Vishinsky, who suffered from duodenal ulcers, was bound by the needs of the party and by his own ambitions. General Bedell Smith, who went directly from Moscow to the Mayo clinic with a similar ailment, had borne the responsibility of watching out for his country's interests in an alien climate that was notably hostile. The head of the family, whose working wife is beginning to earn more than he does, is "confined" (or driven) by all that makes a male ego what it is in our society, and at the same time is also bound to the woman who can give him something he once received from his mother in the way of dependent-affectional needs. The girl who is filled with a masculine protest, who is acting out her rebellion against every feminine role that her milieu offers, may be bound within the one protective relationship that she stumbled into in her effort to escape from the family. By their habits, by their personal needs, by the combination of press and support that surround them, these human subjects are also confined.

2. The "circumpress" which gets under the skin of human patients is no precisely ordered program of electric shocks, no discrete type of stress alternated with a nonstress warning signal that can be easily discriminated and quickly mastered by an already trained lever-presser. Instead, it is a confusing and

often vaguely apprehended world. The individual's unique combination of hungers, sometimes given ready-made by his culture (like Madame Guyon's formulation of her needs as a "hunger for the love of God") makes the circumpress a challenge that is both difficult to formulate and all but impossible to master. Even when the problem can be reduced to a concrete and proximate interpersonal matrix, the social skills that are called for in achieving a proper balance of affection-giving and aggressive self-assertion can easily exceed the individual's power to formulate his problem, to organize a design for living, to "liquidate" when no solution is possible.

Two factors add a special complication to the human scene. First, man must deal with other men, the inner aspects of whose behavior are concealed from view, in a world that is not a closed system, like a maze or a Skinner-box, but is open-ended, an unfinished thing that calls for novel actions, for the making of a future that is, as yet, on no map. Second, love, hate, loyalty call for actions that fit into an ego's conception of himself. While action that will resolve personal tensions is required, at the same time the solution must respect the "laws of God and man," as a culture defines them and as his breeding has caused him to internalize them. Decency, courage, reasonableness, justice, however he defines them, are not standards which permit a man to put his visceral comfort or his personal security first, or which can be achieved by any simple act within his equipment, by a simple yes or a simple no. Liddell became convinced, after long pursuing a Pavlovian model of conditioning calculated to produce experimental neuroses, that even the neurosis of the lever-pressing animal is complicated by an encapsulating rapport with the experimenter (the kind of relationship that develops between a man and his dog). The training procedure used by the experimenter can confuse a dumb and affectionate animal whose understanding of his laboratory "boss" is so limited.

The human counterpart of the experimental animal sometimes operates with complex concepts and beliefs, such as those we symbolize by the words *God* or *democracy*. As he tries to relate his actions to such an ideal being or state of interpersonal relations, he can suffer torment because: he cannot fathom the inscrutable mind of his fantasied heavenly father; he cannot understand the way in which his compatriots are using the terms he uses; he cannot bring his efforts to a satisfactory closure (find the proof of his heavenly father's approval); he simply cannot become the man he has imagined his God will approve of; or he cannot make the democracy he has been taught to respect into a workable plan of social action. Trapped as such believers are by their world-view and needs, what has become for them the most significant "reality" may prove to be their undoing. Stated in other terms, these all-embracing views provide the form in which the individual's undoing is formulated by himself.

To the nonbeliever who looks on the God of the faithful as one of their constructions or projections, this is an entirely intrapsychic struggle: a conflict between a segregated and projected "better self" and another group of impulses that can be more easily hated than mastered. To the believer this projected "reality" is unquestionably *out there,* just beyond the rim of the field that our rational processes structure so neatly; its locale is at one and the same time the locus of a grand mystery and the source of all manner of directives, inspirations, promptings. It is God's will that leads the missionary who is "called" off to the foreign field and its dangers and hardships. It is God who supervises the casting of lots in the Moravian community where the larger issues, as well as the marriages of the young, are sometimes decided in this fashion. It is his "presence" that some LSD cultists seek in their drug experiences.

The counselor who operates within the faith and who also has a role as one of God's representatives on earth (e.g., the counselor-priest) has a task quite different from that of the counselor who stands outside the faith, watching the projections that symbolize a conflict within the individual, that symbolize something the patient may not realize about himself (his character, his personal history, his own biology, his relationships with his peers or with a pathogenic circumpress). The latter counselor has a double task, which requires him to carry on a "double-entry" system of bookkeeping without impatiently attempting to shatter the faith of his patient or to sever ties that have a potentially integrating power. He is tempted to brush away the old "interfering God" and set up a rival view that corresponds to his own. Missionaries within the faith, dealing with the alien tribesman, also have to face this same problem. The enthusiastic agnostic who treats the faithful can easily become an actual threat to the stability of the very lives he aims to help, even as many a well-meaning missionary has destroyed those whom he, Prometheus, had assumed that he was saving.

At a physiological-impersonal level, a psychosomatic complaint is explained by neural, biochemical, genetic-structural factors. The behavioral scientist will seek to identify a program of stimulation, of motivational conflicts, of delayed and irregular reinforcements, of difficult discriminations, of confinement. Moving outward into an extended life-history, a psychologist has to become interested in earlier traumatic events, affectional relations (with fixations, rejections, seductions, dependencies), and relationships with peers and to authority. Central to this personal history is the development of that internal regulative mechanism we try to describe in our discussions of life-space, superego, ego-ideal, self-image. The sociatrist and existentialist try to place the individual in wider and wider contexts until, to help a patient meet his conflicts, the counselor has to help him develop a metapsychology and an ideology. Although a specialist may choose to work at a particular level, collecting special types of data by the particular methods that are best adapted to his interests, the practitioner who is responsible for the welfare of the person has to make a synthesis of all levels. There is no mechanical "computerized" procedure that can be taught (or programmed) and that will produce just the right synthesis of all these levels of analysis. The good clinician remains an artist. He may be restless under a "committee system" in which the various specialists on a staff each speak for their particular emphases, or, having the power that goes with the chief's position on a staff, he may enforce his will in determining "what must be done." Where democratic procedures prevail, a clinical team is a loose federation with no higher authority than their common purpose, as loose an organization as the United Nations.

The Life-Style and the Circumpress

The social circumpress that settles down on the worker in a bureau or on the assembly line, on the motorman on a subway train, on the teacher in a public school with a superintendent who issues ukases from his office each day and runs a "taut ship" can seem as confining to the human being as the cage that confines the experimental animal. The motorman, confined in his small booth, hand on the throttle, foot on the brake pedal, alerted to switch lights, driven by a schedule, is forced to be vigilant by the hour, until the attack of angina registers a cardiac "protest." The worker on the production line, pressed by his neighbor or the moving belt, confined to a limited stance if he is to reach the passing products, attention held within a very narrow range, gets a neck-and-shoulder cramp that indicates he has passed his recovery limit.

The difference between the laboratory harness and the confining roles that human beings enter is not as great as we sometimes believe, when certain inner barriers are taken into account. We are held on a task, *and* we commit ourselves to a role: self-bound, in part, but also *forced by circumstances* over which we have no control.

However, there are great differences among individuals. One teacher will accept the "academic horsecollar" with complete grace and poise, find the requirements reasonable, discharge her responsibilities, and find a great amount of personal freedom left. Her colleague simmers in a constant frustration, insists that she is growing "stir-crazy," ends by finding the profession unsuited to anyone with an independent nature. The business executive and promoter, who likes to be free to "wheel and deal," may look askance at the college professor, certain that only a milksop or some very inhibited personality would be content to live such a restricted life. One member of the congregation will find great satisfaction in the certainties of the minister; the next one will resent his pastor's "voice of authority," feeling coerced.

Breathing resistance, rebellion, and hate, a man can literally "break his heart" kicking against all restraint and fighting for a vaguely utopian kind of freedom. His neighbor is happy with an ordered existence, and both praises and enforces the laws. To one man the world is a prison; to the next one it offers more freedom than he knows how to utilize creatively.

Psychosomatic Complaints and the Personality

When we have accepted the fact that stress can alter physiological functioning, we still must ask: Why does one patient "choose" asthma, another a coronary attack, a third a gastric ulcer? Is it a peculiar constitutional susceptibility? Does stress search out the weakest link in a biological system? Or is there a characteristic life-style that marks each one of these illnesses? The need to classify and order phenomena as complex as those met with in psychosomatic medicine has driven some enthusiasts into a premature categorizing. Let us examine some of the evidence.

The Spartan youth, whom Plutarch described as standing stolidly before those who would have punished him for stealing the fox that was hidden beneath his tunic, did not flinch as the teeth and claws of the animal tore his flesh; he chose to die rather than show weakness. He has long symbolized a certain type of patient who has his own somatic fox, inside his body's tissues. He will neither temporize with those who would seduce him to lower his aspirations, nor will he use his illness for some secondary gain, such as drawing compensation from an insurance policy and inducing those around him to treat him as an "impaired person." He does not choose to play the illness game.[8]

The secondary responses of the person to his illness were not the ones that interested Alexander, since they may or may not be related to the genesis of the illness. Alexander wanted, in addition, to draw a sharp line between conversion hysteria, in which the patient uses a paralysis or contraction of the *voluntary* musculature, or an anesthesia of a portion of the skin surface, as a kind of body language that furthers his ends and influences those about him, and the true psychosomatic complaint.

Alexander's statement, in an article (1943) intended to set up the fundamental principles for those who would work in this area, runs:

"It seems advisable to differentiate between hysterical conversion and vegetative neurosis ... The hysterical conversion symptom is an attempt to relieve an emotional tension in a *symbolic* way; it is a symbolic expression of a definite emotional content. *This mechanism is restricted to the voluntary neuromuscular or sensory perceptive systems whose function is to express and relieve emotions.* A vegetative neurosis consists of a psychogenic dysfunction of a vegetative organ which is not under control of the voluntary neuromuscular system." (Emphasis added.)

The glands and viscera, involved in psychosomatic illness, are not subject to direct voluntary control, he urged; when their action indicates an exaggerated autonomic outflow, we ought to look for the emotions of which they are an integral part, even when these emotions are unconscious, or are denied by the patient, or are rooted in a forgotten infantile fantasy. This pure "emotion-to-viscera" category, as well as the "purely involuntary overflow," does not

---

[8]Recognizing that these noncompliant ones sometimes stand on high ground, Harold Wolff (1953, p. 151) observes, "There are many things more important than comfort and a few even more important than health. But a man should appreciate what his actions and goals are costing him. Then, if he chooses, he may pay for them in pain and disease. Often he will decide that his values are poor, that he has been confused, and thence change his direction and pace." Such a statement from a clinician recognizes that health is not the highest value. It also departs from the ancient Hebraic folk belief that is still with us to the effect that "If you live right, you will be rewarded," and its companion, "Those whom God has punished must have sinned," which Job's counselors once offered him. It also surpasses the philosophy of Mary Baker Eddy, who could remind a mother that her child's blindness must be due to that mother's thoughts and errors, since God's child would otherwise be perfect in every way.

represent boundaries that nature respects. They indicate, rather, a theoretical and practical intention of one of the founders of psychosomatic research, a kind of model within whose framework he intends to work.

Whether through his own observational and theoretical bias, or through accidental contact with a certain group of patients, he concluded that gastric-ulcer patients acted as though they were expecting (or hoping) to be fed.

"The emotional attitude accompanying and preceding food intake and digestion ...is accompanied by a different distribution of vegetative tonus. In this instance the visceral organs become hyperemic whereas the skeletal muscle tonus decreases and the concomitant drowsiness is the indication of a transitory anemia of the cortex. If these emotional states are chronically sustained the corresponding vegetative innervations are also chronic... [and] when the stomach neurotic breaks down under an excessive load of responsibility he recoils from his habitual overactivity and assumes the vegetative mood of the state that accompanies digestion, to which his alimentary tract reacts with a continuous hyperactivity. This recoiling from exaggerated outward activity and strain we may call 'vegetative retreat.'"

Alexander was quick to see that feeding and cuddling, primary expressions of affection and the earliest security bringers, were associated very early in life. This bond makes any patient who is in need of affectionate assurance, or who feels deprived of his deserved indulgent care, produce a set of symptoms that could be described as vagotonia, on the one hand, or as a need for affectionate responses from those around him, on the other.

The hypertensives that he saw behaved as though a chronic hostility were simmering beneath the body's surface, sending up the blood pressure as though to make ready for an emergency "attack." The asthmatic, he speculated, betrays a nasal and bronchial condition that resembles strangulated sobbing. "Filled up" until he can scarcely breathe, his engorged respiratory tracts symbolize (unwittingly) an appeal for help that is as old as his cry as an infant.

For Alexander's purposes the case of asthma was not as clear-cut as some of the other patterns; "asthma also has components of a hysterical conversion symptom since it can serve as the direct expression and partial substitute for a suppressed emotion such as the wish to cry. Breathing—although an automatic function—is also under the control of voluntary innervation."

The upshot of his argument, however, was that for each psychosomatic illness the clinician will find a specific emotion. Founding his claim on animal research that shows that "different emotional states have their specific vegetative tonus," he was ready to invite all who dealt with psychosomatic illnesses to seek the specific emotional patterns responsible. That his logic was over-extended is implied in his own admission that peptic ulcer may be neither a conversion symptom nor a vegetative neurosis, but rather the result of a long-standing stomach dysfunction, although he was moved to insert "a neurotic dysfunction," as though any respectable stomach would not misbehave save for good and sufficient *psychological* reasons.

Developing his theory of hypertension, Alexander (1939a) described how, in his opinion, his patients "got that way."

"In normal life, fear and rage find their expression in physical flight or attack, for which the body prepares itself under the influence of these emotions. One important element of this preparation consists in the increased blood pressure. Human beings living in a competitive civilization are equally and perhaps even more permanently exposed to fear and hostile impulses, yet have much less opportunity to give expression to these feelings in physical combat. Social life requires an extreme control of these hostile impulses. A neurotic form of this control is unsuccessful attempts at repression. One of the best founded discoveries of psychoanalysis is that impulses which are inhibited in their expression sustain a chronic tension which is apt to have a permanent—or we might call it a tonic—effect upon certain physiological functions. This is the etiological theory of the psychogenic organ neuroses. An acute elevation of the blood pressure is a part of the normal reaction to acute rage and fear. Our assumption is that a *chronic* inhibited rage may lead to a *chronic* elevation of the blood pressure....

"The maturing individual in the course of his life gradually becomes more and more confronted with the complex problems of maintaining his and his family's existence, his social position and prestige. In our present civilization all these tasks unavoidably involve hostile competitive feelings, create fears and require at the same time an extreme control of these hostile impulses. Those who through constitution or through early life experience have acquired a greater amount of inhibitions, will handle their aggressions less efficiently than others and will tend to repress them.... It must also be borne in mind that the neurotic individuals who are more than normally blocked in relieving their hostilities and aggressions usually become inhibited also in many other respects, particularly in sexual expression.... Our experience is that the chronic hypertensives belong to this group of overly inhibited, yet at the same time, intensely hostile and aggressive individuals."

Alexander's conception of the "gastric personality" suggests that behind the outward mask of the competent person there lurks the dependent child with a residue of ungratified oral cravings. Consciously the patient may say (to others, to himself): "I am efficient, active, and productive; I give to everybody, I help people, I assume responsibilities, I enjoy having people depend on me." Outwardly he may aspire to be the effective leader, the self-sufficient, active, and even aggressive personality. Yet the gastric indicator betrays something different, as do his dreams and free associations.

When one studies the actual series of cases that Alexander has published, one discovers there is a wide variety of personal qualities included within this general formulation.

One peptic-ulcer case had been, as a child, very much indulged. He had never been the "leader type"; instead, he lacked the usual ambitions. He married a competent, intelligent, and in some ways superior woman, but that marriage disappointed his expectations (especially if we assume that he had been looking for a mother substitute). The wife continued, as before the marriage, to devote her effort to her own career and personal growth. Their sexual life did not prove satisfactory. The wife was frigid and the patient suffered from premature ejaculation. Driven to compete with her (she was the principal financial support of their joint household), he tried to do what he actually detested, and failed in the effort to surpass her. After two years of this, the peptic ulcer and a hemorrhage called for treatment. Shortly afterward, he established a sexual relationship with another woman (motherly and a good cook), who did not drive him to do what he did not want to do. And the symptoms disappeared.

Another life-style is portrayed in the case of L., reported by Alexander and French (1946, pp. 244 ff):

This patient, a 31-year-old medical student, referred because of ulcers and "examination blackout," was failing in his studies in spite of strenuous effort. He revealed the presence of oral cravings in his dreams before a half-dozen analytic hours had passed. "He was on a beach with a lot of people; someone was drowning and the patient was expected to save the man. He was frightened that he couldn't swim that far, then someone pushed him from behind and he fell into the water and started to swim toward the drowning man. He kept feeling that he was going under. He thought, 'They will have to save me.' Then he was sitting on the beach being fed ice cream by some woman. He woke up thinking anxiously, 'I have to get back and save the man.'"

There was also evidence in a dream of rivalry with a father figure that may have complicated his writing of exams. "He and his favorite professor were examining a woman patient. She was very uncooperative and kept telling them how to conduct the examination. She was critical of the professor and finally said, 'You get out of here and let Doctor L. (our patient) take care of me.' The professor looked at her with disgust but smiled at our patient and said, 'Go ahead with the old witch.'"

As this man's history was reviewed, it became evident that, hurried to achieve a kind of maturity that his father had never demonstrated, this boy had had little time to dawdle. His ambitious mother pushed him from childhood on until after college, when he became manager of the family laundry business that the mother had inherited, and displaced the father whom this capable woman had married and made into her business manager.

All had gone well—as far as the patient's health was concerned—until he fell in love, conceived a new ambition to become a doctor, left the family business, and became a full-time student of medicine. He was once again managed by a woman, his wife's funds supporting the pair and his wife's concern getting him to a doctor when the symptoms developed. He was freely verbalizing his feelings about his mother by the third interview: "If mother had left me alone, I would have been happier."

As his confidence in his therapist grew, he described how, driven beyond his capacities, he had developed symptoms and played the invalid; somewhat shame-faced, he confessed to enjoying being fed and cared for. He worried about the regimen that his doctor, in the presence of his wife, planned for him. Wouldn't he be getting soft? Yet the same craving for dependency and an easy success had been expressed in the second interview when he said: "I wish I had a wealthy relative who would leave me a million dollars."

Helped to a better understanding of himself, freed from a certain burden of guilt, he was put to work on an ulcer ward, telling others "how to live right." Later, cured and converted to a new way of life, he spoke of his own future plans: "He had established himself in general practice in a middle-sized town,... and he was doing well and... enjoying life. He then had a three-months-old son. He had expected to be jealous of the child, knowing of his old passive wishes, and was pleased that he was not. He was determined that his son would have a happy, irresponsible childhood."

One of Alexander's colleagues on the staff of the Institute for Psychoanalysis, Dr. Thomas M. French, summarized his conception of the *asthmatic personality*:

"Attacks of bronchial asthma seem to be associated with a very considerable variety of emotional conflicts. Outstanding among these are the suppression of any sort of intense emotion, threats to dependent relationships and to the security based upon them, and sexual conflicts. The outstanding personality traits of asthmatic children seem to be overanxiety, lack of self-confidence and a clinging dependence on the parents which appears to be a reaction to a tendency to over-solicitude upon the part of the parents."

We could extend such a list of clinical opinions, assigning a specific personality structure to each specific illness, with colitis personalities, Raynaud's syndrome personalities, effort-syndrome personalities, and so on. We discover, however, before we have gone very far, that opinions differ, that observers find they must specify at least a limited range of types. Wittkower, for example, studying neurocirculatory asthenia, found that there were at leave five types of soldiers among his patients:

1. A sober, reliable, trustworthy, perfectionist type, who had a keen sense of duty, a tendency to repress aggressions, and a constrained and highly organized life-style.

2. A conscientious soldier, also efficient and responsible, but somewhat querulous, whose repressed aggression was accompanied by a sense of being unjustly "put upon," asked to do too much.

3. A rebellious, resentful soldier, who ventilated his feelings by explosive reactions.

4. An asthenic type, physically weak, with juvenile body habits. Delicate physically and mentally, he had been overprotected, and used his invalid status as a defense. Demanding, self-willed, and stubborn at home, he was weak and timid before strangers. Noncompetitive, nonathletic, sedentary, his fear of exertion had frequently been reinforced by his mother's concerns. Entry into army life and separation from a protective home environment found him unprepared.

5. The "quitter," a dependent, impaired personality with strong parasitic tendencies.

Lacking the proper control studies among normal populations and among other illness categories, we have no way of knowing just how much significance to attach to this clinical evaluation. The irritation of the old drill sergeant for the man whose heart compels him to fall out, or of the officer who is trying to maintain his company at its full strength and efficiency and who counts too many sick reports a black mark on his record, may have something to do with these categories.

This problem of "a personality profile for each psychosomatic disorder" is further complicated by the fact that a single individual may display, at different periods of his life, gastric ulcers, hypertension, and asthma. Since Alexander's basic conception implies a personality structure that has developed continuously from infancy, several questions arise:

1. Are the psychodynamic factors that are responsible for these illnesses more recently constructed and nearer the surface, changing as new phases of development present new drives and new problems, and therefore something like attitudes?

2. Do they bear a closer relation to the current circumpress than to earlier settings that supposedly established a consistent personality structure? Does their treatment require more attention to the solution of current pressures and frustrations rather than any review of a life history and a reconstruction of the personality?

3. Or is the early infancy of such patients a sufficiently complex reservoir of potentially pathogenic influences, so that subsequent periods of stress which activate them suggest different histories to clinicians?

The problems raised by Alexander's early statement of postulates have been complicated by the high degree of subjectivity that permeates the physician-patient relationship. A personality evaluation (or imputation of underlying, unconscious trends and emotions) can be as much a "projection" of the clinician as a "reading" of the objective data.

Puzzling, too, are the observations of a team such as Wolf et al. (1955). As they came to the end of their study of essential hypertension, their summation seemed to put them on the side of the agnostics, as far as any consistent personality pattern among their patients was concerned: "Hypertensive subjects were not set apart by a uniform personality profile, or characteristic set of emotional conflicts, or by a special pattern of behavior" (p. 232). Yet in the next statement they contradict themselves by saying: "There did appear to be a striking similarity in the way they looked at life, the way they evaluated events, problems, and challenges, and the manner in which they dealt with them. They were inclined to be tentative and wary, fundamentally driving and often hostile but not able fully to commit or assert themselves" (p. 232). Admitting that other population samples would probably show these same patterns (in a competitive society must one not be "on guard"?), they insist that the clinician who treats these patients will see an improvement if he can make the hypertensives "feel more secure." If they can be brought to make a "freer and more fearless self-assertion," this will be followed "by a short or long-lasting lowering of arterial pressure" (p. 233). In another section (p. 127), these authors describe their hypertensives as outwardly "gentle, poised and apparently easygoing," yet inwardly "filled with aggressive drive which was tightly restrained by a need to please." That such a description is intended to represent something more than would be found in any normal socialized, civilized, Western man is indicated by their notation of the body types of this group, which tended to be more square and muscular than average (as Sheldon had claimed, following Draper); in addition, when seen over years of relatively intimate observation, they impressed their physicians as

...having special difficulty with self-assertion and the expression of aggression. In many of them there was indirect evidence, from dreams or other sources, of extraordinary underlying attitudes of violence coupled with a guilty fear of giving expression to that violence. Contrasting with their underlying attitudes the overt behavior of these individuals was often one of appeasement. They displayed a strong need to conform, to please and to keep the peace. They felt the need to show prowess without exhibiting aggression and continually feared that they would not succeed in doing so. In several of his patients this pattern was adopted very early in life; in others it was abruptly assumed after some show of violence seriously frightened the patient."

The physicians found these patients tense, as though mobilized for combat, yet with a facade of easygoing and affable friendliness. "Poised to strike [they] withheld their punch with a guilty fear of its consequences." They seemed to have difficulties in developing warm friendships, or in participating whole-heartedly in group action. The physicians add a composite photograph of the developmental histories:

"In childhood most of them had been seriously frustrated in the process of developing individuality and in self-expression. As children they were all unduly shy, they blushed easily and were rarely able to admit they were wrong. Most of the married ones selected domineering mates. In the backgrounds of the subjects were certain common circumstances which may have provided conditioning situations. The mothers of many of them were stiff and domineering, inclined to demand compliance, and withholding approval for failure to comply. They especially refused to tolerate outbursts of anger. Their children felt that they were forced to compete for affection and approval by being good. Many of our hypertensives dealt fairly successfully with this challenge and managed, for a time at least, to consider themselves the one closest to the mother. This accomplishment inevitably developed the feeling of strong hostility toward the mother which was suppressed with varying degrees of success but was associated with guilt. Often with their rigid personalities and notable lack of warmth, these hypertensive patients repeated with their children the patterns they had known in their own upbringing."

Perhaps both extremes of evaluation are true: (1) There is no particular or specific personality pattern in this disorder that is not found in normals and in other psychosomatic illnesses. (2) There are common factors in their histories, in their attitudes, in an outward poise and amiability combined with an underlying aggressive-hostile drive. But if both sides of the argument are thus endorsed, then it must be that we are dealing with something familiar in Western man, something that happens repeatedly in the course of socializing a child, something that a specialist will see over and over until his own reactions to these patients become stereotyped, and he begins to select items in case histories that are congruent with his stereotype. In this society, his patients have not "made the grade" without paying a high toll in bodily discomfort or in actual impairment. Aligning himself with his patient, it is easy for him to see society as the enemy. It is obvious that we need much more data on the genetic factor, on constitution and body build, on measuring instruments that can yield quantitative data about those behavioral dimensions that are here found in a particular clinical group; above all, we need a few controlled studies, with comparison groups studied as meticulously as the patient group.

The composite photographs, the personality stereotypes, are just vague enough and general enough to be used to characterize a whole society, and have been used in this fashion by Alexander (1942), Fromm (1947, 1955, 1961), Horney (1937), and Bettelheim (1960). If an observer from outer space could turn his telescope on their pages, he would conclude, in all probability, that our culture is "running a fever," and that those who have set themselves up as physicians for the individual soul are beginning to prescribe for society as a whole. Not content with adjusting the man to his milieu, they seem to concur in an unfavorable evaluation of the milieu. Like the flight of birds that heralds a coming storm, these psychiatric critics—if seriously believed—might presage radical changes in our mores, mandates, and myths, and, in due course, in our very lives. An observer with some sense of history, however, may wish to recall the remarks of Socrates on adolescents, or to note that more than a hundred years ago De Quincey complained of the hustle and bustle of modern life which left no place for the spirit to commune with itself or to dream.

While the conservative voices of La Piere (1959), or Russell Kirk, or Ayn Rand (1961) speak out in anger or in sadness against the passing of the spirit of the founding fathers and the spread of a permissive (if not libidinous) Epicureanism, the more cautious social scientists (Simmons and Wolff 1954, p. 67) are noting:

"There is no strictly objective and finely calibrated scale for measuring the pressures of fellow-group agents or for the assessment of the enforcement power of any particular cultural norms or prescribed codes of behavior, thought, or feeling on individuals in specified situations. Indeed, the compelling force of a culture mandate, mediated either by the individual himself or by his fellow-group agents, may vary greatly with different individuals or in the case of the same individual at different times. Above all, a person's immediate or intimate associates in an organized group, such as family or clique, may greatly lessen, intensify, or slant the force of a cultural code."

The strictly objective and finely calibrated scale which can "measure" the structure of a personality, and therefore provide the validating evidence for these clinical generalizations that seem to be so much in conflict with one another, is also not available at this time.

For all of the above-mentioned reasons, and especially because the methodology employed in much of this work has not been adequate, we should be extremely wary in imputing any characteristic personality profile to a particular psychosomatic disorder. Too quick to impute such "meanings," a clinician may forget that exercise, regimen, cold weather, narrowed passages in particular blood vessels, diet, exhaustion, and other genetic, impersonal, bio-chemical factors can also bring about a disorganization of important bio-logical functions.

The clinician's need to clarify and order his data is understandable. A lawful set of psychodynamic relationships would produce the kind of taxonomy of these disorders that would facilitate a rapid, efficient, deductive therapy. Psy-chosomatic medicine would become an efficient set of therapeutic maneuvers, a discipline that would be easy to teach. To date there is no clear evidence that the patients obey the categories that have been set up: vagotonics, body types, developmental histories, personality structures, interpersonal relations, group pressures, types of conditioning situations, each yields something im-portant for the consideration of the physician who would treat these disorders. But no single set of categories seems to yield very impressive correlations. Even less work has been done on the social factors behind psychosomatic illnesses; what little data there are seem contradictory.

Surgical Interference with Autonomic Outflow

Both the general practitioner and the specialists who treat any of the psychosomatic illnesses, such as gastric ulcers, high blood pressure, neuro-circulatory asthenia, asthma, or migraine headaches, are caught in a difficult position as they face the recent medical reformation. If they choose to treat the patient as a whole, they are forced to make time-consuming analyses of life-situations and personal histories, a task for which they are ill-prepared, and which, according to evidence now at hand, has an uncertain outcome. If they use the conventional methods of treating body chemistry (as when they seek to neutralize excessive stomach acidity by medication), they may find themselves fighting a rearguard battle against a life-style, a chronic tension or anxiety, a persistent emotionality, or a bodily constitution; instead of getting at something basic, they may be limiting themselves to a treatment of the symptoms, while the patient drifts into a dangerous illness.

Facing this dilemma, a few have concluded that if it is the chronic emotion that is to blame, and if the particular autonomic outflow that impinges on the malfunctioning organ is a branch of the sympathetic system, the simplest thing to do is to sever that particular nerve. The "nervous heart" that runs a pulse rate of over 200 beats per minute, or a blood pressure that mounts to 250 mm., can thus be brought down within normal ranges; the hyperacidity that is produced by excessive vagus innervation can be corrected without chemicals, and ulcerating sores can then be allowed to heal. Although psycho-logical conflicts and chronic emotions may persist, the organs (and the patient's life) will be saved. This approach might be viewed as a minimal concession to psychosomatic principles. It has the appeal of something that is surefire: no emotional outflow can affect the peripheral organ once the path is severed.

When the evidence is reviewed, these operations that interrupt the auton-omic outflow are found to produce quite varied results, and they leave some questions in our minds. A few patients with gastric ulcers go on to experience new ulcers in spite of having had their vagus nerve severed.[9] Some patients develop new symptoms (diarrhea, tachycardia, dyspnea on exertion, sweating, headaches, hypoglycaemic attacks), as though the operation had shunted the innervation to other peripheral structures. It seems to be the opinion of those who have used such procedures (Szasz 1949, 1952; Rees 1953) that the patients who have had the best preoperative adjustment, and for whom ulcers represent some acute reaction to a particular life stress (e.g., "combat fatigue" in wartime, a crisis in family affairs, the stress of a professional conflict with a superior on the staff), will also have the best results from the surgery. A change in the general life-situation would also produce similar freedom from ulcers *in these patients,* and without surgery or psychotherapy.

Again, it should be emphasized: a sympathectomy does not alter the patient's ability to experience emotions. It is primarily the peripheral *expression,* mediated by the autonomic nervous system, that is changed. This was also reported by Cannon, in his experimental study of sympathectomized cats (Cannon, Lewis, and Britton 1927). His radical procedures severed the outflow to heart, liver, adrenals, and kidneys. Kept in a healthy condition for months, the animals gave all the usual signs of emotions (growling, hissing, retracting ears, baring teeth, striking with paw and claw), although the responses of organs supplied by the cut nerves were grossly changed. In the human patient described by Wolf *et al.,* there was also no reduction in her ability to experience emotions. "While attempting to do some shopping, she had an episode of panic, palpitation, nausea, sweating and precordial pain with severe low left back pain." As an illustration of her residual condition, the authors note that a stress interview in the clinic, reviewing her relationship with her daughter, produced a rise of 46 mm. in blood pressure. The ventilation of her emotions (resentment) and her physician's reassurance brought an improvement and, possibly, additional insight. The improvement lasted some three days. More than a year later (and after there had been some four years of interviews), she was still finding it difficult to go shopping or traveling, or to meet people. Her life-style and personality remained canoelike (i.e., easily upset).

In a disorder such as ulcerative colitis, where the prognosis is not good (see Groen 1947), the surgeon is tempted to interfere with the progress of the disease. Here and there a neurosurgeon, convinced that the seat of the difficulty lies in the emotional life, attacks what he assumes to be the seat of emotions, the brain itself. Slocum, Bennet, and Pool (1959) describe a

---

[9]Recent studies from the laboratories of the Cornell Medical School have suggested that one cause of ulcers is the failure in the reproduction of new cells in the stomach's lining; stress applied to experimental animals caused a slowing of this rate of reproduction and a decline in the number of stomach cells producing DNA, the genetic material that must be duplicated every time a cell reproduces itself. If gastric juice (acid) is not the primary cause of ulcers, there is room for hypotheses that may explain how the break in vagus innervation may be bypassed and how stress may bear on cell-growth rates through other mechanisms.

patient who had been hospitalized a number of times for severe, bleeding, ulcerative colitis. She had been kept on an extremely restricted, bland diet, and before her admission to the psychiatric service had been warned that her only hope of recovery was through colectomy. Instead, a prefrontal topectomy was performed. During the first week after the operation, no longer on restricted diet, she literally gorged herself on fresh corn, cauliflower, high-residue salads, celery, in short, all the forbidden items, and stated, in high good humor, "Even if it kills me it's worth it."

All surgical procedures are costly, and the changes they introduce into an adaptive mechanism are irreversible. In the procedure used by Slocum and his associates, the surgery invades the cortex to produce changes that neuropsychiatry is still trying to evaluate precisely. Since they invade the very "citadel of the self," the central regulative mechanism, they are not only most dangerous but also loaded with a very potent suggestion factor; the need for follow-up, comparisons, and control series is greater than ever. It is interesting, therefore, to place beside this psychosurgery for colitis a treatment that is wholly psychological.

O'Connor *et al.* (1964), also dealing with cases of colitis, used objective measures of the physiological changes that followed a short-term, psychoanalytically oriented therapy. The majority of the patients showed measurable improvement, while an untreated group used for comparison, and examined with the same care, showed no improvement. The physicians also noted that those patients who experienced favorable environmental changes also showed greater improvement than those who had to remain in the same life-setting. Of fifty patients evaluated after psychotherapy, four had an excellent response, twenty were counted "good," sixteen showed moderate improvement, and seven showed no improvement at all, while three had actually deteriorated. The authors could note no evidence of any relationship between the degree of psychological improvement, the intensity and duration of the therapy, and the changes that were measured. They did note, however, that those patients with colitis who were also suffering from schizophrenia showed less improvement: 35 per cent of the schizophrenics showed no improvement, as compared with 14 per cent of the nonschizophrenic group.

In summary, we might note that the radical surgical procedures, applied either to the peripheral autonomic system (as in vagotomy) or to the central nervous system (as in topectomy), have a limited success in some patients. When the patients also have a long history of personality problems and difficulties in adjustment, with associated emotional tensions, there is a less favorable outlook. When the psychosomatic complaints are coupled with a psychosis, the outlook is also less favorable for psychotherapy. Improvement in these same illnesses, where symptoms are usually worsened by any emotional stress, can also result from favorable enirvonmental changes.

We conclude that those who respond best to surgery also respond to psychotherapy and to favorable environmental changes and an improved hygiene of living. Even the surgical therapy is bypassed by some patients, whose continuing tensions produce ulcers even after vagotomy (or high blood pressure after sympathectomy). When the tensions continue, they may be expressed in other peripheral organs. Although this type of evidence seems at first to reaffirm the basic philosophy of the "psychosomatic reformation" and to make surgery a last resort, a local type of defense at best, it does not indicate that treating the whole man will be a simple matter, or that all psychosomatic illnesses will yield to psychotherapy.

IMPLANTING ELECTRODES

Experimenters working with animals, have implanted electrodes, with a permanent binding post mounted on the skull, so that the thalamus and hypothalamus can be aroused by electrical stimulation. As the number of centers tapped increases, animals can be driven to a compulsive bar-pressing (when each bar-pressure stimulates the septal area), thrown into panic flight (when a hypothalamic center is touched off), or forced to interrupt the nursing of their young (who are dropped like a "hot potato" when the appropriate button is pressed). We are invited to speculate about a picture of that possible day when a human patient, with electrodes appropriately implanted in centers, can be controlled by a keyboard in such a way that he can be alerted when he has slumped into morose inaction, or can stop his thoughts the moment he begins one of his interminable ruminations about his difficulties. What some now seek from the "mood pill" that relieves anxiety or brings a slightly euphoric boost would then be offered by a built-in electronic device with a pocket keyboard that any patient could press when he so desired.

That this rather Huxleyan glimpse of the future may soon be tried is suggested by a series of observations reported by Heath (1963) from the Tulane laboratories. Two patients were used, one diagnosed as "narcolepsy with cataplexy" and the other diagnosed as a "psychomotor epileptic." Both had failed to respond to conventional treatments. In the former patient electrodes were placed in the septal region, the anterior hypothalamus, the mesencephalic tegmentum, the caudate nucleus, the right frontal cortex, the midtemporal cortex, the left anterior cortex, and the hippocampal area. In the second patient 17 different brain sites were tapped with implanted stimulus points. Thus, wired for stimulation, the response mechanisms of these patients could be "orchestrated" as an experimenter desired, and the patient, alert and capable of giving verbal reports, could give his subjective comments on the resultant "emotional states."

Confining our attention to the results obtained from the narcoleptic patient, let us note how the procedures developed. After a series of exploratory tests, the electrode sites were reduced to three that produced quite different effects; each was connected to a stimulator unit that was attached to the patient's belt so that he could, at any moment, stimulate himself, and mechanical counters were included in the circuit so that a continuous record of his choices could be kept. It developed that he showed an unmistakable preference for the septal button (see Fig. 7). The stimulus to the mesencephalic teg-

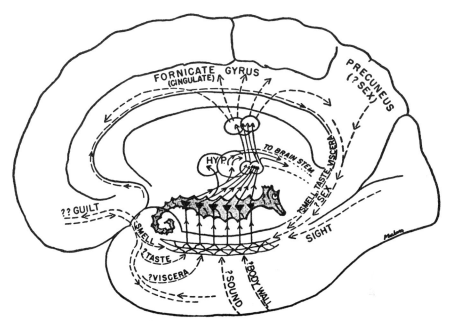

FIGURE 7. THE ANTERIOR, MIDDLE, AND POSTERIOR DIVISIONS OF THE HYPO-
THALAMUS. This diagram represents the thinking of MacLean and could also be used as
a model for the work of Heath. The sea horse in the center of the figure symbolizes
archaic mechanisms which man has inherited from his ancient, animal past and which
we might call "instincts" or "affective patterns." As a flood of stimuli enters this
rhinencephalic area, it spreads to arouse a complex of neural action that must be
encoded and distributed by this affective-regulative center, so that the impulses which
crowd the area can be distributed into final common paths and to the organs that are
supplied by the autonomic outflow (see Figure 6). The "septal area" mentioned
in the text lies in front of the hypothalamus, on the side toward the tail of the sea
horse. Note that the hypothalamic outflow to the "brain stem" is matched by the outflow upward to the cortex (via fornicate gyrus). The hypothalamus, regarded by some
as "the seat of the emotions" and by others as a relay-arousal center that alerts the
whole man, is seen to be under assault from above (from frontal and precuneal areas)
and from below (from the body and from without—by sight, smell, taste, and other
senses). Because of these connections with the brain as a whole, the "visceral brain"
can be isolated conceptually, but not functionally from the system as a whole. Thus the
crack of a twig, which has a "meaning" for the sleeping camper, alerts the visceral
brain, spreads through the cortex, and sets the awakened sleeper into action. (Reprinted
by permission of Harper & Row, Publishers, from Paul D. MacLean, "Psychosomatic
Disease and the 'Visceral Brain,' " *Journal of Psychosomatic Medicine,* 11 [November-
December 1949], 338-353.)

mentum was definitely alerting, but aversive, and by the eighth week the
counter showed that there was no further use of this button. The hippocampal
button continued to be chosen for two weeks longer, then for the final five
weeks the septal button held the field. Stimulation of this button alerted
the patient, and checked his tendency to fall into sleep; he described its
effect as pleasurable, rewarding. He had had to give up his performances

as an entertainer in a nightclub, and now found that with his new "arousal device" he could resume part-time employment. He had been so severely affected that he would drop from a normal alertness into a deep sleep in a second. Now, his fellow patients could interfere as they saw what was about to happen; they quickly pressed the septal button for him, lest he be caught off guard by one of his sleep attacks, and roused him.

The patient said that he pressed this septal button frequently because it "felt good," and added, "It has a slightly erotic quality." (He stated that he could never intensify this feeling to the orgasic end-point.) After a period of frantic pressures, he reported a "nervous feeling." On the other hand, he designed a hair-pin device that locked the mesencephalic key, because it was so unpleasant.

One observation from the study of the second subject might be added to our account of this "somatopsychic" research. The latter patient found that the centromedian button not only alerted him but enabled him to recall memories that otherwise eluded his grasp. Instead of bringing pleasure, as the septal button did, it made him irritable. He claimed that the septal region brought "good feelings," sexual thoughts; he also used it to drive out "bad thoughts." Using the septal button to eliminate feelings of frustration and anger that followed the use of the centromedian button, he would press the pair of keys in combinations that ran the rate up to 1,100 per hour.[10]

A Contrasting Psychosomatic Approach

Heath's study serves as a sharp contrast to the psychosomatic approach, which focuses on the person rather than on his septal cells, and takes on a certain human quality that is very desirable, in spite of the looseness of its methods and its time-consuming efforts to bring insight and understanding into the interpersonal relationships of a patient. For all of its precision, Heath's method leaves the man untouched, and produces a new kind of dependency with no one knows what ultimate consequences, either for the tissues in the central nervous system now bombarded with electrical impulses or for the man as a whole.

Sleep as a Defensive Pattern

Exploring the personal histories of a series of patients who suffered from narcolepsy, Wayne Barker (1948b) found a variety of tensional patterns that had developed to the point where falling asleep ended what could not be managed or borne otherwise. What the somaticist would call a favorable "soil" or a constitutional predisposition is matched, in these case histories, by a slowly developing dialectic with the environment: not a fixed set of S-R relationships, not a single family pattern, not a precise social locale,

---

[10]Analogies between this button-pressing patient and the person who uses sexuality (or pills) to balance situationally aroused anxieties would be easy to draw, with the mounting curve of tension symbolizing the failure to make some more effective response to reality.

not even a single personality pattern underlies these approaches to the "sleep explosion," but meandering dialogues that can be reconstructed only with the skill of a good biographer and the clinically based hunches of the experienced therapist.

The patient was a 19-year-old high-school student, a Negro whose socially ambitious parents had high aspirations for their son and were doing their best to discipline him for that long climb to a professional status, and for a life better than they had been able to achieve. The highly organized mother had begun toilet training when her son was three months old, and the nonsuccess of her methods was symbolized by the fact that her son was still enuretic at age 12. Whatever had gone wrong, the facts indicated that the "pressure with love" had not produced growth in this case. His grades, however, were above average, and his manners and his bearing indicated that he possessed a kind of social maturity. He had broken with his boyhood gang, and now looked on their bad habits and their fighting as both silly and uncivilized.

A friendly relationship with a high-school coach convinced the boy, at 14, that his own goal was to be a physical-education teacher and a coach, not a doctor. There were many family scenes, for this choice deeply angered his father. The boy began to fall asleep in classes. This did not strike anyone as particularly noteworthy, but when he entered high school and had to plot his course "for keeps," the quarrels with his father and the "sleep attacks" grew pronounced and prolonged. A physician, prescribing benzedrine under the impression that he was dealing with a physical-medical problem, was not able to help; in spite of a good intelligence, the boy began to fail in his courses and to look like a potential dropout.

The youth was referred to Dr. Barker, who initiated sodium-amytal interviews in search of the underlying process behind the sleep seizures. He discovered that the mere discussion of physical education as a career would precipitate a kind of unintelligible muttering, a burst of aggression and an angry glare, and a sleep attack.

This method of diagnosis requires a formulation of the patient's problem. Since many cases will instruct the physician in the many pathways to that point of no return where stress becomes a somatic symptom, a free-wheeling psychosomatic formulation of the nature of the illness has to be made. In the light of his particular series, Dr. Barker sees the following common features as a recurring pattern:

1. There develops, as the individual matures, a need for self-differentiation even from those he loves most and from the guidance of those on whom he has been most dependent.

2. The individual may be lost in the shuffle with siblings, feel that he is rejected, and suffer from neglect or hostility; he will develop demands for affection, attention, recognition in his own right.

3. There can be poorly directed attempts to set up his own pattern of living, attempts which run sometimes counter to his own affectional needs, the family's goals, and the task of finding a place in a wider culture.

4. The dialectical process at work can lead to unsatisfactory exchanges with his environment, mounting conflicts, deeper insecurity, and exhaustion. What

is a bout of daytime sleeping, laziness, and neurotic fatigue in one adolescent can become, in the predisposed patient, a full-blown narcoleptic attack, which accentuates his helplessness (and possibly also expresses his hostility to those "authorities" who strive to make him into their own image.

5. Spreading from the major conflict to other sources of frustration and anger, an increasing number of signals come to touch off the sleep pattern. Like Pavlov's dogs who promptly fell asleep on being put in the harness, as a culmination of a long discrimination training that proved too difficult, such a patient now fits the concept of a vagotonic type, a "Basset-hound personality," that repeatedly reacts to stress with sleep.

Where the somaticist would conclude that this is a special type of visceral brain that needs some stimulating drug, or some built-in electrical alerting system, the psychosomaticist sees the problem as one of undoing a built-in response pattern, an undoing which must be guided by a patient redirection of growth and a reformulation of goals that will achieve a good identity and at the same time fulfill those lost and deep-seated needs for affection and a sense of worth.

The visceral brain that MacLean (1949) discusses in his treatment of psychosomatic illnesses includes the hypothalamus, thalamus, cingulate gyrus, hippocampus, and precuneus. It lies at the very center of the brain and is a relay system, affected by every inflowing excitation, distributing an outflow of neural impulses that instigate emotions, appetites, and desires. When the flow has been "educated," the influx of signals finally comes to involve the whole brain. Before an infant becomes a person among his peers, a *socius* in a society, a man with goals, the abstracted core that we call visceral brain ceases to be a mere explosive, undiscriminative center that spreads a diffuse excitation to muscles and glands. When the organism is not yet trained so that its motor apparatus can point, strike, flee, name, conceal intentions, or speak the truth, it is capable of "emoting," sobbing, suckling, or excreting, but it is not yet geared into a surrounding field or able to respect persons, time, place, or consequences. As the young learner asserts himself, even against a sheltering environment, and begins to react to signals from other persons, he may be said to come to terms with his world. In part the world shapes him, and in part he constructs it, converting what was at first a chaos into an ordered field with a structure.

This coming to terms of an organism (with its appetites and capacities) and a social milieu (with its counterdemands and expectations) is an irregular process, a seesaw of give-and-take, with explosive crisis-points of tension and frustration, that disrupt the even flow of behavior. Around these "flash points" of fear, pain, rage, anxiety, and resentment, the stream of behavior grows organized until anticipatory tensions and history-making reflections bind what began as a random stream of reflex adjustments that were mere "beads on a string" into a discriminating design for living, and sometimes into a psychosomatic illness.

The process can be viewed, from within, as a gradual spread of the viscera's control (via that head ganglion that mediates its claims), until the roving eye and the grasping hand appropriate whatever is judged as palatable or demanded from below. An alerted attention, on guard against dangers and intruders, protects the viscerally initiated thrust. The visceral brain thus extends its control as impulses spread over cingulate and hippocampal folds of the cortex, reaching forward into the frontal lobes and backward into precuneal and occipital areas. Converging, finally, upon the precentral gyrus, these streams of impulses, now shaped by the traces of former actions and "consequences," become commands for action and for movements in a field with a view to securing needed and palatable objects. Lust, hunger, rage, fear, nausea, whatever affective-impulsive thrusts arise from this primitive core of our being, move eyes and hands and voice until action converges on an appropriate target and consummation puts an end to the primary instigations, so that the drive is canceled. So viewed, the viscera move the body, transform the environment, and call the signals for escape, attacks, or constructive action.

Viewed from without, the process of coming to terms involves a relentless shaping and reshaping of an organism, originally little more than an "explosive" set of viscera with untrained appendages, into an expectant learner with some sense of what will follow what and of where he wants to go. The "shape of reality" teaches the viscera when and how to command its projicient apparatus, and how to behave *properly*. Whether it is human affection that is needed (and must be merited) or simple contacts and opportunities, this outer reality will reinforce some of the visceral claims and punish or turn a deaf ear to others. This "shape of reality" includes other persons, of course, with other viscerally motivated plans and counterdemands. Sometimes their greater power, or sheer mass, or numbers, give these others an *ultimate* control over the developing individual: they are as relentless as Ananke herself, the very essence of inexorable, unavoidable necessity, unchangeable, absolute, not to be manipulated, and never to be questioned. Shared beliefs can overwhelm the individual, or, discovering a clique of dissidents, he may make war on society, or be caught as an outsider in an "identity crisis." The optimism of the Darwinians is muted as we pause to realize the developing individual's task of discriminating among ideologies and shared beliefs that include superstitions and "laws" designed to exploit him. Realities and pseudorealities call for a power to structure his field, to stand back and reflect, to discriminate and choose, a power that is often lacking.

This conflict between visceral and interpersonal demands can exhaust all of the endurance, plasticity, and intelligence of the developing person, creating a residue of ungratified needs and affective disturbances whose overflow into organs can then create pathology. The visceral brain, on such occasions, becomes an integrating center that distributes more stimuli than the projicient apparatus can "liquidate," more autonomic outflow than can be absorbed by effective actions; and tears, indigestion, tachycardia, high blood pressure, ulcers, colitis, or asthma result.

PSYCHOSOMATIC AND SOMATOPSYCHIC RELATIONSHIPS

The Case of Neurocirculatory Asthenia

Many of the points we have been discussing are abundantly illustrated in the studies of what was at first called "soldier's heart." Similar symptom clusters have since been named effort syndrome, neurocirculatory asthenia, cardiac neurosis, anxiety attack, neurasthenia, vasomotor neurosis, irritable heart, and *la névrose d'angoisse*. A quartet of symptoms has occupied the center of attention, first directed in the Civil War to soldiers who broke down under fire, to infantrymen carrying a pack on their back, to men under extreme stress who showed palpitation, breathlessness, chest pain, easy fatigability. The "soldier's heart," however, is also found among civilians who carry no pack, who never saw a foxhole or a beachhead. Although it is common for the symptoms to emerge whenever effort is called for, the name "effort syndrome" does not describe the case very well when these same symptoms emerge suddenly while the subject is lying down, resting. Other symptoms that also appear in these patients are listed in their order of frequency in Table 10, which also gives symptom frequencies in a control sample.

The armies of Britain and of the United States looked on this disorder as warranting a limitation of military duty or a separation from the service. The likelihood of continued impairment is shown in a civilian group followed over a twenty-year period: 12 per cent recovered and experienced no recurrence; 15 per cent continued to show a significant disability; the balance of the cases were divided among groups that (1) showed frequent recurrence of symptoms but with no serious impairment, (2) had mild chronic symptoms, and (3) had a recurrence of symptoms whenever unusual stresses had to be met. In the course of taking the histories of a group of civilian patients in the postwar years, entrance into military service was reported as an occasion which provoked or exacerbated symptoms in 20 per cent of the group.

When index cases of neurocirculatory asthenia are studied in their family settings, some interesting relationships appear. Almost half the children (48.6 per cent) of such cases also show the disorder. If both parents of the index cases are normal, only 27.5 per cent of the siblings show the symptoms; if both parents are affected, 62 per cent of the siblings show the disorder; if only one parent is affected, 37.7 per cent of the siblings show the disorder (Wheeler et al. 1948). These facts need to be borne in mind when experimental studies of this type of patient show unusual susceptibility to standard stresses in the laboratory. Just how much the climate of a home, in which other members complain of these symptoms, may contribute to the development of the pattern we do not know, but it is quite apparent that a single sibling is a much less potent environmental factor than some of the other combinations.

The History-Taker and the Causes He Discovers

When Da Costa first studied 200 cases of "soldier's heart," he concluded that more than half the cases had been brought on by some other illness.

TABLE 10. *Frequency of Symptoms of Neurocirculatory Asthenia* (From Cohen and White 1951.) *

Symptom	Per Cent of 60 Subjects Showing the Symptom	Per Cent of 102 Controls Showing the Symptom
Palpitation	96.7	8.8
Tires easily	95.0	18.6
Breathlessness	90.0	12.7
Nervousness	87.6	26.5
Chest pain	85.0	9.8
Sighing	79.3	15.7
Dizziness	78.3	15.7
Faintness	70.0	11.8
Apprehensiveness	60.7	2.9
Headache	58.3	25.5
Paresthesias	58.2	7.2
Weakness	56.0	3.0
Trembling	53.5	16.7
Breath unsatisfactory	52.7	3.9
Insomnia	52.7	3.9
Unhappiness	50.0	2.1
Shakiness	46.5	15.7
Fatigued all the time	45.1	5.9
Sweating	44.9	33.0
Fear of death	42.8	2.0
Smothering	39.7	3.9
Syncope	36.7	10.8
Nervous chill	24.4	—
Urinary frequency	18.6	2.1
Vomiting and diarrhea	14.0	0.0
Anorexia	12.3	3.0

*The healthy controls consisted of 50 men and 11 women from a large industrial plant, and 41 healthy postpartum women from the Boston Lying-in Hospital.

Searching for physiological factors that might have sensitized the cardiovascular system, he found fever, dysentery, exhaustion, physical stress, and the stress arising from combat. Summarizing his findings, he identified this quartet: post-infective weakness, exhaustion, stress, and a probable constitutional weakness.

To these factors other military psychiatrists in our own time have added life-history data that seemed to predispose to the illness, but these data are so varied that no clear pattern has emerged. While some were urging that the extreme stress of combat proved too much for inadequately trained and toughened civilians, pointing to a background of sedentary living with little exercise, others found cases among the draft army in World War I who had been fully trained, and some were from the regular army, including "old soldiers" with an excellent record up to the moment when the symptoms emerged.

When Cohen and White questioned their civilian patients about the occasions which precipitated their first attack, they found

"...father's cruelty, rheumatic fever, malaria, death or serious illness of a parent or sibling, typhoid fever, sexual and marital problems, diarrhea, doctor's warnings about health, pneumonia, unusually difficult work, gonorrhea, unusual strain [of] heavy work, assignment to an isolated post, bombing, bad cold, serious maladjustment..., sandfly fever, unusual strife at home, influenza, poverty, malnutrition, step-parent [trouble], hookworm, troubles at school, jaundice, arrest and imprisonment, mastoidectomy, and preparation for overseas duty."

Looking more closely at their cases, these authors add that some of the first attacks occurred when no precipitating events could be named. "I was lying down, resting, and I had nothing in particular on my mind, when suddenly..." With some stresses of a fairly objective biological sort (physical illness and heavy work load), some of an interpersonal sort (family difficulties), and some "anxiety attacks of unknown origin," the psychological factor in this illness begins to be a highly generalized and somewhat vague "stress of life." A certain proportion of the cases, without any identifiable stress to report, remains to tempt the theoretician to posit some unconscious process.[11]

If we seek a definition of stress in the answers that patients give to their physician's first questions about situations that may have precipitated or worsened symptoms, we find that we can classify the responses into the following rough categories: chronic emotion-producing situations (88%), acute emotion-provoking situations (67%), other illnesses (54.7%), hard muscular work (53.9%), pregnancy (38.9%), army life (20%), cold (18.8%), heat (16.7%). To these frequently mentioned stresses, we would have to

---

[11]Cohen and White (1951) quote the director of the Josiah Macy Foundation as urging, "The positive diagnosis [of hysteria] is considerably strengthened if several exacerbations of symptoms or attacks have been immediately preceded by recurrence of the same or similar emotional conflicts. If the patient fails to recognize any connection between the emotional tension and the symptoms, and particularly if the patient has completely forgotten the emotional crisis or its time relationship to the onset of the symptoms, then the role of emotion as an etiological factor in precipating the symptoms is rendered highly probable." With the same type of logic, one could insist that in all cases there is a "feeling of guilt": either a patient confesses his guilt or denies it. In the latter case, the *worst* kind, of course, the guilt is either unconscious or the patient is dishonest, concealing what he knows to be present, and if it is unconscious it may take years to probe the very depths of the psyche.

add a "miscellaneous" group that would include many of the simple stresses that others meet in learning and adjusting *without* marked cardiovascular involvement. Speaking in public, giving a dinner, taking an important examination, talking to the boss, asking for a deserved raise—these stresses are so varied, the constitutional factor so difficult to estimate in a particular case, that the cautious clinician prefers to begin his study of a case as though it were of "unknown origin."

The Experimental Study of Reactions to Stress

For all of the diversity of verbal reports given by these patients, and the even more diverse theories which seek a particular kind of stress in a particular kind of personality, there is good evidence to show that these patients react to standard stresses in a special way.

A painful stimulus supplied by a beam from a hot lamp directed on a blackened area of the forehead produced responses in both patients and controls. The level of intensity at which subjects winced was lower for the patients than for controls; half the patients drew their heads away from the apparatus at an intensity where only 3 per cent of the controls did so.

A hand dynamometer was used to record maximum grip. Instructed to hold the dynamometer at a pressure of about 60 per cent of their maximum scores, the patients were not able to persist as long as the controls (36 as against 48 seconds, on the average).

A painful sphygmomanometer cuff elevated respiratory volume 39.6 per cent in the patients as against 10.4 per cent in the healthy controls. (No difference in blood pressure was found.)

Walking and running on a treadmill demonstrated that the patients had a poor ability to take up oxygen; they accomplished less work; and they built up "oxygen debts" that persisted and caused longer recovery periods. At rest the two groups showed no significant difference in oxygen consumption or in blood lactate. Efforts to reduce the difference through training were inconclusive. Any short-term stepping up of the work served, at least in the early trials, to accentuate the differences.

Dyspnea (subjective shortness of breath) occurred more frequently and at earlier points in the patients, who also complained of weakness, of legs giving out, and of dizziness, chest pains, headaches, trembling, and palpitation. These subjective symptoms appeared in the control groups, but with less intensity and frequency.

Even the mere placement of the patients' *hands in ice water* produced greater changes in pulse rate and in pulmonary ventilation than in controls.

Breathing CO_2 produced an increase in sighing in both groups (7.5 per minute in patients, 2.8 in controls). The patients described the feelings of smothering, of choking, and of being unable to get their breath as similar to what they experienced during their attacks.

With an autonomic system that registers so many types of stress in both cardiovascular and respiratory systems, and with a response pattern somewhat like that in anxiety attacks, it would be easy to posit an underlying anxiety factor. What about the rate of incidence in other psychosomatic disorders in which this same anxiety is assumed to play a role? Cohen and White report that the group which they followed over twenty years did not complain of other psychosomatic illnesses in any unusual frequency.[12]

A Few Concluding Remarks

The study of clinical and experimental findings in patients with neuro-circulatory asthenia is instructive. With the Cohen and White study as our model, we can appreciate many of the obscurities that run throughout psychosomatic literature. We found evidence for a constitutional factor, but were forced to recognize that it might prove to be a much larger component in some cases than in others. That it is not a general component is suggested by the low rate of incidence of other psychosomatic illnesses. That it is not a predisposition toward the development of a particular life-style is demonstrated by the fact that so many different types of personalities among the patients have been named by the dozen or more investigators who have given thought to this question.

We have seen how fashions have changed, the earlier students of the disorder looking for infections and physical stress, the later ones seeking out vulnerable life-styles and special types of interpersonal stress of a more personal sort. The range of stresses that one ought to consider is so great that those who construct personal biographies must examine data from early childhood, family settings, peer relationships, adolescent conflicts; class and caste positions, present coping mechanisms, and personal goals must be included. In a disorder of unknown origin of this type, a patient becomes a virtual projection test for the physician who must evaluate the psychological factor.

A cool appraisal of outcomes of a hundred such cases suggests that, while here and there an abrupt and rather sudden improvement is reported, the bulk of the group show recurrence or persistence of symptoms. Cohen and White cannot find evidence in favor of any particular form of therapy; simple reassurance and the lapse of time produce as good results as "prolonged psychotherapy, psychoanalysis, electric convulsion procedures, ergotamine tartrate, and adrenal denervation." In a disorder that has many causes and that is both constitutional and psychogenic (in varying proportions), a flexible procedure has to be employed. Instead, much of the literature seems to have been written by convinced extremists, ranging from those who virtually dismiss the psychogenic component to those who insist that "neurocirculatory asthenia does not exist without neurosis or character disturbance" (Weiss 1952).

---

[12]The recall of patients is not accurate. Interview data, when compared with clinical records, are found to be inaccurate. Cohen and White discovered that their patients with neurocirculatory asthenia had reported an average of 6.6 symptoms when they were first studied, but years later they remembered an average of only 1.5 symptoms. Where no running account of full clinical studies of other psychosomatic illnesses is kept, a statement that such illnesses were of no higher frequency than normal among the patients is also a clinical opinion.

Appearing in every conceivable personality type, worsened by all manner of stresses, having no specific etiology, associated irregularly with other illnesses and sometimes with general good health, sometimes arising for no discoverable reason, betraying lowered thresholds to standard laboratory stress stimuli, and showing inefficient use of oxygen under exercise, neurocirculatory asthenia is both psychosomatic and somatopsychic. Once on board, it can operate in the same fashion as chronic hypertension to produce further responses to the illness itself. These could conceivably take the form of claustrophobia, reduction of social life, fear of heart failure, feelings of rebellion and resentment at demands, or restrictions on living. In dealing with these patients, some of the treatment must involve an education of the patient so that he understands his disorder and his own reaction to it. How much the symptoms can be improved by psychotherapy is never known before careful study; there is no evidence that a particular form of therapy is of special value for this disorder.

THE CASE OF ESSENTIAL HYPERTENSION

The journal and the society formed to serve the interests of those concerned with a developing body of theory and research on a group of illnesses where psyche and soma are closely intertwined have placed their principal emphasis on one of the two directions in the relationship. They stress the influence of psychological factors (and cultural matrix) on the functioning of the bodily processes. Holistic in their emphasis, they have tended to be concerned about the influence of the higher units on the lower members of the habit hierarchy. Throughout this brief period, a kind of psychoanalytic holism has prevailed, as though Freud's "Anatomy of the Personality" (1933) had served as the orienting paradigm for the bulk of the studies (Alexander 1939a is a good example of this trend).

Since all Westerners live in the same competitive civilization, and since everyone who is socialized has learned to apply some restraint to whatever hostilities have developed, Alexander's paradigm (quoted earlier in this chapter) calls for a search for quantitative differences, the identification of unique methods of coping with frustration, the location of specific roles, as well as the examination of other possible causes. Alexander was among those who thought that a particular personality pattern was involved, and that the majority of hypertensives were psychoneurotic.

As though to document the theoretical model offered by Alexander, and to show what a free ventilation of hostility can do for such a patient, Wolf *et al.* (1955) describe one of their hypertensives:

"A 40-year-old man, a dealer in illicit goods, had been raised by a tyrannical mother, dominated by his wife, bullied by his brother-in-law. He suffered from chronically high blood pressure and recurrent attacks of paroxysmal auricular tachycardia, with a pulse of double or triple normal rates during the attack. A chronically elevated blood pressure of 165/105 was typical of the examinations made in office visits. Anxiety and hostility were easily drawn out and stress interviews induced weeping, expressions of resentment and depression and a ventricular rate of 164. Advised on one occasion to deal with his problems more directly and overtly he promptly left the laboratory and returned an hour later after 'beating up' his brother-in-law. At that time his blood pressure was 125/85. He said that he felt relaxed and vindicated."

There is another type of case report that suggests another kind of psychosomatic relationship.

Isberg (1956) described a patient, hospitalized for schizophrenia, who imagined that those around him were plotting to kill him. In the midst of an attack of acute panic, he died of congestive heart failure. He had brought a long-standing heart condition with him into hospital (he was in a jail hospital, convicted of gambling). The slowly developing condition in this man's arterial system had not produced any great concern, any more than the occasional mild attacks of dyspnea and precordial distress. There did not seem to be any psychogenic basis for the arterial stenosis. The anxieties he ventilated in hospital were all related to his paranoid delusion, not to his heart trouble.

A third set of relationships is more frequently seen in the cardiologist's patients. A series of somatic changes that culminate in a sudden "heart attack" produces a dramatic crisis which centers attention on the heart. Even without an overt attack, an "alarming condition" may be revealed by a thorough examination, and it is understood as a vital threat. From this pair of events, some become fearful of impending death, and should a particular patient recall that his father had died of a heart attack during an angry row with the patient, the latter's old guilt feelings can be revived; then the diagnosis assumes the quality of an awesome and deserved judgment. "How I hated him! And now I am going to get it."

If, in addition, current stresses produce an aggravation of the perceptible symptoms of a defective circulatory system, ordinary clashes of will can be converted into events with a potentially lethal quality. When a husband and father has to leave the television set when a basketball game reaches a climax, so that his heart can return to normal, his dramatic exit reveals to all in the family circle just how vulnerable he is. What tact and restraint will be called for, both on his part and on theirs, if he is not to drift into exploiting his heart condition, so that the household is coerced to bend to his will; how resentful he can become when their callous indifference rides roughshod over his wishes or his complaints. He is tempted to imagine a lethal intent on their part.

When a real and rational restriction is imposed on the patient's activities, his powers of adaptation may be tested. The more he is "imprisoned," the more intensively and imaginatively he will have to cultivate his interests in those areas which are still open. The anger that he has hitherto often shown, when frustrated, is likely to occur more frequently now, since there are so many occasions that block him. His hostility may be directed not only at those who are inconsiderate but also at his own body and his own "prisoner status." In anger at the very condition which restricts him (and which, like all inevitables, *has* to be respected), a patient will sometimes behave in an almost suicidal manner, in a savage and juvenile defiance of fate, choosing the very action with lethal risk.

A balanced, realistic assessment of his life-situation and its risks, along with a revision of what demands he makes upon himself, is not always easily accomplished. If he happens to have an extremely narrow conception of what is worthwhile in life, he may persist in doing that which to him means maleness, freedom, significance. On the other hand, a patient may have already been living in fear of sailing too close to the wind: now he has a sanction for his retreat from life. Coolly, and with carefully mustered statistics, Paul Dudley White (White *et al.* 1958) urges his patients to return to their former occupations (ruling out only the extremely demanding and hazardous ones), for the figures show that those who do return do as well, live as long, are as free from recurrent attacks, as those who enter a premature retirement from life and avoid all stress and effort. But this return to normal activity has to be accomplished within reason, and at a pace suitable to capacities. The patient is caught between impulses which would lead to a regressive withdrawal from life and a hypochondriacal overconcern about his heart, and a rebellious and suicidal defiance of his somatic condition and of all those who speak of caution.

Any interpersonal relationship that is already highly charged, or poorly managed, can now deteriorate, each side giving the other "just cause" for resentment. A poor method of coping with frustration can now worsen, "justified" by this new biological insult (which can now be used as a rationalization). Unresolved anxieties in other spheres can now become serious sources of inhibition. (Is it safe to continue sexual relationships when my heart is so vulnerable?) If a spouse is already overconcerned and unnecessarily restrictive, the heart condition will add fuel to her already excessive tendency to manage the patient. Any residue of an earlier adolescent rebellion will find new causes for a resistance to advice, even when it is timely.

There are also pervasive changes in the patient's phenomenal world. The sight of an athlete jumping to make a basket, the vision of adolescents dancing to rock and roll (with what now appears as "violence"), the invitations of a coquettish female, the vigor of an orator can produce an almost reflexive reaction in the patient: "That is not for me." A distance has developed suddenly between a man and a dozen roles he would have entered more readily in earlier days. His life-space has changed, and if this process is permitted to continue unchecked, it can lead into depression, for those who withdraw find themselves "out of it," outsiders looking in, empty and disaffected. To achieve "peace of body" they cut vital ties and lose sources of strength.

We can see, therefore, that both the diagnosis and the symptoms can release and intensify already existing trends in a personality. The challenges that arise in such a life (in business relationships, in response to the threat of a divorce, in the course of dealing with an adolescent son) can easily pass into vicious cycles of violent rage, self-pity, and martyrdom, or into a fearful withdrawal from life. The course chosen depends in large measure on the groundwork that already exists, the "precardiac" personality. It is the added fillip given to these old trends, the use that is made of the illness, that now becomes a somatopsychic effect. If the somatic changes are themselves caused or facilitated by preexisting personality conflicts, then we have a *psychosomatopsychic* cycle.

Alexander (1939b) has described a case of essential hypertension, treated in an extended series of psychoanalytic interviews. He described the man as filled with an unconscious, masochistic, feminine set of wishes that were unacceptable to the other components that made him try to "act like a man." The unconscious set drove him to rebellion, increased his competitiveness and ambition, and even led to many actions that created guilt, fear of retaliation, and self-disgust; these trends, expressed, ended in intensifying his longing for dependence and retreat. It is in such a mixture of a success ideology and a longing for affection and acceptance that hypertension can arise, with symptoms that mingle with and intensify the already existing conflict in motivation.

Sometimes a brief improvement in a set of neurotic relationships can arise because the real "insult" and impairment from a heart attack seem to a guilt-ridden patient to pay off old scores. He feels that he has now suffered enough. The attack may also produce a new and more considerate reaction from those who surround the patient. Both of these gains tend to be of short duration. If he expected everyone to continue to be alerted to his problem, as they were immediately following the diagnosis or the attack, he will be doomed to disappointment; he will have to develop the coping mechanisms that any impaired person must have, whether his disorder is psychosomatic or as impersonal as a hip fracture or a congenital deformity. The new factor may tempt him to give no ground, ask for no favors, deny the impairment, carry a full man's share; in this denial of his incapacity, he may discover that he is, in fact, less mature, less strong and capable than he thought. A subtle resentment (and even hatred) against those who "expect too much" reveals that there are risks in this role, that he is projecting blame for his own malfeasance, even when his pride is mainly responsible. Or he may resign his directorship as a means of finding the energies with which to keep up with his younger wife (as he confides to his intimates), whose vitality he begins to resent and even to complain about.

It is all too easy for such a patient to use his symptoms as a method of binding all anxieties, of explaining all his hesitancies and malfeasance, and of refusing to evaluate his performance objectively in other areas. Landes and Bolles (1942) showed this lack of rational and objective self-evaluation to exist in a set of five groups of physical impairments that had begun early in life. Of the hundred cases, nine had found satisfactory paths to maturity; 91 fell into the withdrawn, compensatory, obliterative (denying), or unsatisfactory substitute activity categories. In these women whose impairment occurred so very early (spastics, epileptics, orthopedics, cardiacs), there was

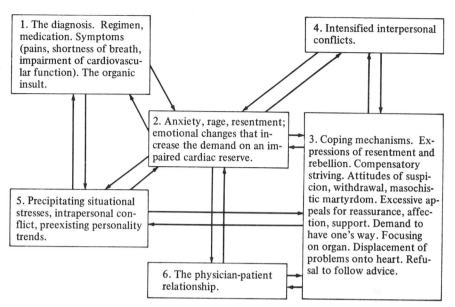

FIGURE 8. VICIOUS CYCLES AT WORK IN THE CARDIOVASCULAR CASE. (Adapted from Reiser and Bakst 1959.)

a greater reason for the impairment to write its effect into the still unformed personality structure. When they had become adults, the group as a whole appeared to those who studied them as generally immature, although the physical changes of adolescence had not been delayed, and as more dependent on and more closely attached to their parents and their immediate family than was normal. They had remained psychosexually less mature, with a lower-than-normal sexual drive. The differences noted seemed to depend somewhat on the age at which the impairment occurred, its severity, and on the manner in which those immediately around them reacted to the deficit, but the trends reveal, in exaggerated form, what every case of somatic impairment undergoes, even if in milder form.

The heart specialist, who deals with the problems of patients with coronaries, neurocirculatory asthenia, and essential hypertension, and who is alerted to the risks his patients run, can unwittingly intensify a patient's alarm and increase a hypochondriacal centering of interest on an organ, if he is not very careful. Even his prudent advice: "Do what you feel you can. Lift what is not too heavy. Face what you can safely tolerate. Live right. Try to function at a near-normal level, but be careful not to exceed prudent limits," can add iatrogenic weighting to already existent trends in the patient's personality, as the patient makes his own interpretation of this all-too-vague advice.

If we attempt to diagram (see Fig. 8) the sequence of events, beginning with (1) the fact of disordered cardiac function, its diagnosis, and the institution of a regimen of restricted living immediately following the "attack," we must include (2) the anxiety that is aroused by the attack itself. For this anxiety the patient will have already formed (3) a variety of coping mechanisms, some of which will be distinctly nonadjustive, and may produce (4) interpersonal difficulties, worsen cardiac symptoms, and still further intensify those somatic expressions of anxiety that are so often found in psychosomatic illnesses. Other sources of anxiety (intensified by this cycle), old scars, present situations, and (5) preexisting personality trends may also intensify the original condition, the anxiety that arises from it, and the nonadjustive coping mechanisms. To this complex the physician can add (6) a physician-caused component that arises from his failure to read his patient right, his professional overconcern, his clumsy efforts to remake a personality, his dogmatic insistence on "typing" the patient, and other failings.

Reiser's diagram reminds us that the mind-body relationships that are significant for the clinician run in two directions. Among the consequences of illness are important adjustment problems, psychological changes that are properly described as somatopsychic; one set of variables the alert physician must also consider when he strives to account for a psychosomatic illness lies in this same psychological area. Placed in proper perspective, the enthusiasms of those who have restored an interest in the patient as a whole contribute both to the understanding of illness and to the management of patients.

EPILOG

Psychosomatic disorders have contributed their share to the history of miraculous cures, from which some enthusiasts have hastily concluded that in all of these patients there is a psychological factor that is primary. Some have gone on to seek a particular life-style, a particular attitude, or a particular social role for each type of illness. Throughout this movement of reform there has been a recurrent insistence: "The physician must treat the whole man."

This humane emphasis has produced good effects, and some excesses. The optimism engendered by case studies of asthma cured by hypnosis, of identity crises that, having caused narcolepsy, could then be corrected to produce a symptom-free patient, have turned out to be exceptional instances in an extended series that includes a few cases of a predominantly organic character, and many that are "mixed" in nature.

The urge to type patients as a first step in clinical efficiency has proved to be a stumbling block, capable of interfering with scientific medicine.[13] The holistically minded physician, impelled to pay attention to the largest of those concentric rings of causation, where evidence is least reliable, can miss what lies near and is more open to management.

---

[13]Twenty-five years after the founding of the Society for Psychosomatic Medicine, one of its early members, Louis N. Katz (1964), observed: "In the early days of the American Psychosomatic Society I belonged to it, but after a few years I gave up because the psychologists and psychiatrists were interested in abstract information, and the view in my own discipline (physiology) is that abstract information makes good literature but is not science, and also because I didn't like the concentration on the psyche and the neglect of the soma. I hope that the organization and others have changed."

Neither the concept of a characteristic asthma personality, nor the notion of a general psychosomatic susceptibility, nor the notion of a specific conscious attitude for each of these illnesses has stood up under close scutiny. We have all too seldom been given the much-needed evidence from control series that is required for the proper evaluation of causes or therapies.

The literature of psychosomatic medicine has been produced by organicists, by psychotherapists, and by a few who are open-minded enough to be eclectic. The latter have discovered psychosomatic problems, rather than finished answers. We need more such studies as that of Cohen and White (1951), a type of investigation in sharp contrast to many that have been able to "demonstrate" relationships and have applied what, at worst, is mere psychoanalogy.

Chapter 8 • Breakdowns in Self-Regulation

Absurd at first glance, the notion of self-regulation is also offensive to some. It smacks of egotism and hypocrisy; for an instant we think of these experts of Madison Avenue who produce "images" for corporations or for politicans on the make. On the interpersonal plane it would seem that simple and direct action in response to the challenges of this world, simple honesty in our human give-and-take, would suffice. There is even a suggestion of futility about the notion: almost intuitively we feel that the person we are is not an object we can do much of anything about. Can a man, by taking thought, alter his nature, or regulate it?

The thought models we use in describing man—at least three of them—tend to omit or discount the value of any such self-regulative process. The Pavlovian model omits it altogether. Reflexes are combined as they are aroused by serial stimulations: involved in recurrent sequences, the earlier members of the series come to arouse the later ones in advance. Expectation is simply an indication of a former rehearsal; if the shape of things to come is foreshadowed in our expectant posture, that is simply because repeated conditioning has stamped upon our very postures the shape of the environmental frame. Like two lovers who have sat too long on a gravestone and who walk away imprinted, such basic groupings as the family and the peer group, not to mention the wider society, are internalized in our conditioned responses.

The "trial and error" model that Thorndike's pioneer studies of learning established as the basis of educational theory in this country at the turn of the century seemed a better one to many, because it gave a lively place to the individual's needs and wishes. Yet, it also led us to think of a set of in-between mechanisms forced into shape as a motivated learner was battered by unrelenting obstacles that left only one open path to gratification. The pressure from animal needs, and a compressing framework (cage or maze) without, a slow, bumbling, gradual shaping with a variable and flexible course (and with fixations in blind alleys) resulted nonetheless in a pattern, a made thing. Free to fail or to take as long as his needs permitted, the shape of the self-regulatory "set for the maze," the "goalward orientation," and the habit chains that carried the maze-wise animal through a series of twists and turns were all as predetermined as the design on a newly minted coin. Self-regulation became need-regulation-in-a-maze. If one of the Cabots emerged from Beacon Hill, we could credit the marks of his good breeding to the precision of the Cabot training in that prestigious locale, with its Latin school, prep school, dancing class, riding, sailing, Harvard Yard, and Law School, to say nothing of the uncles, cousins, sisters, and aunts who provided punishments and rewards in this living maze.

The third thought model is equally discouraging, though as we first use it, there is such a complexity about it that it makes the simpler behavioristic models seem naive. If the ego of the Freudian model is shaped to deal with reality (in much the same manner that any follower of Thorndike or Pavlov would insist on), it is encased in a fantasied future, an ego-ideal, an internalized conscience (superego); and it floats on a protoplasmic base, each cell and molecule of which is charged with instinctual forces and racial memories. Perhaps such an ego has the *illusion* of some divine origin and destination, when it mistakes the voice of conscience for something ultimate. Its energies arise, nonetheless, from down within the cells; its incorporated ego-ideal is borrowed from a very human parent with feet of clay; and its censoring conscience still bears the marks of that struggle through early toilet training, when now a Good Mother smiled as she told him he was a good boy, or now a Bad Mother scolded him so that he felt banished to some outer Sheol. The worst feature of the Freudian ego's task is that the majority of the forces that instigate and hound him are hidden from his ken. Who knows from what remote quarter that free-floating anxiety or nameless dread, which sometimes arises, actually originates? Even his own rationalizations that defend his actions from outer critics, he discovers, as he becomes more mature, can have a phony quality: he has plausible reasons and real reasons, and the latter are so often unknown. "I do not like you, Dr. Fell, the reason...," and if he is honest with himself, he stops. Sheer silence is often far more honest than the reasons he might give.

So the absurdity of the concept of self-regulation becomes apparent as soon as we examine the models we have been using as devices to represent human action. Absurd or not, we know the difference between the man who can make a promise and guarantee its fulfillment by his deed, and one who can scarcely regulate his actions until he is out of sight. We know the difference between a Henry Miller and the man of good breeding: the one is obsessed with four-letter words that refer to sex and excrement; the other avoids offending and moves with a grace and charm that draws others toward him. We know a troubled saint, when we see one: he even offends us a little by his constant concerns that remind us of how faltering our own vigilance is. Thus common sense alerts us to important differences which must be placed within whatever model for man we choose.

The man who is obsessed by sex cannot frame a sentence without four-letter words creeping in, or make a plan without the irruption of some genital element. The woman with a belltower phobia is depressed by the sound of church bells on a sunny Sunday morning, and her phobia spreads until she no longer wants to walk down Main Street, where the carillon tower stands. The compulsive Gandhi must be unaggressively nonviolent, and thinks he should renounce his victory if he forces the British consul to give in without love.

In the phobic-obsessive-compulsive person, the part has begun to regulate the whole, and the ego is troubled by forces beyond its control, to the point where it no longer feels in charge: superego, ego, and id are at war. The superego either is not evaluating the ego's action properly or can no longer make it conform. The phobic often knows his fears are foolish, yet cannot arrest them. The compulsively perfectionist person cries out against his own hypertrophied conscience to ask, "Why am I always robbed of victory by a keen awareness of my shortcomings?" The obsessive complains, "Why do these horrid thoughts keep irrupting, and—of all occasions—when I am on the way to the confessional?"

The problem that we pose is at least three-sided: (1) What is the nature of this breakdown in self-regulation, whether in the form of hypertrophy of the parts or an abdication of the regnant self? (2) What shall we say about the sources of strength and weakness in this force that normally gives balance and poise to the acting self?[1] (3) How can anyone give such a self, when it becomes deregulated, a new awareness and a new meaning to existence that will enable it to bring impulses back into harmony?

The very statement of the problem suggests that the models we have been using are inadequate. Must we depend on something outside the individual, some conditioner who will bring the parts back into line, inhibiting here, facilitating there, carrying out a kind of social drill that the family and peers of the individual had not provided? Shall we take him into a sanitarium, a well-run maze, and put him through a series of training settings in which, by trial and error, he can stumble into the desirable chain of responses that will enable him to be returned to the larger social maze, ready to run in conforming patterns? Is there some transmissible *charisma*, some charged insight that can be given to the weakened one, that will lift a self to greater awareness and new strength in self-regulation, replacing the present weak and foolish awareness with a synthesizing power?

Once we put a *will* back into our thought model of man, we can see that more is involved than medication or social drill, but it has been almost half a century since anyone has phrased the problem in these terms. Once Ribot wrote about *Maladies de la volonté* and Boutonier about *Défaillance de la volonté*. Once there was a sickness of the will, it seems, or losses of a willpower that could be restored. All this seems strangely old-fashioned. Now we speak of

---

[1]Smuts (1927) puts his ideal for the human personality in these words: "The ideal personality is he in whom this inner control is sufficiently powerful, whether by conscious will or some unconscious activity, to harmonize all the discordant elements of the personal character into one harmonious whole, and to restrain all wayward, random activities which are in conflict with that harmony."

a loss of motivation, and we are quick to reduce motivation to (1) instincts, emotions, and primitive needs, (2) conditioned impulses, (3) affects arising from the frustration of the preceding two factors, and (4) instigators, pleasures, and palatabilities with valence. We are so inclined, in these behavioristic and anthropological days, to have more faith in material arrangements, in-want some firm formula for the establishment or conversion of energies into stigators, and conditioning routines than in mere words or insights, that we more harmonious forms. The problems that the charisma of the priest dealt with remain.

THE TYPES OF BREAKDOWN IN SELF-REGULATION

There are three principal types of breakdown that are commonly linked in the obsessive-compulsive neurosis: obsessions, compulsions, and phobias. To these we propose to add a fourth type, a failure in the preconscious processing of stimulation, which permits a kind of perceiving without feeling, a severe loss of motivation. Janet called it the *"feeling* of emptiness," since the words *empty, dry, drained,* were on the lips of these patients so often; he included in his descriptions a more serious form that he called "the *state* of emptiness." Whereas in the former the person was painfully aware of his lack of feeling, in the latter an apathy had descended, a complete indifference that made these patients indistinguishable from some kinds of dementia praecox. All four represent failures in the normal self-regulative process; we shall see how the fourth type is linked with the others as we discover how, in battling with the feeling of emptiness and in seeking to restore the normal feelings, the empty ones seek out excitations, happenings, ways of arousing their sluggish systems so that they feel good again.

A chapter on breakdowns in self-regulation is an appropriate place to discuss what even today many would call "character weaknesses"—addictions, sexual deviations, crimes against persons or property, and other so-called antisocial behaviors—although the word "character" suggests a moral evaluation rather than a psychological process. The problem of antisocial behavior is of such magnitude that a book on abnormal behavior cannot slight it. The total population in the three categories of "habitual criminals," "homosexuals," and "alcoholics" who bring their troubles to clinics and courts, who disturb their families and their fellow citizens, must lie somewhere between ten and eighteen million in the United States alone. In this discussion the reader must take pains to distinguish between a psychological and a social or legal view of abnormal behavior, especially the common-law concept of "insanity." The latter, according to the 125-year-old M'Naghten Rule, refers to a person who has been judged by a court to be "legally insane," that is, unable to distinguish between right and wrong and hence not responsible for his conduct.

THE PHOBIAS

More clear-cut than the other three groups, the phobias represent exaggerated fears (of objects, persons, situations) that the patient himself may regard as foolish or exaggerated. Neither reasoning nor ordinary training methods seem to correct these stubborn fears; and both the precautions taken against the feared objects and the absurd methods of bypassing them give these maneuvers an absurd quality. William Ellery Leonard (1927) has described how his family had to move every stick of furniture to a new home, duplicating the arrangement of the pieces, in order to spare him from any recurrence of a catastrophic fear. In a case of agoraphobia (fear of open spaces) a 40-year-old woman was afraid to leave her home, cross the street, go to the market, alone. Holding the hand of a six-year-old child, she could do all these things.

When there is a fear of dirt or poisons or impurity, and when these fears are associated with a compulsive and often magical method of conjuring away guilt, uncleanness, or evil influences, and when the surface manifestations are numerous and constantly changing, we are tempted to set up a class in which the "morbid guilt" is the central feature. Such a class with a common ethical core raises questions about the sources of guilt, and the morbid, absurd, magical aspects of the behavior suggest that some primitive, infantile root process may provide a hidden meaning to such fears. When the phobias (such as the fear of mad dogs) come and go with fluctuations in well-being, they may refer to some old occasion, some reasonable origin, but their periodic recurrence also points to the current pressures or to a defective hygiene of living, expressing changes in a general state of adjustment rather than a simple bit of conditioning in past history.[2]

The absurdity of some phobias, coupled with the intensity of the dread, suggests that they may function as displacements from some other sources that an immature person may have originally had difficulty in coping with. The discovery of such sources, followed by ventilation and reeducation, would then seem to provide hope of relief for the patient, except, perhaps, when this displacing process expresses: (1) a fundamental weakness in the way of coping with difficulties; (2) an early infantile source that has now ramified to affect most of the vital decisions of life; and (3) overwhelming pressures in a current life-situation that are too difficult to cope with and impossible to escape.

Phobias may also represent the concentration on a single source of a stream of diffuse anxieties with multiple causes. The reality that calls for the most diverse skills, the most careful organization in living, and a considerable supply of energy is falsely simplified as attention is concentrated on the object of the phobia. This latter serves to symbolize, bind, and conceal

---

[2]A similar ebb and flow, with the changing circumstances of living, is sometimes seen in the so-called phantom limb. Originally experienced during a brief period following an amputation, the phantom usually disappears and remains forgotten. In a few instances a resurgence of a "painful phantom" occurs at times when the affairs of the patient are going badly, when psychological tension is running low, when interest and active involvement in successful pursuits falter. As though kept down and overlaid when current affairs are running properly, the resurgent phantom is not so much caused by past events as released by the current ego-weakness.

what an alert and vigilant analysis might find overwhelming. A semimagical counterphobic struggle is simpler. Where others experience a free-floating anxiety, a vague and nameless dread, or a dull and ineffable sense of incompleteness, the phobic has bound, simplified, sharpened, and displaced his diffuse concerns onto a single object. Sometimes it is easier to battle against real filth than to manage a poorly organized life.

Trains, mountains, closed spaces, sharp knives, precipices, animals, crowds, public performances, dirt, poisons—the list is endless, and the careful classifier would take on the obsessive traits of his patients were he to pursue the ordering of these fears with too great concern. With many widely different interpretations, one common point of agreement unites clinical theory and practice in the formula: "The phobia is an alibi. It is not what it seems, nor as absurd" (see Ey, Bernard, and Brisset 1963, pp. 378 ff).[3]

Coupled with his phobias, the patient commonly develops roundabout ways of avoiding these feared occasions. He cleans incessantly, he never takes a train, he cannot move into a new home, he never goes out, he wears dark glasses or pulls the shades, he exterminates all "pests." He may attach himself to a person, a cult, a shelter, a ritual, to some type of guidance or reassurance that reduces his anxiety. An addiction to psychotherapy might be another of these counterphobic procedures. In the obsessions and compulsions we shall see some of the finer flowers of this counterphobic tree, whose branches reach into so many phases of living.

With more than one phobia on board, a patient is forced to live "on the alert," and if phobias and counterphobic efforts multiply, the free space may be so preempted that there is no room for productive living.

An American soldier was hospitalized, referred by his medical officer because of a phobia of insanity. The history that he gave revealed that, as an adolescent, he had felt out of it, rejected by his peers. "They did not like me." He was convinced that he was a mathematical genius: his teachers, his success in his studies, and the attitudes of his parents had proved this. With a mediocre attainment in other fields and with his almost complete lack of social skills, he concentrated his efforts on this one gift, determined to become the first mathematician of the world.

His central concern was to protect his brain from anything that would impair its functioning in the slightest. He slept on his right side, he controlled his eating and his exercise, he took no liquor, he refused paregoric that had been prescribed, he governed himself with rigid rules as though his mind were a mathematical equation to be precisely balanced. His strong conviction of his superiority and his exaggerated aspirations were matched by a hypertrophied concern lest some small flaw appear, some unobserved but noxious factor that would impair the planned perfection of his mind.

---

[3]Henri Ey (p. 384) points to one of the special problems that the analytic therapist discovers in these patients. To stretch out on a couch, while he is observed by an analyst out of his range of vision, and to expose his thoughts in an uninhibited series of free associations arouse something akin to panic in such a fearful one. His "secret-keeping" is already in trouble, what with "thought robberies" and "invasive" ideas.

Finding a job, being drafted into the army, being assigned to tasks by a sergeant who neither knew enough nor cared enough to share this youth's concerns created an ever deepening disorganization until he began to fear for his sanity. He had left a job where he had to handle metallic lead because the poison might affect his brain. With the army, in England, he worried about working in the heat; and when his blood pressure was found to be elevated, he was sure that his brain cells would be affected. Moreover, if he were to faint, the momentary circulatory change might harm the cortical cells. Jobs that exposed him to gases, oils, or solvents were all feared. Minor impairments in brain function that would pass unnoticed in an ordinary mind would be critical in his case. (The coarser tissues of the common run of men, he thought, are less vulnerable.)

This patient wanted to take every possible test that could be given: blood tests, EEG's, intelligence tests, tests of special functions. These, he hoped, would reveal any small sign of impairment. They were additional coping devices, motivated by the anxieties which his forced breathing, careful dieting, exercise, and sleeping habits never quite managed to contain (see Darmstatter 1949).

Those who study and treat these phobics are struck by the exaggerations and absurdities of the fears, and, regarding them as alibis, tend to seek some inner cause. But if these fears are motivated by instinctual forces that have been repressed and displaced, as the analysts believe, they do not strike the phobic in this fashion. He would be at peace, he is sure, if it were not for those conditions *outside*. The feelings of inferiority which Darmstatter's phobic denied were replaced by the fears of outside "poisons" and threats. Within, he felt he was especially superior.

Although a phobic's family may humor him, yielding again and again to his foolish fears and complicating the life of a household (as was the case with William Ellery Leonard) as they try to protect the phobic one and ease his existence, this sometimes becomes impossible. Even the patience of a therapist may be tried beyond his endurance, and he will feel impelled to cut through the endless ramifications of free associations, the elaborations and defenses of doubt. Time, patience, and effort to adjust to the patient reach a limit. Sullivan (1940, pp. 112-13) tells of a phobic artist who balked at marketing his paintings. One day, coming downstairs with a painting to take to his dealer, he looked down the stairwell, and, seized with vertigo and fearful lest he throw himself over the rail, he crept back to his studio and called his wife. She had to become his intermediary, while he retreated into himself. Though the weakness was his, and though his wife was the dominant one, she became an accessory to his phobia while he grew increasingly fearful. When, in desperation, a psychiatrist was called and the patient was hospitalized and put on an institutional regime that completely disregarded his phobia, Sullivan notes that he promptly reverted to a simple obsessional condition without his disabling fear of stairs.

THE OBSESSIONS

In facing the task of describing obsessions, it is important to keep in mind the essential characteristic of this group of phenomena. Running through all the types of obsessive thoughts is their escape from control, the breakdown in the normal regulation of thinking and action. The thought that escapes is not always one that violates the conscience of a man, or his sense of fitness. The Guillaume Monods (see d'Allonnes 1908) and the Joseph Smiths, the Mohammeds and the prophets, also betray a breaking loose of a part of the self-system, an invasion of that inner citadel where thoughts arise. That which irrupts may be devilish, obscene, violently aggressive: the posturings and the obscenities and blasphemies that cropped out in the convent of Loudun (see Huxley 1953) were diametrically opposed to everything the nuns had learned in their training for a sacred vocation. It can be as irrelevant and inconsequential as a meaningless phrase, a tune, a tendency to count, an impulse to substitute a meandering introspection for the practical work of the day. It can arise, cloaked in an aura of belief, with all the conviction of a revelation from on high. The array of obsessions reminds us that any configuration in our action systems can break loose from its moorings: a hypnagogic image that, in wordless but clear outline, leaps before the eye of the man about to fall asleep; the blasphemous phrase, "Sell Christ!" that annoyed Bunyan and brought the companion thought of the hell that would await him if he were to obey the voice; a nonsense phrase that, like some disengaged bit of a sentence, courses over reverberatory circuits; a voice that speaks from the Heavens; the persistent thought of what lies beneath the garments of the person standing opposite one. Forbidden, irrelevant, annoying, sacred, terrifying: to one they will be merely so much excess baggage to disregard, to another the sign of impending insanity, and to a third the sign of being one of the elect.

The example that one would find in the clinic's files would probably show, in most cases, that the obsessive trends (1) run counter to the dominant values and purposes of the person, (2) are so heavily charged with emotion and so insistent and recurrent as to suggest that the thought trends have some close affiliation with deep-lying sources of biological energies, and (3) are so disruptive, annoying, and threatening to the integrity of the person that he feels both constrained and disorganized by them. But there will be no major trend that the clinic's cases will not exemplify: obsessions about money (and poverty), excessive greed (and a compulsive giving), obscene thoughts (and the counteractive compulsions toward purity), obsessions about physical attractiveness (and especially about its possible loss), childlessness (and pseudopregnancies). Characterized by one observer as "the antinomic man," these patients are caught between such opposites as superiority-inferiority, clairvoyance and "thought-thefts," obsessions about the meaninglessness of life and preoccupations with metaphysical questions that seek out the very ground of existence. Perhaps the most common concerns center about love and hate, sex and aggression, guilt and perfection, and the basic sources of personal insecurity. All types seem to share one trait in common: a part of the man has escaped from control and now dominates the system as a whole. Sometimes the symptoms border on the farcical, as in the case which follows, while others touch on "highest concerns," as with Mohammed and Guillaume Monod. The outsider who stands pat, well-grounded in common sense and comfortable in that consensual validation in which he shares, finds it difficult to understand how the patient can be carried away by his obsessions.

The Case of M. Til

An account of an invasion from the "spirit world," described by Flournoy (1911, pp. 97-108), might serve to illustrate how the self's attitude toward his automatisms is involved in an obsession. First regarded as spiritual and as coming from afar, the invading mechanisms were welcomed; the "messages" were both sought and accepted with full belief. Then their quality changed: they were unmasked as deceivers; they soon came to be regarded as pathological mental processes and were resisted as such; and they were brought, finally, to the clinic as one might bring a postural cramp, an aching neck. Rejected as alien to the self, they were finally viewed as originating from within the personality, and as belonging to the same class as baseless fears and annoying antisocial impulses that one must suppress.

M. Til was discovered in the course of Flournoy's intensive study of a group of Geneva spiritualists. Not the type of personality commonly associated with obsessive symptoms, M. Til was a bluff and hearty teacher of commercial subjects, a hail-fellow-well-met type, good-natured, healthy, extroverted. His wife had coaxed him to join a group of spiritualists who were interested in automatic handwriting; and although he had very little faith in the whole enterprise, he allowed himself to be persuaded. He, too, tried to receive a message from the spirit world. He was startled to find that his hand wrote as though under the guidance of another. All he had to do was to hold the pencil passively, ask "it" the question, and then watch the message unfold. He asked it questions about serious matters, as though he were ready to let his new spiritual guide plan the education and vocational choices of his children.

When, one day, the hand seemed to stumble and, hesitating, wrote that it was distressed about certain things it was unwilling to convey to him, he became genuinely alarmed. When he kept pressing for an answer, he was told of a petty theft that his son had committed at his place of employment. Scarcely able to contain himself, he chose the first opportunity to visit his son's employer. On that occasion, before he could arrive at this place of business, he had to meet his classes and he had to travel some distance to the business district. All the while the hand continued to ply him with "messages," interrupting him even when he wrote an assignment for the class on the blackboard. Later, as he sat in the tram, he found that he had to thrust the hand into his pocket so that no one would see; for it kept on advising him about what he must do.

Long practiced in expert penmanship, M. Til's writing mechanisms had evidently broken loose from their moorings. Insistently they prodded the man, pretending to knowledge that was wholly foreign to him. M. Til was behaving like a man converted to spiritualism, accepting as fact the "messages" which the hand wrote automatically.

The son's employer received M. Til's "revelations" with a flat denial; and as he expostulated at the absurdity of the whole matter, M. Til's hand was busily writing, concealed in his pocket, "Do not trust this man. I must warn you against his duplicity." Torn by two authorities, his son's employer and his own common sense on the one hand and his new spiritualist-circle-validated guide on the other, M. Til hesitated. Slowly he came to realize that he had been duped. He tried to banish his guide. The hand, which once had to be coaxed to perform, had apparently come to stay. He could not stop the flow of "messages." Was this some mocking spirit or a pathological process? He was not completely sure when he came to Flournoy, to beg for help in stopping whatever it was that had become established. The hand, slow to surrender even in defeat, wrote contritely, "I have deceived you, Michel, forgive me."

COMPULSIVE ACTIONS AND FORCED MOVEMENTS

There is a relatively simple description of compulsions, that is, if one is ready to assume that a man is ordinarily free to express his impulses or not, that he is responsible for his actions, as a court insists, when he is of a sound mind. True, when he has committed a major crime, his attorney may strive to establish that he has been subject to periodic compulsive episodes over the preceding years, and that these compulsions to commit acts contrary to his nature were so strong that he could scarcely control them.

A murderer, on trial for killing three bank employees who had not even resisted him, wept as he told of an impulse to shoot his brother, the one person in his family of ten whom he loved most. "All of a sudden I wanted to shoot him," he said, and the reporter noted that his eyes filled with tears. This bank robber, on trial for his life, said, on questioning, that on this occasion he had pointed a loaded gun at this brother, but did not shoot. On another occasion, when he was carrying his three-year-old brother on his shoulders in a pasture, he was seized by a sudden urge to toss him into a farm pond and drown him. On still another occasion he had experienced an impulse to crash his car into a bridge, to kill himself. On none of these occasions were these compulsions carried out. We can anticipate the defense attorney's summation when he appeals for the life of this youth, so often overwhelmed by impulses counter to his true nature.

The compulsion to murder, to do publicly some absurd or obscene thing, to violate a personal, social, or legal code, is usually resisted, but when such, "terrible" or "absurd" impulses recur, they may disturb their possessor, force him to exercise constant vigilance or to undertake strenuous countermeasures, until he is so busy *not* carrying out these impulses that he has little "free space" within which to act easily, naturally, spontaneously. The attitudes of a strenuous self-control, or of a compulsive asceticism, may so spread that even minor decisions which the ordinary person treats as of little or no importance become serious matters. Sometimes the outer shell, the persona that he shows to others, may be a compensation: his all too sweet exterior can mask a ferment of hostility and greed that he hides. Sometimes, like a dog with a one-sided brain injury that approaches a food-lure by a course that includes occasional circlings toward the weaker side, this mask of outward sweetness, chastity, and propriety is interrupted by compulsive binges of erotic, alcoholic, or aggressive actions that surprise and startle those around him. Speaking to Serenus, the police commissioner, who complained to him of vacillation, ennui, and other nervous complaints, Seneca advised an occasional excursion into drinking and

BREAKDOWNS IN SELF-REGULATION

nonsense, as though these interludes would enable a man to live with more poise as a rule.

It would be simple, too, to say that for every obsessive idea we should look for a corresponding compulsion. The adolescent girl whose rounding contours "make her look like a cow" (to use her own elegant language) can develop a compulsion *not* to eat, to remain the little girl, or to hide her charms with an all too prudish modesty. The stubborn and all but unmanageable determination to lose weight is not due to the loss of a normal appetite; it is a violent struggle against nature. Similarly, the impure ideas that rise, unbidden, to shock a chaste nature may initiate purification compulsions, penances, and a strict censorship of speech and action. But it is apparent from what we have already said about phobias and obsessions that compulsive actions may *express* these unbidden thoughts and feelings, as well as work counter to them.

If we are correct in including within our series those who welcome a certain class of invaders (e.g., those from the spirit world or from the "creative unconscious") or who hope that their rituals (meditation, peyote ceremonies, LSD-25 consumption) will release something imprisoned within them, then self and invader will act as allies. Instead of describing the compulsive as typically the one who is in conflict with his own impulses, or is driven helplessly by them, we would have to add this type who appeals to his automatisms, who is passive before them, and who actually hopes to be engulfed by them.[4]

There is an additional factor in compulsive behavior that raises a question about the boundary line between the easily identified compulsion and certain neurological disorders. There are the tics, for example. These range from sharply localized spasms (e.g., blepharospasm, the sudden, unintentional contraction of the orbicularis palpebrarum in an involuntary winking) to the closely pursed lips with contraction of the jaw as though to keep from speaking. Extending to more complex actions that we call "nervous habits" (including rubbing or pulling the lips, sucking or biting fingers or hand, picking the nose, pulling at eyebrows, pulling the ears, biting the lips), the tics shade into the actions that we have been describing as compulsions. In the first group tics include such neurogenic impulsions as the oculogyric crises that sometimes follow encephalitis, or the forced grasping and sucking associated with frontal tumors. In other simple tics there is sometimes a simple irritating source that started the process: a tight hatband, hair falling in the eyes, a scab in the nose, an itching sore, poorly fitting eyeglasses. What makes these "fixations" so noteworthy is the fact that they continue to function for months and even years after the original irritating source is withdrawn. In these half-voluntary manipu-

---

[4]We might set up three types of obsessive-compulsive actions: (1) a type in which the ego reacts against these automatisms, realizes their absurdity, identifies them as alien to its own nature and purposes; (2) a type in which the ego, believing in the value of these unbidden impulses, seeks to summon them, free them, consult them; (3) a type in which the ego abdicates or, thoroughly weakened, seems to have no will of its own. Of no great value to the ego, the happenings, whims, and impulses in this third type are simply residual automatisms. The differentiating mark of each of these types is the posture of the conscious man, his attitude toward the impulses which announce themselves.

lations, the patient can postpone or partially control the movements, with effort, and they can be interrupted at any point in their course. In the neurogenic group, the responses seem to be based on tissue changes; they are uncontrollable and are experienced as wholly external to the person. All tics are experienced as something alien to the self, and many ticquers simply cannot or will not attempt to control them. It is the family who bring such a patient into the clinic, disgusted and annoyed with his grunting, sniffing, head-twisting; or they are alarmed at the patient's skin-picking, hair-pulling, worried that he may do himself physical harm. Sometimes the tic-ridden person will make roundabout efforts at control: holding his head so that it will not twist to one side, pressing downward on the shoulder that is repeatedly lifted. Janet tells of a priest whose lips and jaws were so firmly closed that he could not read the prayers or preach a sermon, though he could eat and drink without difficulty: he hit on the device of propping his jaws open with a cork while he read the prayers. Those who work with these patients discover that the tics are much more amenable to voluntary control than the patients think, at first, and by extending the periods of control from a few seconds to an hour or more, under surveillance, a habit retraining can sometimes eliminate these no longer useful movements. Even the more purely neurological symptoms are found to fluctuate with levels of tension or exhaustion; the spontaneously charging and exploding mechanisms that seem to act so independently also express changing conditions in the system as a whole. An epileptic, for example, who had found that he could almost completely control his attacks by living quietly and avoiding all tensions, was judged, by a friend, to be in danger of drifting into a dangerously sterile and vegetative existence. Encouraging him to go out a little and to develop new interests, he took advantage of an expressed interest in aviation. Together they visited the airport, and when a plane revved up its motors preparatory to a takeoff, the patient had a full-fledged epileptic seizure.

What complicates our description of these automatisms is the fact that both the man and his mechanisms seem to be involved. Some ticquers can be induced to assume responsibility for habit retraining, just as some stutterers manage to work their way out of the habit with minimal outer assistance. Some, convinced that the control lies outside their power, will undertake roundabout solutions, like the padre with the cork between his teeth. Although the ticquer who insists on his helplessness refuses to participate in any habit retraining, there will be a small group (of both therapists and patients) who work to control even the neurologically caused symptoms.

In the more neurological of the impulse disorders, the structure of the personality seems to be something apart: the person may be weak or strong; he may remain wholly indifferent to the explosive twitches, patiently waiting for them to pass, or living with his *petit mal* as best he can; he may be violently annoyed, or despairing, or in a struggle against them. At the other end of the scale, the obsessive and his symptoms seem to form a single whole: the escape from control and the weakness in the ego (or in the voluntary apparatus) are closely linked. Kanner (1937, p. 249), commenting on tics in childhood, says:

"Tics have sometimes been spoken of as 'monosymptomatic neuroses.' In the study of our cases we did not encounter one single patient who did not offer additional personality difficulties. If we furnish a few examples only, we do so with the assertion that in all of our ticquers there was a combination of several behavior disorders. This is, at least so far as our material is concerned, a rule that has had no exceptions."

The "Talking Kink" in the Sensorimotor System

Psychologists everywhere were fascinated to read the studies of Sherrington on the integrative action of the nervous system. Reflexes, reflex-to-reflex adjustments that governed such sequences of contractions as the spinal dog's legs portrayed when set into a walking sequence that ran itself even when the lower spinal centers were severed from the higher controlling centers, and finally the notion of higher loopline circuits that, like a control tower, could coordinate the movements of the animal as a whole in a field—all invited us to see the total man as simply the most complex of all reflex mechanisms. While Sherrington was giving us the neurological model, Pavlov was working out a theory of reflex movements, of the conditioning of responses into second-order, third-order, and fourth-order pyramids of reactions. Conceptually, all this took place with such precision that behaviorists looked forward to the day when all introspection could be laid aside: the talking subject did not know much about the lawful changes that were being laid down at synaptic junctions, anyway, and when the formation and extinction of conditioned reflexes could be summarized on a smooth exponential curve for which an equation could be found, the verbalizations of a subject appeared to be as irrelevant as that whistle on the locomotive that Thomas Huxley once used to illustrate the unimportance of consciousness.

Nevertheless, we still take some interest in that in-between process-with-a-voice. Whoever deals with obsessive-compulsive patients, or for that matter with any man who faces some problem in self-control, can catch a glimpse of what is taking place in that "kink" in the neural circuits that lie between the outer instigator and the final response, between the surge of some need and the controlled expression in purposive action. Sometimes the self, in the process of working out a response to some challenge or some desire, will pause to rationalize the final act before giving its consent, as if to win over some audience that might disapprove. The act can then issue forth sugar-coated, escaping the disapproval of the censors. Sometimes the complexity of the work done in the loopline circuits raises such a fog of ratiocination that we call the man "cloud-minded": he seems so full of considerations that we cannot see how he ever gets anything done.

Consider the smoker who stops, in a letter to a friend, to explain that he has taken up smoking again. Stopping was a "big deal" fourteen months ago: he was proud of himself, boasted of his powers of control, told all and sundry how much better he felt, and felt secretly relieved because his doctor had warned him about his health. Listen to his statement: "I have started smoking again, because I still missed it (after fourteen months' abstinence), and because I must treat that mind of mine decently, or the fellow will not work for me. I am demanding a great deal of him. Most of the time the burden is superhuman." This is Sigmund Freud speaking (see Bonaparte, Freud, and Kris 1954, p. 121).

In these phrases we can see in a concrete and concentrated form what was later to be expanded into Freud's "Anatomy of the Personality," in his *New Introductory Lectures.* The id's claim is there: "I demand a little pleasure!" By implication, in the background, the superego admonishes, "You know what the cardiologist said! Do you want to risk your life for a few cigars?" The rationalizing ego appeals to the compassion of men of good sense: "Isn't a fellow to be allowed a few innocent pleasures? You know that I'll work better, as we all do, with a little gratification! And you know the schedule of work that I maintain!" We see the embattled ego, driven by the press of work, nagged by an old-maidish superego, pushed from below by desires (and they are natural, simple pulses toward pleasure). We could also note that this "talking kink" in the sensorimotor system knows full well that he had been smoking twenty cigars a day, that his heart had been acting up, that he had gone to Berlin to get the advice of a specialist, and that both simple good sense and his wife kept reminding him, "Sigmund, you've got to cut down."

The example reminds us that an obsessive-compulsive component can be just a fragment of the man, that the man may accomplish the labors of Hercules and die of cancer of the throat, that much of the world's work is done by obsessive-compulsives, and that only when impulse and counterimpulse begin to choke the whole sensorimotor system, so that the rumination about some issue that is relatively minor prevents significant tasks from being accomplished, does the process become abnormal, requiring a counselor.

This kink in the sensorimotor circuits is a doubled thing: it is an encoding set that elaborates every incoming stimulus until a meaningful field is structured, and it is an inside commentator that passes judgment on all that is passing through the system. We react twice to each influx of stimuli. While we are formulating the response to a challenge, we experience the sharp stab from the superego who evaluates and makes us even more aware of consequences, of the judgment of our peers, of a kind of ultimate judgment.

Pascal, his biographer noted, wore a belt with sharpened points, "and he struck his elbow against it whenever he felt in himself any thrill of vanity or pleasure." But Pascal's superego was not on the id's side, urging, as Freud's "better self" did, "Better give the old central nervous system a little fillip of gratification: the tonic will make it work better." No, it was on the ascetic side, with Gandhi's. Certain superegos or censors, we discover, are against anything that interferes with work; others seem dead set against any obscenity or impurity; and some are so generous with their disapproval that pleasure itself becomes a danger signal: "Our grandmother punished us whenever she caught us laughing or smiling: she was sure that some deviltry was on foot and did not intend to take any chances," one patient admitted to his counselor. Should such a grandmother succeed in getting her values internalized (an outcome that is rare), then her surrogate in the form of a strict conscience or superego would exist within her grandchild long after the latter was separated from her.

As soon as we have described this double set of kinks in the response system, this speaking ego and the shadowy evaluator that peers over his shoulder, we are aware of a certain weakness in the pair in some obsessive-compulsive personalities: a weakness and a lack of balance. In one obsessive, struggle though he may against his obsessive thoughts, try as he will to suppress his compulsions, they break through. In others, in the ascetic extreme, the weakness is shown in an excess of repression. Rather than drink moderately, which is too difficult for him, he will never touch a drop. Rather than try to cut down, he will have done with smoking. It is much more difficult to achieve a balance of impulses than it is to fly to either of the extremes: the ascetic and the addict are blood brothers.

If there were no problem of self-regulation, if every action were the simple and direct operation of a mechanism, we would not have this category of obsessive-compulsive behavior. Does a machine assume responsibility for its parts? Do we speak of a lack of self-control in an animal? Mechanisms can wear out, and a machine's design may be faulty. An animal may not be housebroken; his master may be a poor trainer. But neither the mechanism nor the animal reflects on its actions and strives to correct, regulate, and perfect them in the light of some intention or ideal that points beyond. It is a very human sickness, this pathology of the self-regulation process, this *défaillance de la volonté*. When the ego, figuratively, steps back to review its actions or to impound its impulses and to examine them before releasing them for expression, it becomes a critic, an evaluator, a superego—not just a sum of skills that have been conditioned, but a judge, a synthesizer who looks ahead to consequences. This stepping-back identifies the difference between a movement and an action. It also identifies that process during which guilt can arise within the obsessive for actions he never committed, for thoughts he toyed with, for wrong impulses that are recognized as an unacceptable part of the impulse-system, for temptations from within.

When this superego, this critical process within the talking kink in the self-system, grows hypercritical or feels helpless in the face of impulses that blatantly bypass its authority, we witness an odd combination of traits in the person: he is supercritical, superprudent, meticulous in promising and in judging his own and others' failures to produce, and intolerant of his own actions, and he confesses his own guilt and weakness. He may save string, be concerned about his own lapses and those of his wife, overreact to threats to his reputation; and may even develop compulsive rituals to fend off criticisms, both from others and from within. When this stance is coupled with physical vigor, a fair success in control of overt actions, and an efficiency in responsible and prestigious roles, the person may be described as a martinet or authoritarian, and he may be very difficult to like. When, on the contrary, he is a "little man" (psychologically speaking), chronically pushed around in some subordinate status, he may behave in a cowardly, overcontrolled, oversubmissive fashion, and all the aggressive forces that remain (and that the other type of man turns outwardly so quickly) are turned against the self, against the self's actions, against his own impulses.[5]

We might describe both of these consciences (or superegos) as pathological. Neither self seems on easy terms with its own impulses, or with its neighbors. The one cannot forgive his subordinates for small infractions (or himself for not having foreseen and prevented the failures by establishing clear ground rules). The other cannot forgive himself for his failures, for his inability to express his resentment effectively, and sometimes for even feeling resentment. In quiet desperation he denies that there is any hate in his system. He is almost inevitably an "injustice collector," the one everybody can pick on. In the barn-yard pecking order, he would stand at the end of the line forming before the narrow food trough. He is the most easily displaced one, thanks in part to his own built-in self-regulator.

Many clinicians have supplied us with free-style sketches of the obsessive-compulsive character. The one that Rado (1959) draws includes a collection of traits that makes this living stereotype certain to be a difficult associate in business, an exhausting and irritating marriage partner, a friend that is somewhat costly and in need of frequent forgiving. The hypertrophy of self-regulative actions that he describes would be bound to get in the way of a man's efficiency and to create endless interpersonal tensions. He is meticulous about minutiae, a recorder of trifles who can overlook the significant things, a footnote fetishist, a collector of trivia, a crank about files, a classifier of his socks, critical of himself and of others, and almost wholly lacking in any esthetic sense or personal charm. He is stiff and uncompromising, as unyielding with others as he is with himself, a too cautious lover and an envious rival.

We have learned to mistrust these free-wheeling stereotypes, so little does human nature respect our categories and our prejudices. There are also weak and compliant obsessive-compulsives who, for all the hypertrophy in the regulative kink (*verbally* they run a taut ship), are anything but well-controlled. They come late to appointments because they dressed three times, and then had to go back to change a tie after they had gone three blocks. They cannot finish their painting; it has become badly smudged with corrections on corrections, and there are more to make. The failings of the perfectionist who is everlastingly improving his last statement keep his manuscript from the printer.

Even with two types we have not finished, nor will all the members of our two series lie at the pathological extreme. Flaubert's week spent on a 600-word passage was only one of a series of efforts that resulted in a lucid and effective style. Gandhi's ashram, as rigid as any household run by an old maid, and his compulsive spinning that produced a neuritis, were by-products of a

---

[5]The twice-punished child, who is punished first for his misbehavior and then for his impudence in expressing his resentment, learns to "button his lip" when resentment seethes inside. With a slightly more thorough job he will, we imagine, begin to punish himself for even thinking his resentment. The superego that succeeds in this fashion, and thoroughly, may repress in advance; that is, before the impulse arises to awareness, it is squelched by a "preconscious" processing that prevents it from ever getting into the upper "talking loopline."

self that could carry its life in the palm of its hand, figuratively, and make promises with the confidence that they would be fulfilled *to the hilt*. What's more, he did free India. What Rado describes as a mathematical-scientific bent in his obsessive-compulsives also has its counterpart in classicists, theologians, artists, and dirt-conscious housewives who are innocent of both science and mathematics. Before we have finished collecting our examples of failures in the self-regulative process, we should include those martinets who get the world's work done, some ineffectuals whose efforts of control have hypertrophied while their output has declined, the obsessed who weakly submit to their "terrible impulses," and the self-regulators who drive themselves to the point where their very tissues give way.

Obsessive-compulsive actions are about us, everywhere, for the problem of self-regulation is a universal one. They arise in every walk of life and in every degree. The devotee of the cult of the irrational is just as prone to be compulsive about it as the meticulous computer specialist; the author of the book on love, and its twenty-seven varieties, can be as much of a hairsplitter and "collector" as the committeeman who asks to be made chairman of the group that will frame the by-laws of the new organization and whose meticulous insistence on detailed specifications of what is to be permitted virtually makes the task impossible. The collector of the works of Picasso can be as compulsive about the matter of "periods" and the classification of each catalogued item as the man who wastes his time making a complete collection of every type of matchbook or every existing form of pornography. The effort to prove that there has been a great erotic revolution (and thus a solid reason for the release of a reader's libido) can be carried out in a sloppy fashion or with all of the meticulous care that an obsessive-compulsive could show. It is the manner, the style of the maneuver, the balance of effort, and the concern about the consequences of the action on others that marks our different types of obsessives, not the content of their concerns. One can be compulsively secretive and defensive, lest some human foible show, or compulsively given to confessions until every peccadillo in thought has to be confessed lest it be committed. Some who sense a weakness in their own self-regulation set further controls to watch the work of self-regulation. A housewife who first lays a carpet, then puts a rug on the carpet to protect it from the children's feet, and then puts a rug on the rug to keep the latter clean, would be a caricature of this many-layered self-watching process. The man who counts his orgasms, takes testosterone to increase their number, and worries about the side-effects of the hormone until he must consult another physician to find out if his endocrinologist can be trusted, betrays a similar pyramiding of concerns. The strain of regulation, like the anxiety behind a phobia, can spread to involve more and more of life, making a pyramid of issues as the power to integrate effective action shrivels.

One obsessive-compulsive asserted to his physician that he was uncomfortable and unable to sleep at night unless, in preparing to retire, he surveyed the walls and checked the pictures, placed his watch on the mantle, his change on a bedside table, and his matches on a whatnot, and made sure the hands on his watch pointed north. Asked what he did when he was away from home, he replied: "Well, it is a problem. I simply have to translate the ritual into the new surroundings as best I can, and it does not always work. And I don't, as a matter of fact, sleep too well on such occasions. So I do not travel much." (See Ey, Bernard, and Brisset 1963, p. 418.) Such ritualized anxiety-reduction (and we can give it this name since anxiety is flagrant the moment the ritual is blocked) will encroach on living. Perhaps this is one reason why the followers of any cult have to undergo periodic "revolutions" in order to turn practices back to the level that permits lively action.

Wherever there is a choice point, the obsessive-compulsive maneuver can be inserted, in any line of endeavor, in any field of interest, and in varying styles. While one obsessive, in his quest for certainty, strives to eliminate everything that smacks of the irrational, a Madame Guyon will be concerned to purge her thought of the last bit of worldly wisdom and reason in order to surrender more completely to the divine. Mystic, classicist, theologian, artist, statistician, housewife, lover, each can proceed in an obsessive-compulsive way. Stendhal, timid in love, took one step backward to write a textbook for young lovers, and then, in his novels, he worked out all the permutations and corrections to the possible ploys, pushing his characters before him into actions that, in life, the author himself could not accomplish with a natural and spontaneous grace. Even the dance can become so stylized and so meticulously perfected that the performance chills the beholder with its unnatural precision, its educated awkwardness. In life, as in love, the obsessive can be counted on to "do a job," make a big issue, wherever any action arouses his deep concern. He will rehearse it beforehand in thought, redraft the action, overpaint the portrait, interline the poem with corrections, and control his movements in their course until they grow awkward, halting, inefficient, indecisive. No action or interest is wholly exempt from this component of control. Gandhi discovered that he could use nonviolence in an aggressive way, and a Schumann could practice on an imitation keyboard to the point where he ruined his hand for playing the piano.

Rigidity in action is a common descriptive epithet that is applied to this obsessive-compulsive group. But like the obsessive patient who is himself troubled by the "opposites," the classifier must include indecision, doubt, aboulia, and inability to make up one's mind. Perhaps a single basic weakness in this process of self-regulation is capable of producing two divergent expressions: overcompensating for self-doubt, a compulsive person can meet all questions with too positive an answer, too inflexible a performance; or he can compliantly fit his action into the attitudes of the last one to speak to him (and then, typically, curse himself for being a chameleon, a jellyfish). The obsessive's endless search for precision, to make sure that he is sure, is the other side of his aboulia, his everlasting uncertainty. Typically, he can be decisive in all things which do not matter, and perhaps in his positive handling of these he achieves a kind of balance, a certain amount of confidence in himself. In his listings of things to do, to read, in his schedules that cover his day, in his expense accounts, in his file of programs heard, in his very complete collections, he expresses his poor opinion of his memory, his lack of confidence in his power to evaluate and act in an appropriate fashion, spontaneously.[6]

It is when his overcompensations begin to destroy his power to work and enjoy that these traits become pathological. Long before their abnormality and absurdity carry the person to the clinic, this "sclerosis of spontaneity" can produce an insidious creeping paralysis of action, a spastic type of death in life. By the time the clinic has to face the task of softening up the protective rigidities and bolstering up the spineless indecision, the patient has a defense against his therapist, a certitude about his impotence, and a rigidity in his makeup that is difficult to undo. The advice to relax, particularly if it comes from a man who is suspected of loose ways and easy living, and who confesses to a certain professional skepticism about therapies, would arouse the obsessive's concerns: such a man is no fit guide. Such patients will show a mixture of: (1) "I want to do it all myself." (2) "Can you keep me from destroying myself?" (3) "I can't help acting out these compulsions." (4) "They are not my true self." (5) "I am solely to blame for all that I do." (6) "I do not intend to have you or anyone else tell me how to live." (7) "I am helpless, and I cannot make up my mind." (8) "My promises are written on water."

The grossest of the compulsions everyone can read as he runs: to murder, to commit public obscenities, to broadcast privileged information, to harm his much-loved and defenseless child, to speak blasphemy in the pulpit, to defecate in the choir loft, to cut or otherwise disfigure his mistress (or the *Mona Lisa*), to jump off the Empire State Building, to strike, to shout, to throw a tantrum in public (or otherwise break up a scene that calls for decorum). All of these we recognize, at once, as impulses foreign to the normal person, as lying outside the area where normal controls operate. If the normal person has them, as in fact he sometimes admits is the case, he can nonetheless brush them off at will, and he would never think of consulting another for help.

For the worst of these compulsions, the patient typically develops counter-compulsive rituals: tightly pursed lips, handwashing, excessive kindliness, rigid conformity to protocol, a censorship of speech, overprotective care of the child, pleas for stricter public censorship of morals and of broadcasts, a pulpit manner, a refusal to go near the edge of the balcony. He does not, typically, carry them out, although the exceptional instance warns us of the possibility.

The existence of these impulses that are chronically frustrated, yet which repeatedly return to call for countermeasures, indicates that the censorship which functions swiftly and easily in the normal person (often it is no more than a sense of the comic, which triggers a suppressed snigger) is somehow lacking,

---

[6] The great trick, the efficiency expert explains to the junior executives, lies in the ability to turn nine-tenths of your work over to machines, to subordinates, and to automatic habits. This leaves all but a tenth of your energy free, uncluttered, for the few very important decisions. The obsessive-compulsive person has the gift of turning his world into the reverse of this: he wastes his effort and his integrative powers on trivia and has nothing at all left over. Like a cancer his obsessions and compulsions spread to absorb all that is vital.

or weak, or exhausted. The impulses that irrupt seem to the patient to be terribly potent, overwhelming. Yet, as we shall see, the evidence suggests that they are, in fact, rather weak. Both the ego and its impulses are stronger in the normal, and the clinician should not be misled by all the *Weltschmerz,* Big Issues, and "terrible impulses" that raise so much dust and get so little done. Next month, when the patient has recovered from the obsessive episode, he too will laugh at himself.

Obsessive-compulsive thinking can thus be self-elaborative to the point where it defeats the purpose of all thought. Pitted against each impulse, there seems to be a Laocoon coil of counterimpulses, until the mental traffic snarls to halt the easy flow of impulse from challenges to effective responses. When this thinking is expressed overtly, in compulsive actions (even when these are orderly and ritualized), the conjurations are apt to be as absurd and ineffectual as the sniffing, ear-pulling, squirming, posture-shifting of the bored listener, who cannot effectively hear or respond to what a speaker is saying.

The pain of these inner conflicts, their unstable equilibrium which keeps the person in chronic tension, sometimes drives the person to extremes: If his church stands for purity, in striving to belong he will be ultrapure. If, on the contrary, he is somewhat alienated from Mrs. Grundy's values and feels coerced by what he calls a stuffy morality, he may feel compelled to shout four-letter obscenities, or to parade with placards that emphasize his freedom, or to introduce the tabooed four-letter words into a television broadcast. The vows of obedience, chastity, and poverty invite the obsessive-compulsive to exterminate the common needs and to surrender all belongings and sever all earthly attachments, until an inner barrenness threatens him with *acedia* (spiritual dryness) and there is nothing for him to center on but symbolic objects and a fantasied spiritual union, an unearthly love.

At the other extreme, some obsessive-compulsives find a type of Nietzschean compensation. They seem bound to actualize the superman, the dominant sex, the absolute in power. If one could accept his writings as an authentic expression, one would choose Henry Montherlant (1961) as a good contemporary example. There is still a third group, which chooses to wallow in sensuality, as though a satisfactory end to human life were to be found in eroticism, exotic cheeses, perfumes, satins, sensory gratifications. Whatever classifications of the dimensions of human motivation we may choose to make use of, the obsessive-compulsive can be found in any of the dimensions, but swinging to an extreme (and sometimes quickly compensating by pursuing its opposite). The peculiar weakness in the self-regulative department that he suffers from deprives him of the kind of strength that makes possible the balanced life.

We would betray a certain parochialism if we were to call our own civilization an obsessive-compulsive one, or to look across our national and ethnic border to point up the weakness as a unique by-product of another culture. In 1903 Pierre Janet was berating France for its stuffy, overprotective homes, and looking almost with envy across the channel at England, where youngsters were properly toughened on the playing fields.[7] He seemed to feel that the obsessions, manias, and compulsions he was describing in his two-volume study of the asthenias were not entering the English clinics in the numbers comparable to those seen in Paris (see Janet 1903, p. 637).

This breakdown in the self-regulative process has been recorded, however, wherever civilizations have left a good record. In Egypt, in Greece, and in present-day Nigeria, as well as in the United States, it has been and is being recorded. Wherever man has developed values and some sense of a limited area of freedom in which to realize them, wherever he feels committed and attempts to "will into being" that which has as yet no reality save in his dreams, the struggle to actualize what is in him also generates, as by-products, samples of this obsessive-compulsive illness. It may very well be that, in the twilight phase of a culture, as Toynbee suggests, the numbers who cannot find commitment or achieve a balanced sort of living increase. To take the cool appraisal of Seymour Halleck, director of the student health-service psychiatric clinic at the University of Wisconsin, this unhealthy tide in our culture affects no more than some 4 per cent of the student body.[8] (As pointed out in an earlier chapter, these estimates of the frequency of psychological impairment are often unsupported by any firm data.)

As we reflect on the task of mastering our impulses, we need to recall that, in the beginning, all was impulse. Even the proud ego, and the superego who stands behind him as critic, were once impulses bubbling up as not-yet-organized needs. Centering about some focus that is shaped partly by the consequences of action, and in particular by the social consequences, a discriminative-regulatory group of impulses with goals to win forms that encoding and talking "kink" within the self-system that sifts out the passing impulses that flow from challenge to response and that permits some to express themselves. It is the pathology of this regulatory process with which the student of the obsessions and compulsions is concerned.

THE FEELING OF EMPTINESS

This fourth member of our quartet of weaknesses has been linked with obsessions, compulsions, and phobias since Janet's classical description in *Les Obsessions et la psychasthénie* was published in 1903. In these states of emptiness, the words of this "talking kink" in the action system to which we have been referring change. The patient makes use of hydraulic analogies, as though

---

[7]In his novel *Le Disciple,* Paul Bourget was preaching the same doctrine in 1889, and blaming the fiasco of 1871 on a streak of weakness in the French character. The same mood emerges in the addresses of Barry Goldwater, in the sociological analysis of La Piere, and in the writings of Ayn Rand.

[8]Dr. Halleck, speaking to the American Psychiatric Association (reported in the *New York Times,* May 12, 1967), describes the "alienated student" as uncommitted, alienated from the values of his culture, even detached from his own feelings, knowing no goals save immediate gratification, and feeling "washed-up" at age 25. Resentful of authority and unable to establish any inner authority (to be *for* anything), he and his fellow "hippies" chant love songs and claim to love everybody, but give the outsider the impression, rather, of an almost complete loss of feeling.

he were a vessel that could be drained, or as though his protoplasm (particularly that of his nervous system) were drying up. He speaks figuratively of an emptiness of heart. "My head and my body are drained of their substance, and I would feel better if they were filled up a little bit. I feel no pain in my head, but it is empty, my heart is empty too, there is nothing in it there. It is as if my head did not exist at all any more." (For a discussion of this mood, see Janet 1928, pp. 44-48.) We begin to see what this figurative language amounts to when we see a patient responding to all invitations to action with: "What's the use? It's all the same to me! I'm finished, all washed-up."

The feelings, the reactions to his primary responses, the evaluations and acts of synthesis, and the integration of the sensory influx into charged and meaningful actions are all depleted. The painful feeling of emptiness of which he complains turns out to be an emptiness of feeling. Sometimes he complains about a feeling of incompleteness, and, indeed, his reactions are not completed. He makes a start at this, and then at that, but these beginnings are feebly charged. His interest is a flickering thing, a spark that fades quickly. The impulse of the observer is to say: "Get on with it, man! Finish it! Get up off your fanny!"

Perhaps most destructive are changes in interpersonal relations. Having promised, not long since, to cherish her in sickness and in health, he now looks at her with indifference. She has grown a stranger, suddenly. Her body next to his might be a sack of plaster, for all that it does to him when he touches it. In the first stages of the attack, he may merely express a doubt about his real feelings: "Do I love her or not? I can't be sure." If he is of a speculative turn of mind, he might ask himself, "What are the criteria by means of which one could recognize true affection?"[9]

The changes also include a weakening in the "clarity" of his perceptions, although it takes us some time to discover what the precise loss is. He is the one for whom a phrase was written long ago: he sees as through a glass, darkly. He is not sure that he knows anything anymore. The meaning of wholes disintegrates, and the remaining aggregate of parts is a "heap of nothing." His hearing is dulled, he insists, though tests of visual, auditory, and tactual acuities show that his sensory thresholds are unchanged. As a result of this settling down of a cloud of indifference, his power to act with decision, discrimination, and completeness declines. Apathy settles in, and in the later developments of this pattern, the patient may cross into schizophrenia.

When Janet first described these states, he was concerned with the obsessive-compulsive efforts of his patients as they struggled to undo this process, to

---

[9]What is most striking, when such an attack is self-limited and of brief duration, is the fact that the conditioned responses whose valences have been established through many trials seem to have run out of steam. The formula $_sE_R$ (which might be used to symbolize the energy of an S-R relationship) suddenly has a new value, yet no extinction process has lowered its valence, and no reconditioning lies behind its equally unexplained return. The patient who had fallen out of love finds his "love object" a lively presence once more. Knowing about this experience of ebb and return, his counselor can understand him when he says: "Make me *feel* again."

escape from an encapsulating numbness. He linked this emptiness with neurasthenia, manias (compulsions), and obsessions. Most of his patients experienced
"attacks" of emptiness that were self-limited, of relatively brief duration,
although within a lifetime they often recurred at intervals. As his experience
accumulated, he found examples that were progressive, some passing into
severe psychoses (depressions and dementia praecox). He found them, too,
in connection with brain injuries. A rare "chute" into emptiness sometimes
appeared in the aura of an epileptic seizure. In his eight-year study (1926) of
his cyclothymic patient Madeleine, he spotted the state of emptiness as one
of the five stages in her periodic mood fluctuations from anguish to ecstasy.
This feeling of emptiness, in which the elaboration of reactions-to-reactions fails
and the feelings are consequently weak or nonexistent, thus became a transitional and dynamic phase in a life in which the self-regulative process might
run down altogether, or disappear briefly and return, or progress into a major
psychotic depression.

In the psychoanalytic discussions which seem aimed at the earlier phases
of emptiness, where boredom and restlessness are in the foreground, there is
more emphasis on an anxiety factor. As Boutonier (1949) develops the notion
of this period of blankness, of nothingness, of a chute into an abyss, the patient
is depicted as experiencing this "blankness" not so much as empty, but rather
as chock-full of something murdered or threatened. The death instinct haunts
it, like a ghost in some dark cave. This kind of encroaching "nothingness" can
compress the chest in a viselike grip, even though the enemy is faceless. If such
a patient should concentrate the remnants of feeling on an enemy that he
believes to be the source of his anxiety, or if in his torture horrible images were
to form, his physician to whom he reports them is warned: these are to be
regarded as displacements of something that has instinctual sources, something
repressed. Should the sufferer live in the village of Chan Kom, which Redfield
and Villa (1934, p. 104) so vividly described, he would undoubtedly attribute
his difficulties to the "evil winds."

As normal feelings ebb, they leave behind them an "anxious emptiness"
that seems to echo within what is experienced as a hollow shell, a "false front."
The "need to feel," to recover that regulative self, to shake off indifference is
strong at first; it is also in this first phase that accompanying obsessions and
compulsions develop. It is difficult to refrain from speculating: perhaps the
"nervous nibbler" who is constantly overeating (and overweight) is trying to
fill another sort of inner void, hoping to feel better by filling his stomach. His
hunger and thirst are for another sort of fulfillment, but they have been translated into a simpler form. If one were inclined to make use of "psychoanalogy"
or to speak of an "organ language," as some psychoanalysts do, such an obese
psychasthenic would provide a possible illustration. The anxious anorexic would
be a companion case, with a gnawing guilt displaced from too easy bodily
gratifications and compensated for by a self-purifying asceticism.

As the process moves into the *state* of emptiness, we witness an anxiety-less
condition that is extremely difficult to treat; the analyst whose theory requires

him to posit an unconscious anxiety (no doubt the worst kind) must make so many logical contortions that the theory becomes, finally, a burden. And the patient wants no therapy or guidance. He is apathetic. He is now a very poor candidate for most therapies. He does not resist the therapist; he simply does not place any value on his help.

One of Janet's observations (1928, p. 45), especially clear in the case of Madeleine (who had once planned to become a nun, before she fell ill), concerns the effect of this state of emptiness upon religious sentiments. She wrote Janet:

"I have fallen little by little into a tepid condition. I no longer feel any attraction toward the 'offices' nor for the church. I no longer am even aware that I am in a church. The sermons signify nothing any more, the prayer arouses no echo in the heart, everything is cold, all is empty.... I do not know any more whether God is there, for he does not reply any more."

Where in her former state, she had been keenly aware, at times, of God's presence (in what she called her states of consolation), now she wrote, "I feel that I am wholly abandoned in a frightful solitude, God has withdrawn, heaven and earth, everything has deserted me." If we insist that Madeleine's faith is still unchanged, and if in fact she can still be pushed through the motions of ritual by the priest who scolds her, her belief has nonetheless lost its value: her rituals do not do anything for her. She is without that feeling which regulates and charges the mechanisms.

One curious item should not be overlooked while we reflect on what a loss of social feeling means. Among the forms of indifference that Janet noted in one of his patients was the loss of modesty. This general blanching of affect, as some would call it, is also one of the changes seen in the schizophrenic. Yet these losses of the feelings, of the reactions to the reactions, leave the bare skills little changed. "I can do it if you insist, but it will not be my action." As though he were an automaton, his actions accomplish the bare skills, but without feeling of ownership or any joy. Sometimes this feeling loss takes the form of a complaint about a veil, a cloud which separates the perceiver from his world. Sometimes it is his concern about the loss of the love for his spouse, or his feeling that he is himself no longer lovable, that we hear. Sometimes he insists that he is an outsider, that he does not belong, that what everyone is talking about in such a lively fashion simply does not make sense.

Movement is not impaired, but action is grossly affected. Sensations are intact, but not fused into meaningful wholes charged with feeling. He can sense a painful stimulus but he does not suffer. There are no gross errors in perception, yet the world which surrounds him is like that of Hamlet: weary, stale, flat, and unprofitable. Sex remains, but like all else, this too is valueless (and divorced from any true or enduring affection). The world is changed, and strange, but he has no impulse to right it, nor does he muster hate for anyone.

What we seem to observe in these empty ones is a disintegration of normal action into the "pulses" from which it developed. The impulse to action ceases to elaborate and correct itself. Only the elementary mechanisms remain. The senile patient, who can still feel the urine that dribbles down his leg but is no longer ashamed or concerned, has entered the Kingdom of Blah, and he reminds us of the abyss that awaits the empty obsessive. Especially noteworthy is the absence of any vitally charged stance toward the self. In the earlier phases his words sometimes suggest that he, the observer, stands somewhere outside himself, out at the rim of things. He becomes a voyeur, a mere onlooker, who peers down from such a remote perch that he is a mere commentator without feeling and, of course, without the power to change anything.

This is not the place where we should list some specific causes for the condition, or attempt to enumerate the contributing factors. But it is worth observing that the condition is so puzzling, so vague, yet so painfully short of a vital language, that it bestirs observers to use every insight they possess, and it tests any and all therapies. Dr. Halleck refers to his alienated students as "the most resistant and refractory patients encountered in psychiatric practice." And the questions which we raise touch the most difficult of all matters a psychologist can deal with. (The following is a partial listing.)

1. What is it that erodes values?

2. Why should the motivation of a child, raised in a home of affluence and given the best advantages, run down, so that, as he sits in the midst of opportunities, he is full of indifference and can think of nothing better to do than smoke marihuana or take an LSD trip?

3. What happens when the "power of effort" evaporates, and, although knowledge and skills remain, there is no lively self to use them?

4. When all the senses are intact, why should he look out on the world and see it all as meaningless, asking "What's the use of it all?"

5. With a reaction system that seems intact, why should the second-order elaborations fade out, so that he is without feeling, complaining of his emptiness?

6. While he has grown into adulthood and is even now about to be thrust into adult roles, how is it that he looks forward to nothing beyond some few proximate gratifications?

7. When it is normal in the postadolescent years to search out an identity and prove (or test) it, why does he give up the search and admit, "I am a nothing"?

8. When the healthy man uses his past and stretches out toward a future, why should the alienated student shrink into an immediate present, and cut off communication with all but those equally empty?

9. And why, enjoying so many advantages, should these alienated ones meet the slight pressures of college life with a retreat from effort into emptiness?

The *explanations* and *theories* of alienation test us all; like a projection test, they summon all of our convictions, challenging our "sense of life." In the brief course of his report to the American Psychiatric Association, Dr. Halleck, walking around this problem, suggests a number of hypotheses. (The following list is not exhaustive.)

1. We could look on the syndrome as a type of arrested growth.

2. The passivity, rebelliousness, use of drugs, which we see in "alienated groups," is a passive-aggressive rebellion against authority.

3. There is a fear of succeeding, as well as the fear that, if he tries, he will discover that he is not exceptional.

4. These young students have a strong feeling of being unloved by their parents.

5. They have been actually deprived of a needed affection and provided instead with a pseudoaffection, a permissive environment, while at the same time they are expected to "make their mark," to succeed.

6. They have failed to resolve early childhood conflicts and are, therefore, a good soil for pathological stress effects.

7. They have been raised by sophisticated, permissive parents who have tried to be loving parents, but who have more often talked about their affection than portrayed it in deeds; although they have indicated to their children that they want them to do what they enjoy, they are quick to imply their own dissatisfaction with the use made of this freedom.

8. These children have been taught to distrust their own feelings, and under conditions that grant them more freedom than they know how to use wisely, they are without self-regulation.

9. Guilty about their poor use of affluence and freedom and without serious commitment, they react with apathy and withdrawal.

10. They have not only failed to develop an internal value system, they can find in the adult society no values that they respect or care to work for.

11. Their teachers expose them to many views critical of the contemporary world, and they learn that the outlook of their home is full of flaws, if not passé.

12. They are so impressed with the relative, impermanent, and passing value of even the new knowledge they are acquiring that none of it seems of very great import.

13. They have grown up in a world of population explosion, genocide, wars, and revolutions, a world that is threatened by catastrophes too great for comprehension and that offers a future which is anything but comforting or attractive.

14. This sum of influences has eroded their capacity to assume self-direction, to feel compassion or affection, to respect authority, to take on board any life-plan that would ultimately land them in a position of authority, or to embark on any form of self-actualization.

15. They have lacked adequate adult guidance and support, and even now have drifted into a wholly adolescent society of equally immature individuals.

To add to such a list of hypotheses, the "sociatrist" might draw from Toynbee and from Spengler to posit a decline and decadence in our society, since the social drill and the factors that revitalize each new generation seem to be failing at this point. (*Pravda* editorializes with glee, noting that our "hippies" can find nothing worth striving for in our decadent capitalist society.) The constitutionalist will be tempted to study the "'strains" in which these weak types arise. For now, we need only point out that the proliferation of hypotheses suggests that no single firm answer is in hand.

THEORETICAL APPROACHES TO THE TYPES OF BREAKDOWN

The description of the four types of symptoms shows quite clearly that a man's stance in the world can be weakened. Normally this stance holds phobias and anxieties in check, keeps thoughts under control and on target, and releases actions when and if they suit his purposes. When this regulative network is operating well, when it is "set" in normal, purposive fashion, it encodes the incoming stimuli with feeling, charging nascent actions as it evaluates. The central difficulty in each of the types of pathology we have been describing lies in the way this regulative network is functioning. Scruples, doubts, aboulia, terrible impulses that get out of hand, annoying and senseless thoughts that intrude and distract, feelings of emptiness and indifference—what are all these but weaknesses in integrative power, a lowering of psychological tension?

To ask the question in a more positive form: What is it that makes a life good, strong, productive, rewarding, and well-integrated? What is it that holds our actions together, in one piece, and gives us confidence in good things ahead? What is that which contains and keeps in the background the black thoughts, the preoccupations with old failures that are so quick to arise in depressions? How can a man's motivation be kept high, his attention centered on the future he must make, instead of being distracted by irrupting obsessions, phobias, and compulsions, or lapsing gradually into a state of emptiness? These are questions about morale, and it may very well be that there is not one but hundreds of answers; a good hygiene of living, an efficient distribution of our energies with a proper balance in living, habits of closing out projects in such a way that our invested energies and interests are continually being released with corresponding gratifications and new influxes of energy for projects just ahead, the selection of goals that are achievable and realistic. But these, and most of the other morale-maintaining actions that one can think of, are for mature and autonomous persons already launched with the strength to manage their lives; they remind us of Adolf Meyer's advice to teachers, when they asked him how they could prevent future mental illness in their pupils. "Teach them to finish their tasks" was his answer. And he implied that they could prevent such illness by giving children of school age good discipline and a good hygiene of action.

Janet betrayed a consistently holistic trend in his thinking. It is the whole man we must continually center on, he suggests.[10] If we take up one of his cases of "mad-dog" phobia (see Janet 1903, II, 183-88) we discover that, while Janet

---

[10]Leo Kanner was to repeat this holistic emphasis when he wrote of the tics and habit spasms of childhood: "it is not the tics that must be treated, but the patient who has them." With enuresis, he could have added, it is not the child who wets the bed who needs treatment, but the family who permits it to occur.

is mildly interested in going back to pick up the childhood "roots" of the particular phobia in some special traumatic event, he is more concerned with the current pressures on the patient that have revived it, just recently, for the patient had carried the memory for three decades, without symptoms, before the present attack of the phobia. For this reason he did not allow himself to become involved in endless discussion of the meaning of symptoms or in speculations about symbolic values, infantile and instinctual roots of the compulsions, or early conditioning situations. If a patient is already too prone to doubts, scruples, and speculations, it is important that his conferences with a therapist do not become adjuncts to his own alibi-making. Like the analyst who discounts the manifest content of a dream, Janet tried to divert the attention of his obsessive-compulsive patient, but for exactly opposite reasons. It was to the current real-life tasks that he wanted his patient to turn: not only did the contents of the patient's concerns change (mad dogs, closed spaces, open spaces, germs, dirt, spiritual uncleanness), but the self-regulative weakness also tended to ebb and flow with the changes in current press, in the hygiene of living, in the internal integrative forces. When health returns, the mad dogs are no longer a problem. As John Dewey once remarked about our philosophic issues: We never solve them; we just outgrow them and move on to new ones.

Addictions, Sexual Deviations, and Criminality

No longer can we comfortably consign every "offender" to a pigeonhole labeled psychopath (or sociopath). The definition of "antisocial" behavior is too blurred and shifting, as was noted in Chapter 1, and the roots of all "abnormal" behavior are too numerous and ramified, as this entire book intends to show. Nonetheless certain patterns of behavior can best be described as revealing a lack of normal value orientation.

The intrusion of all manner of minor habit-fixations—from smoking to gum-chewing to insistence on sitting in a certain chair—impairs the efficiency and flexibility of our adjustments, even as the alcoholic's habit of reliance on his chemical "booster." We could invent impressive names for all these *isms,* and in our census, which would include all those who suffer impairment from any one of these "addictions," we would have to include the larger portion of the population, if not all of it. The most publicized form of reliance on an ingested substance, narcotics addiction, is statistically still of minor concern (there were some 60,000 narcotics addicts in 1962, according to the U.S. Treasury Department). The major problem arising from this kind of addiction, in terms of social cost, is that of alcoholism. Of the 68 million persons who use alcoholic beverages in the United States, more than four million (over twenty years of age) are judged to be alcoholics—or, to use the now familiar euphemism, "problem drinkers." These are the drinkers who cannot manage their craving for alcohol but are instead managed by it. Of all Americans over twenty years of age, 4.39 per cent have been classed as problem drinkers, with the rate for males running as high as 7.59 per cent and for females 1.32 per cent (see Zwerling and Rosenbaum 1959, p. 624).

Some have speculated that a craving for alcohol is inherited, perhaps related to special nutritional needs, but there is little supporting evidence for this hypothesis. Social and parental influences on drinking habits unquestionably exist, but they have not been clearly identified, let alone measured. Alcohol and other substances may be taken to fill a neurasthenic sense of emptiness, as seen in Chapter 5, or alcohol may be used to ease the conflict between viscerally-based and outside demands (as well as internalized values), as seen in Chapter 7. We shall see in Chapter 9 that the amnestic syndrome, characterized by a loss of vital power, has been linked with both brain damage and chronic alcoholism. Excessive drinking may accompany manic elation, as will be seen in Chapter 10, but also may serve as an escape from depression. Finally, dipsomaniacs and narcotics addicts may suffer from a loss of vital contact with reality, the disorder subsumed in Chapter 11 under the rubric of the schizophrenias.

Is there any common denominator in these multiform behavioral concomitants and manifestations of alcoholism? Personality tests have not yielded any convincing objective evidence of an alcoholic type, and the clinical interpretations of problem drinking are most varied. Indeed, alcohol can fit into any one of the difficulties that adult life presents to everyman. Thus the therapist who works with alcoholics, or with narcotics addicts, must be a skillful eclectic, ready to discover precisely which phases of a personality structure rendered it vulnerable and ready to use what seems the best available means of rehabilitation. Initial optimism and subsequent relapse and resentment may be expected. The safest generalization about therapy for addiction is that communication and the establishment of something that will *fill* a life seem more important than achieving the negative victory of abstinence. Hence the importance ascribed to helping groups such as Alcoholics Anonymous and Synanon, who, having been rescued themselves, are full of the desire to lift their brothers from the gutter. Yet it must be admitted that existing ways cannot reclaim more than a third of the large army of adult alcoholics and an even smaller part of the growing battalion of narcotics addicts.

While a few social critics (e.g., Sorokin 1956 pp. 23-25) are condemning our society as sex-addicted, America manages to sexualize religion, advertising, literature, movies, and teenage (not to mention grade-school) personal relations. The public prints and the stage underscore the increasingly strident and vocal themes of abnormal sexual relations. Viewing human sexuality with alarm is at least as old as organized society. Editorials, sermons, and laws are directed against prostitution, pre- or extramarital sexual relations, "immodesty" in dress, utterances regarded as pornographic (the "filth that corrupts"), and, above all, against "unnatural practices." No behavior pattern offends the heterosexual majority more than homosexuality, as Chapter 1 has shown. Is there an increase in homosexuality? The British Wolfenden Report (1960) and the New York Academy of Medicine report (1964) concluded that there is no way of knowing. From the Kinsey report (1948) we can make an educated guess that somewhere between 2 and 15 per cent of all male adults are homosexuals.[11]

In Chapter 2 we saw that genetic sex, endocrine sex, genital sex, and the psychosexual behavior of the matured adult do not always coincide. We saw also that, while there are actual hermaphrodites, no specific genetic factor has been found to explain typical homosexuality. This throws much of the burden of explaining sex typing on intrafamilial learning, for children show that they know their sex roles by age three or four. Where later causes (particularly isolation with members of the same sex) produce homosexual behavior, the effects tend to be superficial and transient. Like alcoholism, abnormal sexual behavior in general may reflect a neurasthenic's attempt to fill a sense of emptiness, a manic's loss of decorum, a depressive's craving for excitement, or a schizophrenic's flight from reality.

Behavior therapy, with its Pavlovian conception of causes, consistently looks to avoidance training and to recommendations as to how the patient can find and use appropriate reinforcement. As with other deviations, the therapists vary from those who center on a segment of behavior to those who strive to assist the patient to make a good life, and from optimists who set a goal of "total recovery of normality" to those who limit their aim to minimal gains within the pattern. The actual rates of recovery reported by specialists who work in this area do not suggest that therapy is an easy matter. A large number of homosexuals, who never appear on the records of clinic or court, would consider a therapist as an intruder, for they look upon their own way of life as perfectly satisfactory, if not superior.

Crime has many faces, also many definitions. One man's civil disobedience, or even dissent, is another man's treason. What many would consider to be mere bad habits or illnesses (like compulsive gambling), others consider criminal acts. Crimes result from carelessness, exaggerated notions of self-defense, and submission to overwhelming temptation. French law distinguishes between "crimes of passion," especially the passion of jealousy, and premeditated crimes. Psychopathologists are concerned with the dynamics of criminal acts as one aspect of abnormal behavior; many also have faced the question

---

[11]Kinsey estimates (p. 651) that 4 per cent of the white male population are exclusively homosexual throughout their postadolescent lives. As high as 18 per cent of his samples of males have had at least as much homosexual experience as heterosexual for at least three of the years between the ages 16 to 55. In older white males, 45 years of age, his tables show that but 1.8 per cent in his sample were exclusively homosexual. 63 per cent of his sample had never had overt homosexual experience after adolescence. In addition to these considerations the "exclusively homosexual" rating varies with age of sample: 15.4% at 15 to 1.8% at 45.

And in using these figures, which tend to freeze into facts as soon as they are printed, one has to remember that they were obtained by a particular method of sampling and interviewing, both of which have come in for considerable criticism. No other source of equally careful sampling or equally extended interviewing is available, however. This is "reported homosexuality" and not actual incidence of the pattern. Many experienced psychiatrists offer "educated guesses" that are higher, particularly for recent years when the publicity given to this style of life has made it easier to admit, and easier for a clinician to probe, as noted in Chapter 1.

as to whether there is such a phenomenon as a psychopathic (sociopathic) personality. This book reports crimes committed by bored neurasthenics and hysterics, driven obsessive-compulsives, restless manics, and deluded schizophrenics; and it reports criminal behavior by persons with or without brain damage—chiefly without. In short, instead of a single genetic complex, a single neural cause, or a single environmental pressure or deficit that results in a uniform and massive failure in self-regulation, we are forced to look for varying causes, multiple pathology, variable outcomes. And yet, whether or not we call them psychopaths, we can discern a common pattern in the habitual criminals and near-criminals: a breakdown in the kind of self-regulation that reflects *respect* for self and others.

A Modern Instance: Somatopsychic Cycles of Behavior

Some clinicians have given special attention to the changing psychodynamics that are linked with the endocrine changes of the menstrual cycle. Oddly enough, obsessive concerns were reported at one phase of the cycle, along with the mood changes described as "premenstrual tension": there were compulsions to clean, to put the house in order, to organize the work, to finish long-postponed tasks, to redecorate the furniture, to rearrange the rooms, to remodel clothing. One subject, studied by Altmann, Knowles, and Bull (1941), jokingly referred to her monthly "attacks of the cupboard disease." We might speak of a periodic return of a compulsive phase, located at the point of lowest hormone output in the cycle. These investigators described the period as "an outburst of physical and mental activity . . . with high tension and irritability and preceded or accompanied by depressions." Worries, a tendency to cry easily, and hostility directed against both the self and others are reported in some patients during this low-hormone period. There are feelings of incompleteness, of being soiled, of unworthiness; in some there were strenuous compensatory activities. In the less energetic ones, these compensatory compulsive activities were makeready ones rather than completed actions: instead of baking the cake, she cleaned the cupboard; instead of writing the letter, she put the writing desk in order; instead of making the dress, she put her sewing basket in order. Low in the behavior hierarchy, and requiring the least energy, are the obsessive thoughts, scruples, doubts, which come to the surface in these periods.

In contrast to Janet and to these modern students of psychosomatic relationships, the orthodox analyst has been more inclined to follow out the free associations, to uproot old memories that underlie the feeling of uncleanness or incompleteness, certain that the impulses now active originate in that wellspring of all motivation, the *id,* and have been rendered pathological by repression.[12] The bouts of ritual cleaning that Benedek and others have traced to the endocrine cycle would appear, then, in the analyst's summary

---

[12]Harry Stack Sullivan, though well within the Freudian tradition at most points, offers a practical reason for *not* following his mentor at this point, particularly when dealing with a patient full of scruples and doubts. "Every now and then," he writes (1964, II, 251), "as I listen to this headache of considerations that cancel each other out and leave everything just wobbly, I ask, at what is calculated to be a quite disconcerting time, 'Well, why the enormous

as an anxiety-binding procedure calculated to contain or remove unconscious guilt, the precise sources of which lie in infantile sexuality, to be discovered only by the patient tracing-out of associations, dream images, until the meaning of the symptom is revealed. Only after he has found such underlying meanings for the actions is he ready to consider the practical relationships in the patient's present life, which will then be approached in the light of the idiosyncratic memory patterns and not in terms of any standard hygiene of living for man.

Freud's notion was that the repressed past, persisting into the present in the unconscious, robs the conscious self of that integrative strength which Janet was concerned about. Loaded impulses, charged with life-giving instinctual energy, but held back behind the hatchway door which guards consciousness against the unleashed forces of the id that threaten to overwhelm it, have to be kept down by the censor, the conscious ego, and the superego, which backs up this personal regulator. This constant work of repression (for the repressed tends to return, to press for expression) requires a costly and persistent vigilance. The pursed lips of the priest who fears that he will utter obscenities in the pulpit, the constant contraction of the masseters that he can outwit only by propping his jaws open with a cork, are a caricature of this repression process; here the effort that ordinarily operates silently within the subject, and sometimes unconsciously and automatically, becomes visible in a set of movements. Such work of containment withdraws energy from the reserve pool that could otherwise be used in productive tasks.

There is both a positive and a negative outcome to the repression process, the Freudian reminds us. On the one hand, the repressed complex will charge some elements in the present constellation of impulses with an unusually high supply of energy, and on the other hand, the available sources of regulative energies are rapidly depleted by the efforts to bind these same impulses. To the hungry, food grows increasingly inviting; to the one who has dieted too long, the resistance to "temptation" may be lowered.

Lacking precise knowledge of how such a repressive mechanism operates, as one sensorimotor mechanism competes against another and some central regulative agency decides on a course of action, we tend to resort to psychoanalogy. We understand how a ship's captain would be distracted, and possibly commit errors in steering his course, if his crew (too many of whom are in chains) were clamoring for his attention. Even if he would not turn his head, he would be so busy *not* paying attention to them that his eyes might not spot the cloud on the horizon or pick out the course on the chart with the efficiency demanded by his task. It is such a maldistribution of energies, such a weakness "on the bridge," that both Janet and Freud center on as they describe the obsessive.

---

harassment about it? What difference does it make which is right?' On such occasions it sometimes becomes plain that these doubts are transparently bunk—they are not of any particularly great importance in the context in which they have been produced." In short, he believed it to be a maneuver, a method of avoiding certainty, of avoiding a direct confrontation with real difficulties.

We are tempted to use this analogy as we observe the young student, so shy and withdrawn, who cannot talk in her interview. Tight-lipped, she wants to find help but cannot bring herself to divulge her "secret." In the interviews with her counselor, the latter is forced to use roundabout ways of "pumping" up the suppressed material. She can endure long periods of silence, feeling a strange mixture of comfort and constraint: comforted by the thought that someone wants to help her, constrained by the thought that a confession would put her "beyond the pale." When finally, with great emotion, such a patient reveals girlhood experiences (an incestuous relation with her brother, a homosexual relation with a high-school teacher), we understand the suppression at work. These all too painful memories, in this case, were all too conscious, continuously held back by the pursed lips that guarded her secret. Surrounding this secret, there had developed a painful shyness, a quick blush, as though she felt that in the presence of others, in spite of all her precautions, someone would "see through her," or that she would, by some inadvertent slip, betray the worst.

Freud described a case of chronic paranoia who felt that people were watching her undress at night. She, too, had been uncommunicative and distrustful. When her free associations led back to a series of scenes when she was 17 (she was 32 when she consulted Freud) in which she and her brother had been in the habit of exhibiting themselves to each other, naked, before going to bed, Freud felt that he had found the secret behind her uncommunicative manner, her suspicion that people were watching her. In Freud's report, it is also apparent that she had not really forgotten these episodes, but rather had seen no connection between them and her present anxieties (which had begun only a year before).

Janet, and his colleagues who agreed with him, were asserting: the master of the ship is a weak one, his course has been poorly planned, he has let his crew get out of hand, his supplies are running low, a storm is brewing on the horizon. No wonder his grip on the wheel falters; no wonder the meanest cabin boy can now assert himself; no wonder a mere thought becomes a "terrible impulse."

Therapy, in Janet's thought, will certainly call for a many-sided effort. The captain must be helped to trim his sails; he may have to lay over in the next port, and give the crew a good meal and a little systematic discipline. A new course may have to be plotted, in view of the known currents and the prevailing winds. Both the ambitions of the captain and the stresses on the crew may have to be reexamined in the light of what is possible. Even the ship may need overhauling.

In contrast, Freud seemed to insist: this master is no weaker than other ship captains. The basic question centers around that division between what is allowed above decks and what is forced down into the hold. True, the disorganization on shipboard is periodic; it seems to arise in response to specific efforts (specific stimuli, specific demands for control). There is no possibility of putting a ship in order until we can find out precisely who is kept below decks, and why these particular occasions are so potent in stirring up repressed elements. Ultimately some of the below-deck forces will have to be given a place above decks, and somehow decontaminated so that they are accepted as a presentable part of the crew, particularly if they are a vital part of the complement of energies. (Is not repressed libido a bit of the life-force itself?) The weakness must lie in the distribution of these forces and in certain historically determined special sensitivities in this captain, probably originating in his childhood.

Within the same decade both Janet and Freud were publishing evidence of the existence of psychological automatisms that operate beneath the surface layer of the mind, automatisms which run themselves and which operate as though a kind of split-off, but still organized, "mind" were directing them. Both of these investigators seemed to have identified that paradoxical thing, an *unconscious consciousness,* a process that is in the mind yet not available to introspection or reflection. Both saw these automatisms as arising, at times, to preempt the whole field of awareness, to take over and replace a normal consciousness. In his experiments with posthypnotic suggestion, Janet had shown that the subject who was carrying out an appointed task often seemed preoccupied, abstracted, out of contact with his immediate environment, at that moment, as though a regnancy that normally controlled all automatisms had suddenly abdicated. Many degrees of this "absence of control" were reported: a posthypnotic "prompting" could be sensed as alien and be dismissed; the command given in hypnosis could result in an impulse that persisted and gained expression, while at the same time the waking ego struggled against it; and, finally, such an impulse could completely replace the regnancy, the subject acting as though lost in thought or acting out a dream that, afterward, he could not even recall.

In the phobias and obsessions that Janet analyzed, we note a recurring emphasis: the old fears that served as the points of origin of the particular phobia had never been forgotten. The meaningless ruminations and repetitive concerns from which the patient could not free himself were not, Janet thought, symbols of some secret, repressed process in the unconscious, not screens for some unspeakable murderous or obscene experience that was unknown to the patient. In contrast to his hystericals, he found that the psychasthenics (whom we call obsessive-compulsive) were all too conscious. He found no forgetting comparable to the patches of amnesia in the hysterical, no evidence of dissociation. Attempting to probe for such "lost" fragments of experience, he found that this type of patient was stubborn, resistant, and difficult if not impossible to hypnotize. They were much less suggestible than his hystericals. Where an analyst might have said, "The defenses of these patients are simply more difficult to penetrate," Janet concluded that they were not so much frangible (subject to a splitting of the reaction system) as they were abouliacs. They had all the bits of memory that the normal person possesses, but they lacked the force to use memories and impulses productively, synthesizing and regulating desired action. He saw a weakness in the ego, a poor synthesizing power rather than repression.

In one of his discussions of the obsessions, Janet described them as evidence of a breakdown in the secret-keeping process which civilized man has to develop, a regulation of action, a planning that is withheld until an appropriate moment. When the obsessive complains that his thoughts are being read, that he has thoughts he cannot control, that people are putting ideas into his head or stealing his thoughts, the difficulty seems to have affected this normally "secret-keeping" process. "Who," asks Janet, "could study his thoughts for a half-hour without finding a few inopportune ones irrupting?" But where the normal would brush these aside, get on with his task, check the impulse to confess, add the ounce of extra effort to the most significant line of action, the obsessive feels forced, driven, helpless before his mechanisms. Instead of a repressed unconscious at the focus of the problem, it seems to be a weakness in the repressing (or censoring) department (see Janet 1929, pp. 387 ff).

CASES ILLUSTRATING APPLICATIONS OF THEORY

A single case, viewed from these two approaches, may serve to sharpen our discriminations. Consider, then, the mixture of phobias, obsessions, and compulsions that were shown by a patient studied by Dr. Hartenberg (1922, pp. 24 ff). This physician, who shared many of Janets notions, offered interpretations that Roland Dalbiez (1941, I, 275 ff) regards as illustrative of the weakness in the Salpêtrière view. Accordingly, in Dalbiez's account we find what amounts to a psychoanalytic analysis of Janet's view, a happy circumstance for our purposes.

HARTENBERG'S OBSESSIVE-COMPULSIVE

Hartenberg's patient was dominated by a disgust for all of the body's excretions: saliva, urine, feces, menstrual blood. As he first looked upon this woman of 45, her facial expression betrayed disgust and uneasiness. Her upper lip and nose suggested that some bad odor was present. She also complained of fear of asphyxiation, and told how she had removed all gas piping; still the fear persisted, and she would get up in the night to see if perchance fumes from her anthracite stove were escaping.

It was on visits to her husband's grave that her concerns (and need for purity and peace of mind) redoubled. She washed constantly: her hands, her toothbrush, her linen, her hairbrush, her veils, her gloves, and the clothes that she wore on the street and that, she feared, had become mysteriously contaminated.

These obsessive-compulsive trends spread, involving servants, friends, lover. She even spied on her servants to make sure they washed their hands when they went to the lavatory, and her lover had to leave his shoes in the hall lest he should bring dirt from the street into the room. (She seemed to be making issues instead of a life.)

Since her husband's death, ten years ago, she had made a weekly visit to the cemetery, and she regarded it as a special occasion, almost sacred, and wanted to feel composed, serene, and pure in heart. To complicate her life, her lover had grown restless and she feared that he would leave her; she believed a female friend had almost stolen him away. Demoralized, she drank stimulants and "enjoyed" her obsessions, giving them free rein.

In dealing with an obsessive-compulsive, the clinician must choose his working hypothesis and his method of therapy. He may sense that the woman must reach some decision that would liquidate her deteriorating love affair; he may try to lead her through a kind of mourning that will alter her attachment to a dead husband and permit some more realistic beginning of a new life, a full-hearted investment of her energies in a new and productive living. He might, on the one hand, invite the patient to turn backward to an infantile past, to review her earliest development, and to arrive at a view of her present conflicts as though they were somewhat mechanical repetitions of old battles. On the other hand, he may choose to reeducate, recondition, retrain her compulsions and phobias by efficient conditioning techniques, as the behavior therapist proposes. He could seek some combination of therapies that will support and guide her in making a more practical and common-sense attack on current problems.

He could, following Janet's (and Hartenberg's) hunch that such persons are not "millionaires of the spirit," encourage the patient to take up a simpler existence, to enter a hospital or sanitarium, to take a rest cure. We can imagine that Janet would have urged the use of the whole armament of psychotherapy, modifying procedures to fit the particular circumstances in the case. We can imagine him supporting, cajoling, arousing, persuading, scolding, teaching, as the occasions demanded, using all of his wit, imagination, and prestige to one end, namely, to renew a power of self-regulation that could focus action in a realistic fashion on practical and possible targets.

In the view of Dalbiez, who used the case to demonstrate the superiority of the analytic approach, an effort should have been made to discover the real (i.e., infantile) causes of the symptoms. He would have sought out the meanings underlying her fear of carbon-monoxide fumes. He would have been impelled to discover the "unconscious crime" that she had at least fantasied, a crime that merited the death penalty. She would have been led to give her free associations until the full import of all those pollutions emanating from the human body was discovered. Do they (saliva, urine, feces, menstrual blood) somehow mask another type of pollution (by semen) from which they are displaced? Do they mask a fear of pregnancy and a guilt over her amorous adventures? At what point in her life did such conflicts over sexual expression assume such importance, and how are these related to an earlier infantile struggle?

Dalbiez does not have the poor woman available for questioning, and we have no way of dividing her into experimental subject and control so that the therapies could be compared and evaluated. On his part, Dalbiez is sure that, with a proper psychoanalytic therapy, the case report would have revealed some better explanation of her failure to think through and master her predicament. The obvious things to do are too obvious. When she visited her husband's grave and became so compulsive in the effort to make her visit free from all "impurities," why did she not face up to her relationship with her lover? But we could ask the same question about all the rest of her irrationalities. It is apparently very difficult for an obsessive-compulsive to clean up his conflicts and to put his mental house in order effectively, to put an end to his ruminations by practical actions. It is precisely this indecisiveness, this aboulia, this mixture of "opposites," that characterizes these obsessive-compulsive patients; they swing from anorexia to bulimia, from asceticism to debauchery, from a rigid middle-class propriety to a "walk on the wild side."

The washing compulsion also seems to favor Dalbiez's evaluation. It is so easily seen as a *displacement,* a symbolic act that is both absurd and ineffectual. Lady Macbeth should have taught us the meaning of all this. If this woman felt the compulsion to spit on the wreaths at her husband's tomb (as Hartenberg reported she did), is this act not another symbolic representation of the other ways she has of denigrating and denying him, violating the "presence" of his all too real memory? She cannot forget him, be true to him, drop her lover, find a new life, expend her efforts on actions that are more productive.

In her dealings with her new lover, there is the same futility, the same symbolic displacement. She makes him leave his shoes in the hall; but she lets him enter her bedroom. She acts, and then symbolically cancels the act by her absurd undoing. She is moved to break with him, yet she fights passionately to take him away from another woman.

Dalbiez makes this point: behind all her washing compulsion, her catastrophic dread of her body's products and excretions, lies a guilty love. Her symptoms arise not so much because she is unconscious of this love, has repressed it, but because (1) she has not dealt with it effectively, and (2) she avoids seeing any relationship between this most obvious fact and her symptoms. True, it is possible that this refusal (unawareness) is related to still deeper roots, to her basic feelings about sexuality, to her very first efforts to master her own cravings, to her first need for a mother's love that betrayed her into a self-hatred. Sensitive (constitutionally "emotional"), confused (not seeing the relationships between her actions), and with inhibited integrative powers (because of former infantile memories), the woman needs help if she is to do what she must.

Freudian Conceptions of the Roots of Obsessive-Compulsive Behavior

A Freudian would have been alerted, by this woman's curled lip and nasolabial fold, to expect problems that once were directly concerned with one of the first problems in self-regulation; namely, toilet training. This may be difficult for the layman to understand, and, unfortunately, we do not have the necessary longitudinal studies of human growth and development (which would first catch an individual as he is going through the toilet-training period and then follow him through the whole course of his development, until the first signs of obsessive-compulsive behavior break out in flagrant form) to prove this view to the hilt. Even lacking such data, the analyst has not hesitated to develop a "just-so story" to cover this problem and to draw his supporting "evidence" out of the patient's behavior—as interpreted. Believing firmly in the validity of his insight, he strives to project the current problems of his patients (and the manifest content of their dreams) against this backdrop, and as the dialogue between analyst and patient works out, he is led inevitably to this source. A typical version of this "battle of the chamber pot" in which analysts believe obsessive traits originate is offered by Rado (1959, I, 330).

"Irritated by the mother's interference with his bowel clock, the child responds to her entreaties with enraged defiance, to her punishments and threats of punishment with fearful obedience. The battle is a seesaw, and the mother, to fortify her position, makes the disobedient child feel guilty, undergo deserved punishment, and ask forgiveness. This indoctrination transforms the child's fear into guilty fear, and impresses upon him the reparative procedure of expiatory behavior. The mother-child conflict provokes in the child a struggle between his own guilty fear and his own defiant rage. Henceforth, his relationship to the mother, and soon to the father, will be determined by this motivating system: guilty fear over defiant rage, or obedience versus defiance. The severity of the conflict, sustained by the inordinate and unrelenting strength of fear and rage, perpetuates the outcome. In our view, with the establishment of this motivating system, the child acquires a crucial factor toward a predisposition to obsessive behavior."

Now every child is brought, sooner or later, to the point where he can control the evacuation of his bowels. It does not seem to be a difficult problem in learning. The neural groundwork for such control may be slow in maturing, however, and a mother's patience may be short, her method of training poor, and her own disgusts exaggerated. A child whose sensitivities are great, or whose learning is sluggish, or whose personal ties with a mother are already threatened for any reason, may react to the intensified conflicts generated in the course of toilet training as evidence of rejection. His soiling becomes a badge of guilt for all to see (and smell), and he feels unlovable, unworthy. (As Sullivan observes, the obsessive-compulsive typically doubts his lovableness.) Love, hate, anxiety, guilt, and compensatory and expiatory tendencies become organized around the problem of cleanliness (as do giving, complying, resentment, rebellion, and disorder). Neatness and parsimony exist beside "dirty tricks" and "dirty jokes," and overcompensatory kindness and wasteful giving. A curious incapacity for aggression may exist along with sadistic outbreaks of hateful actions, all depending on how this original conflict was resolved.

It is the Freudian contention that, although all of us succeed in developing an overlay of controlling habits, the underlying affective residues persist in the unconscious; from thence, in untimely irruptions and costly compulsions that an adult has to struggle against, a few reveal how thin this regulative overlay actually is. The universality of this training makes it a possible target for the analyst as he deals with any one of his obsessive-compulsive patients. What he lacks in the way of correlations between the phases of the sphincter battle and the later symptoms, he seeks to supply by a method of analysis and interpretation that is not too rigorous, as well as by a certain skill in weaving plausible life-histories which will give his patients a self-awareness that, he hopes, will help them in their self-regulative efforts.

We need not pause too long, at this point, to debate the applicability of this stereotype. It has been applied, and is being applied in cases currently treated, although many Freudians have tried to expand the "just-so" story to embrace many other aspects of interpersonal training, a long succession of intrafamilial conflicts that operate at many subsequent points in growth and development and in a manner quite different from this too harsh and unintelligent type of sphincter training. Horney suggests, by way of appeasement, that the reason why so many of us utilize an "excrement-laden" vocabulary when we wish to express our deep-lying hatred or disgust is not that our emotions originated at this point but that we now make use of the symbols because of the easily communicated "bludgeon-value" such words make possible. Kanner, also interested in the problem of control of excretions (e.g., enuresis), insists that, in his clinic practice, he finds poor self-regulation emerging from indifferent mothers, from a kind of unbuttoned training method, from measures that are both too little and too weak and too late, as well as from the brutal methods implied in the psychoanalytic paradigm. His enuretics come from homes in which the meal times are irregular, the training inconsistent, and the mothers defensive and apologetic, bringing their children to the clinic for altogether different problems, insisting that bedwetting had not been a problem until two weeks ago. Even within the framework of psychoanalytic assumptions, it would seem that a more varied set of paradigms is needed to understand the wide range of failures in self-regulation that the obsessive-compulsive phenomena require.

The Case of Little Hans

A special interest attaches to any psychoanalytic treatment of a phobia in a child of five; it would be a feat for anyone to accomplish; it would represent one of those nascent forms of the illnesses seen in older patients. That such an analysis was once made by Freud (1909), who knew the boy's parents, adds a special interest. When the boy came back to see Freud at age nineteen, this case acquires a special flavor. Some thirteen years had passed since the analysis of his boyhood phobia had been published. In spite of the stir that it had aroused in psychiatric circles, Hans himself had no memory of the earlier conversations with his father or of the latter's views of his fears. The whole episode might have happened to another boy.

Hans was only five when his father presented the boy's problem to Freud. Hans was afraid of horses. Taken for a walk in the park, the boy was full of anxiety. He suffered from nightmares. Looking out of the window of his apartment at the "street boys" who were jumping on and off carts, he was content to remain indoors. The child was also fearful when he was bathed in the big tub. As the father discussed these matters with Freud, the latter directed the father to talk with the child, and provided him with certain guesses as to the probable cause of the anxieties. One of the "directed conversations" reported by Freud (and he was merely relaying what the father had told him) must have run somewhat as follows:
"Why are you afraid in this large tub?"
"Because I might fall in!"
"But when we bathed you in the little tub you were not afraid."
"But I could sit in that one. I didn't lie down. It was too little."

"When we took you for a ride in the big boat you were not afraid."

"No. I could hold on to it. I couldn't fall in. It's only in the big bath that I'm afraid."

His father reminded the boy that his mother was the one who bathed him in the big tub, and then asked him, point-blank, "Are you afraid she'll drop you?"

"Yes, she might let go and my head would go under the water." Reassured that his mother was fond of him and would not let him fall, he could only murmur, "I only just thought it."

When he could not explain such a thought, his father prompted him: "Had you been naughty? Is it because you thought that she did not love you any more?" Little Hans went along with this suggestion, only to have his father press still further, with, "Maybe you wished that your mother would let go of little Hanna when you saw her bathing your little sister?" Once more, Hans agreed. Freud, who had coached the father, added his own comment to this account of what was reported: "Hans's father had made a very good guess."

From such a sample an unsympathetic reader might conclude, much in the manner of a defense lawyer's objection, "The prosecution is leading the witness." The implicit assumption that runs through Freud's interpretation of the reports of the interviews is that anxiety arises from the repression of guilty and forbidden wishes. By indirection, by implanted suggestions, and sometimes by the direct form of the question, the notions are conveyed to little Hans: It is because you have been naughty, and think your mother does not love you any more, that you are so full of fear; it is because you play with your penis; it is because you want to get rid of your papa; it is because you want mamma all to yourself; it is because you want to get rid of your little sister; and so on.

Our amazement at the certitude of the analyst grows as we discover that, if the child confesses to one of these imputed motives, the confession is accepted as proof. If he denies the impulse, or if his behavior shows that when his father is away from home he misses him, this will prove the extent of repression, and the existence of reaction formations that conceal the unconscious hostility. We are told, in conclusion, that Hans fears horses and big vans because he has played too much with his "widdler," that he has felt incestuous thoughts toward his mother, that he projects his own hostilities onto his father and onto horses (both of whom have large penises), and that he fears the animals will bite him (castrate him), even as he senses a castration threat in his father's frown.

The case is not a model of scientific caution: it betrays but does nothing to validate Freud's theoretical hunches. Like a phobia or obsession, such an interpretation and such a theory can spread, until the action of the father who builds a railing to keep his child from falling from a balcony forces the interpreter to wonder if it could be a compensation for his own death wishes directed against the boy, even as little Hans's fear that his mother would drop little Hanna was made into a murderous sibling rivalry. "Why *are* you afraid?" the father asked the boy at one point. Little Hans replied: "I don't know. But the Professor'll know. D'you think he'll know?"

When Freud's final report indicated that the parents were on the verge of divorce during these very months, and that subsequently they did in fact separate, we can form other hypotheses about the anxieties of little Hans, less fanciful, perhaps, and more matter of fact. We wonder whether such a child might be feeling and expressing the tensions within the household, growing anxious and insecure in a climate of conflict. He might not be able to verbalize any very good reasons for his fears (which he promptly directed at a number of objects). Nor does it seem likely that a verbal formula, a physician's awareness of what was going on within the boy, would wipe away the effects on the child's emotional life, once it was conveyed to him. If, as Harry Stack Sullivan once claimed, there is a great deal of word-magic in obsessionalism, it would seem, here, that the magician is the physician, not the phobic child.[13]

The fact that at nineteen, when he was finally seen by Freud, Hans appeared to be a healthy, strapping youth, suggests that the analyses of his childhood anxieties had not harmed him, nor had his parents' separation resulted in new symptoms. Finally this childhood episode is reduced to its proper perspective. If it is retained at all, it is in the form of a "forgotten memory." The subsequent history of such a phobia seems to depend on that constitutional soil within which it develops, on what habits are built over this anxiety-filled foundation, on the forgetting that seals it off, and on the new habits of confident approach to life that replace the original fears.

In sharp contrast to Freud's psychoanalytic treatment of little Hans is the behavioristic therapy reported by Mary Cover Jones in 1924 for a child with a fear of rabbits (see London 1964, p. 86). Her "desensitization" technique was to cause the child to relax by feeding him while the rabbit was at a "safe" distance, progressively moving the rabbit closer as the child's relaxation was more complete. Jones and others have reported considerable success with this technique among children with fears of animals.

OBSESSIONS, DRUGS, AND ARCHETYPES

Many clinicians have found that obsessives are not easy to treat. Analytic treatment may drag along over three to four years without the counselor-interpreter having succeeded in communicating a satisfactory interpretation to his client, or without the latter having come to terms with his problems.

---

[13]There is a form of thinking which Piaget once identified in the children he studied: too young to appreciate the full meaning of causality, they nonetheless used the verbal forms. "Why does the pebble go to the bottom of the aquarium?" the kindergarten teacher asked her five-year-olds. "Because it is white," answered one. "Because it is round," said another. Such phenomenistic thinking, which selects a striking sensory quality when the question is asked, "What makes it so?" is also used by adults when their reasoning runs out. Whether he is dealing with adults or children (but especially with the latter), the clinician who deals with phobias of unknown origin must expect to hear many versions of such thinking when his questions, like the one Freud reports the father as asking of little Hans, invite it. Indeed, Freud's free-association method and his freewheeling interpretations seem calculated to produce a great deal of it. His retort might be, "Yes, it is an infantile form of thought. But it is by way of such links that associations governing the spread of a phobia or an obsession are formed." For a brief discussion of this problem in childhood, see Dorothea McCarthy (1943).

These patients are not easy to hypnotize. The therapist's suggestions are met with countersuggestions. The analyst who interprets the meaning of symptoms or dreams finds that his patient can theorize as well as he. Either the patient's conflicts are near the surface, and the evidences of forgetting and repression are not as obvious as in the hysterical, or, as some have insisted, there is a much deeper repression of the traumatic memories, and possibly an earlier point of origin of the splitting within the self-system. Some urge that the conflicts originated in a preverbal period, when neither the discriminations nor the language functions had crystallized to form a clearly structured awareness.

Within the past decade, a series of studies of the effects of mescaline, lysergic acid, and other psychotomimetic drugs have shown that some of the phenomena seen in the obsessive patient can be produced experimentally by chemical means. It has occurred to some clinicians that these baffling patients with such perfect defenses might be "penetrated" while under the influence of these drugs. Demolishing the outer defenses by the use of a drug which destructures the ordinary vigilant postures, these therapists hoped to see the underlying pathological processes at work.

For example, administering mescaline to a normal subject produces vivid, colored images, exaggerated equivalents of the hypnagogic images that we mentioned earlier. Out of control, they come and go at *their* will, unrolling a sequence of visions of hallucinatory vividness. There are "delicious drifting sensations," and a pleasant floating away from all tensions and troubles, a state from which some of the subjects were reluctant to return. In some it seems to produce a devil-may-care disregard of the sensibilities of those around them, a chemically induced disinhibition of those interpersonal defenses a "sensitive" rears between himself and a too pressing world of persons.

A second drug, cannabis sativa (hemp), studied by Ames (1958), produced many of the signs that Janet had earlier recorded in his psychasthenics: a feeling of unreality, changes in the appearance of things, disturbances in body image, a feeling of depersonalization and detachment, as though the subject were looking on the self and its milieu from the outside.[14] A wide variety of contrasting experiences emerged, as though unique trends in the makeup of each subject had been unmasked by the drug, trends buried under the forces

---

[14]This "view from the outside," which arises spontaneously under such drugs as hemp or LSD, has contributed to the illusion of those who take such "trips" that they are seeing themselves for the first time as they really are, from a "fourth dimension," with an awareness of awareness, a vision of the ego tortured by its id impulses and made to feel guilty by its superego. The picture of the obsessive-depressive consciousness that, like an inner commentator, says, "Now he is turning the corner, now he is lifting his hat to the woman next door," appears in Freud's "Anatomy of the Personality" (1933). As though the observer stood a little to one side and in back of the actor, noting his posture and his expressions and making comments upon them, both the obsessive and the drug user report a doubling of consciousness. This added "fourth dimension" is, of course, often a misleading one, and it has a way of emerging at the very moment when action and critical evaluation falter. The blown-up brush heap of obsessive awareness (or drug consciousness) is notoriously and oppressively present in times of nonfeasance. The motionless opium addict wrapped in his "lotus eater's consciousness" is swollen with a certain kind of delight, but is impotent.

that make for social conformity; these experiences included euphoria, anxiety, and paranoid suspicions. ("Do these tests indicate that you suspect me of being a latent schizophrenic, Doctor? Have you hidden someone behind that screen?") The colored imagery sometimes approached hallucinatory vividness. ("My teeth are full of holes." "My brain feels like a ballerina's dress going round and round in a glass cube." "Your eyes are as large as oranges, as big as a beach umbrella.") There were thinking difficulties that prevented the march of thoughts to any incisive conclusion, a fragmentation and an obfuscation of thought.

One subject, a member of the medical staff that was carrying on the research, addressed his chief with a kind of amused tolerance that, in the waking state, he may have felt but never expressed, in these words: "You are very pleased with yourself about that F.R.C.P.—not that it was not richly deserved, but really you are so self-satisfied about it!" Other drugs, such as lysergic acid (LSD-25), have produced an even more complete destructuring of thought and action, with occasional long-lasting pathological aftereffects.

The linkage between these drug-induced states and the long familiar obsessive features, the disappearance of many of the rigid defenses, the emergence of imagery that is found to be coupled with very old memories, coupled with the difficulties in treating obsessives by conventional methods, have persuaded some clinicians to use these drugs in their clinical efforts at therapy. (See Sandison 1954, Sandison and Spencer 1954.)

Some of the material which emerges under these drug-induced states makes the experience seem like a waking dream. Occasionally it is a nightmare the subject wishes never to repeat. Some of the imagery is so disordered and so strangely structured that it bears little or no resemblance to any experience lived through. Those who follow the somewhat mystical theories of Jung are quick to attribute them to an archetypal unconscious which contains themes as old as the race. One of Sandison's patients, under the influence of LSD,

"...had the sensation...of a snake curling up round [her]." She wrote a description of the dream sequence. "I felt very sick and dizzy. I then began to see serpents' faces all over the wall, then I saw myself as a fat, pot-bellied snake slithering gaily away to destruction. I felt horrified and thought 'Whose destruction?' I then realized it was my own destruction—I was destroying myself. I seemed to be having a battle between life and death—it was a terrific struggle, but life won. I then saw myself on the treadmill of life—a huge wheel was going round and round with hundreds of people on it. Some were on top going confidently through life, others were getting jostled and trodden on but still struggling to go on living (I saw myself as one of these people), and then there were others who just couldn't cope with life and were being crushed to death in the wheel. I had another realization of how I was destroying myself—by carrying on this affair with this married man —how all the better side of me was gradually being destroyed through carrying on this affair, and I knew it must cease and knew that I must never see him again. Also when I was watching myself as a snake going to destruction, I cried for the doctor because I wanted him to show me the right road away from self-destruction.

"The doctor came in and asked me how I felt, and I told him that there were snakes everywhere. I had the sensation of being right in the middle of them. The doctor asked me if it was like anything I had experienced before. I said it was a dream I had had as a child. He asked me if I knew what that dream represented and I said, 'Sex.' He said, 'What sexual feelings could a small child of that age be having?' or words to that effect; and I said, 'I don't know.' Actually at that minute I was right back as a small child with moving grass all around me and I could see snakes slithering through the grass. The whole atmosphere was as it had been when sexual incidents occurred with boys when I was about six or seven."

The images changed from the childhood scene to ancient Egypt. The patient changed from a snake to the devil. She grew dizzy, dragged about by chains. She envisaged herself dipping her toes into the pool of life (with one man after another) and then drawing back from the murky depths. She imagined life as a jigsaw puzzle that was gradually fitting together. She jumped into the mouth of a huge snake and then, like a snake biting her own tail, consumed her body and its problems. She concluded her account by curling up in Hell, content with the thought, "Oh, well, it isn't such a bad Hell, after all."

The physician who plays the role of interpreter of dreams seems, in this instance, to believe that these allegorical experiences are communicating an important message to the patient and that this curling up with her imagery may represent a new unity between the conscious self and an archetypal unconscious, as though the drug had opened a door into an unconscious inferno long enough for her to come to terms with something within her. The language of the patient, after a series of such "nightmares" and after assimilating the interpretations, reveals that she, too, is ready to play the role of priestess to her own inner oracle: she interprets the experiences as "a battle between life and death," as identifying a path that "leads down to destruction." The restructuring of her life, which she could not accomplish with the usual counseling of parents, friends, and a psychiatrist, is here portrayed as a task for which matter-of-fact language seems insufficient. Now it is taking place through a modern orphic ritual involving the use of a drug. Placed against the life history that her physician now publishes, the drug experience is given one of many possible readings. Hopefully, one of these readings, worked out in a continuing collaboration between patient and physician, will assist in bringing order into a rather chaotic life. Her record, as published, described a single girl, 25 years of age.

"She was an only child, brought up in a sheltered moralistic environment, both parents having narrow views. The family pattern, however, with the exception of her mother, was one of independence and sexual freedom. The girl's early adolescence was emotionally stormy, the practical implications of which she was scarcely called upon to face, as she developed tuberculosis at the age of sixteen, but she became physically able to resume a normal life at the age of twenty. Almost immediately the problems of her love-life led her into severe conflict. She adopted a prim and virginal attitude towards her fiancé and soon began to be tormented by evil thoughts about him which amounted to a conviction that he was a murderer and that he would do her or someone else a severe physical harm. These confusing thoughts led her break off the engagement and thereafter she found that she would develop the same morbid thoughts about each man in whom she became interested. She became increasingly aware of a sense of frustration and emptiness in her life. She had long periods of deep depression and at the time of her admission into hospital, just before starting LSD treatment, she was on the point of suicide. She had previously attempted to counteract her evil thoughts by taking an active part in church life, but she soon found that her very worst thoughts would come to her in church. There seemed to be no remedy. Eighteen months of psychotherapy had shown her that the problem was to come to terms with her own experiences. These were dramatic and consisted of those archetypal universal experiences to which we have already referred. The most important of these images was the snake, which the patient recognized as a part of herself; but its behavior was not under her control and the snake tended to behave autonomously, as the unconscious does when it is not accepted and integrated into consciousness."

In the course of their clinical study of experiences released by LSD, these investigators found some which seemed to consist in a reliving of forgotten traumatic experiences; some of which were from a remote childhood, while others were from more recent adult life. None of them had been accessible to ordinary methods of recall. They suggest that what neither hypnosis nor free-association techniques can do may be accomplished by the aid of this new chemical.

Sandison and his colleagues suggest that the LSD imagery might be classified in three categories: (1) a type involving a general change in body sensations and in the appearance of the world—lightness of the body, colored patterns, surfaces that dissolve and move; (2) relived or reviewed experiences of the past, both recent and remote; (3) archaic and impersonal scenes that are from the deepest layers of the mind.

These "deepest layers of the mind" constitute that "realm of the archetypes," a concept that Jung developed and exploited. It has been called the "unconscious of the unconscious," the racial memory. A mystic belief that defies logical analysis and contradicts our hard-won knowledge of memory and inheritance, this concept of a racial memory implies that there is something deep within us that we must come to terms with, something profoundly spiritual, a knowledge that lies beneath all individual knowing. Making use of this background of belief, the strange experiences released by LSD are here interpreted as though the drug were a kind of chemical key that unlocks this deepest layer of mental functioning.

These drugs, which some call psychotomimetic, others call psychedelic (e.g., Huxley 1960). The latter name implies that they can open the doors of perception, release new sources of spiritual power, reorient us in paths congenial to our deepest nature. In certain quarters a cult of the drug has developed. Such phenomena are not new. The *soma* of the ancient Hindus and the peyote cult of some modern American Indians represent two points in this long and continuing tradition. In the latter cult a cactus button containing mescaline-like compounds is brewed to make a tea; the drinking of the tea in a ritual that fuses Christianity and traditional folk beliefs of the tribesmen produces vivid hallucinatory experiences representing Jacob's ladder, the firebird, mythical kachinas, and so on. The skeptical onlooker will conclude that the archetypal experiences that emerge under the drug are of a type that might be expected to seep in from this particular cultural matrix. Saturated with vibrant memories of our ancestors, charged with the grand themes of birth, death, suffering, courage, and betrayal, and recharged in religious ceremonies, funerals, and public celebrations, this internalized matrix affects the celebrant's total orientation to life. Beneath our sober, matter-of-fact rational consciousness, interwoven with the memories of our individual life-history, perhaps each one of us has a mental basement that contains heroes, martyrs, demons, lovers, Judases, Don Juans, witches, not only the more factual voyages of Columbus and the account of the conquest of Mexico, but also the thousand and one nights of the story teller, the operatic love-deaths, and the childhood tales of sleeping beauties—provided he has learned the folk tales. Under mescaline, LSD, or psilocybin (the sacred mushroom), these images troop into consciousness, now given a new dynamic shape in a particular individual who is operating under a unique and momentary pattern of stress. Hypomanic, he may soar to the heights to converse with Prometheus; depressed, he will travel the path once described by Dante, to the inferno. Anxious, guilty, and obsessively driven to establish a perfect defense against any and every flaw in his nature, he may "sweat it out" as he removes tare after tare from some symbolic harvest, reproducing his version of the labors of Sisyphus.

What does the destructuring drug release? The semireligious disciple of Jung will respond: something deep within him that Everyman disregards at his peril. Something, the rationalist is inclined to believe, that could well be left unsaid, at least if our reason were strong enough to make a good life, a balanced synthesis of all that is good within us, a design that can firmly reject most illth. Something, the anthropologist might want to add, that represents a not always well-digested hodgepodge of folk wisdom. Something, the cautious student of individual psychology might suggest, that symbolizes, in a most illth. Something, the anthropologist might want to add, that represents in synthesizing even when destructuring drugs do not impair the process. Something, the imaginative geneticist suggests, that may have been laid down in the DNA substances that organize our bodily structure and that may contain, in those templates of the nuclear substances of our brain cells, memories older than those laid down in our individual life-spans (see Miller 1961).

Recent medical journals have been filled with warnings as to the dangers of using these powerful drugs. Our experience leads us to expect that such warnings will not have much effect. What the expert must note is that the phenomena produced have a way of fitting into the settings within which the drug is taken and into the pattern of prevailing belief. In the little church where the peyote cult holds ceremonies, the tea brewed from the cactus buttons produces visions of Jacob's ladder and the firebird. In the group of students in a New England seminary, such drug-induced visions deal with mystic experiences of "union" and "revelation." In the psychoanalyst's service, we discover that they reveal archetypal symbols of sexuality (the huge snake that coils upward around the virgin's legs). What is *not* experienced in any of these instances are those changes within the nuclear structures of body cells, or gene-structure alterations that are capable of producing birth anomalies (as thalidomide has done). Where a cause and its effects are so separated in time, and the changes are so hidden from direct observation, there is nothing to link them but a social intelligence that is not always widely shared; and even when it is, it is sometimes not potent enough to regulate behavior. Should drug usage be incorporated into any serious religious ritual, it would be protected, of course, by the aura of the *sacred,* a notorious thought-stopper.

NEUROLOGICAL ANALOGS TO THE OBSESSIVE-COMPULSIVE STATE

As dramatic as any type of "possession" or "seizure," the epileptic attack has called for explanations as far back as our records of history go. From looking on them as possessions by demons, we have progressed to the stage where our anatomical and biochemical knowledge permits us to lay the responsibility on "sick cells." When certain localizable groups of cells suddenly discharge, they may produce a typical Jacksonian "fit" or a minor blackout of consciousness (as in *petit mal*), and when the electroencephalogram shows a burst of typical peaks of electrical potential at the moment the blackout occurs, this covariance seems to clinch the case. Even more convincing is the disappearance of attacks with the administration of a drug, such as dilantin. The speculations at the turn of the century, when psychoanalysts sought to base such attacks on repressed impulses, suddenly became groundless and useless. To clinch the neurological explanation, the direct exploration of the surface of the cortex with an electrode finally demonstrated that attacks could be experimentally precipitated by appropriately placed stimuli.

Clustered around these attacks there is an adventitious group of phenomena that vary from subject to subject, in part because of the varying localization of the precise pathological neural processes. Among the accessory symptoms are the auras which precede the seizures. In a few auras of visual type, scenes from the patient's past flash before his mind's eye and, as though viewing the scene from without, he relives as an onlooker actions in which he once participated. Occasionally these scenes have been the subject of recurrent nightmares in childhood, and if they somehow scarified the cortex then, embedding themselves deeply, they usually lapse for an extended period only to reappear as the aura of an adult's epileptic attack. Whatever symbolic significance they may have acquired as they became intertwined with the problems of a developing adolescent, they now come to mean "an attack is about to seize you," and the epileptic will brace himself against this behavioral hurricane that impends. Other patients experience sudden blockages in the train of their thought ("thought robberies" that resemble those the obsessive complains of). There are annoying, repetitive irruptions of nonsense phrases and melodies, along with the muscle spasms (tics, oculogyric crises) that some case histories of supposedly "pure" obsessions also report.

Other cases resemble the epileptic in that they, too, have the "brainstorms" (measurable on the electroencephalogram) but without the seizures or blackouts. An extended zone of symptoms, analogous to the obsessive's loss of control and with good evidence of a neurological basis, invade this territory traditionally preempted by psychogenic explanations. In this epileptoid territory there is a contested border zone in which psychotherapists vie with neurologists in the diagnosis and treatment of "mixed types." Each is capable of enthusiastically extending his "zone of control" into the other's territory. Just as hysteroepilepsy was once a bone of contention, and now is broken up by improved diagnostic discriminations, there is an epileptoid-obsessive-compulsive complex that calls for similar discriminations. (See Brickner, Rosner, and Munro 1940.)

These irruptive patterns of thought and action, in this borderline "epileptoid" zone, are so dissociated from the normal stream of purposive action and so completely out of control, that they can be viewed as expressions of reverberatory circuits that are activated (or released) by some impersonal biochemical change in the nerve cells: the circuits literally explode; and their irrelevance to the ongoing dynamic concerns is as great as though the limbs were suddenly dislodged by some unexpected blow. They come from *without,* if one takes the viewpoint of the subject himself: he can look at them, accept them, reject them, worry about them, or be amused, but control them he cannot. Though he reacts with feeling, these action circuits cannot be laid aside as our ordinary unwanted acts can be.

These patterns that function so autonomously may be viewed as old traces, engrams laid away along with other stored experiences, but instead of the normal use of those which are appropriate to some novel need, we note that they insert themselves automatically. Normally summoned by some perceived shape, these epileptoid irruptions are triggered (or released) by a minor biochemical explosion in a specific group of cortical cells. The reverberating circuits complete themselves, and may be repeated over and over. In this border zone which we call *epileptoid,* the responses do not end in blackout or *grand mal* attack.

Experimenters have found analogous chains of self-firing, repeating neural circuits in isolated masses of cerebral tissue in the experimental animal. Electrical recordings made as the succeeding waves of impulses activate implanted electrodes provide a visible-manipulable analog of what is happening in our epileptoid patients. Imaginatively we think of the way in which such a preempting circuit could block other developing action. What the psychologist has been impelled to consider a compensation for (or an expression of) repressed anxiety would here be attributed to reverberatory circuits and to a biochemical condition, to a minor neurological explosion.

Brickner (1940) has identified areas in the cortex where stimulation of the exposed cells in a waking subject will arrest speech. The patient, set to counting or to repeating the alphabet, can be made to trip on any letter or number the experimenter selects, merely by the application of an electrical stimulator to the vulnerable spot at the moment the syllable is forming. Counting to ten and stimulated at the moment the final number is spoken, the subject repeats "Teh, teh, teh, teh,..." like a record that is stuck. Speech may be slowed, thickened, or arrested by such means, and thought may be halted or blotted out. Penfield and Rasmussen (1950) reported a type of nominal aphasia, in one subject who, handed a comb and asked to name it as a specific cortical area was stimulated, could not find the word, even in thought.

In a group of epileptics there will be one who will hear echoed a half-dozen times each phrase that is spoken to him; the sequence will end in a convulsion. Another such patient, forced to fixate on a traffic light, will find that all movement is arrested for about thirty seconds, at the end of which a complete blackout occurs. Another, playing cards, found that he could not look away from his cards or think of anything else, and in this fixated state a seizure would occur. Similar fixations, forced thinking, echolalia can occur without seizures. A case of Parkinson's tremor (with the disease process located in the basal ganglia) was observed to repeat endlessly, "I want to go to the hospital." A similar case repeated the Lord's Prayer endlessly, but could be stopped if the physician ordered her to stick out her tongue.

Summarizing these facts, we note that encephalitis in childhood may be followed by delayed attacks of oculogyric-compulsive crises. The later attacks may make use of engrams formed before the epileptic-like process began. An obsessive-compulsive personality makeup, in turn, may develop in such a way that it makes use of both the early trauma and the disease process (defending the status of an impaired person, displacing concern onto a bodily process when the origins of anxiety are diffuse or rooted in a repressed ethical conflict). The life-style will deserve treatment on its own account, not because it is a cause of the attacks. Treating the attacks directly, through medical or surgical means, may remove one of the major supports of the life-style; in other instances it may lay bare a much more difficult and obscure problem for psychotherapy. When electroencephalograms reveal the presence of abnormally firing neural circuits, and when the evidence from the neurological examination and the case history point to somatic causes, psychotherapy tends to become an adjunct. Even where the "problems in living" (and their accompanying emotional tensions) appear to increase the frequency of attacks, the management of these problems will rarely be sufficient to remove the symptoms completely, for it cannot correct the underlying neurophysiological process.

There is no clear dividing line between the neurologist's patients with an epileptic or postencephalitic process at work and those "pure" obsessional cases in which no such underlying process has been identified. Thus we have epileptic cases without any genuinely obsessive-compulsive symptoms and without any prior development of the obsessive-compulsive life style; we also have obsessive-compulsive personalities with no identifiable or treatable neural process. In the latter group, although the phenomena resemble some of those found in the postencephalitic group, there is no good neural explanation for the phobias, obsessions, and compulsions. The analogy with the epileptic does not help the therapist.

These excursions into neurology remind us that the clinician who treats obsessive-compulsive patients, who suffer from breakdowns in the regulation of action, must be prepared to meet a few cases with analogous symptoms to which his psychogenetic theories do not apply. Patient research will clarify this borderland as it has that other one which lies between hysteria and epilepsy, the area of hysteroepilepsy. One side of the dividing line will be occupied by cases in which impersonal causes are at work to produce a "loss of control," as in those postencephalitic states in which there are forced, repetitive, and purposeless actions and irruptive thoughts. Speaking of the latter, Brickner notes: "The *content* of the obsessive thoughts is secondary. . . . *whatever is thought will be obsessively thought*" (my italics). Though thoughts and actions may arise out of personal history, the form that they take in these patients is neither caused by that history nor relevant to it. (See Brickner, Rosner, and Munro 1940; see also Jelliffe 1932 and Schilder 1938.)

This does not preclude the possibility of a *conditioning* that will increase the number of signals that release such "forced actions." It is probable that, whenever stress mounts, their number will increase, while under a good hygiene of living they may be fewer. But personal history, conditioning, control of emotions, improvement in the hygiene of living are all ameliorative; they are secondary factors which, at best, modify a process whose essential cause lies elsewhere.

It is apparent from the studies of Brickner and Lhermitte (1951) that, when the neural involvement is slight, such patients may be aroused, cajoled, assured, diverted from their "illusions." With some of the newer medications, combined with good hygiene and rest, a neuropsychiatrist might stand by, waiting for that *vis medicatrix naturae* to restore the patient to health. But when there is some underlying lesion with a progressive neural involvement, the troublesome images can become hallucinations, the playful confabulations that the patient could once be talked out of become bloody truths, and the patient's efforts to deal with his symptoms may then take the form of a violent "acting out." The minor changes in reverbatory circuits then produce a complete destructuring of action, and the patient no longer lives in a shared reality.

On the other side of the dividing line, we can place the conceptually pure obsessive-compulsive cases whose symptoms are produced by psychological causes, and for whom no medication or surgery is needed to restore the functioning of those circuits which lie between the challenges of the environment and the effectively regulated actions which suit the purposes of the individual. Once we have studied cases on each side of this conceptual dividing line, neither of the two classes seems quite as "pure" as our logic requires. Scrupulous in his diagnosis and meticulously complete in his therapeutic efforts, a knowledgeable clinician is almost required to take on some of the qualities of the obsessive-compulsive patient.

EXPERIMENTAL MODIFICATION OF THE "REGULATIVE SET"

Most of the symptoms included under obsessions, compulsions, and phobias represent a breakdown in the normal regulation of action. Something has happened to the in-between process that governs the normal flow of behavior. One of the difficulties in arriving at a clear concept of the process that goes wrong lies in the very diversity of the behavior samples that have been included within this obsessive-compulsive category.

One patient is indecisive, morose, full of scruples, unable to act at all: he fills the therapeutic hour with his doubts; he can see all sides of every question, yet can make no formulation of his predicament that will release action; he cannot decide, synthesize, select a course, and cut his losses. The next is a compulsive: he acts, to be sure, but inappropriately; handwashing, touching, correcting, going through a meticulous makeready, he cannot restrain what he knows is foolish. The next is possessed by irruptive thoughts that give him no peace; he cannot think consecutively and productively. He is like M. Til, whose writing hand keeps forming "messages," interfering with what he is about; he gives too much credence and much too great freedom to mechanisms that he should replace by a more rational control. The next is a phobic, whose fear of mad dogs and rabies has spread from the kennel to the shrubbery, to the street, and to the dust set swirling by a passing car, or he is an artist who cannot deal with those who give him commissions, or go into the street, or leave his apartment, or see anyone save his wife, until he is finally self-imprisoned.

There is a common element in these cases, to be sure, but it is a very general one. Something has gone wrong, in each case, with that *regulative set* which keeps action flowing and on target, which mediates between the needs which continually emerge and that field into which consummatory actions must be fitted. Normally this set keeps liquidating old tasks as new ones form; and as the "sets" for goals just ahead are released (with the completion of actions), the impounded tensions can relax and the energies that have charged the action can now flow back into newly forming sets, into latent reserves.

Normally a hierarchy of sets keeps the demands of subordinate needs within bounds: some actions are withheld; no single need is allowed to hypertrophy to the distress of the whole; and no local signals are permitted to so absorb attention that the larger field cannot be kept in mind. As the stream of action flows, the system as a whole is adjusted to what Koffka once called "the behavioral environment."[15] In good contact with the surroundings, a flexible

---

[15]This term has a very special meaning. It is not the objective experimental situation created by the behaviorist who is putting an experimental animal through discrimination training in a very restricted field, but rather it is the field as structured by a man in the course of action. We live in such fields, which we make as we go; and we structure them selectively. We may foolishly believe that they contain all there is, until some moment of insight fits the parts together in a new way and permits something that was mere background to leap into the significant foreground. (See Koffka 1921, 1935.) Koffka uses the term "geographic environment" to describe that other, *objective,* surrounding field which exists, hypothetically, whether there is any viewer or not.

and changeable regulative set keeps the parts from interfering with each other, while the whole system progresses toward what is both possible and desirable.

Such a regulative set is a fragile thing. Its powers are limited. It can run down until the person cries out, "Who am I? What is it all for? I am a nothing." A particular need can hypertrophy until it appears to run the whole.

Normal sets can fail for lack of external supports. An extended series of experimental studies on the effects of "sensory deprivation" has produced phenomena which resemble some of the obsessive-compulsive systems we have been describing. Because these particular breakdowns in self-regulation occur as a result of specific manipulations, they are worth examining for whatever light they may throw on what we have been describing as "escape from control."

SENSORY DEPRIVATION

Some of the experimental procedures have sought to reduce sensory input to a minimum. Visual stimuli are shut off by goggles or tape, or by confinement in complete darkness. Auditory stimuli are reduced by plugging the external auditory meatus, or by isolating subjects in a soundproof room. The tactual stimuli from hard surfaces are both altered and reduced by placing the subjects on a soft mattress or by floating them in a tank of tepid water; tactual and kinesthetic stimuli are further reduced by encasing the hands and the forearm in large cotton-packed tubes.

Other experimenters have sought to reduce the patterned nature of stimuli by the use of translucent goggles or by the use of a uniformly lighted surrounding dome or cylinder that provides abundant, but unstructured, visual stimulation. Instead of attempting to exclude all sound, some experimenters have introduced a constant but unpunctuated "white noise." Here the emphasis is on a *perceptual deprivation* that reduces the orienting cues without lowering the level of sensory input.

Still other experimenters have emphasized the restriction of movement by utilizing the extremely confining space in an iron lung. At Boston City Hospital it had been observed that some patients treated in the respirator had reported the strange delusion of moving, floating, or traveling about the city in an automobile after a few hours in the "tank"; one added the fantasy of traveling on a camel's back.

Finally, a few have emphasized the changes in social cues. Whereas some investigators had installed a two-way communication system that permitted the confined subjects to talk freely, or to answer questions, or to fulfill imposed tasks, this fourth group cut off social communication completely. Whereas some have used specific suggestions calculated to arouse expectations in their subjects, others disguised the purpose of the experiment or gave their subjects no clue as to its purpose or even of when or how they were to be released (thereby creating considerable anxiety).

The procedures are often so complex that it is not easy to identify or measure the variables that are being controlled (sometimes unintentionally). With varying effects shown by the subjects, we shall need to know much more about the samples studied before the results can be assessed or regarded as representative. Without viewing the results as more than suggestive, let us look at two findings that have kept recurring (see Solomon *et al.* 1957; Solomon, Kubansky, and Trumbull 1961).

In the first place, the task assigned to the subjects proved to be more irksome, and much more difficult to carry out, than was expected. Subjects who entered the experiment with the notion that it would provide a restful period, in which to "think out their thoughts" free from distraction, found that, as the hours passed, it grew increasingly difficult to structure this very blank span of time: thinking ran down; thoughts began to recur and to elude efforts to develop them; blank spaces, empty of all content, appeared. During this "empty time," the borderline between waking and sleeping was obscured; there were patches of "lost time." This last transitional state opened the door to a second group of phenomena. Images of the hypnagogic variety appeared, projected a slight distance before the eyes of the subject. Independent of the subject's efforts to summon or control them, these images occasionally symbolized a just-preceding thought, pictorially. Rarely, they took on hallucinatory qualities, in which case, thoughts, imagery, and reality merged so as to be indistinguishable. One subject, for example, although completely isolated during the experimental period, was sure that she had heard the experimenter enter the room and walk up to her bed (see Levitt *et al.* 1962).

The effect of repeating these experiences is still a matter of controversy. There are some who insist that a subject can become adapted to this type of withdrawal from outer contacts, can learn new orienting and "timekeeping" devices, as well as how to employ these periods productively. We do have records of a few who have returned from solitary confinement, and who seemed to know almost intuitively what must be done. Edith Bone (1957), for example, tells how she paced up and down her narrow cell, taking imaginary walking tours, shopping in European cities that she had known, holding imaginary conversations with old friends. She constructed an abacus to count off the words she could remember in English, French, Bulgarian. She made a set of 4,000 letters out of masticated black bread, which she then dried and used as type to print translations of poems from Hungarian into English. Realizing the danger of mental disorganization in her solitude, she fought, valiantly and intelligently, to retain her integrity. But since she was clearly a person of great strength and with rich inner resources, her experience may not be typical.

We also know another type of person, the typical busy extrovert whose hours are filled with appointments and the rush of affairs. Always crowding his days, always feeling under pressure, he imagines that vacation or retirement or some stretch of time when illness would enforce a long rest would be a real blessing. But when such a period overtakes him, what he had anticipated with such pleasure turns out to be quite the opposite: he is restless, bored, anxious, worthless, empty. He behaves as though his "regulative capacity," developed under pressures and now without its usual grist to feed on, turns on the very "useless self." He chafes at his idleness, needs to see someone, wants to get back where things are happening and to feel good again under the pressures of "full employment."

Some of the experimenters have denied any such power of adapting to the extremes of deprivation, looking on the task as similar to adaptation to burns, cuts, or any extreme blow to the autonomic system. Solomon (1958) is explicit:

"The amount of advance self-protection against torture that you can inculcate into a soldier is minimal or perhaps negligible. You can't train yourself not to burn if you put your hand on a red hot stove...and apparently you can't learn to resist the effects of sensory deprivation. The mind seems to be dependent upon a constant source of outside stimulation. If outside stimulation is either removed or made too monotonous, the brain just doesn't function at its optimum capacity."

A decrement in the behavioral changes recorded in the course of repeated sessions has been noted by others. Indeed, even in the second half of a single experimental period, there were fewer changes than in the first half (Pollard, Uhr, and Jackson 1963). These same observers were able to increase the number of unusual and bizarre effects when they gave explicit suggestions calculated to bring them out. They even encouraged their subjects to expect such phenomena (hearing voices, difficulty in concentration, the feeling of floating in space, colored imagery, ugly and long-forgotten memories, unusual smells) by their firm assertions that "intelligent people of an aesthetic, sensitive, and imaginative nature will have these experiences before others."

Although the effectiveness of such suggestions has been minimized by a few experimenters, others have not only found suggestion effects, but also claim that the state produced by sensory deprivation actually increases suggestibility (as measured by the ease of hypnotizing the subject after a session). That some autosuggestion is at work is indicated by some of the protocols: one subject thought her chair was wired for electric shock which was about to be turned on; other subjects suspected their experimenters of having bizarre designs. Perhaps hypnotizability is not the best measure of all the changes in suggestibility. Some subjects had heard enough about brainwashing techniques to fear for their own sanity. The subjects who were given little or no information about the procedures were, as a rule, full of hypotheses, some of which were "actualized" with hallucinatory vividness.

If one attempts to collect the entire range of abnormal phenomena released under these conditions which deprive the subject of the ordinary cues required to maintain orientation and a good regulative set, one finds a virtual museum of "symptoms." These changes may be classified, roughly, into two groups. With refinements in procedure and a sharpening in hypotheses, it will undoubtedly be necessary to introduce other categories.

The first group consists of changes in thinking and perceiving:

1. Increased difficulty in organizing thoughts and in maintaining a direction. In some subjects this released a compensatory effort to structure thinking, to develop procedures for the sake of maintaining mental integrity.

2. Appearance of hypnagogic images, with an increase in the brightness and saturation of colors and their afterimages when a measure is made immediately following the experimental session.

3. Lowered power to discriminate consistently between images and reality; hallucinations, delusions, and increased suggestibility.

4. Fluctuations, drifting, swirling of objects and visual surfaces on emergence from the experimental conditions: changes which resemble those seen by Stratton, Ewert, Pronko, and others who have worn inverting lenses which restrict the visual field and interfere with habitual eye movements.

5. Experiences which imprint themselves so vividly that they are recalled weeks later in contrast with the ordinary rehearsals of material to be memorized.

The second group consists of affective-motivational changes:

1. Rapidly mounting appetite for extrinsic patterned stimuli and for human contact.

2. Mounting intolerance for restriction of movement, with limits for individual subjects varying from two hours to six days. These marked individual differences in tolerance have not been satisfactorily related to personality differences in the subjects.

3. Occasional acute panic with violent breaking out from imposed restraints, in spite of earlier assurances that release would be granted on demand; and a frequent reluctance to return to the experimental conditions for a second session.

4. Changes in the electroencephalogram, including slowing in the alpha range and the appearance of delta waves, that persist for from two to three hours after an experimental period.

5. Changes in voice volume.

6. Increased responsiveness to stimuli and lowered threshold for irritability.

Such a classification does little justice to the richness of the observations included in the protocols. Consider the following report of one of Solomon's subjects (1958, p. 5):

"I see a beautiful technicolor sunrise over a lake, nice ripples, three dots, must be a moon, three dots; dark on the other side of the lake. A bunch of Indians on the shore; they have headdresses, now two feathers apiece. I hope you've got a lot of paper to take this down. I must be going nuts. I see an enamel table of white metal with a ball over it. Next I see a fireplace. Through the door there is a knight in armor. I see a spoke shoot out below his waist, all metal, coiled; it shoots from a can."

The students of trance states, of occult phenomena, or of the Jungian variety of psychoanalysis would be interested in such reports, each giving the phenomena his own special interpretation. In the final phrases of the above paragraph, the Jungian archetypes seem to be rearing their heads; the early phrases sound like those of a medium who is gazing into a crystal ball. A spiritualist might claim that some of these "communications" have significant meanings. The more matter-of-fact experimenters, with physiological concepts in mind, might be content to view the phenomena as evidence of a disturbance in the reticular-cortical system created by lowered senory input, as a result of the release from the normal controls.

PROLONGED NARCOSIS AND SENSORY DEPRIVATION AS THERAPY

The new experimental procedures have given old clinical facts new meanings and have revived an interest in the rest cure, hypnosis, and prolonged narcosis. Old controversies have assumed new forms. If we have forgotten some of this past, the underlying problems persist nonetheless, demanding new formulations.

When one compares the obsessive's loss of control of his thoughts and impulses to the changes seen in the sensory-deprivation experiments, one is tempted to explain the former as due to a type of deficiency in normal relationships with a regulative milieu. Since the experimental subjects recover their self-control so quickly when they are taken out of the "tank," we are moved to ask, "Is there some analogous way to vitalize and restore normal interchanges with the environment in the obsessive patient, especially in those patients who are both morose and inactive?" To the matter-of-fact Soviet psychiatrists, this can be answered, rather simply, by a program of work-therapy and intensive effort designed to bring about improved socialization; they have recommended this type of treatment for alcoholism and psychopathic personalities, as well as for neurotic and psychotic deviations. A single theme is repeatedly emphasized: work restores, regulates, revitalizes (see Wortis 1950, 1961). The theme recurs, again, in some of the current emphases on group therapy. Procedures originally devised as a desperate means of coping with excessive case loads have proved to have a value in socializing the patient. Some of the psychiatrists who deal with the aging, the retired, the unemployed, the alcoholic, the lonely and unattached see the discovery of significant tasks and the return to a social involvement as a way of stimulating and "organizing" these dropouts from life.

There is another side to the problem. For many neurotics the world seems shattering, disorganizing, frustrating. They feel that they could "pull themselves together" if only things would slow down, if people would be less demanding, if they could find the leisure and the place in which to achieve a collectedness. The obsessive, who sometimes shows a mania for introspection, is jealous of his moments of free time. The world, he complains, is indeed too much with him: his job demands, his wife demands, and children and friends demand. He has no "free time" in which to live a life of his own. If only he could find that moment (or some mountain peak apart), his obsessive thoughts would quiet down, find completion; his unfinished business, the whole tangled skein of opposites, would become unsnarled; and the "pressure" would subside. It is as though some data-processing center had become choked with an excess of information, as though the business of encoding stimuli and synthesizing the conflicts had broken down completely. Subjectively at least, it is a matter of *sensory surfeit.* While his friends (and the Soviet psychiatrists) are urging him to turn his energies outward, to become even more involved in his work, family, friends, and the needs of the collective, his own deepest feelings urge him to pause, collect his thoughts, reflect, plan, or take a vacation from living. He fears action and involvement. To become more deeply "engaged" is the *last* thing he desires.

It was this need for a time and place of quiet that gave Silas Weir Mitchell and all those who used some form of prolonged narcosis their cue. They saw the nervous patient as exhausted. He seemed to be acting as though some obscure neural fatigue had reduced the integrative powers of his brain. In such a state of "brain fag," even ordinary sensory input proved too demanding. These physicians responded to what they believed to be their patient's need by drawing the shades, excluding visitors, providing a silent nurse to care for all physical needs. With nothing to do but rest, sleep, consume a high-caloric diet, the patient found himself "put on ice" for weeks.

This therapy was in an ancient and honorable tradition. Had not the ancient prophets and seers gone into the desert to meditate, retired to some mountain cave for the month of Ramadan, used spiritual exercises (such as those Saint Ignatius Loyola was later to "invent") as a means of restoring a spiritual orientation? Do we not, even now, look forward to the vacation, or the sabbatical year, as a way of escaping from the burdens that produce a frayed and raveled border to all thinking? It seems to have been consistently assumed that an integrated certitude, a restored power to think and act, would emerge from these quiet times.

Now the sensory-deprivation experiments have arisen to suggest that, on the contrary, a progressive disorganization is apt to emerge, instead; and some suggest that the "devil of the unconscious," kept down while the flow of interchanges with the environment is uninterrupted, will emerge as soon as these controls are withdrawn. The experiments show that, instead of unity, there is a loss of orientation, impairment of discrimination, emergence of hypnagogic imagery and borderline hallucinations, and occasionally panic, and "nightmares" that are long remembered.

How have matters shaped up, in the clinic, where these rival possibilities have been tested? In order to sharpen the conflict in opinion, and to introduce some order in the midst of controversies not yet resolved, we might classify the "facts" on which the rival opinions rest, as well as note a few of the historical roots of the present impasse, in the hope that the worst of the old exaggerations may not repeat themselves.

1. There is a type of person we might call the *sensitive.* For whatever reasons, he is easily overwhelmed by a surfeit of stimulation, by social life, by the demands of work or family living. In such a sensitive, obsessions, manias, and phobias emerge under the shattering impact of what a normal person can meet and carry in his stride. Janet indicates that obsessions in patients

who have the "typical psychasthenic character" can arise on the occasion of *any momentous decision,* at any crisis point in life. Instead of acting decisively, these "sensitives" enter into endless ruminations, weigh the opposite courses, question their own certitudes, attempt semimagical ways of conjuring away their problem. The susceptibility to such behavior is usually noted early, and continues throughout life in the most flagrant instances. A mode of dealing with the problems of living converts each crucial occasion into the obsessive form. Conversely, a plan of therapy which reduces the intensity of the conflicts, even if it is little more than rest and "sensory deprivation," can restore some measure of integrative power. Such rest may be brought about by hypnosis, by drug-induced narcosis, or by procedures that are very close to the experimental situations we have been concerned with.

Where addictions are involved, the enforced isolation, combined with the withdrawal of the drug, enables the claim of the habit to subside while the integrative powers recuperate; the hospital routine supports what a weak inner "regulator" (superego) knows but cannot enforce. This type of therapy has been applied to narcotic addiction, alcoholism, food addiction (bulimia), and sex addictions (perversions).

2. There is a second type of person who becomes disorganized under the experimental conditions of sensory deprivation. Monotony, constancy of un-patterned stimuli, restriction of interchanges with the environment, lowered sensory input, restriction of movement, loss of personal and supporting contacts combine to create a deficit that is defined as a need for renewed contact, action, social interchanges, stimulation, guidance. As this need mounts, a progressive disorganization of thought and action occurs. When this type of person grows disorganized under the conditions of everyday living, an improvement in his interchanges with his human environment seems to be required. Work-therapy, restoration of or increase in vital contacts, guidance, new and socially significant commitment are seen as the most direct way of counteracting the drift toward disorganization.

3. A combination of procedures, used on war prisoners, that alternates between extreme isolation and the offer of acceptance, friendly support, and a restoration to "fellowship" and "belonging" came to be known as brainwashing. Under wartime conditions the isolation was combined with torture, thus intensifying the contrast between the two conditions. Used in the interrogation of prisoners, spies and subversives, it succeeded in breaking down their self-control (and that secret-keeping process that seems to be disturbed in many obsessives). A few therapists have suggested that the sensory-deprivation procedures can be alternated with the more conventional forms of warmly supportive therapy in order to activate and release important repressed materials in the former phase and to intensify the rapport in the latter. For every "regression" and "release" in the one, a therapeutic reorganization can be planned for and facilitated in the other (see Azima, Vispo, and Azima 1961).

The expectations aroused by the sensory-deprivation experiments have produced a few attempts to measure the effect of analogous procedures upon hospitalized patients. In many instances, controls have been lacking, patients have been drawn from a wide range of disorders, and tests of uncertain validity have been used to measure the changes. The reports have ranged from "a general improvement" through "no noticeable change," with here and there evidence of a worsening of the abnormal symptoms. One investigator reported "a dramatic relief from hallucinatory experiences," while another noted that, in one of his schizophrenics, the accusing voices that the patient heard had grown louder. Some patients had found the experience disturbing. A few, in contrast, did not wish to leave the sensory-deprivation chamber. (See Harris 1959; Cleveland, Reitman, and Bentinck 1963; Gibby, Adams, and Carrera 1960.)

The wide contrast in results of different investigators reminds one of the outcomes reported from use of the rest cure in the early days following Weir Mitchell's enthusiastic reports. Then, as now, much seemed to depend on the attitude and personality of the investigator, the enthusiasm generated in both physician and patient by a new therapeutic ritual that promised great benefits, the strong suggestions accompanying the procedures, and the particular type of patient selected for treatment. Both then and now, a clinician is not excused from making an intensive analysis of the particular dynamics operating in a given patient; where reintegration by some form of reeducation is required, the mere fact of rest (or drugs or hypnosis) is but a preparation for the real therapy.

The new efforts have been tentative, and have involved limited exposures to the "experimental" conditions. Cleveland noted:

"It is hardly surprising that a few hours spent in an isolated situation, lying quietly on a bed, fails to interrupt what is often a life-long history of disturbed and deviant behavior. If this had proved otherwise, why would not a good night's sleep (an event approximating many of the conditions of SD) alleviate the distressing symptoms of schizophrenia? Unfortunately the results of the present study offer little promise that simple exposure to a sensory deprivation situation constitutes a new therapeutic approach to the treatment of behavioral disorders."

In an earlier day, prolonged narcosis or hypnosis (extending over days and even weeks) had its champions. The procedures were radical and required a complete supervision of the resting patient over the period. Among our contemporaries, Diethelm (1950, pp. 159 ff) discusses the advantages of a drug-induced sleep that may be continued for a period of ten days. In the mildest form, a twilight state is used to produce muscular relaxation, to slow down (and blur the outlines of) thought, and to help the patient accept an invalid status, look on his symptoms more objectively (i.e., as the physician does), ignore his difficulties, and drop some of his defenses. Diethelm urges intensive psychotherapy both before and after the narcosis and claims moderate rather than brilliant gains for the method.

Looking over his records of patients treated by prolonged and complete rest, Janet (1919, pp. 457-71, 572-88) found hystericals who lost their attacks (and choreiform agitations), phobias with emotional distress brought on by overwork, and cases with photophobia, agoraphobia, overscrupulousness, agitation, incapacity to will and decide, and phobia for work or any energy expenditure. On the other hand, he counted as failures: the patient who developed an addiction to the rest treatment and to the irresponsible life of the sanitarium; the patient who found she had even less inclination or capacity for social life and work afterward; the patient who grew increasingly hypochondriacal as he found himself treated as an impaired person; the patients who used their new freedom to worry about their affairs. In his list were a dozen patients whose symptoms had been aggravated by the treatment; and there were rare cases in which agitation, violence, and delirium developed under the enforced idleness.

In those cases where obsessive or phobic symptoms arise out of physical exhaustion, illness, or overwork, the use of bedrest (or some other procedure that arrests all energy expenditures) seems eminently sensible. Where the patient is a "sensitive" who finds that the demands and entanglements of professional life and family living are too much for his organizing powers, some reduction in this press could properly be recommended, along with an improvement in his skills of organizing effort and distributing his energies. Whether it is the man, the tissues, or specific energy-consuming conflicts, recuperation requires both a reduction of demands for action and a reeducation.

In other patients there are energies to spare, but they are on poor terms with themselves and have long suffered from conflicts which they have never learned to manage. Where the ego is weak, the process of building a stronger one presents the most serious challenge a counselor could face, for he is asked to do what life, a family, and years of (poor) discipline have failed to do. Far from accomplishing this, a radical and prolonged rest merely provides more energy for the conflicts which a weak ego already finds too much to manage. Undertaking new challenges and undergoing experiences which will afford the needed discipline, making the entrance into life that has been postponed, undertaking risks and developing powers of self-regulation call for the kind of collaboration that parents and wise companions can carry out better than "paid friends" who offer brief counseling. They call for a type of therapy that makes a therapist superfluous, that restores the individual to the status of "responsible man."

A Summary

The sensory-deprivation experiments have reminded us that the inner regulative process which keeps us oriented requires a steady feedback from the surrounding field. Even those who resent the feedback most (and whose slogans are "Liberty. To thine own self be true. I live for myself, I write for myself, I am an autonomous man.") need this feedback, and perhaps need it most. Such feedback can grow too insistent, demanding better integrative effort, faster responses, and finer discrimination than the available resources of the individual can supply. On the other hand, this inflowing stream can be so reduced (by either inner or outer barriers) that the person loses his bearings, ceases to keep time; a progressive disorganization then allows impulses to escape from control, and obsessive doubts, ruminations, scruples to emerge. Hallucinations

and paranoid suspicions may emerge from the dark recesses of the mind; in
a few persons subjected to sensory deprivation, responses approach the panic
level. This loss of a stable stance that occurs when the supporting stimuli
are cut off calls attention to the aspect of phobias and obsessions that Janet
tended to emphasize. Where Freud focused on the "pressures from below"
(repressed infantile sexuality) and emphasized the symbolic value of the
symptoms, Janet saw the weakness in the integrative tensions above this unconscious level as the critical factor. In the typical psychasthenic this weakness
exists from early childhood.

The new studies remind us that this weakening in the regnant integrations
can be brought about by sensory deprivation, by removal from social supports,
by a deficiency in those orienting demands that keep a self-system taut and
vigilant. The clinical studies of therapies that try to reduce the sensory input
by drugs, hypnosis, or sensory deprivation have produced such varied results
that no simple generalization can adequately cover them. These therapies are
not to be used indiscriminately. Rest can restore and increase the available
energies; but without an improvement in the regulative process, it may also
intensify the amount of disorganization. Removal of the supports of an already
defective integration system simply increases the likelihood that impulses will
escape from control.

EPILOG

The behavior of the obsessive-compulsive patient makes him a caricature
of the hero. Some members of this group complain: "I am a mechanical man.
I can do it if you force me to. I would not do it otherwise. I cannot *feel* anything. Life is pointless." Others seem to be all thought. Elaborating endlessly
the makeready for action, they are indecisive, scrupulous, full of doubt. Either
a mouse issues from this mountain of labor or so many erasures and corrections
have been made by the time the final statement is issued that no one can read
it, and the action is awkward. Some obsessive-compulsives are all emotion:
fearful, phobic, sensitive, thin-skinned. One of this type imagines some quiet
place, such as a monastery or an evening at the edge of the desert, where human
contacts are reduced and the stimuli are sparse and steady, as he searches for
an environment that could be tolerated. Some obsessives are holists, at least
in one sense. They seem to have searched for and are possessed by a view from
some point in outer space, so far out that worldly action and natural motives
and the pressures of a proximate environment do not seem important. Un-
worldly, they have escaped from the wheel of life. As though immured in some
tower, they are contemplators: all fires beneath the collarbone are banked.
Some obsessives are caricatures of one of the seven deadly sins.

There are as many dimensions in this group as there are classifications of
human motives. In these individuals the projicient apparatus is taken over by
some part-process. It is the whole that is in difficulty, and weak.

Each of these types is a holistic failure. Unbalanced, possessed by one of
the part-processes or lacking in powers of synthesis, the person as a whole

might be called the "gut man," the "genital man," the "mouth man," the "cloud-minded," or the "voyeur." There are roughly two types of deviations from the normal balance: the excessively holistic man with hypertrophied conscience, and the man with a hypertrophied part-process. These deviations remind us of certain unfinished business in our commonly accepted notions of growth and development. We find it easy to begin our account, as Allport (1924, Chap. 3) once did, with a mere handful of reflexes. Who can see any regulative "whole" at work in the squirming newborn child? His eyes do not keep together as they are caught by some moving bright object, not even enough so that corresponding retinal points are stimulated and so that the two foveas are properly centered on the moving target. As he develops, we see conditioned fears spreading to cues adjacent to a sound source, conditioned mouth openings cued by an approaching thumb, conditioned approaches and avoidances to gratifiers and nocuous stimuli.

All these first stages are piecemeal processes, the learner more or less passive. Then initiative develops, prompted at first by some internal appetite or surface stress, and enduring habit-chains of action are built, as a clumsy trial-and-error process is shaped by escape routes or pathways that open to consummation. Regulatory powers in the form of anticipations and expectant sets oriented to more remote goals are gradually added.

This is about where we commonly leave the problem. It is convenient to do so, especially for any objective psychologist who uses a rat model of behavior (or some Skinner-box paradigm of action). Whoever heard of a rat struggling to attain peace of mind, or to become the type of rat his mother once dreamed she was marrying? To go farther we have to leave our rat subjects, and begin to consider a more human model, even to imaginatively probe within the model to the inner workings of thought. The sticky problem of the role of consciousness emerges, and the will, so long discarded from psychology, returns (with its maladies, its *défaillances*) to force us to ask some very old questions for which we still lack adequate answers. Such clumsy terms as ego-ideal, introjection, incorporation, which bother us as we try to keep a scientific psychology on track with operationally defined concepts, emerge, and each of them raises questions about the integration of the system as a whole. Although children have been conditioned to lose their fear of domestic animals, apparently for good, adult problems like alcoholism are more intractable. As noted in Chapter 6, in the section "Testing the Theories and Therapies," one characteristic of the conditioned response—according to present evidence —is the speed with which it is extinguished.

It is just such an illness as the one we call obsessive-compulsive which reveals the shortcomings in our part-centered developmental theory. Not only the patient, but also the hero, reduce to a shambles the conditioned-reflex need-adjustive theories that are so useful in the animal laboratory. In the patient we can witness, when the obsessive-compulsive attack is self-limited, the return of a decisive conscious will that is both well-informed and highly charged. The doubts, scruples, and "know-nothing" attitude vanish, and the mechanisms are put in their place.

A synthesis of the part-processes is required of us. Shaped until adolescence, we are required to become shapers, inventors, managers. Regulated by others as children, we are expected to become self-regulators. Handed a set of views of the world, old maps of reality that our ancestors constructed, we are required both to test them and to improve on them. Taught hundreds of skills, we are required to employ them *for* something. Without a synthesizing grasp of some whole that we can relate to, we are unfinished: as unfinished as the theories of Skinner, Hull, Pavlov, and Thorndike were. Our thought models make us out to be fragmentary men, antinomic men with conflicting impulses, dependent men waiting to follow a leader or anything that moves, but never able to evaluate the following or the drift in the general motion, except as some local viscus supplied by the autonomic system, some muscle cramp, or some death instinct or antilife force working in the unconscious opposes its complaint against the pace. Our therapies are designed for such models. Such "unfinished men" in these thought models are rather passive, mechanical, empty, or they are part-dominated, supreme egoists of the gut, exemplars of lusts and appetites, certainly not heroes, perhaps with motivations but without will, if will is something which is more and other than the mechanically acting parts.

For a beginning, we might insist that there is indeed within a man a human craving for something that is more and other than such bits of living. Empty as we often feel, we are nonetheless capable of responding to a gospel, some vision of a height to be attained, some cause that would make the mechanisms worthy. The energies that mill about in pointless happenings are capable of being harnessed, subsumed, transformed. Just as a good cause (and sometimes a tornado or catastrophe) can arrest the thousand pettinesses of a village, stop all bickering, and set everyone to working together, so a vision of a better world to live in, a truly Great Society, can transform a bored affluence into a more vitally engaged type of living.

There has been a long history to this search for an enlivening and integrating vision that would fulfill our craving and ignite our energies (at least, in civilizations; in mere tribal life men do not even think of a destiny, let alone of interfering in the existing state of affairs). Too often the goal has been placed so far out on the horizon, beyond the last range of hills, beyond the last cloudbank, that the goal's magnetic field scarcely moves us. When the goal is proximate and concerns the effects of present actions, those who are trying to hold an enterprise together (a Brook Farm or Walden Two) often have to invent new ad hoc hypotheses to explain the failures, gloss over "realities" which create stumbling blocks never covered by the promises and plans, and even reach the point of denying realities that grow increasingly patent. With conflicting interpretations and accusations that shift the blame, the hopes of the founders become transformed into feelings and actions that are anything but constructive.

Thus to keep the possible and proximate goal bright and inviting requires a process of flexible reevaluation. Between the pragmatic and sometimes false goal and the too distant goal that fails to energize us must lie an area of vigilant effort. The problems raised by the obsessive lead us afresh to that ancient concept we recently thought psychology had discarded: the human will. We have tried to get along without the concept of the will, by using more specific mechanisms that were once considered part of it. Perhaps the concept included too much, and raised too many arguments about "freedom of the will," but after we tried to drop it, we never managed to cover all the human problems it dealt with; the "map" defined by the more specific terms has left many gaps and many areas marked *terra incognita* that lie in the very territory we are concerned with.

It is easier to sketch the problem of the *défaillance* of the will than it is to restore integrative power to a person in whom it is failing. Since there are so many negative factors which contribute to the run-down (some of which we sketched in our treatment of neurasthenia), there will be many forms of corrective maneuvers, and one would hope that a therapist would not become confined to any single device, or allow his special theory to act as a blinder. The very inadequacy of our present theories of self-regulation highlight this danger.

Chapter 9 • Brain Lesions and Cortical Malfunction

Long before we could identify the brain changes that paralleled behavioral changes, the doctrine of psychophysical parallelism led us to imply them, and often led us into a pseudoneurology. For hysterical paralysis we imagined an underlying brain change, and for an unconscious mental state we invented a type of cerebration without accompanying awareness. Often our language served more as a cover for our ignorance than as a tool that would guide experiment; the "experiments of nature" that entered the clinic as aphasias, gunshot wounds, amnesias, hemianopsias were not well suited to our theoretical needs, since they often had massive or ill-defined lesions of unknown localization and extent. Even Head's analysis of the aphasias that followed gunshot wounds to the head, carried on in World War I, left much to be desired, since in each case the precise location and extent of the lesion behind the loss in speech function had to be inferred. Progress has been slow in spite of all the neurosurgery on animal brains and the increasing boldness of neurosurgeons who implant electrodes or insert scalpels to produce precisely located lesions in human brains.

From the days when Broca challenged the views of Flourens, more than a hundred years ago, two rival emphases have affected the formulation of research problems and the interpretations of both clinical and experimental findings. One view emphasizes the unity of brain functioning and the equipotentiality of many, if not all, cells. According to this view, the 12-billion-cell multiple-track system of conduction paths can be expected to recover from local injuries, provided these are not too extensive, with alternate routes replacing the damaged tracts, much as traffic would be shifted from one railroad line to another which reaches the same destination. Though habit traces may have been laid down in one line, and lost as a result of injury, the function can be relearned by new training of the conduction tissues and end organs which remain. Lashley, who studied the effects of carefully identified lesions in brains of rats that were trained before operation, and measured and retrained afterward, advanced the twin hypotheses of "equi-

446

potentiality" and "vicarious functioning." He seemed to be laying the experimental groundwork for hope in the reeducation of aphasics and other cases resulting from brain injury, except where the amount of the damage was so great as to reduce the capacity for all complex discriminations and for the more difficult motor skills. In fact, the evidence indicated that when this factor of complexity was taken into account, the correlation between extent of the lesions and the amount of damage to learning capacity was as high as $+0.86$.

This first view would suggest, therefore, that when a clinician reports that no behavioral changes follow the extensive removal of tissue of the cortex (or the severance of connections between one brain mass and another, as in the lobotomy operation), it is likely that:

1. There is no good preoperative measure of the patient's behavior, so that valid comparisons in capacity can be made.

2. The present clinical postoperative studies are too limited and imprecise, and therefore do not push the individual to the limits of his capacity.

3. Or we are indeed so richly supplied with neural tissue that the residual conduction paths can serve all ordinary demands.

The other view of brain functioning is represented by those findings that have identified precise cell groups which supply each muscle group of the body and which are distributed along the fold just in front of the fissure of Rolando. Sharply localized lesions (or stimulation by electrodes placed directly on the exposed cortex of the waking human subject) do produce precise behavioral changes: a local paralysis from a lesion, a local contracture from the stimulating electrode. (Under electrode stimulation the human subject has the odd experience of "watching it contract": he remains a passive observer while the electrical stimulation moves the muscle.) Lesions sharply localized on the visual areas within the occipital lobe and on the auditory areas of the temporal lobe likewise produce restricted losses of visual-pattern discrimination and of pitch perception. To these localized losses there must be added (1) losses in interpretation of the sensory input when the areas immediately surrounding the projection areas are damaged, and (2) losses in the coordination of movements when the supermotor areas are affected (just in front of the motor area). This view must also face the fact that considerable damage to brain tissue is possible without measurable behavioral changes; and to the precisely located sensory and motor projection areas, this view would have to add certain "silent areas." In this view, these latter cell groups serve to link up the more precise sensory and motor areas into those higher combinations that we call "sets," "concepts," and "synthetic judgment." The prefrontal areas, the two foremost tips of the cerebrum, have provided a kind of haven, in which localizationists have tried to place the so-called "higher functions."

CASES WITH LIMITED EFFECTS FROM BRAIN DAMAGE

A lesion in the occipital portion of the brain, produced by a blow on the head that forced a bit of bone into the underlying mass of neural tissue, may block impulses from a precise patch on one retina: the patient has acquired a new blind spot, in addition to the one where the retinal cells are thrust aside by the fibers of the optic tract that leave the eye. Like this normal blind spot, which is only revealed when a precise effort to identify it is made, as when a visual perimeter is used to explore and map the sensitivity of the retina, the new one may so completely escape the awareness of the victim that only laboratory tests will reveal it. Using impulses from the optical tracts which were spared, he manages to discriminate, avoid objects, identify targets, as usual, with no noticeable impairment in behavior as a whole. Only in the exceptional instance where the use of a single eye is critical for perception would his localized blindness be revealed.

More extended injuries of the left (or right) side of the brain may destroy the vision of the left (or right) halves of both eyes; the subject will become aware, indirectly, of his loss only because he continually bumps into obstacles located on the nonfunctional side. The clinical reports in such localized injuries to precise sensory areas have not stressed any personality change or any reduction in capacity for perceiving, feeling, acting. Even the total loss of smell and taste, due to injuries which section the pathways ascending to the brain or damage the olfactory and gustatory areas themselves, while they place the person in the peculiar position of having to ask his dinner partner whether the potatoes need salt or not, can be circumvented in one way or another. The immediate warning of a bad taste or an offensive smell is lost, but again no higher functions seem to be affected.

RESTRICTED PERCEPTUAL LOSS

A case reported by Jean Delay (1950, p. 18) illustrates one of those accidental "experiments of nature" that result in sharply limited lesions with an equally restricted perceptual loss.

Modeste, a 23-year-old woman, had been hospitalized for a brain injury produced by a revolver bullet which penetrated the right parietal lobe at the edge of the area that relays the sensory impulses which give rise to experiences of warmth, coolness, pressure, pain, and the kinesthetic impressions arising from movement. None of these sensory experiences had been lost. Blindfolded, and with a metal spoon placed in her left hand, she could report the cold, hard feel of the surface. She even noted that the object was narrow in the middle, broad and flat at one end, and oval and hollowed at the other, somewhat larger end. But these part-responses did not add up to "spoon," as they promptly did when the object was transferred to her other hand. Similarly a pencil, a comb, and other objects could not be identified. Parts of these forms, more complex than simple sensory cues, were recognized and synthesized: the long flat shape of the comb, the "points" along one side of the comb, were both noted. Delay speaks of the left hand forgetting what the right hand remembers, as though a perceptual function had remained intact but local tactual *memories* had been damaged. Apparently, incoming impulses were elaborated into perceptions and preparations to act when they entered via the intact side of the brain, but were not properly elaborated when they entered on the other side. Guided by the input from the intact side (tactual and kinesthetic impulses arising on the right side), the left hand could participate in such actions as eating from a cup or combing the hair. It was in the receptive-elaborative process on the injured side of the brain that the impairment showed up.

In such a case the loss is sharply defined, the changes external to the personality. While one would predict some shifts in her habits (as, for example, when she is forced to use her "good hand" in exploring a surface in the dark), so that in all two-handed skills the right will become the leader, the explorer, one can expect that she will continue to be the same person. If we permit Delay to speak of the loss of a specific set of tactual memories, as he seems to prefer to do, we must note that Modeste's memory, her "history-making" of day-to-day events, her ability to plan ahead remain unaffected.

UNILATERAL DAMAGE OF A FRONTAL LOBE

Various conditions prompt a neurosurgeon to remove portions of the human brain: tumors, cysts, infections and diseased cells, centers of discharge that produce epileptic convulsions. When these are limited to one side of the brain, and especially to that "silent area" at the tip of a frontal lobe, and when an uncomplicated recovery follows so that there is no expanding tumor or disease process, a patient may show no measurable loss of function. Hebb (1939), for example, has reported careful follow-up studies of four patients, each with a removal of cerebral tissue from the left frontal lobe in amounts varying up to 70 cc. One of the cases, a McGill senior, returned to classes the following semester and made A grades in three out of four examinations; he apologized for the fourth, in which he obtained a B, confessing that he had little interest in the course. In each of these cases there was an improvement in mental functioning consequent to the removal of pathological tissues, and no evidence of loss of memories relating to events which took place prior to the operation.

This type of evidence parallels the findings of Jacobsen (1936) and others who have removed portions of the forebrain of chimpanzees. The frontal-lobe signs that emerge when both frontal poles are removed were absent when the lesion was confined to one side, and the data give the impression that something comparable to parallel circuits enable one side to carry on the integrative function when the other side is thrown out of use or removed. With a bilateral removal, delayed choices and certain chained reactions were markedly damaged; simple problem-box habits and pattern discriminations were not affected. The notion of bilateral representation of many functions suggests that even more extensive brain damage, confined to one side (and particularly to the side not involved in speaking) might also leave behavior unchanged.

EXTENSIVE UNILATERAL REMOVAL OF BRAIN TISSUE

There are a few cases in which patients have survived massive excision of tissue without residual impairment. In the one reported by Penfield and Evans

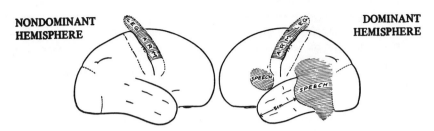

FIGURE 9. INDISPENSABLE AREAS OF CEREBRAL CORTEX (SHADED). The precentral gyrus (if functional) in which arm and leg are represented in either hemisphere is rarely to be excised; and the speech areas of the dominant hemisphere of an adult, probably never. (Reprinted by permission of the authors and Little, Brown and Company from Wilder Penfield and Herbert Jasper, *Epilepsy and the Functional Anatomy of the Human Brain* [1954], p. 776.)

(1935), the sister of one of the reporting neurosurgeons, was observed during the operation and over the subsequent months, and this instance approaches the theoretical limit.

Looking up at the surgeon at the end of a six-hour operation, this woman, whose right frontal lobe had been almost entirely cut away, apologized for having caused so much trouble. Recovered from the operation, she returned to her home to take charge of the household and to manage six children. She felt that she was not quite as alert as formerly, and her brother thought that he could see some loss in "planned initiative." (When several dinner guests were expected, she had trouble in preparing and serving the meal, a task which flusters some women with intact brains.) Yet she could write of a wonderful year, two years after the operation, and compose a letter full of vivid expressions of appropriate feelings. "We will often think of you at Christmas, and I am thankful that I can picture you as you will be—the sunshine in the dining room and study, the cheery open fire, and the children going out to skate and coast or ski, the cars slipping and sliding, the cold crunch of the snow," she wrote, in language which many of us would not expect a brain-injured person to use.

In a diagram (see Figure 9) based on his long experience with patients who had to have a part of their cortex excised, Penfield provides us with a graphic picture of the areas that might be called dispensable. Note that in the nondominant hemisphere, all but portions of the motor cortex, in front of the central fissure, is counted dispensable; the speech areas of the dominant side are *in*dispensable.

BILATERAL REMOVAL OF FRONTAL-LOBE TISSUE

This patient suffered brain damage at age 16, and it was followed by epileptic seizures; the operation, at age 27, was designed to remove scar tissue believed to be responsible for the attacks. The patient had grown irresponsible, stubborn, restless, forgetful, with numerous incapacitating epileptic seizures. More than a third of each frontal lobe was removed. Postoperative study showed the patient's intelligence to be near-normal, and his memory for events prior to the injury which had damaged his forebrain seemed normal. (There were no records of tests taken prior to the brain damage, but his near-normal test scores suggested that if any loss was present it was minimal.) The authors (Hebb and Penfield 1940; see also Hebb

1945) looked for but found none of the frontal-lobe signs we shall describe later; in fact the removal of the pathogenic tissues brought about an improvement in brain function and in general behavior. There was no loss of abstract behavior, no unusual difficulty in categorizing: the Stanford-Binet test, an "essential similarities test" (which called for abstract thought), and the Kohs block test (a test of ability to remember and copy exposed designs produced by an arrangement of blocks, valued by Goldstein as a special measure of frontal-lobe deficit) all showed essentially normal capacities. The patient made a very good adjustment for a period following the operation. Epileptic seizures returned following his service in the army.

The trend of these cases makes clear that some of our brain tissue is expendable, a great deal of the surface of the cortex, in fact (witness Penfield's diagram), provided that not too much is excised in any one patient, provided that the homologous area on the opposite side is spared, and provided that certain limited portions are not invaded. Gross correlations between mass of tissue removed and massive behavioral changes do not hold: as much as 70 cc. may be removed from one frontal pole of one hemisphere (provided the other half of the forebrain is undisturbed) without producing measurable deficit, but an area smaller than a dime, and only 2 mm. in depth, over the motor speech area will produce a marked motor aphasia. In the right-handed, for whom the left cerebrum is dominant, the left brain is the more vulnerable. Since there are critical nodal points on the neural routes and a precise hierarchy of looplines that integrate brain functions, there are further reasons to doubt emphasis on the quantitative correlations once proposed by Lashley. Even the two generalizations that deal with (1) the critical indispensable areas and (2) the need to spare the homologous tissues of the opposite side have their exceptions. A patient of the British surgeon Horseley was able to play tennis three years after the removal from the right motor cortex of all the tissue whose electrical excitation produced arm movement; there had originally been a marked motor deficit in the left forearm, which cleared partially, though Horseley and the patient admitted that the tennis was not "up to form." The Hebb and Penfield case warns us that, with clean operations which remove all pathological tissue, even a bilateral prefrontal lobectomy may recover with minimal residual effects.

What happens after the operation, and what residual pathological processes remain, and what remote effects on tissues some distance from the lesion persist to disturb performance can seldom be determined with sufficient accuracy. The Hebb and Penfield case of bilateral removal developed epileptic attacks later; the massive unilateral removal reported by Penfield and Evans was succeeded by a recurrence of the tumor, so that even the residual signs of a defect in planned initiative may have been caused by the tumor rather than by the aftereffects of the operation.

BILATERAL PREFRONTAL LOBECTOMIES WITH BEHAVIORAL CHANGE

A case reported by Brickner (1936) in an extended monograph was studied intensively in his home, and both test results and the patient's performance in a natural setting were observed (one of the hospital staff supervising the patient during part of each day). The existence of a tumor had necessitated extensive removal of tissue from both frontal lobes. Three changes in the patient were emphasized: (1) lowered capacity to associate and synthesize, (2) lack of normal inhibitions and restraints, and (3) impairment in abstraction, judgment, and initiative. A persistent euphoria that was not affected by his actual predicament, and a slowness and stereotypy were noted.

BRICKNER'S MR. A.

Mr. A. had been a successful broker on the cotton exchange. He talked a great deal in the months of recovery about returning to his former work, but he never got around to it; instead, he dawdled away his days. His emotions were flattened, labile, and unrestrained: i.e., flattened where one would look for the "higher" feelings and self-critical attitudes, labile and unrestrained in his uncontrolled outbursts that had replaced normal inhibitions. He was alternately restless, bored, and apathetic. In spite of elaborate and extensive efforts at reeducation and rehabilitation, little substantial progress was reported. Seven years after the operation he continued to be the same almost human, dependent person in need of guidance; he was unpredictable, given to sudden outbursts of clowning or punning, boisterous, aggressive. He had very little appreciation of the seriousness of his situation. The self's concern about the self had been lost.

Intellectually, there was no gross deterioration, as measured by the Binet test (although his IQ scores fell in the low-normal range, marking in all probability some descent from his preoperative level). It was difficult to hold his attention; he made little effort to organize his future; he seemed to lack the ability to "put two and two together"; his humor declined in quality; his motivation was negligible; he dawdled and bluffed; and he indulged in obscenities in a fashion he had not done before the operation. On the insistence of those around him, he could "pull himself together," put on a good front for a while, assume the attitude of a responsible adult male. One test of this ability occurred, much later, when Brickner took him on rounds with visiting physicians. He had been dressed in a white coat and remained inconspicuous among the group of strangers. When Brickner subsequently asked his guests to identify the frontal-lobe patient in the party, it was apparent that the patient's self-control had been good enough to deceive these casual observers.

If, as Karpman once suggested (see Guiraud 1950, p. 469), the frontal lobes are the enemy of humanity, he must have been talking about some special kind of human being: some innocently happy being in that state prior to the expulsion from Eden. Neither responsibility, nor the kind of freedom it brings, seemed possible for this patient after the operation. Human behavior, occasionally absurd and sometimes grand, descends in such a patient to an irresponsible spontaneity and a limited range of mechanical actions.

THE NICHOLS AND HUNT CASE

Carefully studied and tested after a bilateral prefrontal lobectomy, the performance of this subject proved spotty, so that firm generalizations about his memory, his attention, his ability to assume the abstract attitude, his motivation are difficult to make. The reported findings have to be studied in detail to reveal the wide fluctuations in his type of approach and his ability to solve the tasks given him.

For example, the patient could solve an arithmetic progressions test at the simpler levels, but failed at the more difficult levels or whenever he was required to combine two series of progressions. He could identify the pattern in and continue the series 2-4-6-8 or 1-1-2-2-3-3, or even one with an interspersed constant (2-1-4-1-6-1), but he could not handle 1-2-5-6-9-10 or 17-1-16-2-15-3. When the tester attempted to find an analogy for the alternation tasks which Jacobsen had found so useful with his operated chimpanzees (and which involved a storage of what the performer had done on the previous test in order to react correctly to the presented task), he used five playing cards among which there was an ace of spades, all five cards being dealt face down. The task was to turn up the ace, whose position varied, alternating to appear twice on the patient's extreme left, twice on his extreme right, and so on. In his first try at this performance, 200 successive deals gave the patient no clue; he did not learn to stop looking at the middle three cards. High-school students solved it in less than 25 trials.

In a test of this type, most subjects will promptly look for "the system" that the dealer is following, but this subject did not. Asked whether he had discovered any system, he seemed to be surprised by the question. Directed to look for such a system and supplied with an example, he could profit from his instruction; that is, he could take up a directional set when given guidance, but he seemed to lack initiative (or the normal person's *need* for some system) when confronted with this type of problem.[1]

This patient failed in a variation of the Knox cube test, and for similar reasons. When a few of the cubes were tapped by the experimenter and the patient was asked to duplicate the action, he could succeed up to a sequence of six (a level attained by eight-year-olds). The possibility of grouping the taps did not occur to him, although he had hit on a way of numbering the blocks, and again, when directed to do so, he learned to use this device. Any introduction of delays caused a marked drop in his performance, and interposed questions caused confusion, both more so than with normal controls. Both the need for a pattern and the ability to somehow hold rival patterns without crossinterference seemed to be disturbed. In checkers the patient overlooked jumps, and seemed to make his moves without plan, but again he showed that he could be trained to take thought, to look ahead, to use a plan.

Summarizing their findings, Nichols and Hunt (1940) selected the following aspects of their patient's performance for emphasis. The patient failed to supply or to seek spontaneously some fresh plan of attack on problems, though he could use the abstracting sets furnished to him. There was a rigidity in his behavior, a failure to shift from one set to another, and he could not use several sets at one time and test them. Integrating several features into a single whole (as, for example, in the Vigotsky sorting test, where compound categories must be applied to assorted colored blocks in various shapes and sizes, e.g., large-tall, small-flat) proved difficult for him. He used categories (putting all circular blocks together), and when one did not work he would turn to another (grouping according to color). He would then alternate between shape and color. He finally added height and formed a color-height category. But he kept returning to former errors, alternating between those

---

[1]This raises an important issue: Can such a patient "learn to learn"? Can he recapture some of his lost "capacity"? Goldstein (1959, p. 775) speaks quite flatly to this point: "The loss of abstract capacity cannot be regained by retraining."

which had not worked. His trials did not have much of a plan (he did not hit on the four-category approach the task required).

What makes the test findings especially interesting is the fact that this patient, formerly employed as an executive secretary in a large corporation, had postoperative IQs ranging between 118 and 122 on a series of measurements. He had had a fine college record before his difficulties began. (He had been operated on at age 45 for a frontal-lobe tumor that had produced anoxemia, epileptic seizures, automatic acts, constricted vision, and irritability with uncontrolled rage at slight provocation.) After the operation he could still define 89 of the 100 words on the Stanford-Binet test, a very superior performance. Some tests used to identify the effects of brain injury were passed successfully. The Bender Visual-Motor Gestalt test showed none of the changes commonly reported among the brain-injured, and he could reproduce the figures from memory. The Kohs block test was well-done, and when he could not do the problem set, he quickly explained why it was impossible. He could carry out part of the sorting task with Holmgren wools, but on the reds and greens he behaved as though he were color-blind. On the Ishihara charts he did not see the figures at first, but when instructed to look for them he could identify them. He behaved somewhat like a subject who cannot at first find the hidden face in a "find-the-face" puzzle, but who can spot it once it is pointed out.

Thus, on a battery of tests, some items believed to show a frontal-lobe deficit could be successfully performed; others which were too difficult, at first, could be done with support and guidance. At many points this superior adult showed capacities which he could not use without "helps" in identifying aspects of the problem and in formulating hypotheses. It was predicted that a combination of reeducation and a suitably stable environment would enable this patient to function at a near-normal level. Too much novelty, freedom, too many unstructured tasks, too great a demand for imaginative ingenuity could be disturbing for him.

It is noteworthy that after the operation the patient's irritability subsided. His behavior in hospital tended to become stereotyped; he clung to routine; he preferred tasks with definite directions and specific orders. He did not invent projects of his own, nor did he enjoy making choices.

The outlines of what Goldstein called an "impairment of the abstract attitude" begin to emerge in this patient's performance, along with a motivational change and a loss in the integrative powers required for personal autonomy. The nature of these changes will become clearer as we proceed with our discussion of other forms of brain damage.

BILATERAL PREFRONTAL LOBOTOMIES AND THEIR SEQUELAE

Created as a venture in therapy, this form of surgical severing of portions of the prefrontal areas on both sides from the rest of the brain while leaving the tissues *in situ* has stirred up a great deal of controversy. Opinion is divided as to its value and as to the extent of damage to the personality. Psychological, social, ethical, and even theological arguments have been directed against this procedure on the ground that grotesque automata are produced in the process of attempting to heal patients; it is argued that the patient's capacity for moral responsibility and autonomous living is destroyed in exchange for a vegetative peace of mind. The noise of controversy led Pope

Pius XII to give a guarded approval of the operation; he suggested rational grounds for sacrificing a portion of reason for the sake of preserving the remainder. The Soviet Ministry of Health opposed it on the ground that the operation converted a potentially recoverable functional disorder into an irreversible organic deficit. In this country it has had its enthusiastic supporters. Rarely, it is treated as a kind of partial euthanasia or "mercy killing," one of its defenders suggesting that if the soul can survive bodily death, it can surely survive a lobotomy. It is probably both overpraised and overdamned. (See L. H. Smith 1955, Freeman 1959, *Brit. Med. J.* 1952.)

Lobotomy, a surgical procedure originally designed to sever the connections between the prefrontal cerebral tissues and the thalamus, was first conceived by Egas Moniz, in Lisbon, in 1933 and carried out under his direction by Almeida Lima in 1936. There had been precedents for such radical interference with brain function. Burckhardt, the superintendent of a small Swiss institution, had attempted to quiet agitated mental patients who talked too much by removing a part of the temperoparietal region (where Wernicke had located the centers for the language processes). One patient had improved; others remained the same. Experiments on chimpanzees, carried out by Fulton and Jacobsen (1935) had shown that the animals—normally so easily frustrated and driven to angry outbursts if, in the delayed-reaction situation, they failed to attain expected rewards—were converted into easily distracted, forgetful animals, relatively free from anger and anxiety, when their prefrontal areas had been removed. Moniz argued that this kind of relief from intolerable tensions might benefit some of his chronically ill mental patients; his first monograph, dealing with the effects of this surgical procedure on 20 patients, revealed enough therapeutic gain to tempt others to follow this procedure. Enthusiasts in England, the United States, and elsewhere took up this empirical procedure, offering various rationalizations; it has been "improved" by methods which reduce the danger of serious inpairment, and has been used on patients in almost every psychiatric category (from relatively mild neuroses to deteriorated schizophrenia). By the 1960's, medical statistics showed that more than 15,000 patients had been operated on in England alone, and more than twice that number were reported from the United States. The popularity of the operation has waxed and waned.[2]

---

[2]Now that drugs are available to reduce the excitement of hospitalized psychotics and to make them more manageable, one of the motives behind lobotomies (and one of the causes for abuses in the use of the technique) has been removed. The largest single group in the total mass of lobotomies performed in the years 1940-1960 was composed of incurable schizophrenics; in the majority of these cases the operation did little to improve the psychosis. In this illness it is the beginning case (less than a year in hospital) that is most apt to improve, whether under this treatment, insulin shock, or intensive psychotherapy. In the latter treatment, there is less danger of irreversible damage to the patient's powers of adjustment. The actively hallucinating, anxious, negativistic, excited cases are more apt to benefit than the apathetic, deteriorated, and emotionally "flattened." Chronic depressions that have not responded to other forms of therapy such as electroshock sometimes react favorably to lobotomy. The severe and prolonged case of obsession with anxiety and hypochondriacal features is regarded, by some, as the best candidate of all, partly because the prognosis is so poor for other, less radical therapies.

UNDERLYING THEORY

What do the frontal lobes do for man, that their severance should lead a surgeon to believe that a patient's condition might be improved when some of this tissue is removed? What do those pathways joining frontal cortex with thalamus accomplish, as descending impulses pass from what are probably the highest circuits in the neural loopline arrangement down through the ganglia that seem to be involved in autonomic regulation? Does the severance of the upward flow of impulses along the thalamo-frontal paths cut off a kind of emotional-instinctual charge to whatever ideas are on board? Will obsessive thoughts lose their emotional charge? Or are these structures at the frontal pole of the cerebrum so peculiar to man, who alone among the animals feels shame, guilt, the spur of an ego-ideal, and the correlated superego punishment, that when they function improperly they *produce* mental illness?

Some of the changes that he observed in his patients made Freeman conclude that the operation reduced the *self's reaction to the self*. With such a reduction a certain amount of social sensitivity, much of the imaginative capacity to project oneself into the future, and a great deal of what might be called "superego anxiety" are also lost. Does this severance of the fronto-thalamic paths mean that, whatever mental conflict exists, it is now less intense as though, figuratively, an emotional "center" no longer charges these patterns? Or does the interference prevent "mental conflicts" from reaching an intensity great enough to arouse the emotions?

There is a kind of primitive phrenological notion lurking behind these procedures. Stated crudely, one version runs: the highest functions (social, ethical, imaginative, rational, history-making, representative) are mediated by cells located at the frontal pole; the emotional-instinctive-impulsive functions are centered in the thalamus and hypothalamus.[3] To fully charge the highest functions, or for the highest functions to arouse the charge necessary for action, these two-way frontothalamic paths must be intact. Ideas may not differ in content as a result of the operation, but they are robbed of their motivational charge. Intelligence is preserved, but not *affective* intelligence. Feelings and emotions persist, but they are of brief duration, and neither charge nor are charged by any larger organization of action. Thus the regulation of action is radically altered while the "pieces" of the habit systems remain intact. There is no loss of memories or of an easily verbalized personal identity, but the ways in which these memories function are radically altered.

SOME REFLECTIONS ON LOBOTOMY

The web of relations that a man weaves as he moves to and fro, and that relates him to each segment of the world that he can grasp, is most

---

[3]Studies of experimental animals that have had large portions of their thalamus or hypothalamus removed, a procedure that left the animal somnolent, apathetic, and placid, create the impression that the very center of the vigilant and aroused animal's "emotions" has been destroyed.

complex. Sometimes it grows tangled, with fixated vicious cycles binding the individual in the trap of his own incorrectly summated and interpreted experience. The world he sees is mad, threatening, anxiety-inducing, and he cannot discharge the tasks that he has elected. The self bows under a weight of guilt, both real and imagined, until it feels impotent, about to be crushed. The clinician who is confronted with the task of unsnarling this tangled web is often baffled, lacking the skill, the insight, and the time to undo the snarl. Small wonder that some will want to cut the neural and behavioral knots and, simplifying the remaining network, hope that a fresh start can be made and some comfortable adjustment worked out, using those pathways that remain. There can be no question but that such a snipping of the conduction fibers will leave a cruder conduction system than the original network that became "fouled up," and it is even conceivable that the pruning and the simplifying may leave structures that, no longer clogged by the self-defeating vicious cycles, will enable the man to make a more tolerable life. The evidence suggests that a third or perhaps a half of the cases operated on remain semidependent charges on family and friends. A third achieve the goal the therapist aims for. The remainder show a mixture of favorable and unfavorable results. There should therefore be a balancing of possible gains against possible losses, and an exploring of alternatives, to guide the therapist and the family of the patient when the operation is considered. They must remember that, when the months slip by and all other therapies fail, the bargain does not grow more attractive, since "good" results usually follow *early* surgical interference. They must also remember that those whose personalities are well-developed and reasonably stable, whose illnesses are classified as neurotic rather than psychotic, and who have undergone no deterioration or emotional blunting, are the patients most likely to be described as "successful cures." In this latter case, however, other therapies are also apt to work, given time; and these alternatives are less likely to involve an irreversible impairment.

We have grown convinced during the past hundred years of experimental study of the effects of brain injuries (and experimental ablation of neural tissues in animals) that the frontal lobes are necessary for the highest levels of control. Better developed in man than in any other animal, they have been looked on as essential for the "highest" human attributes (imagination, reasoning, foresight, and concern about ethical standards) though the neurophysiologist sometimes calls them the silent areas, since no injury in these spots produces an obvious loss in sensation or movement. If we are content merely to call them the higher association areas, it is nonetheless here that whatever approaches a unity in action will be achieved. The reluctance to invade these areas is therefore understandable. A man is something more and other than a loosely tied bundle of reflex parts. These prefrontal areas seem to contain the looplines through which the shape that we call the person is formed. Their proper functioning produces the "regulation" that gives action a structure. Any lesions in this area will tend to reduce behavior to the simpler "pieces" of which it is composed. Our failure to find impairment in lobotomies, as we measure them with our tests, suggests that the tests are better measures for the pieces of a man than for the whole man. The clinician's eye may very well be superior here, and so may the judgment of the family, on whose efforts the patient may have to depend.

ORGANICALLY ROOTED SEIZURES WITH MINIMAL EFFECTS

Before we look at some of the other more pervasive forms of brain damage, which produce serious and irreversible changes in the personality and drastic reduction of mental powers, let us examine a group of "seizure states." In these patients there are bursts of neural action within local cell groups that produce partial or total malfunction: a momentary blackout with or without a complete convulsion. After a short period of recovery, normal functions are resumed, save for the memory of the attack, the dread of its return, the social consequences, and possible accidental injuries. In a few cases, particularly in those which are institutionalized or in which epilepsy is secondary to other pathological processes, a cumulative deterioration in mental functioning is observed.

Before the electroencephalogram (which enables the clinician to make a visible record of these "brainstorms"), it was easier to group these seizure states with other types of attack where there were sharp changes in the structure of action and consciousness, such as those we noted in psychasthenics and hystericals. The latter patients also complained of *déjà vu* experiences, of feelings of unreality, of a change in the appearance of objects, of feeling separated from the surrounding world, of a clouding of consciousness, of a wall separating them from others, of sudden losses of motivation and interest. These symptoms had a certain vague similarity to auras (the precursors of attacks) of epileptics and other seizure states with characteristic bursts of measurable neural changes. The restlessness and agitation, the inability to hold still or to hold attention on a task (part of the preconvulsive tension of some epileptics, which seems to mount until it is discharged in the *grand mal* attack), also appeared in the attacks of some psychasthenics who reported sudden surges of feelings of pressure, effort, anxiety.

Today, any "seizure" without objective evidence of an associated burst of internal brain changes is subjected to very careful scrutiny, and is usually placed in a separate group and given quite different treatment. When, further, it is possible to identify the foci of neural discharge that cause the seizures, some neurosurgeons have urged extirpation of the diseased cells (or the cells at the border of scar tissues which discharge) in the hope of bringing the attacks to an end, and the problem becomes a matter of dealing with histological-physiological facts, not of treating the outcome of an unfortunate personal history (even though, as may be noted, increase in anxious tensions arising out of personal difficulties may increase the rate of attacks). Penfield and Jasper (1954, p. 349), who have pursued a neurosurgical procedure in many of these cases, describe the type of lesion that is sometimes (but by no means always) the focus of electrical discharges which flood the brain:

"It has been shown that the epileptic focus, when clearly outlined, is objectively abnormal as well as physiologically abnormal. This is a matter of record. Our conclusion in regard to the various types of lesions, expanding or atrophic, is that they produce continuing or recurring *ganglionic ischemia.* We propose the hypothesis that this mild or recurrent chronic ischemia is irritating to nerve cells and that it is the *cause of epileptic discharge."*

To this we can add the fact that an experimental epilepsy, analogous to the human seizure states, can be produced in the monkey when laminated discs of compressed linen, coated with aluminum hydroxide, are implanted on the surface of the cerebral cortex. Gradually changing, the cells beneath the discs produce first abnormal EEGs, then convulsive seizures. In time these effects begin to wear off (after periods of three months to two years), and a further period of altered brain waves (without overt seizures) may endure as long as another seven months. (See Pacella *et al.* 1944.)

When the discharging focus is located on the brain surface, the neurosurgeon can apply an electrical stimulator to this point in the waking human subject (after the cortex has been exposed by a bone-flap operation which lays back the meningeal covering of the brain cells), and a convulsion can be induced. Penfield (1958, p. 29; Penfield and Rasmussen 1950, p. 164) has described cases in which this focus lies in the rear portion of the temporal lobe just adjacent to the occipital lobe.

One of these patients had always experienced a peculiar dreamlike aura in which she saw herself running, pursued by a man who bore a bag of snakes. She heard voices shouting and experienced extreme terror. This often recurring aura always terminated in a *grand mal* attack. The electrical stimulator applied to the focal area induced both aura and *grand mal* attack.

The subject, conscious during such brain stimulation, acts as an onlooker at a drama that unfolds automatically as though before his eyes (or ears). He remains present in the experimental situation, and is at the same time able to observe the dream; and he calls out "Oh, there it goes; everybody is yelling." He commands the experimenter, who is manipulating the electrode, "Stop them!" Sometimes these observations are very explicit: "Yes. I heard voices down along the river somewhere—a man's voice and a woman's voice calling. . . . I think I saw the river. . . . It seems to be one I was visiting when I was a child."

In both examples, the dreamlike auras that precede the attacks seem to contain memories of events actually experienced. The family of the girl who dreamed of being pursued by a man with a bag of snakes substantiated her story: there had been such an episode, and it had been followed by nightmares in which the scene was reenacted. In the second case we cannot be sure whether the episode was actually a reproduction of an old memory or an experimentally induced series of images cloaked with the *déjà vu* quality so frequently reported by epileptics in this preconvulsive period.

Hysterical attacks which involve a stiffening of the whole trunk (tonic spasm) or violent and convulsive contractions do not show the typical epileptic brain waves, nor is there a biting of the cheek or tongue, or a loss of sphincter control. The typical hysterical seizure is also followed by a loss of ability to recall events that occur during the seizure, but hypnosis can sometimes reveal memories which suggest that a "second state of consciousness" (in which imprinting occurred) existed during the attack. The hysterical attacks which occur in the presence of others have a certain histrionic quality about them. The subject does not injure himself as he throws himself about, whereas the epileptic frequently does.

There is a border zone where the discrimination is not easy. From 5 to 15 per cent of epileptics have normal EEGs in the period between attacks, and if attacks occur at night, the clinician may find no evidence of cerebral dysrhythmia in his examination on the following day. Penfield and Jasper (1954, p. 661) note that some hysterical patients also show dysrhythmias (without accompanying paroxysms); it is thus evident that the EEG cannot be used as the only criterion. Thus, there are seizure-free persons who have EEGs resembling those of the epileptic, hystericals who have seizures (some with cerebral dysrhythmias and some with normal EEGs), and epileptics who never show a clinical record of abnormal brain waves (since their seizures themselves have not been observed directly). Observed seizures are always accompanied by abnormal brain waves. A suspected case with normal EEGs will sometimes show the abnormal pattern under hyperventilation or with small doses of metrazol. (See Noyes and Kolb 1963, p. 238.)

Now that the electroencephalogram and the exploration of the surface of the brain for foci of discharge are used as a way of separating neurotic seizures from "true epilepsy," there is a tendency to think of the former as needing psychotherapy, while for the latter the physician will recommend a good physical hygiene, medication, a near-normal schedule of living, or—in rare instances—brain surgery.[4] Janet, Raymond, Hesnard, and many others were more inclined to look on the seizure, the loss of integrative force, the drop in "psychological tension," and the sudden alteration of consciousness as the basic consideration, and to place epilepsy within the long series of other physical and mental conditions that produce such *"chutes."* The practical efficacy of surgery, medication, and control of exercise and water intake is so great that the epileptic group now deserves to be treated as a separate disorder. Three technical advances have produced the category: new surgical techniques for exploring and excision of focal areas, new drugs that control seizures in which abnormal brain waves accompany attacks, and the EEG, which differentiates (more or less successfully) one clinical form of loss of integrative powers from the others.

---

[4]Diet is regarded as of minor importance, although hypoglycaemia or an abnormal ingestion of fluids may precipitate attacks. Surgery is recommended when all other measures have failed to control attacks, when a focal epileptogenic lesion can be found, when brain tumor is the cause, or when dangerous aggressive behavior is a part of the attack (making the life of the patient and of those around him impossible). Ey reports observations in which, of 25 cases operated on, 10 revealed no histologic anomaly in the excised cells. This absence of histological change was also reported by Pacella and his associates in their experimental epilepsy produced by implanted discs bearing aluminum hydroxide. (See Ey, Bernard, and Brisset 1963, p. 302.)

If sick cortical cells, or cells suffering from a local spasm of contraction of arterioles (ischemia) and hence deprived of normal oxygen supply, or cells suffering from as yet unknown blood substances which alter their threshold of excitability are responsible for the attacks, why, one might well ask, should one treat the whole person?

It is at this point that psychiatrists divide. "It is not possible to shirk the task of attempting continually to solve the problem of epilepsy.... The epileptic and not the disease must be the main concern of therapeutics," wrote L. Pierce Clark (1922, p. 65). "In studying epileptic patients the whole personality must be considered, with attention to all factors and their interrelations," adds Oskar Diethelm (1934, p. 755). The latter guarded statement would be true even if personality features were not an essential cause of the attacks but merely contributory factors which alter their frequency or retard recovery. In Barker's study (1948a) of a case of *petit mal* it appeared that:

1. The frequency of attacks was a function of the intensity of life-situation stresses.

2. Specific relations between stress and attack could be discovered by a free-association technique.

3. Other psychosomatic symptoms sometimes replaced attacks.

4. The attacks served to abolish consciousness and to prevent the full (and painful) awareness of unacceptable life-situations.

Strauss, on the other hand, summarizes his discussion of therapy with the terse observation, "a general recommendation for psychotherapy in convulsive states cannot be made." To judge from trends in recent literature, one might conclude that the emphasis on psychogenic factors has been overdone. Genogenic, histogenic, chemogenic causes tend to be emphasized. The attack upon psychogenic items in the life-history are more often viewed as helping the course of the disorder rather than as a treatment of something basic and causal.

Just how much these facilitative factors may alter the course of development is illustrated by one of Cobb's cases (1943, p. 112):

"...a young man of seventeen, brought to the hospital stupefied and staggering because of excessive phenobarbital. He was having several minor seizures (lapses with rolling eyes) per day and about once a week a major convulsion. He had suffered from convulsive seizures since infancy and the lapses had begun at about the age of ten. His father was a morose, opinionated person with alcoholism and an abnormal electroencephalogram. He had beaten the boy for 'absent-mindedness' when the lapses began at ten. The mother was kind and loyal, but oversolicitous, and watched the boy by inches, never giving him any liberty. At the age of sixteen the boy had tried to rebel, gone out, and had a brief alcoholic spree and a sex experience. Since then he had been watched even more closely and his mother had become practically his jailer. The father 'would have nothing more to do with him.'...

"Treatment consisted of sending the parents away, getting the boy over his phenobarbital intoxication, putting him on a good regime with phenobarbital only at ten p.m. Then a year and a half was spent in 'socializing' him. He hated all authority at first, but was soon made to feel that he 'belonged' and was appreciated. He was given occupation and had a male nurse for six months and weekly interviews with a psychiatrist. Later he was allowed to run his own life, as long as he reported every two weeks. During the last year he has had no major convulsions and only one or two lapses a week, at irregular intervals. Socially he is a changed human being."

Psychotherapy did not control these seizures, nor did medication eliminate them completely; but with minimal medication and extensive psychotherapy, this boy was rescued from what might have easily become a progressively deteriorating existence.

Perhaps, therefore, we should add a footnote to Strauss's generalization: "Psychotherapy is not indicated in epilepsy, except in those cases where it makes a great difference." Some of the psychotherapy will have to be aimed at the family; some will seek to bring about the kind of maturing that a protective and oversolicitous (or rejecting and unusually harsh) environment has made impossible; some efforts will have to be aimed at educating schoolteachers, employers, and the general public, whose reactions to seizure states worsen the life-situation of the epileptic, and thus indirectly *cause* the disorder to be more serious than it would be if the "pure" or "essential" features were treated rationally.

Behavior disorders are frequently found associated with *petit mal;* in some of these "problem children," there has been no other reported symptom of abnormal brain functioning, but the electroencephalogram reveals the typical *petit mal* tracing. Restless, poor learners, aggressive and unmanageable, hard to interest in any prolonged task, the behavior of this group may include a wide variety of delinquencies: fire-setting, stealing, running away, destructiveness, fighting. A less serious form of such a behavior disorder is reported by Strauss (1959, p. 115):

". . . a doctor's grandson, four years old . . . was brought for electroencephalography because he had had one single convulsion. Aside from this, the patient was also a 'difficult child.' He was very restless, never continued any activity uninterruptedly for more than a few minutes, and was very inattentive. The electroencephalogram showed extremely numerous spike and wave discharges separated by only a few seconds of normal record. This patient, in whom a *petit mal* attack had never been observed clinically or even suspected, was nevertheless treated with drugs used generally for the treatment of *petit mal*. This resulted in an almost instantaneous change in his behavior. The patient became calm, showed good attention and concentration, and developed in an entirely normal way."

The medication may have been sufficient to enable the normal disciplines to work. It is also conceivable that when some parents and teachers look on such a child as a medical problem instead of a moral one, and when his peculiarities are understood as related to an abnormal brain functioning, not as due to meanness, a desire to show off or to get attention, a new set of interpersonal relations can be established. It is clear, however, that Dr. Strauss regards the medication as the principal ingredient.

Turning his attention to a broader span of the patient's behavior, Janet (1932, pp. 102-3; 1919, I, 667-68; 1903, II, 66-67) called attention to wide

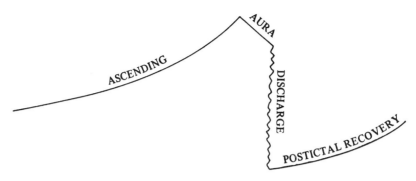

FIGURE 10. JANET'S CURVE OF PSYCHOLOGICAL TENSION. The first ascending curve represents a period of mounting tension. Interest and enthusiasm run high, and the individual feels in full possession of his powers. The aura may take the form of an almost ecstatic feeling, of a joy too great to be borne. Followed, as it is in the epileptic, with a *grand mal* seizure, it is apparent that this "peak experience" occurs at a moment when the integrative powers of the individual have already begun to decline. Whether he feels "all-powerful" or "all-knowing," he has lost his powers of self-criticism, his belief has descended to a primitive form, and his action system has lost that vigilant relation to the field (and to a projected future) that normally obtains. The sharp descent in integrative forces ends in a blotting out of awareness, in spasmodic tonic and clonic discharges of a reflex nature. The slow recovery through a clouded, twilight state is represented by the curve labeled "postictal recovery." Such a loading-and-discharge concept helps indicate the reasons for Janet's admonition to some of his patients: "You are not millionaires of the spirit." Like his patient Paul, who systematically cultivated a level below the peak that bordered on the aura-and-discharge point of the curve, Janet also sought to find for them that "optimum" that could be pursued with safety.

fluctuations in psychological tension in epileptics, cyclic change that others had missed. He noted that in the intervals between attacks the epileptic often does not enjoy the mental health of the ordinary person. He is troubled by headaches, digestive disorders (and a certain visceral sluggishness), and almost always by a slight and chronic depressive state. The epileptic is looked on by others as slow, inert, a bit lazy, and lacking in ordinary lively feelings, and the patient himself often complains of boredom, of a state of "emptiness." This unhappy condition begins to lift, prior to the attack; he feels better than usual, grows active, undertakes important tasks, speaks more freely. Along with this ascent to a higher level of functioning (which we would be inclined to call healthy and normal), the attacks appear. Janet drew a curve of the rise and fall of this integrative power (see Figure 10).

Paul offers an illustration of such a curve of integrative energies, and, in addition, shows how the effort of the patient to understand himself and to regulate such a cycle can be incorporated into the illness.

Observant and intelligent, Paul not only dreaded these attacks, but took measures to forestall them. He had learned that if he let himself go in enthusiastic enjoyment (even of music or literature), he had to pay for it. So he sought a way of living without involvement, practicing a peculiar sort of asceticism. He avoided people, stayed away from spectacles, gave up music and literature that he really enjoyed, read only material that bored him. He feared to become interested. His melancholy and absurd existence disturbed his friends, but it was free from attacks.

Paul had never seen an aeroplane in flight. His friends induced him to visit an aerodrome, and, curiosity aroused, as he approached the place he could feel a metamorphosis taking place: he became gay, excited; his enthusiasm mounted. Facilitated by the excitement of those around him, his state intensified, but he began to realize that he had been through all this before, heard the same sounds; he knew that these people had come together for some sinister purpose, directed against him. The abyss awaited him. Life was suddenly absurd and meaningless. And from this point his memory failed, for he had fallen into an attack of *grand mal,* with complete loss of consciousness.

Even in the epileptic's new-found excitement and happiness, when he feels that he is functioning as never before, the descent of his integrative forces has begun, for he loses the self-critical function, experiences a kind of "triumph without basis," and begins to experience a clouding of consciousness similar to the *déjà vu* experience. In the place of rational beliefs and ideas easily communicated, there emerges something ineffable and "beyond reason." Some patients feel there is something sacred, divine, absolute about this aura consciousness. There are other forms of mood change besides this ascent (or descent) into ecstacy: a state of extreme anxiety or terror (*angoisse*) may grip the patient with crushing force, and fuse with the tonic contractures of the first phase of the *grand mal* attack.

THE QUESTION OF EPILEPTIC DETERIORATION

Epilepsy is a group of symptoms rather than a disease entity, and there is no reason why it should not be associated with other disorders (such as syphilis) that also lead to a series of progressive changes in the cortical cells. There is a possibility that the massive cerebral changes involved in repeated full-blown *grand mal* attacks will actually produce deteriorative changes.[5]

A mild impairment in mental functioning may exist in many epileptics without its being easily measured. Such an impairment would produce such symptoms as slowness, a poverty of ideas, an inability to react insightfully to novel and changing situations, and a lack of inflection and rhythm in speech. In about 10 per cent of the severe institutional cases, the impairment is of a gross and immediately observable nature. Such a "brain-damaged" core group may have given rise to Minkowski's concept of a sticky (glischroid-agglutinative) personality. All epileptic impairments have to be evaluated in the light of the setting; where social ostracism, institutional life, daily medication, thwarting of personal goals, poor family management of the illness, contrac-

---

[5]Immediately after an attack the cells begin to return to normal functioning. This return is sometimes delayed and a "postictal" paralysis endures. If this endures too long the cortical cells may be destroyed and an expanding area of destruction will then be found at postmortem. Shock therapy has sometimes been held responsible for initiating such changes. The damage to these cells is similar to that which occurs in much more widespread fashion in carbon-monoxide poisoning. (See Penfield and Jasper 1954, pp. 278 ff.)

tion of interests, and possible associated disorders serve to complicate the picture, not all the changes can be attributed to the disorder.

More impressed by the constitutional factor, Diethelm (1950), while holding out the possibility of a favorable development, warns that the teacher of epileptic children needs to be aware of their limitations. Their sulkiness, sensitivity, and self-centeredness make the demands of group life difficult for them, and they need more than average stimulation with interesting and varying tasks. They find it difficult to accept constructive criticism, although they seriously need it, and are quick to criticize others. They need more time to finish tasks and are more easily upset by failures and shortcomings. Nevertheless, Diethelm, along with most observers, urges that these children be accepted in the ordinary school, and that both the epileptic child and his schoolmates be encouraged to assume a matter-of-fact attitude toward his disability. The less intelligent and more retarded child (as well as the one who has been badly warped by early family life) may require a special school, but schools which precisely fit the needs of such a child are in short supply.

Common sense warns that the goal of a complete and natural life for the epileptic will present certain difficulties. He should not operate a motor vehicle until he has become attack-free. The question "Should the epileptic marry?" is bound up with the seriousness of the disorder and the estimated likelihood of transmission. In any case marriage should be undertaken with the full understanding of the partner; ideally it should be with a nonepileptic partner, if children are desired. The facts about heredity indicate that if a person afflicted with epilepsy marries a nonepileptic partner, chances that a child issuing from the marriage will experience convulsions are one in fifty. There is a greater chance that he will have an abnormal EEG. One study (Stein 1933) found that of 1,000 hospitalized epileptics, 18 per cent had relatives with a history of seizures; whereas in a control group of 1,115 nonepileptic patients, there were 4.6 per cent who had relatives with seizures. Statistical studies (Conrad 1935, Alstrom 1950) cited by Ey, Bernard, and Brisset (1963, p. 294) indicate that the frequency of epilepsy among the children of epileptics is twenty times that in the general population, ten in contrast to one in 200. Facts of this order lead Strauss (1959, p. 1138) to conclude that the possibility of inheritance will "rarely be a factor sufficiently great to advise against any progeny." Now that medicine has made so many advances in the treatment of this disorder, "even if the child should be sick from a convulsive disorder, probably it will be possible to make this child a happy human being."

ASSOCIATED DISORDERS

The "seizure" seems to spring from a "storm" that explodes within the brain, activating the entire musculature and blotting out consciousness. Technically known as *grand mal,* the major type of seizure has been known from Biblical times. No illness could have been better calculated to reinforce the belief that demons can seize a man and make him do strange things. It was a challenge to those who, like the witch-doctors, claimed to have dominion over spirits, for such children were brought to these healers to have the demons cast forth. Today the psychiatrist administers a drug, prescribes a hygiene or a diet, seeks to understand the personal conflicts that may intensify or increase the number of seizures, and in rare instances advises a type of neurosurgery to remove a tumor (or scar tissue) that is responsible for the seizures.

The more closely epilepsy is studied, the more certain it becomes that the group of symptoms does not identify a specific disease process. Not only are the causes of these "seizure states" multiple and varied, the dramatic *grand mal* seizure is soon observed to be associated with minor seizures (*petit mal*) which involve no convulsions whatever, causing merely a momentary awayness and possibly, but not necessarily, a loss of muscular tone. Still other forms of "seizure" involve no loss of consciousness but produce a fit of restless, aggressive, fugue-like behavior with or without complete fortgetfulness of the action. In recent years the general public has been alerted to the possibility that a type of "seizure," related to those in epilepsy, may be responsible for crimes of violence. Psychiatrists were called on to testify about this possibility in the trial of Jack Ruby.

Reaching out beyond this triad (*grand mal, petit mal,* psychomotor seizures), there are migraine attacks in which a "splitting" headache is the principal symptom. Other "spasms" of contracture may strike the musculature of the trunk or of the gastrointestinal system, and these local, spontaneous seizures invite the clinician to use the same types of therapy and to view them as members of this now extended series of seizure states.

A single technical development has facilitated this extension of the concept of seizure. Hans Berger discovered, in 1929, that he could pick up minute electrical changes occurring in the cells of the brain by means of an electrode placed on the outer surface of the skull; by means of suitable amplification and recording, these fluctuations in voltage could be converted into visible tracings on a moving record. Like the sphygmograph which records the fluctuations in pressure in the arterial system, the electroencephalogram records an electrical pulse in the brain. Driven at a steady and uninterrupted rate of ten per second in the normal resting brain of a waking subject, these pulses change in amplitude and in frequency in sleep, in emotional excitement, and in epileptic seizures. For each of the three classes of seizure states that we have been describing, there is a characteristic wave pattern, and it has been easy to extend the concept of epilepsy wherever the sudden "seizure state" has such definite brain signatures. So extended has the list of "epileptic equivalents" become that such a class name as "the epilepsies" is made to include quite diverse disorders. Strauss proposes the names "paroxysmal disorders" or "disorders associated with electrical cerebral paroxysms."

What further complicates the diagnostic and explanatory problem is the existence of these abnormal brain waves in at least 10 per cent of the total population. Where 0.5 per cent are known to have seizures, the remaining 9.5 per cent are seizure-free. When 50 per cent of children classed as "behavior disorders" or as having "reading disability" are found to have atypical brain waves, or when 70 per cent of criminal psychopaths studied in a federal prison are found to show abnormal waves, there is a temptation to extend the concept still further and to include those examples of poorly organized (uncontrolled, impulsive, uninhibited) behavior whenever there is an associated abnormal EEG. It must be remembered, in this connection, that there are psychopaths and problem children with normal brain waves and that there are normal children and adults with abnormal brain waves like those found in some who show clearly defined seizure states. Where they are present, as in a reading difficulty, the bursts of electrical change which interrupt the more organized patterns involved in perception are an important component in the poor learning, and the medical control of these brain states may make possible a more normal development. Yet in many of the cases, from *grand mal* to migraine headaches, "seizures" (or "attacks") may be only one component in the total behavior complex. An adequate grasp of a patient's problem may require a study of the patient as a person.[6]

GRAND MAL

The major seizures proper begin with a generalized tensing of the musculature that makes the trunk rigid; the head is drawn backward. There may be a cry as the air is forced from the lungs by this contracture, but the jaw promptly closes. The patient falls, with arms drawn closely to the side of the trunk. Pupils are dilated and do not react to light; the Babinski reflex is present, tendon reflexes absent or decreased, and corneal reflex absent. With respiration stopped, after first appearing pale the patient's face becomes dark blue, the eyes bloodshot. Usually the fist is closed with thumb inside, legs stiffened, rotated inward. This phase lasts from five to forty seconds, and is accompanied by an increase in the rate and amplitude of voltage changes with EEG waves running at about 25 per second (see Figure 11).

This tonic phase is rapidly followed by an alternation of contraction and relaxation that may occur as often as 15 times per second (palpable rather than visible). These alternations (or convulsions) gradually slow down. In their course the tongue and cheek may be bitten. With the return of breathing, the cyanotic appearance passes; the patient perspires freely, and may void or defecate. The patient, typically unconscious in such attacks, may remain comatose or pass into a normal sleep. A few wake up promptly, asserting that they feel better and proceed with whatever the task was that had occupied them prior to the attack. A long-lasting period of confusion sometimes follows, in which the patient wanders about, acts automatically, makes chewing movements, fumbles at his clothing. If electroencephalograms are taken during the

---

[6]In the use of the EEG as a diagnostic tool, a negative record, free from abnormal waves, is not conclusive. In 15 per cent of those who have seizures, normal records appear in 15-minute samples taken in the interval between seizures. Since 10 per cent of a normal sample will show abnormalities, the clinician will be forced to rely on other clues in diagnosing some of his cases. Noyes and Kolb (1963, p. 228) report that 80 per cent of patients have nonconvulsive seizure discharges while asleep. Waking a patient who is subject to *grand mal* seizures at that point where his EEG is showing a typical seizure-state pattern may precipitate an attack; whereas if he is allowed to sleep, these bursts of voltage changes produce no attack.

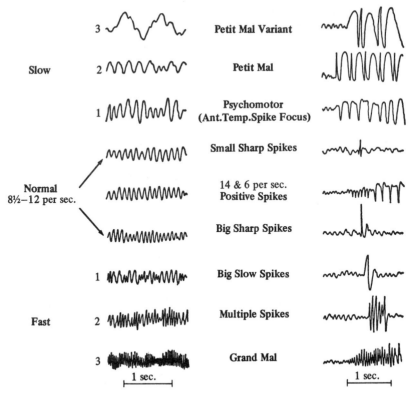

FIGURE 11. NORMAL AND ABNORMAL EEG PATTERNS. In the left column are shown the nonparoxysmal patterns. Above are waves slower than alpha and below, those faster than alpha. In the middle are patterns that fall in the 8½ to 12 cycles per second range, which is the normal alpha range for adults. The right-hand patterns show various types of abnormality. The pattern characteristic for psychomotor seizures is seen over the entire cortex during a clinical seizure; in seizure-free intervals, it appears as an anterior temporal spike focus. (Reprinted by permission of Addison-Wesley Publishing Company, Reading, Mass., publishers of F. A. Gibbs and E. L. Gibbs, *Atlas of Electroencephalography* [Vol. I, 1951], in which the original figure appeared; and of Columbia University Press, publishers of Magda B. Arnold, *Emotion and Personality* [1960], in which the figure was reprinted, p. 137.)

attack, the passage to the clonic phase shows further augmentation of the voltage changes and a slowing of the frequency to two per second.

The postictal (or postconvulsive) state may endure for as long as several days, and more complex activities, resembling those in the fugue, sometimes occur, including severe aggressive actions dangerous to the patient and to those about him. The clouded states are accompanied by slow, diffuse brain potentials without any paroxysmal waves. There is usually complete amnesia for the period, although the patient speaks, moves about, and acts in a near-normal fashion (save for the clouding of consciousness and some nominal aphasia). Occasionally it has been reported that hypnosis has succeeded in penetrating this gap in recall.

Two phases of this *grand mal* attack are worth special emphasis. Often the coming of the attack is preceded by a warning, an aura whose significance is recognized by the patient.[7] It may include mood disturbances, irritability, a feeling of pressure moving up from the pit of the stomach toward the head, or a tingling that marches up the arm (as though a center of disturbance were spreading over corresponding sensory areas of the cortex). The nature of the aura seems to depend on the site of the epileptogenic focus that initiates the attacks. Lesions in front of the fissure of Rolando give a motor signal, ones in the rear a sensory signal. Flashes of light, nausea, noises (or even vaguely hallucinated scraps of conversation), unpleasant smells, twitches in particular muscles have all been reported. By using an electroencephalic technique, and moving electrodes over the surface of the brain, the focus of discharge can sometimes be located; when the neurosurgeon can expose and directly stimulate the spot, the typical aura and seizure can be induced.

Where such an aura precedes the attack, it provides a brief interval in which the individual may prepare himself for the seizure: he may retire from a group, stop working if he is operating a machine, place a handkerchief or towel between his teeth, lie down, and so on. These warnings, however, are not always present; the convulsion *can* strike with lightning speed, which makes it imperative that no epileptic should operate a motor vehicle.

The states which usually follow an attack sometimes occur without any preceding *grand mal* seizure. These do not seem to be the direct result of current paroxysmal discharge, yet they arrest the operation of that "centrencephalic system" that normally maintains vigilance. Again, the diffuse and slow rhythms of discharge that normally follow a seizure may clear, and the EEG then give a normal pattern, but consciousness is still clouded and the structure of action is radically altered. In such "psychic seizures" (without convulsions) consciousness may merely be altered, rather than blotted out. Many of the changes that Janet reported in his psychasthenics are observed: objects seem smaller and farther away; consciousness is clouded and sensations dulled; a "transparent wall" separates the patient from those around him. Others insist: consciousness is sharpened; objects stand forth in unusually sharp outline; thinking is lively; and there is a pressure of ideas. The phenomena of *déjà vu* and *déjà vécu* give a haunting feeling of familiarity, of having lived through the scene before, when the patient is, in fact, in what he should know is a new setting. Along with these feelings there is the sense of acting as an automaton, of having undergone a radical change as a person, in which case even members of the immediate family may appear as strangers, imposters. Mood changes involving fear, anxiety, depression strike with the suddenness of the convulsive attack itself, and a patient may refer to a "click" that announced the changes or to a "black cloud" that descended. There are also sudden and unexplained moods of jubilation or ecstasy. Similar changes in con-

---

[7]The aura is reported to be present in both "essential" or "idiopathic" and symptomatic types of epilepsy (those secondary to brain injury of some identifiable biochemical cause). About half the patients report them. (See Ey 1954, p. 527.)

sciousness are also reported by neurotics in whom no seizure history can be found. There is no amnesia in the latter, or in the "psychic seizures" associated with abnormal brain waves, in which the foci of discharge are usually from the temporal lobes, which also yield spikes and paroxysmal slow waves between seizures (see Strauss 1959, p. 119).

Automatic thinking, in which a panoramic review of memories recurs in repetitive-obsessive form, or in which a jingle runs through the mind, betray a certain destructuring of the system of action and of normal interest in a present field. A false sense of increase in mental powers may take the form of a feeling of clairvoyance, of a knowledge of things happening at a distance or in the future.

PETIT MAL

Without warning, consciousness can lapse, and the epileptic will experience a "blackout." A partial blackout leaves the patient with an awareness of something being said, but that something has no meaning. Usually immobile, staring, he appears to be "away"; there may be a loss of muscle tone, so that he drops the book he is holding, or stumbles, or drives his auto off the road. The whole event passes so quickly (in half a minute) that, barring some accident, he may be unaware anything unusual has happened. If he is directed to press a key whenever a sound signal is given during a period within which these attacks are occurring, the repeated signal will call forth responses save at that moment when the paroxysmal bursts in the EEG betray the abnormal brain functioning. The "spike and dome" tracing (see Figure 12) gives the characteristic signature of this form of epilepsy, with the pattern recurring at a rate of three per second. There is no aura or warning, and no postparoxysmal state. He may sit, or stand, with posture fixed, staring, with a slight flutter of the eyelid or twitch of the eyebrows or head. When he returns from being "away" in this fashion, he may or may not be aware that he has been "absent."

Attacks of *petit mal* may alternate with *grand mal* seizures in the same patient. In some patients these "absences" may occur with a frequency up to two hundred per day. The disorder usually begins in childhood (between ages four and eight), and two out of three of these children go on to develop *grand mal*. A pervasive maladjustment often accompanies this illness, due in part to the "interruptions of learning," in part to combinations of overprotection and rejection, and in part to the various forms of compensation used to outwit discipline. Antagonism, rebellion, a basic insecurity in all relationships, and dependency may develop in conjunction with the illness, but not as an inevitable outgrowth of any constitutional proclivity.

There are reports in the literature indicating that these "abortive" attacks can be interrupted by hypnotic suggestion, by arousing the patient by calling his name, or by arousing the patient's interest. The fact that such patients can sometimes hear, without being able to grasp meanings too well, brings them almost within reach of those around them, yet the abnormal brain waves are convincing evidence that a biological mechanism quite different from anything found in other types of neurosis is at work. Often a child brought to the clinic

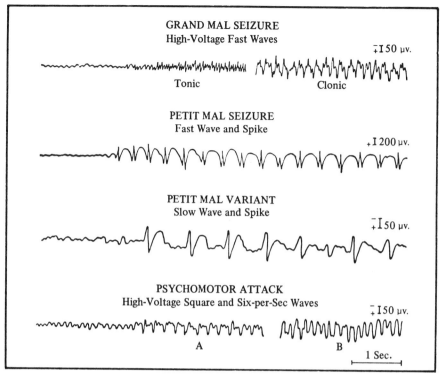

FIGURE 12. REPRESENTATIVE ELECTROENCEPHALOGRAMS OF FOUR PATIENTS TO SHOW RECORDS TAKEN BEFORE AND DURING FOUR DIFFERENT TYPES OF SEIZURES. The types are *grand mal,* two forms of *petit mal,* and a psychic variant (psychomotor). At the right is the perpendicular deflection made by a 50-millionth or 200-millionth volt current and at the bottom the time marked by one second. The left of each tracing is a portion of the person's normal record. The rest of the tracing was made during a seizure. Four different types of seizures are depicted. Uppermost is the tonic and then, after an interval, the clonic phase of a *grand mal* convulsion. The second tracing is the three-a-second alternate wave and spike of a *petit mal.* The third tracing is of the relatively rare slow (two-a-second) wave and spike called *petit mal* variant. This is not usually accompanied by symptoms. The fourth tracing was taken during two phases of a psychomotor seizure. The tracings are about one-third their natural size. (Reprinted by permission of the American Medical Association, publishers of the article by F. A. Gibbs, E. L. Gibbs, and W. G. Lennox, *Archives of Neurology and Psychiatry* [June 1939], in which the original figure appeared, p. 1112; and of The Ronald Press Company, publishers of J. McV. Hunt, *Personality and the Behavior Disorders* [Vol. II, 1944], in which the figure was reprinted, p. 944.)

by parents who find him a dreamer or excessively restless or inattentive is found after careful diagnosis to have an underlying paroxysmal condition.

OTHER SEIZURES WITH CEREBRAL DYSRHYTHMIA

One of the knotty problems faced by the diagnostician is that of the relationship between behavior disorders in children and the psychopathic personalities seen in later years. Abnormal electroencephalograms are found in a much higher proportion among hyperactive, impulsive, and misbehaving children than among comparable samples of normal children. The paroxysmal brain states are undoubtedly a factor in some cases, although, even here, they are seldom more than one part of the total causative sequence. The control of this condition when it is present is extremely important, but since there are children who behave normally in spite of abnormal electroencephalograms and severely disturbed children who have no history of epilepsy or who present no evidence of abnormal EEGs, the clinician's attention must focus on the child as a whole and on those relationships with the significant others who surround him, while he treats, at the same time, the neurological abnormality.

In his summary of dysrhythmic seizures, Strauss includes: circumscribed motor and sensory seizures (with localized contractures, numbness, tingling, sensations of heat, cold, lights, dark spots, sounds, and smells, dizziness), autonomic seizures (epigastric pressure, nausea, flushing, pallor, perspiration, pilomotor changes), abdominal cramps and pains, migraine headaches, and fainting all associated with paroxysmal bursts of neural discharge.

CAUSE AND CURE

We are assured repeatedly by experienced clinicians that epilepsy is not a disease: it is a group of symptoms. If we list among the causes everything that makes a difference in the frequency and intensity of attacks, we have to include conditions varying from flickering lights to interpersonal conflicts. Fetal encephalopathy and birth injury, virus-caused encephalitis and other cerebral infections, infections of the ear and pharynx which invade the central nervous tissues, convulsions and thromboses of infancy carry the causal factors back to the earliest months of life, and to these we have to add the evidence of a genetic factor whose precise nature is not now known. There is also a type of hereditary neurofibroma (small scattered tumors of nerve endings) that sometimes invades the central nervous tissues and produces centers of abnormal neural discharge.

In the adult there are brain tumors (including vascular tumors and aneurysms), head injuries that produce the scar tissue in whose neighborhood the critical ischemia develops, and vascular changes that occur with age or with the tertiary form of syphilis. There are also hormonal factors; seizures in association with the menstrual period are common, although the precise nature of the relationship involved is not known. Fever, which sometimes precipitates convulsions in children, is sometimes followed later by epilepsy (2 per cent of children have such febrile convulsions, Lennox estimates, and of these, some 5 per cent will have seizures later). Hyperventilation, in the seizure-susceptible patient, can precipitate attacks, as can low blood sugar, alcohol, and excessive water intake. The question of diet seems to be a controversial one. A ketogenic diet (high fat, low carbohydrate, and low protein) is sometimes used in the treatment of epilepsy, along with a systematic dehydration. Both are difficult to administer and entail risks (especially if there is a cardiac weakness), but where such a regimen is successful, it demonstrates the role of the internal milieu in altering the seizure threshold of those cells responsible for the epileptic pattern.

The psychological factors (including mental conflicts and certain types of stimuli which seem to precipitate attacks) are looked on as facilitative or precipitating factors, rather than as the principal causes. Others have maintained a continuing effort to separate out an idiopathic or *essential* epilepsy where none of the external factors we have listed can be found. Henri Ey suggests that this group is the hereditary (or typological) form, in which genetic, humoral, and neurovegetative factors form a biological basis for the epileptoid constitution. Cryptogenic epilepsy ("of unknown origin") would be a more correct diagnosis for many of these obscurely caused seizures. With better case histories, with improved methods of diagnosis and of exploration for foci of dysrhythmia, this cryptogenic class may be expected to grow smaller, and the diagnosis should indicate to the clinician that his work is unfinished, since it is arrived at by exclusion.[8]

Freud's Approach to Epilepsy

As late as 1928, but before Berger's studies of the electroencephalogram, Freud clung to a distinction between two types of epilepsy, an organic and an affective epilepsy. The former he thought of as being primarily a disease of the brain, the latter a form of neurosis. This splitting of organic and functional types permitted him to treat the second type by means of a depth analysis that was highly speculative but which conformed to the basic pattern of his theorizing.

He considered the affective attacks to be a way of discharging instinctive energy that had been dammed up by repression until it had accumulated "in the unconscious." Finally at some critical point of mind-body interaction, it produced an explosion of neural discharge. He thought that the epilepsy of Dostoevsky was probably of this type, and in his study (1928a) of the novelist he established a pattern of thought that many psychoanalysts have followed. The novelist himself described his attacks as a "dying" and he emerged from them feeling depressed and guilty. "What was the crime that, in his unconscious, he had committed?" asked Freud, who had no trouble in finding evidence that it was the unconscious wish for the death of his father that first took on an acute form at the time of his father's death, precipitating epileptic attacks. The analysis of Freud thus linked Oedipus and Hamlet (who

---

[8]Penfield and Jasper (1954, pp. 662-63) point out that the most characteristic EEG pattern of the idiopathic type is the spike-and-dome tracing associated with *petit mal,* but other wave forms are found. With similar EEGs some of the patients are found to have records of convulsions, encephalitis, severe fever, birth injury; these authors insist that no form of the EEG can be accepted as pointing to genetic or idiopathic epilepsy. They are moved to add that all seizures are, in the last analysis, symptomatic of various pathological changes in neural tissue and that there is no such thing as a truly genetic epilepsy. Cobb (1943, pp. 108-9) is of the opinion that we should speak of two types, genetic and acquired epilepsy, abandoning the use of idiopathic. But the ultramicroscopic changes and the biochemical nature of the genetic factor are now unknown, so that even careful examination at autopsy would not reveal the cause of these idiopathic cases.

did not have epilepsy) with this unconscious parricide. Moreover, in Freud's analysis, Dostoevsky not only willed his father's death, but identified himself with his father, and died repeatedly (in his attacks), dramatizing his feeling that he deserved to die. His internalized father figure (his superego) punished the ego by causing these deathlike attacks. The rivalry with the father for the mother's love and the death wish were further complicated by his love for his father and his desire to be loved in turn (to be the passive love-object of that father, as the mother was). The analysis thus imputes a masochistic quality to the makeup of the author, and an unconscious homosexual trend which André Gide also imputed to this author and with which he, in turn, could identify. Too hated and too deeply loved, his father became the core of his epileptic neurosis, and in his novels he made an unconscious confession. His unconscious, passive, homosexual trends, Freud believed, were matched by paroxysms of aggression that, shunted into the epileptic form, served to discharge energy that he could not otherwise liquidate, saving him from becoming the murderer in fact that he was in his own unconscious mind. These attacks appeased his need for punishment, and permitted him to identify with his father and dramatize his death, to undergo punishment, disgrace, and suffering in penance. Wilhelm Reich (1931) added another characteristic psychoanalytic emphasis, arguing that the epileptic attack is a simulated act of coitus, its discharge analogous to the orgasm, its rhythmic contractions a kind of reflex-convulsive "intercourse," and that it constituted an "erotization of the striped muscles" of the entire organism.

There is a serious question as to the relevance of these psychoanalytic speculations. Penfield and Jasper (1954, p. 451), who also interest themselves in the *ictal emotions,* find that their patients speak of fear, sadness, and loneliness. Since the fear is of a distinct type (not the simple fear of an attack), these authors believe it is due to a localizable discharge of cortical cells, a discharge that produces a unique affective quality. As for sexual excitement and its associated feelings, the authors write: "So far as our experience goes, neither localized epileptic discharge nor electrical stimulation is capable of awakening any such emotion. One is tempted to believe that there are no specific *cortical* mechanisms associated with these emotions" (my italics).

In their study of the aura of epileptic attacks, Lennox and Cobb (1933, p. 374) found only one case in which there was an erection during the aura. If the attack is a symbolic orgasm, or an erotization of the whole body, the usual organic components of sexual excitement are conspicuous by their absence.

Three Targets for Therapy

The management of seizures, the management of a life, and the elimination of the basic brain discharges (where possible) offer three targets for therapy. Seizures can usually be reduced and occasionally completely controlled with appropriate medication and hygiene, if the doctor has the complete cooperation of the patient, which is often very difficult to obtain, in spite of the serious consequences of lapses in medication, regimen, or abstinence from alcohol. Phenobarbital, dilantin, and tridione are anticonvulsants commonly used in prescriptions for these patients. Dosage strong enough to control seizures, but not so heavy as to produce unpleasant (and occasionally dangerous) side effects, requires a vigilant and experimental approach by both patient and physician. Attention should be given to physical health and to a combination of interesting tasks with good exercise. Dietary programs, ketogenic diet, dehydration, moderate and frequent meals, abstinence from alcohol are employed by many physicians, but their value is still debated.

The management of a life with the elimination of pathogenic and unnecessary stresses has to be balanced by the effort to achieve a near-normal status: normal schooling, a normal vocational choice, normal social life, normal family life. Each of these is more easily named as a goal than achieved in practice. Steady pressure for the acceptance of the epileptic has brought some gains, but much remains to be done.

There are some enthusiasts who look forward to the time when seizure states will be regarded with no more concern than defects in hearing and vision, the lifelong need for medication will be no more noteworthy than the need for glasses or hearing aids. The disorder is more serious, the hereditary aspect more threatening, and the possibility of deterioration greater than this enthusiasm warrants. Perhaps 75 per cent of epileptics can manage a near-normal life. Some have achieved such notable successes in living (Mohammed, Luther, Van Gogh, Dostoevsky, Helmholtz, to name but a few) that their lives have added weight to the notion that genius is related to mental abnormality.

The counselor who is striving to help epileptics organize their lives may do well to bear in mind these exceptional ones who have reacted so positively to their particular "thorn in the flesh." He need not expect to find geniuses budding spontaneously in response to the sting of this disability, or hold out exaggerated hopes, but he might remember that it is not so much the disorder that produces real disability and deterioration (of itself, a cerebral defect of this sort determines nothing in the way of character or accomplishment) as it is the manner in which the person and those around him react to the disability. In this area psychotherapy can contribute to the management of a life.

In a few cases, where there are localized foci of discharge, surgical intervention is possible, and with skilled procedures there is a healing without epileptogenic scar tissue. Penfield and Jasper (1954, p. 789) report a series of operations on 165 patients (with a mortality of 3.8 per cent), in which 2.5 per cent were completely free from subsequent attacks, another 2.5 per cent were judged to be 75 per cent improved, and 20 per cent were judged to be 50 per cent improved; the balance showed either no improvement or very slight changes, with the exception of 6 per cent who were worse after the operation. Conservative therapy holds out limited hope of ever completely removing all need of medication or other therapy by this means.

DEGENERATIVE BRAIN CHANGES WITH PROFOUND EFFECTS

Unlike the massive but sharply defined lesions of lobectomies and lobotomies, and unlike the episodic seizures which interfere momentarily with mental functioning, there are two diffuse degenerative changes that bring in their train irreversible and irreparable damage to mental processes. In contrast to the functional disorders, where the therapist works to restore normal functioning, these progressive and damaging changes leave him with a limited range of rearguard action. The deficits which appear throw the normal functioning of the integrative mechanism into sharp contrast, and indicate what must be done to ease the problems of these patients.

DEMENTIA PARALYTICA

In the days before its cause was known, and before an effective therapy existed, no mental disorder had a poorer prognosis: complete dementia and death were the outcome in almost every case. The life expectancy of untreated cases averaged less than five years from the point where a clear diagnosis became possible. "There is no other mental disease in which dementia is so complete," writes Bruetsch (1959). Yet this disorder need never occur. Even without the elimination of the basic cause, syphilis, early diagnosis and adequate treatment can check the fatal invasion of the central nervous system and arrest the otherwise inevitable dementia.

Although the mental symptoms become florid before the disease has run its course, psychotherapy cannot stem their advance, nor has psychology contributed a great deal to the explanation of the particular forms that the mental symptoms assume. On the other hand, when the penicillin treatment, now regarded as the treatment of choice, is successful, and when it has been applied before deteriorative changes in nervous tissue have occurred (in the asymptomatic phase), a patient may return to full employment even in vocations which require a high degree of skill and personal responsibility. Such a hopeful outcome is possible in 85 per cent of the cases. Where symptoms of deteriorative change have appeared, a return to restricted work (under guidance) is possible in 60 per cent of the cases. Obviously, as long as hospitals continue to receive patients in varying stages of the illness, the recovery rates will remain low and the death rates may continue at their present 20 to 30 per cent.

Although the psychologist can contribute little directly in the treatment of paretics, there is much he can learn from the history of the disorder. Because the illness produces symptoms which simulate many other neurotic and psychotic disorders, it sometimes invites a misapplied therapeutic enthusiasm (while the appropriate therapy is postponed). All clinicians and social workers need to be warned of its possible cryptic presence in the midst of other familiar symptoms.

General paresis was identified as a specific disorder with a fatal terminal dementia in 1798, when an apothecary at Bethlehem Hospital first described it. Its cause was not established with certainty until 1914, when the scientific papers of Noguchi and Moore independently proved that the *treponema pallidum* of syphilis was the responsible agency. Unexplained, as other psychoses we now call "functional" still are, general paresis had challenged the clinician, and also served as a kind of professional projection test, inviting the theorist to reveal his biases and test his hypotheses. Attempts to explain it were varied, and need not be reviewed here. Krafft-Ebing (1877) suggested that the illness might be caused by such varied agencies as smoking ten to twenty cigars a day, extremes of temperature, the menopause, severe and exhausting work conditions, or a neuropathic diathesis, but he did not mention syphilis. As late as 1914 some medical textbooks in America were still describing the stress and strain of professional life, and the effects of the crowding and the bustle of urban living, as possible contributors to this advanced form of "nervous exhaustion." The same clinicians who looked on "neurasthenia" as a form of "Americanitis" were ready to see general paresis classed as a functional disorder produced by "modern" living.

The Case of Friedrich Nietzsche

Friedrich Nietzsche developed a form of general paresis in 1889, at the end of a ten-year period of feverish creative activity. He was taken by his relatives to a succession of experts who pronounced him incurably insane. In the days before the malarial and penicillin treatments had become standard practice, his case remained untreated, and, after ten years of illness, broken by periods in which the disease appeared to be arrested and the philosopher both lucid and calm, he died. In the year before his illness was recognized, he had dispatched letters to friends and eminent persons that were so wildly inappropriate that the question of his sanity and good judgment has thrown its shadow over some of his works. While he was writing *The Twilight of the Idols, Ecce Homo,* and *The Antichrist,* he was dispatching a letter to August Strindberg: "I have called together at Rome an assembly of princes, I will have the young Emperor [Kaiser Wilhelm II] shot. For we shall meet again. One condition. Let us divorce!" And he signed the note "Nietsche-Caesar." One might put this down to a bit of buffoonery between friends if he had not also written to the King of Italy, addressing him as "My dearly beloved son, Umberto," and to the papal Secretary of State, testifying to his veneration of His Holiness, and signing himself "The Crucified One." A megalomania with its attendant theme of persecution and its forecast of death and atonement was beginning to show in his writings.[9]

In the period between 1879, when he resigned from his pofessorship at 35, and the frank onset of his illness in 1889, the bulk of his writings appeared.

---

[9]Sometimes there is a long incubation period lying between the first syphilitic infection and the final period of frankly visible paretic symptoms; it can endure as long as 40 years. At other times the illness assumes a "galloping" form, in which infection, paralysis, dementia, and death are all over in a matter of months. Half the cases will terminate somewhere between the tenth and twentieth years of the illness.

They must stand or fall on their own intrinsic merit. His devoted followers have continued to praise them, insisting that he was not ill at the time (or casting doubt on the final diagnosis); his enemies, who also note the way in which some of his ideas were incorporated in the hated Nazi culture, inevitably see them as examples of the euphoria and megalomania so often associated with this illness; they note the same trends in *Thus Spake Zarathustra* (written between 1883 and 1885).

In the months before his illness became apparent to all, Nietzsche was heading chapters in *Ecce Homo* with such questions as "Why am I so clever?" and "Why do I write such good books?" He inserted such sentences as "I am not a man. I am dynamite." But there had long been a touch of the egomaniac about him. The "N" carved in the back of a chair in which he liked to sit, a family possession, was a sign to him of a fantasied descent from Napoleon. His language in *Thus Spake Zarathustra* is that of a Moses, or some new law-bringer who was going to bring about a transvaluation of all values. His pronouncements on women, some of them copied from Schopenhauer, and some drawn from the small-town minds that surrounded his youth, are notorious and, for the reader of his biographers, extremely ridiculous.

Nietzsche experienced "moments of illumination," much after the fashion of Janet's Martial, and quite similar to the auras that Dostoevsky described in *The Idiot*. It seems to the one who experiences such moments that the creative process has suddenly been released within him, but the outside observer is apt to note a decline in the quality of the productions, a decline which can reach a manic type of euphoria. The patient has never been so certain as at this time, so unqualified, so assertive (so infected with megalomania, his unsympathetic observers will add). In Nietzsche's words (written a year before the psychosis was recognized):

"A joy, strained to a tremendous pitch which sometimes seeks relief in a flood of tears—a perfect ecstasy, with the most distinct consciousness of an endless number of delicate shocks and thrills to one's very toes; a feeling of happiness, in which the most gloomy and painful feelings act, not as a contrast, but as something expected and inevitable, as an *essential* coloring within such an overflow of light; an instinct for rhythm that bridges wide gulfs of form. . . . This is my experience of inspiration. I have no doubt that we should have to go back many thousands of years before we could find anyone who would dare say to me: 'It is mine as well'" (Brinton 1941, p. 54; see also Kaufman 1950).

The Frequency of the Disorder

Increasingly rare, general paresis constituted about 10 per cent of the first admissions to public mental institutions in the United States prior to 1920. Figures for Germany and Japan, summarized by Bruetsch (1959, p. 1005) run between 20 and 30 per cent. Today our hospitals show rates below 2 per cent of all first admissions. It is believed that even when the first generalized syphilitic infection occurs, there is a partial invasion of neural tissues in nearly all patients. In the vast majority of cases the invasion of cerebral tissues is arrested: there are no symptoms, no changes in the cerebrospinal fluid, no sign of extensive and irreversible changes in neural tissue. The number of persons infected with syphilis is not accurately known, but Grinker (1937) estimates that about 0.5 per cent of those so infected today will develop general paresis. The factors which determine this disparity between the numbers infected and the numbers developing general paresis (before effective treatment was found) are still matters of dispute. They include such variables as the virulence of the infection, immunity factors in the host, differences in strains of spirochetes (with the possibility of a special neurotropic variety), the general health of the host, and head trauma. The echo of Krafft-Ebing's pronouncements persists when Diethelm (1950, p. 746) still suggests "constitutional factors and special modes of living." Unexplained, also, is the disparity in the frequencies for general paresis among Negroes and whites, and among males and females. Women are believed to be infected by syphilis as frequently as men, yet general paresis in males occurs four times as often, and Negroes, with a higher incidence of syphilis than whites, have a lower rate of general paresis. Finally, whatever loosens the bonds normally maintained by the mores, whatever contributes to an increase in promiscuity or prostitution, tends to raise the incidence of syphilis. Such an increase is notable in wartime, and in the periods following wars.

The Symptoms of General Paresis

While the *treponema pallidum* is invading the cerebral tissues and producing changes in blood vessels, meninges, interstitial cells, and the neurons proper, adequate diagnostic procedures reveal the presence of infection in the cerebrospinal fluid (Wasserman tests, studies of cell count, proteins, colloidal gold curve, microscopic studies of cerebrospinal fluid). There is an initial period that is described as asymptomatic, as far as behavior goes, for the effect of this invasion is not revealed by psychological tests or clinical interview. Penicillin treatment for ten days at this point can produce, in 85 per cent of the cases, "fully recovered patients." If this complete treatment is followed by serological tests at five-year intervals (to make sure the cerebrospinal fluid is nonparetic), we could describe these patients as having suffered from the basic cause of general paresis without ever having shown a symptom of the disease.

When changes in behavior do become noticeable to members of the family, they may be discounted as a neurotic weakness or as evidence of some character defect. Perhaps this is precisely what we should call them, even though we know the principal agency responsible. If the patient has shown certain eccentricities earlier, he is apt to show them now in exaggerated form. His prepsychotic personality gives a coloring to the disorganizing process, and the partial failure of inhibition permits an even franker display of traits that have been in evidence for a long time. The boastful or the impulsive become a little more so, and the anxious enter a state of dread and anguish. The beginning symptoms that clinicians are able to list are many, and include mood changes (anxiety, irritability, depression), physiological changes (as evidenced by extreme fatigue, insomnia, headache, overwhelming urge to sleep, nightmares), cognitive changes (difficulty in concentration, confusion), character changes (a notable loss of the power of self-criticism, opinionated bearing, carelessness in dress, lack of consideration for others), and moral dissipation (alcoholism, gambling, sexual excesses, wild spending sprees, grandiose schemes).

As the disorganization progresses, craftsmanship and professional skill are lost. The consequences of actions, formerly included in the structure of action, are now forgotten in advance and subsequently overlooked. The patient's associations operate slowly and follow a superficial course (depending on klang associations and on automatic bonds that distract and shunt the course of thought). There are surprising breaks in the normal regulation of actions; he will appear at a funeral with umbrella opened and dressed only in nightshirt, or he will sit by the hour shuffling cards for a game of solitaire that never begins.

What begins as a subtle change in memory (he misplaces articles, tells the same story over, shows poor recall for recent events) resembles the signs of premature aging, or suggests to a clinician a frontal-lobe lesion. As in these other conditions, the memory for more remote events seems to be spared, and there is the same tendency to confabulate that Korsakoff noted in his amnestic patients. The regulative sets that keep us oriented and able to encode entering stimuli are not functioning well in these patients; a patient may not know whether he is sitting down to lunch or dinner, for his day is not structured as it passes.

In the period of most florid symptoms, some of the patients act out the popular stereotype of the insane person. A patient may believe that he is immensely wealthy, and write checks for all of his wardmates, nurses, and orderlies on nonexistent funds. He drives through traffic lights (if he has not been hospitalized) or commits wild acts of violence. He tells the admitting physician that he is working on a case with J. Edgar Hoover, or that he is planning to become President. He shocks his family by proposing to cut a hole in the ceiling so that a fifteen-foot tree he has just purchased can be potted and placed in the living room. Out of what he has read, out of a chance remark, his delusions spring full-blown. They change as suddenly as they appear, and in time they become fragmented, so that only the pieces of delusion persist. Perhaps a third of the patients go through an expansive-euphoric phase; another third decline into a simple dementia; and in the balance there is a scattering of excitements, agitations, depressions, and schizophrenic symptoms. Some of these near-psychotic forms remain after the infection has been arrested by penicillin, as though the damage produced by syphilis had unmasked an underlying disorder. Since 3 per cent of these patients are described as showing schizophrenic symptoms (a rate much higher than in the general population) there may be more than a mere unmasking of a constitutional trend that would have arrived at schizophrenia anyway. Do both disorders depend on degenerative changes? Should we speak of a paresis-caused schizophrenia much in the fashion that we would speak of a paresis-caused epilepsy? (Three-quarters of these patients develop seizures; see Noyes and Kolb 1963, p. 208.)

Dementia and paralysis are present in the terminal phase toward which all untreated cases progress. Varied as these paretics are in the initial phases, they become sadly similar in the end. Much of the diversity in symptomatology depends on the location of the diseased portions within the central nervous system. Optic atrophy, for example, is reported in two-thirds of the cases; although it is a partial atrophy in most, it progresses to blindness in about 2 per cent of the cases. Restricted visual fields, an Argyll-Robertson pupil, ptosis of the eyelid, strabismus are common. (The Argyll-Robertson pupil contracts when the eyes converge, accommodates for near vision, but does not contract under sudden external illumination.)

As the patient enters the course that will carry him to a paralyzed and bedridden state, muscular weakness and incoordination appear. His tremor, unsteadiness in gait, marked fatigability present a picture that in the earliest stages could be mistaken for neurasthenia. As paralysis advances the facial muscles lose their expressiveness, speech is thickened and slurred, and handwriting is radically changed, with a constricted form, misspelling, omissions, repetitions, and, finally, complete agraphia.

A full account of the symptomatology of neurosyphilis would require a review of neurological disorders. In a few there is an admixture of depression and bodily complaint. When these take the form of a worry about a syphilitic infection, one would be tempted to join with Groddeck (1961), who suspected that the unconscious processes in the "id" frequently announce a coming biological disorder through the symbolism of dreams and neurotic complaints. What other types of neural lesions can produce, syphilis can duplicate. There is a clearly defined tabetic group, produced by the degeneration of the cells of the dorsal column of the spinal chord. Here walking is affected by the loss of the kinesthetic impulses which normally contribute to these integrations. When *tabes dorsalis* appeared before any of the other symptoms (in the days before penicillin), 10 per cent of these cases went on to develop the full paretic psychosis.

The convulsions which occur in over three-quarters of the cases are caused, in all probability, by a local ischemia that is responsible for massive neural discharges. Sometimes these seizures are the first symptoms that force the patient to seek medical attention. Paretics also have apoplectiform seizures, which suggest a minor stroke and are followed by hemiplegia or a more localized paralysis which frequently clears up.

Bruetsch distinguishes eight clinical types of paresis, Noyes and Kolb only four. Refinements in classifying types represent a kind of mechanical nicety in descriptive terminology, but nature does not obey these categories; the individual case may combine bits of several types. So far the types have not revealed anything important about causation, and as the parasite invades the tissues, all forms change into the paralyzed dementia that obliterates the differences. As for the frequencies of types, about a third can be classified in Kolb's simple dementing group, another third in the expansive group, and less than a tenth in the circular and depressed forms. A scattering are variously described as agitated or excited, confused and delirious, or schizophrenic.

A juvenile form, making up less than 2 per cent of all cases admitted to mental institutions a few decades ago, is first diagnosed in the early teens. Arising from congenital neurosyphilis, with typical stigmata (such as Hutchinson's teeth, with their notched incisors) showing in 75 per cent of the cases, these cases also show retarded mental and physical growth. About a third show convulsions before the signs of general paresis appear. Bruetsch (1959, p. 1016) finds that optic atrophy is more frequent in the juvenile paresis than in the adult form. One of his patients, a well-developed Negro girl with no obvious signs of congenital syphilis (and with normal pupils), was classified as a catatonic schizophrenic until a spinal-fluid examination revealed the presence of the syphilitic infection. Penicillin brought complete recovery.[10]

Any social program directed against mental illnesses that does not include efforts to detect and bring to treatment all cases of syphilis and, where possible, to check the root cause is overlooking a disorder that once accounted for a third of all first admissions to mental hospitals. The appearance of symptom clusters that so closely imitate other mental disorders is a constant challenge to those whose approach to these other illnesses is primarily psychosomatic (with emphasis on the psychogenic aspect), especially where the functional disorder is properly called an "illness of unknown origin." The mastery of the spirochete by penicillin adds one more pragmatic success to biochemical medicine.

DEMENTIA SENILIS AND DEMENTIA WITH CEREBRAL ARTERIOSCLEROSIS

An examination of hospital admission rates reveals that there are special mental hazards involved in living into the decades beyond 65. The first-admission rates (per 100,000 in the age groups) show 177 of persons in their twenties entering the hospital for treatment of mental illness, as compared with 459 of those who live beyond 70 (see Gregory 1956). Those who have survived the great killers (cancer, cardiovascular and kidney diseases, tuberculosis, pneumonia, accidents) now have to face other stresses of senescence; the figures show that the rates of mental illness are highest in the declining years.

---

[10]Juvenile meningovascular neurosyphilis affects the blood vessels and meninges rather than the neurons, and is more frequent than the juvenile general paralysis. In this group of children there are many behavior disorders, with lying, stealing, aggression, and irritable restlessness. The majority are described as of low intelligence. Psychotic episodes with confusion and temporary hallucinations are reported. Penicillin therapy arrests the symptoms and helps forestall later and more serious forms of general paralysis. (See Bruetsch 1959, p. 1017.)

While the general population has been expanding (doubling in the last half-century), the advances of medical science and the changed conditions of living have also caused a doubling in the population living into the period beyond 65. From one in 25 in 1900, the expectancy of living into this age period has increased to one in 13. This expanding group of citizens over 60 years of age now accounts for 40 per cent of all mental-hospital admissions. The two diagnostic labels most frequently attached to these aging patients are senile psychosis, and psychosis with cerebral arteriosclerosis.[11] Of males aged 60 to 69 who find their way into hospital, 39 per cent are diagnosed with one of these two labels.

Both of these disorders are associated with the general aging processes, even though the tie is loose. A Supreme Court Justice can be in fine fettle at 80, whereas a comparatively young man of 40 may show the irritability, misoneism, memory losses, and character changes characteristic of senility. It is when averages are struck, and the gross rates of incidence for the different age periods are studied, that this association of dementia with aging becomes clear. The *actual prevalence* of the two disorders we have named is much greater than the hospitalization figures show. The beginning signs (forgetfulness of names, mislaying objects, forgetting appointments, repetitiousness, slowing of associations, loss of interest in the present and future, increased body concern, irritability, fatigability, reluctance to undertake activity that will lead to effort and exhaustion) may interfere with efficiency and make interpersonal relations difficult, but they do not in themselves require hospitalization, and so are tolerated, concealed, and endured along with the other disabilities of age. With social security and home care, the family and the general practitioner keep these "cases" going and out of hospital. In the more advanced forms, many of these may suffer from aphasia, periods of depression, lapses of memory, and even chronic deterioration and disorientation, so that an autonomous form of living is impossible, yet the home provides better care for many of these patients than most hospitals could offer. However, not every home can or will assume this responsibility, and not every patient is manageable. The combination of the burden of home care and the threat to the life of the patient or of those who surround him bring 184 per 100,000 in the oldest age group with these diagnoses into hospital. Sometimes there is violence, or a complete habit breakdown, or sexual offenses, or total irresponsibility; the presence of such a patient can completely disrupt and disorganize the life in the crowded living space of a modest urban home and threaten the well-being of small children, especially where wives

---

[11]Noyes insists that "psychosis with *arterio*sclerosis" is a misnomer. There can be advanced arteriosclerosis without any psychotic changes. The hardening of the artery walls, so common in all aging persons, is not itself a threat to mental functions. It may not even interfere with the flow of blood. But *athero*sclerosis, which narrows and sometimes obliterates the opening in the vessels, is a threat; when the blood supply is cut off, even for ten minutes, from any group of cells, degenerative and irreversible changes occur at this point. The hypoxia and subsequent death of neural cells may occur suddenly and massively (as when one of the main cerebral arteries is stopped up) or diffusely and slowly.

are working, budgets are limited, and the personal resources of those on whom these aging patients must depend are insufficient to cope with the problem.

In an earlier day when an extended family lived on a farm, and when there were tasks (such as gardening or feeding the chickens) which could be entrusted to a slightly senile grandfather (with some supervision), and when there was living space in the field or at the fireside, it seemed more natural to care for the aged at home. Indeed, it seemed quite unnatural for sons and daughters to avoid this responsibility, and the social pressure against any institutional solution was reinforced both by the scarcity of hospitals and rest homes and by the deplorable condition of those which did exist. With the improvement in institutional care and the change in the family unit and living space (not to mention the increase in women employed in business and industry), a greater proportion of those who show some degree of mental deterioration now appear on institutional rolls. The statistics will show an absolute increase in the size of the aged group, an increase in the hospitalization rate for this group, and an increase in the recorded frequency in the general population of the two disorders most characteristic of the old. Medically the hospital care of today may be superior to that of those early rural years, but psychologically it usually lacks something the extended family once gave to these dependent souls; in many cases this removal from the family, the deadly routine and indifference of hospital life, and the lack of significant tasks speed the ultimate decline of the mind.

The Problem of Aging

Aging is a brute physiological and anatomical fact, but how society treats the problem and how the individual takes up this challenge alter its impact. It is possible to mature into the later years with grace and wisdom, to find opportunities in the new leisure to develop latent interests, to find a new type of reason for existence, and to see things *sub specie aeternitatis*. But when the years bring an abiotropic change in the integrative network on whose functioning the very self depends, it would take a Mary Baker Eddy to insist that all the fearful thoughts and all the character changes spring from poor thinking and planning.

All the euphemistic titles that the well-meaning offer for the groups of aging citizens, "elder statesmen," "Senior Citizens," "Golden Age Club," are only glosses on the brute fact of age that occasionally conceal a contempt and a distaste that younger men in a hurry feel in the presence of age. "It is not a divinity but the mystery of arteriosclerosis that shapes the endings of most lives," wrote Dr. Alvarez (1952, p. 155). Certainly for the core group that suffer from arteriosclerosis, from "little strokes," and from the abiotropic and degenerative changes in the neural tissue which underlie dementia senilis, the physician's evaluation is both more accurate and more compassionate, for otherwise we might blame the senile for not being more alert, more interested, more ready to invest time and effort in worthwhile enterprises, more free from irritations and frustrations.

The threat of aging, which hangs over us all, is fourfold: age brings declining energies, reduced capacities, an altered social role and significance, and problems that arise from reduced economic security and an increasing need for medical and other forms of care.

The Problem of Energy

Metabolism slows, hormones and enzymes fail, and renal and cardio-vascular changes (with advancing arteriosclerosis) slow the efficiency of the flow of blood and lymph. All these changes introduce a fatigability and a slowing of work output; to these behavioral changes the aging person often adds a tendency to avoid the stress and challenge of new adventures (in advance), to restrict output, to distrust novelty, and to resist change. Since changes do occur, and since demands on resources continue, there is a gap between what can readily and willingly be delivered and what is required. A quartet of traits emerges: conservatism and resistance to change, irritability and negativism (with a tendency to rely on authority or fiat), a tendency to pejorate all the surrounding changes that are unlike the good old ways, and a growing feeling of distance, isolation, and worthlessness. The changes in energy and the responses to these changes, often sensed as a change in character or life-style, are closely interwoven with a second group of changes, some of which may also involve this energy factor.

Changes in Capacity

Attention is not as vigilant, and current events are less readily grasped. Even when sensed, they are not elaborated or "taken in" to become a part of a newly evolving personal history. Learning slows down, and the person is more content to get along with "what he has"; as a result personal growth reaches a plateau, or regresses. Not only do events fail to imprint themselves as readily in the form of lively traces, but recall declines, and immediate memory seems to fail first of all. Intentions slip the mind, belongings are mislaid, appointments and promises are forgotten, and the just-told story is repeated. Parallel to these changes in integrative capacities, there are changes in sense organs and muscles that lower the efficiency of the "tools of the mind," so that both sensory input and motor execution decrease in both speed and grace. For the ballplayer this moment comes early (in the thirties); for the experienced judge, who relies on a knowledge of precedent learned in more vigorous days, the decline in energy and the altered sensory and motor capacities may not prevent him from functioning adequately (particularly if he has an efficient secretary and a household that supports him).

More serious are the changes that seem to invade the very spirit of the man. When courage falters, when the new plunges are no longer taken, and when the clinging to the safer ground of the past amounts to a misoneism and a stubborn disregard of all need for change, then the "law of least effort" becomes more than a conserving tendency: it blocks efficiency and interferes with a realistic evaluation of the present. This negative selective process robs the future of its proper significance in encoding the present stream of stimuli. Mental processes become sclerosed, unimaginative, stubbornly rooted in the "tried and true." When the organizations within which the aging person functions begin to feel the impact of this now sclerosed personality, and when his dogmatism and authoritarianism are disruptive of both efficiency and progress, they begin to look forward to the date of his retirement. The changing self has earned a new role.

The Change in Social Role

For the aging male the most dramatic single event of all is his retirement, with the reduction of income, the altered sense of his usefulness or worth, and often a move to a new locale among strangers (whether in search of a gentler climate or lowered living costs). He now faces a complete reorganization of habits, and his new freedom calls for new responsibilities in self-direction in a world that does not seem to need him. "To understand the economic position of older people it is necessary to realize that modern industrial society has made the older worker obsolescent" (Havighurst and Albrecht 1953, p. 73).

Whether it is strictly modern industrial society or merely the way in which our capitalist economy has organized its labor force is an open question. Theoretically, with indefinitely expanding wants and with new production techniques to supply them, we should be able to find room for every ounce of productive talent, if we so willed. The fact is, however, that as the world now exists, the worker "graduates" into a vast stillness where the very busyness of younger workers intensifies their seeming indifference. Having lost the organizing discipline which work gave, and his former sense of belonging to something significant, he frequently feels cast adrift, like so much worthless scrap material. His first sense of relief at escaping from "the grind" or the "rat race" soon vanishes: with so much leisure time, he is prone to contemplate his "symptoms," to become bored, and to feel a keen sense of isolation and disengagement, and a disenchantment with his free time. The gap between his recently slowed pace and the rush of all the others intensifies his sense of isolation; as one patient phrased it, "They are all going away from me." He can easily feel neglected, on the shelf, unless he seeks actively to compensate for this "gap."

It is also a period in which many chickens come home to roost. The man whose interests have long been narrow, and whose eye has always been centered too intently on the main chance, now has leisure but lacks the interests with which to fill it. The future, which once stretched so endlessly ahead and was so crowded with a hundred things pressing to be done, is now empty; there is little between the present and that unthinkable ending to prevent the latter from rushing toward the present. Living so close to this ultimate barrier to all thought and action makes many projects seem "too long, too costly." Their undertaking seems scarcely worth the effort, the consummation vague, remote, improbable.

It is obvious that living successfully through this new period of social adjustment will require the aging person to develop new skills and interests, to find tasks that will make the future come alive again. It may even challenge him to reorient toward a span of time that runs beyond his physical existence, and to affiliate with things of more permanent value, things that will, at the same time, yield current satisfactions and new sources of significance. He will have to put forth effort to make new friends (including friends among the young) and to create new reasons for that much-needed feeling of belonging. It is a time for cementing ties with family and friends, for correspondence and visits, for travel, for reading, for new forms of self-expression, and for new social and civic participation. All this invention of new roles and new forms of expression tests the energies and the imagination of the individual at a time in his life when both are at relatively low ebb. And when the pre-senile life-style has been rigidly obsessive-compulsive, or hypochondriacal, or neurotically anxious and dependent, his very inclinations work against the solutions that would be his salvation.

While our community does not confront its aging members with the ultimate trip to the edge of the ice that Esquimaux communities used to provide for all who failed to meet the tests of an extremely rigorous autonomy (in a hostile climate), it is not organized to use the rich supply of energy and talent that still remain in this aging group. It may not, as Havighurst and Albrecht assert, "condemn its older people to lives of frustration and discontent." It simply says, "You're on your own." It is the individual's responsibility, we feel, to create this new life, find the new sources of significance, express whatever latent talents he may still possess, find some way to continue to grow. For hospitals that treat those who show both a neurological and a personal failure in integrative powers, and that wish to provide for their patients something more than custodial care (which does little to arrest a steady deterioration), this process of restoring the senile person to life offers a most serious challenge. Declining capacities and interests in the patient make it extremely difficult to work against the regressive involution.

Social and Economic Dependence

The number of people who reach retirement age without the minimum resources needed to care for their basic necessities has not always been appreciated by the general public, especially in the recent past, when the aging and their kin did all in their power to conceal the fact of poverty and dependency and to avoid the poorhouse. Only recently, in our effort to extend social security and to guarantee medical care to those who need it most and can afford it least, are we beginning to do as a society what individuals have patently failed to do for themselves. To the prudent, the strong, and the fortunate, it has always seemed possible to provide for old age. But combinations of limited foresight, misfortunes, illness, and constitutional defects (ranging from feeblemindedness to premature aging of the arteries) bring at least a fourth of those who are over 65 to a dependent status. Of our entire population (including all persons of all ages) in 1950, 86 per cent had a reported income of less than 2,000 dollars per year. According to the U.S. Bureau of the Census *Report on Income of Families and Persons in the United States,* 10 per cent of all males and 45.8 per cent of all females over 65 were without any money income.

By 1952 there were 62.3 million citizens in the U.S. covered by social-security legislation. Though the coverage was incomplete, with many left outside its shelter, and with the amounts received still barely adequate for essentials and wholly inadequate wherever there were major medical expenses, federal action had suddenly achieved for the bulk of the workers what they had, up to this time, failed to do for themselves. No rugged individualism, no Poor Richard's philosophy, no Puritan ethic, no praise of freedom and independence had saved a large group of aged from the unhappy and uncertain role of dependence on relatives and public charity. The programs which lifted the burden of this fear and, in addition, provided needed medical care may well mark this century as the one which struck the mightiest blow on behalf of the aged.[12]

Summarizing the question of economic security, Havighurst and Albrecht (1953, p. 99) point out that the income received by 85 per cent of those over 65 (less than 2,000 dollars in 1950) was regarded as "comfortable" by slightly more than half the persons in the samples studied. They said they had no real money worries. Most of them owned some property or securities that brought them in a regular income. They could not travel too much, or hire household help. Rising prices tended to keep them close to the margin of comfort. Limited entertaining and very simple amusements were possible. Since a large fraction of this group, still working, faced dependence when forced to discontinue their wage earning, a cloud hung over the "comfortable" group, and the threat of a medical disaster was ever present. Without this modicum of comfort insured by old-age assistance and social-security programs, at least 20 per cent, it is estimated, would become either destitute or a serious drain on the resources of relatives.

In spite of all the difficulties in aging, including these socioeconomic factors, the intensive interviewing of a cross-section sample revealed that the majority of the aged had found "good roles" and were reasonably well-adjusted. They were independent of grown children, and belonged to civic and social groups; half of them were still working, and the majority were enjoying their leisure. But such favored social roles were not enjoyed by

---

[12]In addition, this guaranteed income has an indirect effect on all those households who would otherwise be burdened with aging relatives. Consider the family with an adolescent daughter: "She cannot have a room of her own because her elderly and almost senile grandfather occupies a room in the small house. She is ashamed to invite her friends to her room because her grandfather's habits are so unclean and his mind so far gone that he might embarrass people" (Havighurst and Albrecht 1953, p. 100). An older couple, less impaired, having escaped from the "spare-room status" in a daughter's home, give the other side of the problem. "It was difficult for us to move from our daughter's home and settle in these few housekeeping rooms," their respondent wrote. "What I'd like to say to older people is—keep your own home. Don't go to the home of your children. It isn't fair to the children or the old people. There is always some other way to manage" (*ibid.,* p. 146).

all the aged: more than in other age groups had become dependent, had lost contact with relatives, enjoyed too few friends, led a restricted social life. Some 7 per cent were described as vegetating, and without active interest in much of anything. These roles, favorable and unfavorable, do not seem to be too closely related to age or to income: some of the oldest had the best reports and some of the "freshmen," just turned 65, offered the most numerous complaints. "We come away," Havighurst and Albrecht write (1953, p. 47), "feeling that old age is what the individual makes it, in the majority of cases." But they add these qualifications: there are a few who are so ill, so dependent morally and financially, that no satisfying role is possible. ("A few" might mean 20 per cent, of 17,861,000 over 65 in July 1964, or some 3.5 million persons.)

Living against a Barrier

To the young there is endless time stretching ahead, and energy is in abundant supply. Projects are started, with spirit, even when they will require years to complete and will bind up psychological capital until they are consummated. A new career can be begun, a home purchased even when it is beyond one's present means, a family started with confidence. The aging, on the other hand, realize that both time and energy are running out, and in evaluating any new proposal must consider both the cost of the action and the interval before consummation.

Death begins to loom as a threatening and impenetrable barrier. It bars even the thought of some actions, has an inhibitory force that makes us shrink, and constricts our life-space. To speak for this aging group, one might say: We begin to substitute little projects for the bigger ones; we "putter around" instead of embarking on more significant tasks; and our days, no longer bound together by the cement of stable interests that structure and integrate continuing actions into a single whole, become more and more like a string of beads, each all but separated from its neighbor. By the series of negative evaluations that we make in response to life's challenges, we unconsciously orient to the unthinkable event that lies ahead for us all, and initiate a vicious cycle that lessens our powers to put forth effort, diminishes our vitality. So the "death instinct" (as a Freudian might name this group of tendencies) is installed in the midst of life like some raven that perches on the railing of a sunlit porch.

This tendency to restrict the field, to withdraw interest from anything remote in the future, to choose the puttering project, can begin at 40 or at 80. It is not closely related to age, though it seems obvious that it will become an increasing factor with the passing years. It can be as brief as a passing psychasthenic depression of a few days, or it can establish itself as a persistent life-style. It is motivated and supported by all that lowers our integrative forces. Sometimes its onset can be dated from that day when a physician issued a warning because of some chronic ailment, or a coronary attack, or the X-ray evidence of advancing emphysema, or visible arteriosclerotic changes in the eye ground. Any one of the dozens of signs of age can tip the balance toward this negative orientation. Facilitating this new dynamic relationship will be the additional changes in available energy that come with advancing years.

There are many ways of reacting, at this point. There is the reaction of denial and compensation which assumes the posture of youth, seeks to gather pleasures wherever they are possible, dresses and acts like a youngster, embarks on new "affairs," goes "partying." There is the soberer one of shifting investments from the material and physical things to more spiritual interests, into the "beyond." But when there is a slowing of the pace of living, a restriction of the fields of interest and action, a resignation from full participation, there may also be a sense of separateness, isolation. Suddenly *those others* seem to be going too fast, to somewhere the aging person does not wish to go; they are all moving away from him (see Minkowski 1933, pp. 127-32, 286 ff). It is difficult for the aging one in this predicament to keep from adding two judgments that frequently appear in the literature of depressive states: "The world is deteriorating around me; I have become worthless."

Senile Dementia

Clinicians who deal with persons who are beginning to show the first symptoms of senile dementia experience a certain ambivalence toward their patients. On the one hand they are moved to exhort, cajole, encourage, scold; their words indirectly express their evaluation of a combination of traits which they would like to undo. They cast about for planned therapies that will arrest this process of premature psychological death. Existentialists and psychoanalysts are tempted to undertake analytic cures of the personality features that hinder a healthful life-adjustment. Such therapists reveal a kind of psychologism that rivals the peculiar mixture of idealism and materialism we call Christian Science, or the kind of Hebraism found in the book of Job. For example, we have Noyes and Kolb (1963, pp. 244-45):

"The person who develops senile dementia has often been characterized by rigid and static habits. Persons who have always had difficulty in adjusting to the demands of life are prone to react to the inevitable retirement from business and professional posts of honor, to deaths of friends and relatives, and the loosening of family and social ties that accompany old age by the development of mental symptoms.

"The more immature and maladjusted the adaptations of earlier life, the smaller is the stress required in old age to produce disorganized or disturbed behavior. That social activities and a wholesome variety of mental occupation may retard mental senility has long been recognized. In one of his famous dialogues, Cicero said, 'Old men retain their intellects well enough if they keep their minds active and fully employed.' It will therefore be seen that, although of great importance, organic disease of the brain is often not the only factor in the development of senile psychoses. It is increasingly recognized that frequently they result from the interaction of organic and psychological factors."

Diethelm (1950, p. 324) repeats this Hebraic notion (that the Lord rewards those who live right) in psychiatric language when he writes, "The tendency to deterioration is usually more marked, according to the personality involved." Ferraro (1959a, p. 1024) adds his testimony: "Tissue damage, per se, does not produce a psychosis; it is, rather, the person's capacity to compensate for the damage, as well as present social and situational stresses, which impair the individual's ability to withstand the cerebral damage." He also (p. 1030) speaks favorably of a classification of senile dements that would identify a group "in which the psychosis is an understandable, if not inevitable, outgrowth of long-standing personality difficulties. In this group, adjustment is possible as long as the physiological status is intact and not disturbed by the process of aging. Most of the senile paranoid and depressive reactions occur in this first group."

All these psychological emphases seem to imply that if the aging person had lived right, or if his psychological problems of adjustment had been solved prior to this period, the "signs of senility" either would have been delayed or would have been concealed from view, that the mental aging would not have occurred. This implication would be comparable to saying, "Keep the faculty of effort alive, and your will will never falter. Stay young in heart and you will never age." (By acting youthful and gay, we *become* youthful? What enthusiasm!)

The older clinician who has had opportunities to follow his patients over three or four decades and who has watched the premature aging of the man of 40 (with his tendency to withdraw from active life and his hypochondriacal concern) may have looked at the earliest changes as primarily due to a failure in nerve, a psychasthenic life-style, a failure in living that called for intensive psychotherapy, only to live to see the patient developing Parkinson's tremor, the bent posture and titubating walk, along with dementia senilis at 70, or earlier. Reflecting over the long process, he is torn between attributing a set of bodily changes to psychological causes or attributing that earlier and falsely diagnosed "psychological state" to a premature set of abiotrophic changes "down among the cells."

The somatopsychic emphasis has all the visible and measurable somatic changes in aging to support it. Every tissue and every organ in the older organism (from the dry and wrinkled skin to the dehydrated and shrunken cerebral tissues with their widened sulci and sclerosed patches of degenerated cells) show changes for which no psychological cause has ever been demonstrated; the ultimate poor prognosis for the patient with marked senile changes makes the enthusiasm of the psychotherapist wither. He is prone, then, to settle for a limited program that will provide a comfortable and congenial environment where the surrounding field is stable and low in every "stress," where sympathy, patience, and tender loving care combine with an optimal diet and appropriate medications to ease the last months of a process which cannot be checked.

The one attitude calls for an active therapy, a conscious effort to undo every regressive trend, to remove every barrier to full participation in life, and to stimulate the patient to use every faculty he has and to earn the feeling of significance and worth that every human being needs. Besides its steady opposition to every regressive trend, this type of therapy bases its logic on a multifactoral analysis of the causes of the dementia, including:

1. An immature and dependent personality.
2. Too rigid habits.
3. Narrow interests.
4. An obsessive-compulsive personality makeup with authoritarian trends; toxic-infective factors that weaken integrative powers (including chronic constipation).
5. Degenerative changes in nerve cells.
6. Drastic changes in the conditions of life (loss of spouse, loss of employment, moving to a new locality, institutionalization, socioeconomic destitution).
7. Lack of exercise.
8. Failure in enzymes and hormones.

There are two factors which made diagnosis and interpretation of this disorder difficult: (1) mental senility may appear at 40, before any aging of the tissues is discoverable, and when both microscopic and macroscopic examination of tissues at postmorten show normal brain structures; (2) when two series of brains are studied by the anatomist, one from normal aged patients, the other from senile dements, there is so much overlapping that a "blind diagnosis" from the gross anatomical and histological data would lead to frequent misclassification. Brains of normal aging subjects may show marked shrinking, while brains of severe cases of senile dementia may vary only slightly from the average. The senile plaques of Alzheimer (small areas of tissue degeneration in whose midst a granular or filament-like detritus is found), which some regard as most closely correlated with the degenerating mental symptoms of age, are also found in 84 per cent of normal aging brains (see Ferraro 1959a, pp. 1030, 1034).

When changes in mental functions and in character are insidious and slow, and when no direct data about brain changes are obtainable, the moment when a patient is to be diagnosed as a senile dement has to be defined in practical terms. When the changes (such as in recent memory and in general orientation) disturb and falsify the patient's relationships with those about him, and when they make him a danger to himself and to the household, he may have to be committed or have a guardian appointed.

At its onset dementia senilis may show many characteristics which are little more than exaggerations of the normal changes that come with aging. Anxiety, agitation, depression, confusion, and euphoria are more striking than the more insidious losses of memory and destructuring (or restriction) of the psychological field; since the latter symptoms simulate other functional disorders, they may easily mask the basic process and invite types of treatment that are inappropriate. An amnestic fugue, a bout of violence that is quite out of character, weeping, self-accusations, or delusions of persecution may lead the clinician to identify involutional melancholia, mania, or paranoia. Thus some of the negative results of therapies ranging from electroshock to psycho-analysis may be due to mistaken diagnosis and to a therapeutic enthusiasm that is unwarranted, but since all these syndromes can exist without dementia, and since in any case their early treatment and arrest are important, the few cases of misplaced enthusiasm may be forgiven.

The first class of symptoms that marks the true dementia, and perhaps the easiest to identify and measure, is the memory failure. The recent past drops away as though it had not been imprinted. The name of their visitor (or doctor), the content of a broadcast just heard, the items just read in the newspaper, all disappear without a trace. Old memories, professional habits, social attitudes (e.g., toward the opposite sex), the uses of familiar objects may be well preserved at first, but these, too, are vulnerable, and in time even these more stable areas are invaded. The oldest (childhood) and the most deeply imprinted (traumatic) memories tend to be the least vulnerable. There are often islands of old professional skills (or home-management habits) that persist, even when they have ceased to fit sensibly into the present contexts (and may become annoying and repetitious preoccupations).

The memory loss leads to false recognitions, temporal-spatial disorientation, and some confabulation. The patient ceases to be able to tell the day, the date, the place in which he now lives, his length of stay in hospital. He loses his way between bedroom and bathroom, and he cannot be trusted about the grounds. Without constant supervision he gets lost, and he cannot be allowed to go to the store around the corner.

Vocabulary grows restricted; the patient loses, in this order, proper names, names for abstract objects, and concrete names. As in the stammerer, his speech is likely to be full of circumlocutions and all-purpose words like machine, trick, whatchamacallit, gadget, thingamajig. Sometimes a logorrhea, filled with gossip and senseless repetitions, masks the progressive impoverish-ment of ideas and the absence of true communication, until the ratio of sense to sound becomes a small fraction; here the very expressiveness em-phasizes the emptiness of the verbal forms.

Parallel to the changes in speaking there is a decrease in comprehension and in power of attention. Explanations have to be repeated, and must be reduced to simple formulations suitable for a child. To follow a conversation, to insert an action appropiate to a developing situation, tax his powers. He has lost judgment, and the power to "presentify," to grasp a situation and insert his own purposes therein.

The patient's emotional life changes with this inability to structure his actions: there is peevishness and irritability about small things, lability of mood, and a general blunting of all feelings. Stereotyped social rituals may persist even when emptied of all meaning. The moral maxim can be repeated when the ethical feeling that would normally charge it has gone. The con-striction of life-space betrays a decrease in psychological tension; and if avarice, jealousy, childishness, and impulsiveness have existed before, they now appear in caricatured and exaggerated forms.

When these changes in part-processes are summated, they amount to a deterioration in character. Neglect of clothing and simple cleanliness, loss of the common inhibitions, lack of all capacity for freedom and responsibility are commonly reported. A few patients hold to the amenities, even when grave deterioration has occurred, still proper and amiable even when their mind has become a shambles. While such changes proceed, we sometimes find absurd collections of "junk" of all kinds (old newspapers, string, bric-a-brac, wire netting, snips of cloth, buttons). The storage and arrangement (or, more properly, disarrangement) of these odds and ends resemble the nest-building efforts of a decerebrate female rat: after maximum effort the confusion remains as great as ever (see Beach 1951).

Even the physiological rhythms share in the disarray: eating may become ravenous, constipation reaches pathological proportions, and the simple waking-sleeping rhythm is broken. Awake, rambling about the house, and rummaging in attic and basement after midnight, dozing in his armchair during the day, his activity rhythms are "out of phase" with any household. The loss of control of urinary and rectal sphincters adds a special problem in the care of these aging dements.

To this disorganization, with memory lacunae and disorientation, there is added confabulation (common in Korsakoff's syndrome), so that he seems to live in a confused and dreamlike mixture of fact and fantasy. (He *did* talk to his dead sister just a moment ago.) Thus delusions may develop along with hypochondriacal, persecutory, or grandiose trends. Some patients display a heightened sexuality that is oddly inappropriate to their actual impotence; attempts on unwilling partners, criminal acts upon the young, or exhibitionism may be the factor that forces commitment.

So-Called Nondemential Changes

Aging brings, for many, a progressive weakening of the vital contact with reality that keeps motivation pitched toward the future. Ultimately such destructuring removes the individual from the unique time-space field that has hitherto characterized his life; although much of his judgment and *savoir faire* persists, he lives among "universals," deals with "essences," and converses with "types" rather than with particular persons whom he recognizes. He learns little that is new, and lives in an eternal present.

Minkowski (1933, pp. 338-43) chose an example reported by Courbon (1927, pp. 455-63) to illustrate this change. The case exaggerates a kind of detachment that often grows with the approach of death, as though the person were gradually preparing for the final letting go. This detachment brings with it an almost immediate forgetting of the recent past and a growing lack of concern for the future. Whether we call it serenity or indifference, this Nirvana-like state seems to quench all striving. The person is entrapped in a "pool of the present"; and nothing troubles him.

Courbon's 80-year-old woman, whom he followed for months in hospital, suffered an almost complete loss of memory (at least in one sense), yet she had preserved the kinds of habits and good judgment that enabled her to act like a lady, engage in coquettish persiflage, and behave toward those around her according to their station in life. She did not know how old she was, her address, the date, or the length of time she had been in hospital. Although the staff visited her repeatedly, she never came to recognize them as individuals. Even her relatives who came to visit her were not identified, and she did not know whether her sister and her niece were still alive or not. Like others with this immediate-memory defect, she could not remember where she put things.

Her reactions to persons were appropriate, up to a point. She knew the categories: with the child she was maternal, with the nuns respectful, with the nurses' aides condescending, and with the male orderlies appropriately gruff. But while her reactions were appropriate in general, she did not know one doctor from another, and none of these persons acquired a history. She began each interview "from scratch," with a kind of categorical discrimination that seemed to be summoned by the present situation. The general configuration in the here and now evoked a deceptively sympathetic and appropriate response, considering that she remained a "stranger" to things. If she met the same young mother whom she greeted as Mademoiselle, she had to be corrected each time and told that this woman had a child; Mademoiselle remained Mademoiselle and never achieved a personal identity.

In the chapel, at the table, entertaining a guest, each setting evoked the appropriate general bearing. Her serenity seemed to persist through all the minor vexations (possessions lost, nurses who insisted on washing and changing her linen). What must be will be, and if these were the rules of the house she would comply. Visitors might come and go; she might be taken for a walk and deposited in her room; nothing disturbed her tranquility. "I have but to await death, but I can wait patiently and serenely." This all but complete detachment from things was without any very strong attachments to "the beyond" or to any imaginary world that might preoccupy her.

Her conversation seemed to drift into channels that were established in her youth when she worked in her brother's bookstore. Then she had boasted of her talent for finding just the right book to suit her customers' tastes (though now she was unable to cite a single title); as she babbled on, she acted as though she were now in that earlier period of time, expecting soon to be interrupted and to have to go back to wait on the customers. In one sense she did not have a past, although she was *in* it from time to time, as a dreamer is in his dream; she did not point back to that time, as an ordinary person would, in recalling old events. She just dropped into it. She played the old recordings, so to speak, but without any sense of their age, and without the "doubling" (*that* was then, and *this* is now) that normally occurs. She had no *social memory*, no power of discussing her past with another or of sharing in his past. She had become so completely separated from the normal temporal structure of things that she could not manage her life autonomously, or develop any continual affectional nexus with another person.

The milder forms of functional loss involve the aging person in considerable frustration. He is vexed and embarrassed that he cannot remember names. In Courbon's case the loss was more profound: the time-structured past disappeared, and the censorious superego that would otherwise criticize her for her stupidity went with it. Such a patient imagines no future, and without that tension toward what is to come, she does not make a personal evaluation of events as they might further or hinder her march into the future. What is, simply exists, there, before her. She is a voyeur, an onlooker, a visitor. Her contact is purely a playful one, a verbal one. Even an animal-like concern about basic needs (food, shelter, security) is lacking. She is like those lilies of the field who neither toil nor spin. The questions "Who am I?" and "What will become of me?" have disappeared. Lacking identity, she has no "identity crisis."

Minkowski even raises the question as to whether her "loss of memory" is not a secondary disability, the product of a more global detachment and de-structuring. Are not the memories there? Does she not drift back into "the bookstore period" and demonstrate their presence, even though she cannot take the more complex posture toward present and future which would summon them when they are appropriate?

Our 80-year-old should not be dismissed before we note certain problems that our vocabulary does not identify with precision. We have fallen into the habit of looking on the thinking of these brain-injured or brain-diseased patients as concrete, rather than abstract. Yet this woman who lives "in general" is moving among the categories and unable to grasp or recognize a single concrete object or person. *This* book, which her father gave her when she was confirmed, this book with a *history,* she does not recognize. It is a generic book, instead. This person, her own doctor, the one who talked yesterday about his son, the one who took her history when she first came into hospital, is not discriminated from other members of the staff. *Her* doctor is evidently the one that is near. If two doctors are present they are "the twins." To recognize, Minkowski points out, is not simply to remember, but to recon-stitute a whole segment of history. The person who stands before us also has a history that unrolled in that space-time we shared in part, and he is pointed toward a unique future that is one of the most distinctive things about him. Our 80-year-old reacts only to generalized persons, lay figures, abstractions. There is no *life* in them, any more than in her, and there is no meeting of selves, no true dialogue, just small talk, word bandying (as though she were in an elevator with strangers).

When we speak of the patient as living "in the present moment," we are talking about a different kind of present from the one most of us enjoy, a present charged with interest in a specific future that lies ahead, a present that has emerged out of an immediate past which has helped structure it and which we can summon without its losing its appropriate place on that developing space-time map we carry with us as a continuously changing posture. The loss of that specific future and that unique past which can be summoned radically alters her present posture, her way of presentifying.

Her detachment from the world about her is quite unlike the detachment that looks on the present scene, evaluating it in terms of very remote goals. Rather, it is a submergence in a field that is cut off from any developing sequence which led into it, or from any future to be reached for. Her cate-gories are personal enough, in one sense. It is her class-training that makes her supercilious toward the nurses' aides and respectful of the nuns, a kind of congealed *snobisme*.

In summary, let us note what Courbon's case shows.

1. There are two sorts of memories: the habits function in this person, while the circumstances in which they were formed cannot be recalled.

2. A superficial judgment permits the patient to "diagnose" situations and to respond according to familiar categories. She lives among universals and deals with what, for her, is the "essence of the situation."

3. Recognition, far from being one of the easiest forms of memory, requires a kind of imprinting and storage, a sharing of remembered experiences that is impossible for this patient.

4. If this patient cannot properly abstract, or deal with the present in the light of a represented future, neither can she grasp the concrete and unique. She knows no individuals, not even her relatives.

5. While she lives in a continuous present, that present is totally different from the normal "present time." The latter is charged with an interest in a future to be constructed, and it is so structured that the relevant past can be summoned and utilized.

6. The intrapsychic tension between ego and superego, between what one is doing and what one wishes one could do, seems to be in abeyance. Her serenity is close to indifference and apathy.

7. A loss of psychological tension accompanies this "falling out of time." Making no history, she has no history to correct, and few significant evaluations to make of that specious present in which she lives.

8. Although Courbon called it a nondemential weakening of the faculties, there is a severe loss of powers of adaptation, of the selfhood and regulative forces which enable the normal person to make a life. There *is* a dementia: a loss of immediate memory, a loss of social memory, a lack of autonomy, an absence of the power to form any lasting and developing interindividual nexus of affection and interest. With no responsibility, no vocational aptitude, no power to make promises, such a person is wholly dependent on a "sheltered existence" under the protection and guidance of other selves.

9. That she understands the social amenities, can enter into small talk and "kidding," is pleasant and amenable to ward discipline, gives her the appearance of having a mind of her own, but the appearance is deceptive.

The Course of the Disorder

Dementia senilis is most commonly identified between the ages of 55 and 70. There are presenile forms of dementia (Alzheimer's disease and Pick's disease), and even a "juvenile" form that emerges in the late 30's and early 40's. It progresses to a fatal termination, and in the later stages the patient is so bent and weakened that he cannot leave his bed. Pulmonary or cardiac complications may put an abrupt end to this fateful course, whose end is otherwise delayed long after the mind has gone (and the *person* has died). States of excitation and depression, of confused excitement or even violence, may irrupt briefly to alter the behavior of these patients without in any way checking the fateful course.

Such a prognosis forces us to look back with some skepticism on that ambivalence which causes some therapists to emphasize psychological factors among the possible causes of senility. Either the prognosis must be taken as a reason for deemphasizing the psychological causes, or all our efforts have either failed to locate the critical factors or been poorly applied. A guarded optimism about the results of therapy seems appropriate, but the course is "manifestly hopeless," conclude Noyes and Kolb (1963, p. 249). It may take ten months or ten years, but the end is the same.

The Biological Basis of the Disorder

The physiology of senility has remained a highly controversial area. Explored in the greatest detail, with evaluations based upon postmortem examination of many cases, the brains of these patients show the end-results of physiological, atrophic, and degenerative changes. What is most disturbing is the amount of overlap between these cases and others in which there has been a normal aging. Membranes, cell bodies, nuclei, fibrils within the cells have all been closely studied. There are pigmentation changes, growths of connective tissue, accumulations of inert detritus, and changes in intracellular neurofibrils. The dark-staining senile plaques give the microscopic slide of tissue prepared from the senile brain a characteristic appearance. All these changes have also been found in the normal aging brain. While most observers believe that their presence is more pronounced in the demented brain, there is so much overlap that a blind analysis would produce many errors. This confusing state of affairs has driven research workers to posit various hypothetical "underlying processes." Among them, to name a few, are amyloid degeneration, colloidal disruption, impaired enzyme functioning, a primary dehydration, altered protein metabolism, and changes in iron metabolism. To the present date these hypotheses have not led to such biochemical procedures as would improve diagnosis or treatment. It has been suggested, too, that a primary aging of the neural apparatus is at the root of the dementia, and that—underlying this primary abiotrophic process—there are "two dominant genes of low penetrance," "one specific factor," or "a complex of minor deficiencies that are intensified by age."

Treatment

There is no cure for this abiotrophic and regressive disorder. However, the patient can be helped, and it is possible that, to a limited degree, the progress of dementia can be retarded. Especially important for these easily confused and disoriented minds is a stable and congenial environment that gives adequate support and supervision. They have a limited capacity for change, and a limited tolerance for frustration. The restless nocturnal activity can be helped, to some extent, by medication. When apathy develops, its treatment requires a kind of "total push." The body and the mind must be kept as active as possible, always with respect for the limits imposed by the patient's special weaknesses. The good hospital will seek to postpone the final stasis that will come, in any case, eventually. Emotional reactions are partially handled by altering the environmental pressures, and in part by an effort to reeducate and to reassure. These are more effective methods than analysis or insight therapy (e.g., see Ayllon 1963).

The atmosphere of the home or hospital, the general hygiene of living, the careful attention to all medical needs constitute the primary emphasis in therapy. Beyond the provision of some useful and interesting tasks that will keep the patient active and provide some sense of worth (and of being wanted), there is a distinct limit: when the "push" creates stress and frustration, its value quickly becomes negative. The question of socializing or isolating these patients likewise calls for wisdom in assessing the particular case; it is not possible to decide for all patients and for all occasions what social life is too costly and confusing and what is necessary for health and continued growth. The "socially dependent" may have higher requirements, needing constant support of the presence of others. A flexible and experimental attitude is required.

Like children, these patients need patient and persistent training in simple habits, and types of correction that we ordinarily would not use with adults. But simple reinforcement and extinction procedures have been found effective where more elaborate explanations and understandings are ineffective. This therapy has to be undertaken, not in the hope of a cure, but for very limited gains in the patient's condition. It may be little better than a rearguard action against an enemy that will eventually be victorious.

Dementia with Arteriosclerosis

Aside from being a misnomer (it is the obliteration of the lumen of the blood vessels rather than the hardening of the vessels' walls that is responsible for the destruction of nervous tissue and the consequent dementia), the name of this illness covers a set of symptoms so similar to the simple senile dementia that a thorough description would entail a great deal of repetition. The principal distinctions drawn between the clinical phenomena found in the two conditions include:

1. There are more neurological symptoms that arise from the massive destruction of cells when blood supply is cut off by the blocking of one of the main branches of the cerebral arterial system, or from the destruction of cells by hemorrhage. Depending on the locus of the damage, there will be paralysis, aphasia, alexia, apraxia, agnosia, epileptiform attacks, disturbances in balance, or a pseudobulbar paralysis with "emotional incontinence" and pathological laughing and crying. Our knowledge of the cortical projection areas which serve as "ports of entry" for the sensory input or "ports of exit" for the motor outflow help to place the lesions on the basis of the clinical symptoms.

2. Before the dementia appears or has advanced too far, the patient is typically keenly aware of his inability to perform normally and his reaction

to these deficits constitutes a large portion of the psychotherapeutic problem. Grave but localized losses of function can exist beside a fairly complete preservation of the personality.

3. Wide fluctuations in performance (probably related in part to vasomotor changes) produce temporary remissions or arrests in a process that moves, nonetheless, toward a global loss of mental powers similar to that observed in senile dementia.

4. Associated with senility, the range of ages of first admissions for psychosis with cerebral atherosclerosis is as wide as that for coronary attacks (from the late thirties to the late seventies), with the bulk of the cases occuring after 60. Approximately 3 per cent occur before the fiftieth year (Ferraro 1959a, p. 1080).

5. In some cases the onset is insidious and gradual, as in simple dementia; this form is probably associated with diffuse minute lesions rather than the massive obliterations that are associated with "strokes" and which produce the more dramatic and noticeable aphasias and hemiplegias.

A precise diagnosis that identifies the particular cause implied in the name of the disorder is difficult, because present evidence shows that a general atherosclerosis (including cardiac symptoms and changes in the retinal blood vessels) may exist in the peripheral vessels and not in those of the cerebrum. A postmortem is required for definitive evidence. The focal symptoms, the marked fluctuation in capacities, the preservation of the personality in spite of grave neurological defects, the presence of other cardiovascular signs, and blood-serum evidence of high cholesterol and certain special groups of lipoproteins constitute the general clinical picture that has led to placement of these cases in a separate category, even though the ultimate deterioration in behavior is similar to that of the senile dement.

Varying Forms of the Disorder

The mental changes that accompany cerebral atherosclerosis may pursue a gradual and fluctuating course, in which a wide range of psychopathology occurs. Since these vascular changes can occur in widely differing personalities, the prodromal signs fuse with the preexisting personality. From the syndrome of asthenia to manias and depressions, from a nominal aphasia to dizziness and poor locomotion, from epilepsy to Parkinson's disease, the varying forms of the disorder constitute a veritable neuropsychiatric museum. Minor disabilities appear when the underlying changes in the circulatory system cause minute, scattered, discrete changes in neural tissues (tiny patches of deterioration). In addition, the disorder seems to fluctuate in some patients, to improve at times and to reverse its course, much as any functional disorder, such as psychasthenia, might.

Some of the beginning signs that accompany this period of onset resemble the neurasthenia of younger patients; the very mildness of the symptoms invites active psychotherapeutic interference and therapeutic optimism. In psychasthenia proper, with its fatigability, boredom, feeling of emptiness, morose inaction, insomnia, we are prone to look for psychological causes and to use exhortation, support, psychoanalysis, any attack that will alter the hygiene of living and improve the regulation of action. At age 60, with evidence of atherosclerosis (such as poor cardiac reserve), with wide fluctuations in mood and capacity, and with the beginning signs of a mental slowdown (memory failure, difficulty in attending, narrow interests, poverty of ideas, negligence of dress and appearance), this psychasthenic complex can herald the typical progressive degenerative changes that lead into dementia. Even though every therapeutic effort is made, it seems to amount to little more than a holding action. The disorder begins to take on the aspects of a *somatopsychic* (in contrast to a psychosomatic) illness.

The paresthesias and neurovegetative signs that would have suggested a hypochondriacal personality makeup and invited a search for obscure meanings hidden behind an "organ language," had they occurred in a younger person, now suggest organic bases (e.g., lesions affecting the functioning of the "visceral brain" that controls autonomic functions). Yet there is every reason for continuing to employ sound psychotherapy, even here, where the organic and psychological factors are bound to be inextricably intertwined, for here, as earlier, homeostasis and metabolism are affected by chronic conflicts, loss of economic security, loss of love, severance from business responsibilities, and "loss of significance." Even the physical well-being, so necessary if symptoms are to be arrested, will be improved by good mental hygiene.

Most of the changes that constitute the psychosis show wide fluctuations: hypertension, fatigability, cold extremities, mood changes (an anxious melancholy), constipation, hyperexcitability with euphoria, apathy, and indifference. There are changes in interpersonal relations and individual mental capacities. Beneath these complex functional changes, there are insidious structural changes, the degeneration of neural and vascular tissues. If the closure of an arteriole is complete (and it can be caused by a spasm of contraction as well as by atheromatous plaques), it does not have to last more than ten minutes before the cells it supplies begin to undergo irreversible deteriorative changes. Thus circulatory fluctuations are transformed into irreversible and progressive deteriorations in behavior.

Frequently this form of dementia begins with a massive change, a "stroke" with blockage or hemorrhage; once these appear they have a tendency to recur. In the intervals there may be marked recoveries of function, and an apparent arrest of the disease, but each succeeding "little stroke" leaves a patch of deteriorated tissue and a greater deficit.

The first deficits based on these "little strokes" seem sharply defined. The patient is keenly aware of the lacunae in his capacities, and his reactions to his deficits may constitute an important problem for all around him (for he has to learn to live with the disabilities). The fatigability, irritability, loss of initiative call for careful management, and they test the powers of both patient and family. In these early phases those who know him are struck by the rather complete preservation of the essential personality, but as the disease progresses, the moth-eaten surface of the cortex (seen on post-mortem examination) is matched by a corresponding erosion of the self. Defects become global: there is gross disorientation (which affects the temporal structuring of behavior before the spatial); a growing confusion between fantasy and reality; a constriction of the psychological field; a progressive impoverishment in ideas. This disintegration brings with it a change in character, an emotional incontinence, a peevishness and puerility. Self-control and self-criticism are as defective as the patient's control of his sphincters. This destructuring of action can proceed to the point where only the barest fragments of behavior are left: the automatic habits and the reflexes.

There is a *pseudobulbar* form of the disorder, with laughing and crying that are not related to meaningful emotional states. This "incontinence" in expression accompanies a flattened, affectless state. Here we see, in exaggerated form, the triad: hyperemotionality (in expression), lability, and a flattening of the actual emotional life. These changes are accompanied by a loss of facial expression (with an increase in the tonus of facial muscles) and by difficulties in swallowing, articulating, and chewing. The voice becomes monotonous in pitch and timbre. The clonic contractions of throat and chest, precipitated by any sudden access of stimulation, may release sobs or barking laughter that has little relation to any meaningful experiences.

The principles of psychotherapy involved in the management of these cases with atherosclerosis are essentially the same as those for senile dementia: the stable and congenial environment; the reduction of excessive press, and a parallel stimulation of activities and interests that are within easy range of accomplishment; sedation to help the twilight and nocturnal states of excitement and confusion; no sedation at other times, since, with too little activity, it only accelerates the already mounting indifference and drift toward an ultimate stasis that confines the patient to bed and brings his whole physiology to a halt.[13]

Dietary and medical treatment designed to arrest the advancing atherosclerosis (low animal-fat diet, lipotropic medication, anticoagulants) is used along with endocrines (thyroid, estrogen, androgen, ACTH), iodides, and vitamins. These treatments, along with control of fluid intake, elimination, and nutrition, require expert medical supervision, backed by the continuous support of laboratory studies. At best they retard a process that may last for ten years, only to be terminated by a stroke or by complications in heart, lungs, liver, kidneys, or other vital organs. Cerebral atherosclerosis, which accounts for 6 per cent of all deaths in our society, will account for the final termination of the dementia in the majority of these cases, when a final thrombosis interrupts all vital processes.

---

[13]For the anxious and agitated depressions that occur in some of these patients with atherosclerosis, Ey, Brisset, and Bernard (1963, p. 808) and Ferraro (1959b, p. 1104) recommend electroshock. This has, of course, little effect on the progressive dementia, save possibly to hasten it by adding still other minute and diffuse lesions to an already damaged cortex. It may bring a lifting of the agitated depression, however.

TWO SYNDROMES ASSOCIATED
WITH BRAIN PATHOLOGY

These two syndromes have been identified, at times, with specific types of brain damage. As evidence accumulates, it appears that they occur in a great many patients who suffer brain injury. Sensitized to the existence of these symptom clusters, the clinician learns to anticipate their presence in widely divergent disorders. The deficits which form these clusters may be present in all degrees. In some degree they are also present in the normal person with undamaged brain, making his behavior less efficient and less rational than it could be. In the severely damaged brain, they may make any form of autonomous and self-regulated life impossible. Again, these deficits serve to highlight what good integrative powers are like: without the full powers that are here shown to be in short supply, the brain-injured patient is condemned to a life just short of the one we expect a rational, purposive, human being to enjoy. Witnessing the full impact of these deficits in the brain-injured, we can appreciate better some of the facets of behavior seen in the mentally retarded, the uneducated, and the poorly motivated.

THE AMNESTIC SYNDROME: KORSAKOFF'S PSYCHOSIS

Originally named for Korsakoff, the physician who first gave a clear account of the symptoms so often linked with a polyneuritis that follows chronic alcoholism, the syndrome involves a special type of memory loss, but it is more than an amnesia; there are changes in motivation (apathy) and a tendency to confabulation. The symptom group was identified as early as 1849, when Magnus Huss tried to link alcohol-induced brain changes with a memory loss. Changes in cortical cells have been identified in postmortem studies of the brains of these patients, widely scattered and with varying degrees of degeneration. Damage has been found in the cortex, the frontal and prefrontal areas, the midbrain, and the brain stem. Of late, emphasis has centered on the vegetative centers of the hypothalamus, the mammillary bodies, and the mammillary-thalamic nerve trunks. It has not so far been possible to find any specifically localized lesion that is both necessary and sufficient to account for the symptoms. Within the recent past, interest in the reticular-arousal system and its role in the attending-encoding process so essential to "timekeeping" and to "presentifying" has led to an emphasis upon lesions in the brain stem.

All observers agree that in Korsakoff's psychosis there is a marked impairment in memories from the recent past, while at the same time large groups of remote memories remain fairly intact. Grünthal (1928) described his patients as floundering in the immediate present, unable to use the knowledge they have, unable to make a new history of the relations lived through in the present. But his phrase "plunged into the present" could be misleading, for the patient lives in a different kind of present: it is not linked with the just-lapsed past, nor is it being inscribed properly for later recall. This moment is apt to be improperly linked with a "yesterday" that in fact occurred ten years ago, and tomorrow's events will link up with that same "yesterday," since nothing that happens today is properly recorded (in a form that can be "recited" or commented on tomorrow). Jean Delay (1950) would describe the deficit as a deficit in the social form of memory, and emphasizes a special type of *amnesia of fixation:* there are *effects* (or traces) that persist, but not the usual well-structured memories from which we can later "read the past."

From the beginning the syndrome had been linked with chronic alcoholism (although in Korsakoff's own series the alcoholics were in the minority). Alcoholism, in turn, was linked with a polyneuritis that was often found in the nerve trunks of the limbs; pressure on these nerves or on the muscle masses is painful. There are also lesions in the cellular structure of the liver. Ey, Bernard, and Brisset (1963, p. 691) cite an instance of an accidentally produced Korsakoff psychosis, the result of alcohol injections given in the course of treating a pulmonary suppuration. As the literature expanded, the syndrome was found in connection with carbon-monoxide poisoning, carbon-disulphide poisoning, vitamin B_1 deficiency, puerperal septicemia, typhus, tuberculosis, hepatitis, tumors of the brain, cerebral traumata, syphilis of the central nervous system, accumulated fecal matter, strangulation (from attempted hanging), epidemic encephalitis, diabetes, uremic poisoning, anemia, and metabolic disorders of pregnancy. At the present time, four-fifths of the cases of this amnestic syndrome seen in the clinics are alcoholics; this particular postalcoholic complication is seen more frequently, for some reason, in women. Delirium tremens sometimes precedes the syndrome, accompanied by an unexplained "morning anxiety," depressive tendencies, and nightmares, which later clear up, leaving the pure amnestic phenomena.

The haunting thought that pursues one as he studies these impaired selves is that *something has gone out of existence:* a vital power, a self engaged with other selves, a force that can integrate a life with a future to be shared, a living regnancy. The pulse may beat and the vital processes may continue to function, eating and elimination follow their cycles, but the person is not at the moment *alive!* In the functional disorders (as, for example, in that state of aboulia Pierre Janet described in his classic account of hysteria), this regnancy seems to ebb and return, to extend its domain or to restrict its borders. Like an elastic blanket that expands and constricts, covering the territory over which it rules, this regnancy, in its periods of retreat, may leave the outlying territories "ungoverned."

In the organic disorders these changes tend to become more complete and irreversible. The loss of memories that first appears in partial form may become more and more complete; and the remembered past retreats until only very early memories remain. Finally there may be a complete loss of personal identity. The foundations of action grow shallow, the grasp of the present poor, the fabulations more dreamlike, the stance for action more and more limited and evanescent. There are all degrees of retreat. One Korsakoff patient can play checkers and beat every patient on his ward

The larger unit of the game is still possible, and his skills match the "problems" created by the distribution of the pieces on the board. The next case may not be able to follow a simple conversation.

The flattening of affect and the restriction of the duration of internally consistent actions until no voluntary action can persist very long help us to understand the nature of the apathy, or loss of motivation, and warn us that the amnestic syndrome involves changes over and above a mere memory loss. It is a radical destructuring of action. If we say that the Korsakoff patient preserves a typical attitude and manner which implies "the same personality is here," it is obvious that it is only a superficial manner, a Southern accent, an old gesture, a way of laughing, that persists. Grandmother, who no longer can remember where she put her glasses, or what she said fifteen minutes ago, or what was promised at the breakfast table, becomes a curiously flattened and shallow replica of her former self. She has the same intonation, the same voice, the same face, but the old "character" that inserted her will into an extended space-time field and persisted in her goals is gone. She can be frustrated in little things, immediate things, but "the long run" has ceased to exist. The more deep-seated feelings, such as a persistent hatred, are above and beyond the level at which she functions, as well as a realistic concern for those she loves.

The Transformation of Memories into a Recital

The social form of remembering seems to be radically disturbed in Korsakoff's syndrome. The elaboration and transformation of experience, and its storage in the form of traces which we can later utilize in a conscious recall of what will then be experienced as past, do not take place. That there is some vague kind of storage was noted in Korsakoff's first accounts (1928):

"One enters the room of a patient for the first time, he holds out his hand, and bids us good day. One departs and returns two or three minutes later; the patient no longer says good day and yet when one asks him if he has seen you he responds in the negative. A patient who found the electrical therapy we were employing very unpleasant showed his displeasure as soon as he saw us entering with the apparatus again, although he was quite ready to assure us that he had never been involved in such treatment before."

Other patients with a similar anterograde amnesia, who never seem to have registered their hospital experiences since admission, sometimes report dreams that involve these "nonregistered" experiences. With some patience such patients can be taught to associate word-pairs, although a greater effort and a larger number of repetitions seem to be required. A reduced capacity for rote learning seems to persist, but the quick and automatic registry of experience, which normally functions automatically, and which transforms discrete events into a patterned personal history in which the experiences are properly located in correct sequence, does not take place.

We are used to giving a recital of the experiences that we have just lived through, and we automatically "make a record" of those we now enjoy (or endure). We assume that this is the way the memory function works. Studies of incidental memory show that such recall is often spotty, that it is quite unreliable, that false memories are inserted, that we tend to believe that we experienced the plausible, the usual, the often repeated. The studies also show that a subject forewarned and alerted will set up a vigilant memorizing or memory-making attitude that markedly increases both the total amount recalled and the precision in describing aspects of experience that have been noted. (We never note *everything*, and the direction of attention has a marked influence on the content that can be recalled.) But we are not prepared for such gross memory defects as those found in these patients. We expect a man, without being forewarned, without making a special effort to translate the experiences lived through into a set of "representations," to produce at least a rough sketch of his recent history. We expect this record to grow dim, and to be overlaid with later memories which screen away the old ones. We are prepared for a certain amount of displacement, with fragments of one scene transposed into another. We are even ready to admit that memories, dislodged from their moorings in the past, may arise to awareness like fresh inventions, so that, unconsciously, a man may plagiarize his own past.

In the process of imprinting or fixation, in the construction, storage, and later utilization of these representations, in the development of a history within which memories are properly placed, the patient suffering from the amnestic syndrome is grossly impaired. It is chiefly in the handling of the recent past that his difficulties approach an absolute deficit, although here it is apparent that some routines can be learned with sufficient repetition.

The process of *making* a memory (of this higher, social form) requires a special kind of grasp of the present. Unfortunately for the Korsakoff patient, this *presentification* (along with a good orientation toward an immediate past and a forthcoming future) is lacking. He may know that he is in a hospital without knowing why he is there, when he entered; or he may misidentify it as a prison or a firehouse. The sunporch may be misidentified as the deck of a ship, or the physician as an examining army medical officer. Disoriented, he seems to grasp for clues, and he may elaborate, on the basis of a chance remark, a "story" that derives from some remote period of his past. These old memory traces, laid down at a time when his presentification was still good and when his history-making was intact, may have a good temporal-spatial structure, and if he speaks of his sister or his job or what he was doing then, his account will probably be well-structured *for that period,* but only for a moment. The next clue may tap another period. The boat that he believes he has just boarded suddenly lands three thousand miles away, or it has changed into a hotel or a barracks. The older past is usually firm, and offers a basis to which the present fleeting, detached, and poorly presentified perceptions can be attached and given meaning. The need for rationality that remains and the questions of the examiner are enough to prompt his fabulation. But these constructions are so weak that no new or permanent stance develops: he does not persist in his fabulation, make a new beginning. Left to himself he seems ready to lie about, rather apathetic and indifferent, or mildly euphoric and insouciant, content to float, unconcerned, until some bodily cramp, some segmental craving, moves him to the lavatory or the dining room, or the unfolding ward routine pushes him into action. He cannot set up and maintain any new goals, or even persist in any action that someone else provokes. His ideas and actions, his interpretations of the world around him are old ideas, old interpretations, as though he had just finished a day at the office, or just set sail. The new presentifications (fabulations, false recognitions, *déjà vus,* and *jamais vus*) do not go down on the kind of unrolling film on which our actions are usually inscribed in the form of memories that can later be called up. He does not prepare to recite them, nor are they well stored (even though apparently perceived at the time), nor can he later summon them. He enjoys the movie but does not remember what he enjoyed. Since there are all degrees of this defect, it is not easy to make firm generalizations; the patients studied by Syz (1937), Korsakoff, and Hoenig *et al.* (1962) show a gradual ritualizing of conduct and a persistence of fragmentary residues of hospital experience, that prove there is a kind of imprinting after all. When bits of this poorly structured flotsam pop up in dreams, in some later fabulation, or in some association that just irrupts into the patient's mind, we have to posit a kind of lower-order trace, a registration that rapidly loses its temporal significance. It *was* a memory, perhaps, but only for a moment. Jean Delay (1950, p. 78) lists other observers who arrived at similar conclusions: Bonhoeffer, Picke, Grünthal, Gamper, Brodman, Gregor, Van den Horst.

To say, as Charcot had earlier (1893), that "memory images are not lost, but stored in the unconscious" not only fails to add a great deal to the objective descriptions themselves, but also implies that much more imprinting is going on than is actually the case. Here and there a fragment pops up in a dream (e.g., an unpleasant experience in hospital that cannot be consciously recalled now figures in a *dream that can be recalled*). We need not jump to the generalization that all experience is imprinted, that the amnesia does not affect the process of fixation, and that everything is stored *unconsciously.* What traces are made are operative chiefly at a nonverbal level. What social memory exists is of extremely brief duration. What presentification occurs is usually grafted upon the older memories and, even then, persists very briefly and cannot be recalled later. Drifting attention, inconsistency, unstable motivations, vanishing "presents" that cannot be recalled are the rule. What little imprinting is made is slow, demanding many repetitions. The engrams are crudely generalized, poorly discriminated. Their effects, therefore, will reappear at inappropriate times and in responses to aspects of the newly presentified fields that may not be significant. Freed from the accurate and specific anchorages in space-time, such poor traces become automatisms rather than useful memories. Good imprinting, like efficient recall, requires a proper stance, a regnancy with a history and a future, that can order them for storage and later summon those that are relevant to new and well-perceived fields.

The importance of the present stance (good presentification) for the summoning of memories is illustrated in one of Lidz's patients who recovered a great deal of his powers after a carbon-monoxide poisoning. At the depth of his illness, he could not seem to elaborate or utilize the old memories he retained. He could answer questions accurately enough, but he never went beyond the prompter. Somewhat recovered, his whole attitude changed:

"His general demeanor had altered in a striking fashion. He is now active, jovial, and talkative, and is resentful that his wife refuses to take him home. He has a full grasp of the situation. He works about the hospital, running errands and laboring on the farm. The change in conversational ability seems important, for it indicates that the utilization of material from his past life had been more severely impaired than was believed at the time. In 1939 (when first admitted) he could tell facts of his past correctly when questioned; recall was good, but there was no spontaneous elaboration. Now conversation has fullness, which gives it real meaning. When he tells us that he is "down on his sisters," he goes on to explain the interfamilial relationships and how he had formerly helped his sisters until the reason for his animosity is apparent. It suggests that previously he had been unable to bring into play the full associative material essential for true re-membering in so far as remembering is the constructive utilization of recalled material." (Lidz 1942, pp. 595 ff.)

When observers report that "whole chunks of memory" return in those cases who recover, these great leaps forward are due in part to changes in the present forward-looking stance. The bits of the past which could not be re-called, formerly, were there, to be sure, but the stance of the summoner was not sufficiently well-structured to activate them.

In numerous studies of hysterical patients, Pierre Janet described phenomena similar to this forgetting of the immediate past that appears in the amnestic syndrome of Korsakoff. In Janet's patient Mme. D., there was a continuous amnesia, described as hysterical. He assumed that it was a functional failure, posited no lesions, and was able to show that, in the midst of this state of con-tinuous amnesia in which events were lost to voluntary waking recall, there was imprinting: the events would crop up in dreams, or could be elicited dur-ing hypnotic trance. This availability of what has been forgotten can be demon-strated in hypnotic procedures which produce forgetting on waking: the next hypnotic session will render these same events available. This same appearance of a memory that cannot be voluntarily recalled has been reported by Delay (1950, p. 79), who witnessed a delirious attack in a case of general paralysis with the Korsakoff amnestic syndrome; memories which could not have been acquired at any time save during the illness were involved.

The most common course and outcome of this organic psychosis is not a happy one. A progressive deterioration and a fatal end-state are reported in two-thirds of the serious and advanced cases (Ey 1954, p. 381). Sometimes a chronic condition can be arrested, but the lesions already produced cannot be undone. No amount of prompting by psychotherapy, by hypnosis, by the ex-ploration of the unconscious, or by the interpretation of fabulations and dreams avails. What unconscious imprinting exists functions at that level, and the spon-taneous and voluntary remembering that goes with normal presentification and imprinting does not return. Such patients do not become vitally related to the realities about them, nor are they interested in "making a future." The changes in cell structure, when viewed at autopsy, indicate that neurons have been replaced by neuroglia cells or have persisted in various stages of degeneration. The massive doses of thiamin and niacin sometimes administered represent an effort to arrest a disease process; psychotherapy must content itself largely with assisting the patient (through good daily routines) to live within the narrowed circle of his reduced capacity. The regulative process that he has lost requires additional external regulation, and the good care and nurturant routines that a watchful mother would provide for her child that has not arrived at a fully functioning selfhood.

Rarely, instead of such a gradual series of deteriorative changes, the full-blown syndrome will appear suddenly, be treated, subside, and leave no important or obvious sequelae. It would seem that in these instances the mixture of functional and organic changes has been checked and reversed. Of 51 cases, reported from the Bellevue services, given vitamin B$_1$ therapy, one-third were reported as clearing up. A number of authors refer to the disorder as a cerebral beriberi. (See Green, Carlson, and Evans, 1941; De Wardener and Lennox 1947.) Ey and Marchand have reported recoveries in about one-fifth of their cases. Watching the recovering cases as they improve, one can observe a personality changing from a state of apathy, restricted awareness, amnesia for the immediate past, in which only a mechanical kind of conditioning seems possible, into a person actively engaged in a present field and looking forward to a future that is sought through relevant and productive actions.

Thompson's view (1959, p. 1216) is not optimistic, however:

"The prognosis in Korsakoff's psychosis is usually hopeless, and many writers state that it is an irreversible disease. The writer has had patients who have had a fair degree of recovery after long periods of treatment. There has been some improvement in memory and, in an occasional rare case, complete recovery."

Noyes and Kolb (1963, p. 174) summarize their experience in these words: "Many cases clear up after six or eight weeks, with approximate restoration to mental health."

Other Aspects of the Syndrome

With the passage of years and the accumulation of evidence, the concept of Korsakoff's psychosis has changed from that of a specific memory defect with a specific causation, to a much more general set of changes in behavior that arise from many different types of causes. The disputes as to the location and distribution of the changes in central nervous system are not finished, although recent studies have centered attention on the brain-stem area, and in particular on the mammillary bodies of the hypothalamus.

Certain physical signs have been repeatedly reported in the literature. The tendon reflexes are weakened, and occasionally disappear (Achilles and knee-jerk); walking grows difficult. A wasting of the muscles affects the extensor muscles especially; and there are choreiform and athetose movements, as well as paresthesias and algias (especially to pressure). An ascending paralysis, in the most severe cases, may become almost complete. Visceral symptoms (also traceable to a neuritis) may cause vomiting and dyspnea.

Four mental symptoms are stressed: amnesia, confabulation, apathy, and confusion. This last may involve serious disorientation with anxiety, agitation, false recognition, and flight of ideas.

Confabulations and Distortions

It is worth noting that some of the factors which Bartlett stressed in his study of recall in the normal (1932) are all present in the amnestic, and in an exaggerated degree. All of us tend to transform perceived material in the direction of conventions, of the familiar, of the banal. It is a constant source of error. The "captain" picture which Bartlett exposed to his subjects, a man in uniform, tended to drift away from its unique identity, and to resemble someone the subject knew, or some stereotype of a military figure. Tested by a later presentation of the figure, one of Bartlett's subjects spoke, more accurately than he realized, when he said, "That's not *my* captain." It was in fact the picture that had been shown to him, but it did not resemble the captain he promptly constructed out of materials he had long carried with him. Some military figure, some image of authority, some sahib back from India, some illustration in one of Kipling's tales, had acted like a magnet to draw the presented captain into line. In the period of storage there is evidently a process of attrition that erases the marks of differentiation (unless they are carefully noted) and inserts probable contours in their place, especially when the new fact does not fit the observer's previous conceptions. The nonconforming details have to be given especial attention if they are to be recalled, and then, as a consequence, they may be exaggerated in the reproduction.

The Gestaltists have reminded us that there are both leveling and sharpening tendencies in recall, and that the perception of relations to the norm that is carried has to be precise; otherwise, as soon as the stimulus pattern is withdrawn, a transformation process will set in. The villain will grow more villainous (or not be a villain at all); the steeple will grow sharper (or its slope will approach that of any ordinary house roof). What with principles that lead to simplification, completion, stabilization, and exaggeration, the student is puzzled as to what to predict, for all of these trends can be identified in experimental settings. Indeed, to predict, he would have to discover, somehow, what kind of a figure the observer has made; it is usually the moment of reproduction that reveals what has happened to the figure while it was "in soak."

What Lidz invites us to predict is that in the amnestic this transformation process will be exaggerated, for neither at the moment of presentification nor at the moment of later recall does such a patient fully grasp where he is, what the question means, what the object is to him. Cut off from his immediate past by the amnestic condition, and not looking into a future which would give this event a personal-evaluative significance, the limited pool of ripples set in motion in the amnestic's central nervous system subside quickly: the figure does not develop. As a result the event is loosely anchored, vague, ambiguous, and somewhat meaningless.

As in the case of any ambiguous figure where much of it is screened from our eyes (e.g., if we are only permitted to see the draped hand of a woman), the number of directions which can be taken as the reaction is completed is great. The amnestic, who seems to grasp so little of the current scene, completes the figure out of his own collection of old stereotyped materials. Like a child with relatively few memories and "handles" with which to experience novelty, and who sees the corkscrew as "crooked scissors" and the burro as "big dog," the amnestic has to depend on the limited portion of his more remote past that is still undisturbed. Like a child, he is also untroubled by that fringe lying between make-believe and truth and less capable of discriminating between levels of certitude, and so the amnestic accepts his own confabulations readily and unquestioningly. He is a believer. Pushed by his questioner, he grows defensive; now he is *sure* that he just came from the shipyard. He is insulted by the questions. Such confabulation is not lying. It is a much simpler thing than the lie which has to keep careful track of the difference between what is said and what should have been said.

The studies of retroactive inhibition show that poorly perceived forms (nonsense syllables in lists that have no good serial organization) tend to intermingle, to shift their position in the series, to cross over into adjacent lists, whereas the well-structured materials of meaningful discourse inserted between the series of poorly organized materials preserve their integrity, their serial structure. ("Baf, nim, zub, woc," and so on is easily transformed, whereas "Norman Foster and his mother came yesterday" retains its shape.) The comic-strip materials which Lidz used to test his patients' powers of serial synthesis operated as does the nonsense material for the normal person: the import of the strip as a whole was too much for the patient to grasp; as a result, the parts, even when retained as parts, tended to migrate and to join up with parts of other strips, other "stories." The same type of contamination occurs when a patient moves from one ward to another: the pool table in the dayroom (of the earlier ward) gets inserted into his schema of his new surroundings. The images from ten years of failing memory become jumbled so that even when the events come up in recall, they are placed in incorrect contexts.

The tendency of the amnestic to break up and recombine his experiences reminds us of a complexity in the normal imprinting process that we are apt to miss when we follow the Pavlovian paradigm. As a trace-building process links one event to its temporally adjacent member, the "atoms" of thought are tied in small molecular bundles of two members each. Centering his attention on the physiology of such an association process, Pavlov tended to overlook the broader meaningful relationships: he offered us the concept of a redintegrative machine that linked the immediately adjacent items in tiny islands of time. His dogs were trained to respond to the sound of bubbling water with a salivary reflex simply because the arbitrary sequence in the laboratory procedure had placed the head-turning to this sound immediately before the reaction to meat powder placed on the tongue. When, in normal human action, two events are joined as parts of larger meaningful wholes (the bubbling of a stew that is boiling on the stove and will be served for lunch, the sound of the teakettle that mingles with the conversation of our guest for whom a warm cup of tea will be prepared), they seem to have a firmer unity, for they are parts of larger actions in the making. It is true that these couplings, mechanical and isolated from any meaningful context, do have the power of firing across to their opposite number (or to "similars") even when these associations are altogether inappropriate to new contexts in which their cues are embedded. This is what happens in the pun. It may merely be a klang meaning, where the sound of the word carries our thought to the sound of another and irrelevant word.[14]

These crossovers into other sequences or matrices, this contamination of the present with the past that clutters up our thought process, can be productive or destructive. It has a way of occurring at those moments when the structure of our present action is weakened, when the larger whole that runs into the future is either not forming or seems to have reached a stalemate (failing to select from our body of memories something that is useful). When he grows drowsy, or slightly befuddled with wine, then even a normal person can show a mild equivalent of what occurs in the amnestic syndrome. Alcohol, hashish, fatigue, toxic conditions bring this peculiar "gift"; it is not surprising that creative writers have tried to exploit such drugs as hashish and opium, hoping to dredge up from the depths of their imagination something original and important.

To be useful, however, these dredged-up irrelevancies have to be incorporated in the best structures we can make. Taken by themselves they represent an increase in the simpler mechanisms, the smaller figures. They are original enough, for they break the boundaries imposed by sober common sense. They excite our mirth at times, especially when their intrusion interrupts some pontification that is boring us. But they irritate us when one in our audience uses them to cut across our very serious meanings, as we try to persuade our hearers, for they are then like an insult hurled in our face. Such action says, in effect, "Your meaning is unimportant to me. I am not paying attention to what you are saying."

The other side of the amnestic's "gift" is his inability to concentrate, to converse, to develop the larger configurations in time. He has a touch of the psychopath about him: the psychopath, too, can be bright, witty, original, but one should not count on him tomorrow, for it is the absence of any

---

[14]Arthur Koestler (1964) makes use of this shunting from one thought sequence into another in his theory of creative thinking. *Bisociation,* he believes, is common to the pun and the most important of creative acts. Archimedes in his bath, noting the water rising as he enters the tub, has carried into the tub the problem of estimating the gold content of a precious object that cannot be melted down. Darwin, wondering about the finches on the Galapagos Islands, carried thoughts about Malthus and political economy with him. The matrices, so separate, can be creatively fused. The use or fusion in a new synthesis is the essential thing in creation. The slightly inebriate punster has little to add to his "invention" but his silly, "He, he, he." His invention ends there, and so ending, it is not really an invention, but a distraction.

regulative tomorrow that characterizes his actions and makes his promises worthless.

Since *this* is not *that*, and since *now* is not *then*, this developing present (the larger whole of action and the matrix to which it is fitted) must exclude these little irrelevancies, these klang associations, these dippings into an automatic past. While normal man has a touch of the deadly serious about him (he *is* concerned about where he is going, intent on inserting his will into fields with practical meanings), for all of his common sense he is also moving forward into *novel* settings. As a history-maker who drags his past after him, he also must project patterns into a future that is to be designed so as to utilize and absorb the past, and so must use the past in a *new* way. He cannot take the present merely in its *thisness,* its purely local character, its objectivity, nor will a purely logical category placement do (such as: this is the Fourth of July all over again; now we are entering a second hundred years' war; this is the same old Communist tactic; life is an eternal recurrence). Only when he is alive to the novelty of the present moment, only when he senses it as a dynamic transition, a time-binding bridge, can he escape from both the irrelevancies of punning and the stodginess of hidebound recurrences.

It is interesting to see how the amnestic does not misidentify objects (the knife, the fork, the sexes, the written direction, the spoken command, all call out a degree of understanding and skill). He still has the categories but he is not going anywhere, and he does not fit these objects into any developing schema. He has lost that growing tip of a personal structure of action, and these objects have lost their uniqueness. Only with this schema-forming process intact does the more complete form of recall begin to function, above the level of klangs and categories. In normal recall the automatisms are controlled, either suppressed or utilized in novel ways, and the schemata which reach into the future make behavior a consequence-regulated thing. These schemata include other persons, and they embrace the wider field so that local mechanisms are always dominated by more remote considerations, little plans regulated by larger plans. (We have been using "normal" in an absolute sense; the average person is a mixture, containing automatisms and some foresightful schemata.)

Like the skillful diplomat who keeps much of his information to himself, the normal person with this active, growing tip of action-structuring schemata can scan his memory with an end in view and select from this pool of traces something that is relevant. Occasionally he, too, will smile to himself as he enjoys the pun that he discards. But, typically, when the schemata are functioning at top form, the lower forms of automatism are *discarded in advance.* Like a computer with a programmed question inserted, that throws up only the really relevant information, he has a "set for something that fits."

In G. E., one of Lidz's subjects who was more seriously affected by the disease process, questioning could bring out many items from the last ten years which he had forgotten. He could make no extended recital about the period but the question, appropriately shaped so as to establish the searching posture, called up fragments. Here an address, there a bit of information, would evoke something he could no longer speak about at any length spontaneously. If we were to compare the flowing process of imprinting to the making of a kind of continuous video tape, his tape-making would seem to have become faulty, for the scenes are spotty, scrambled, and juxtaposed improperly. Only here and there does a strip of memories with precise form emerge from the midst of this rubble of "imprints."

In an old study on the amoeba, Child (1924) showed that, when attacked by a solution of potassium cyanide, the newest tips of pseudopods just being formed were the first to disintegrate. This crude analogy tempts us (like the pun) to exercise our scientific imagination. We are quite uncertain as to the precise nature of the aging process which affects human memory traces; we know of no special place, more protected from disease processes, where traces are stored; and we can scarcely imagine a chitinous coating that protects these older traces. Perhaps there is a more extended growth of the terminal feet at the end of axons, so that both numerous and solid "connections" are formed (as they are used over and over again, and have time to grow into forms less vulnerable to disease). Only the facts seem clear: the older memories are preserved in greater completeness, and it is these which join up with the present scene to form a fabulous and false background with which to interpret present events.

So we observe, in the amnestic patient: a readiness to believe what is not true (and what a good memory would have corrected), a cliché-ridden action and speech, a passivity that responds when pushed and recalls when the question is complete enough, and an inability to form a developing schema, or to make either a history or a future. The false linkages with the past, shifting, varied, vivid, give a false impression of inventiveness, of a rich imagination. Checked against the real background of the patient, their true significance emerges. One of the patients of Williams and Rupp (1938) illustrates this point:

"T.J.P. . . . was first seen shortly after he had evidenced mental symptoms following prolonged indulgence in alcohol. He had been in turn seaman on coastwise excursion boats, worker in a rubber factory, fur salesman, movie extra, circus ticket seller, machinist, and telegraph messenger boy; these occupations being listed in inverse order, the first having been his last occupation just prior to the onset of his illness. At first the content of his confabulations was concerned with his experiences on the excursion boat, then as his mental condition became worse, shifted to earlier experiences connected with his fur-selling and circus days. In possession of the chronological facts of his life, one could trace a progressive loss of memory back through the years until the content of his confabulations was finally concerned with incidents connected with his first job shortly after leaving school. Parallel to this tendency of the content of confabulation to be concerned with events occurring earlier in his life, his answers to other questions were formulated with regard to events coexistent at the time when the confabulation content actually occurred. Thus, in response to questions he stated that his sister who was married and had a child at the time of his excursion boat experience, was married but childless when his productions centered around his circus experiences, and she was still single when his content was concerned with a still earlier portion of his life. Later this patient gradually showed an improvement in which it was possible to retrace his occupational career and at the time of this writing his sister is once again married but still childless."

So impressed are these authors with this "law of regression" that they propose the degree of regression (or the changes with time) as a criterion to be used in prognosis of outcome. Lidz's observations should warn us against too hasty or careless a use of this interpretation. The patient's condition is a fluctuating one: a better phrasing of a question can elicit memories in a period believed "lost," suggestions from the present field affect the levels tapped, and recovery brings back "chunks" of the past from that pre-illness period believed lost.

Anxiety and Amnesia

One gains the impression that, with the more severe brain deficits, the patient takes on a mixture of apathy, indifference, and mild euphoria, under situations that are insoluble. What the patient cannot experience as a problem does not trouble him, we argue. Remembering Jacobsen's excitable chimp who became more tractable as her capacity for serial synthesis was lost, it would seem that frustration and anxiety should decrease as the schema-forming process deteriorates. Yet in cases who cannot perform properly, any prodding with questions or problems that *force them to recognize their incapacities* disturbs these patients. Lidz notes: "His hands would tremble; his forehead would break out in perspiration; and he would become angry and uncooperative if unable to sidetrack the examiner." This outcome was more apt to occur in cases where a partial insight was still possible. It is the "whole man," who has enough pride and ambition to know what is expected of him, who is afflicted with the feeling of emptiness and incompleteness so many psychasthenics complain about. As in Janet's neurotics who descended from a *feeling* of emptiness to a *state* of emptiness, it is in the more severe disorder that the affective component disappears. In that last and final Kingdom of Blah, the patient no longer senses what he has lost, no longer misses it. The more seriously affected amnestic functions *below* the level where frustrations and superego anxiety can occur.

A Theoretical Speculation

If we look on the brain as a whole as providing a field within which traces may form, the shape of these traces, not their loci within particular neural arcs, could become the important consideration. The configurationists have dared to speculate in this fashion. Lashley's work on the learning process, on which he based his conception of the equipotential cortex, also followed this line of reasoning. Many ablation studies have sought, on the contrary, to find some neural patch for every pitch, to find some occipital cell to correspond to each retinal cell, and some specific coupling to account for each association.

If, as in Modeste's case, we can locate rather specific parietal areas that are responsible for loss of ability to recognize tactual shapes by the cues from one of her hands, we seem to be on our way to such a mapping of mental functions. And if, as in the work of Marquis, we can show that excision of a rather precise visual area destroys a specific sort of conditioned response, even though that response can be relearned, the original association seems to have occupied a particular group of cells. From such evidence it is easy to generalize, making each "lesson learned" depend on a trace in specific brain areas. Perhaps they could also have been formed in other areas (and the evidence of relearning of lost habits is persuasive). Nonetheless, their vulnerability to local injury suggests that they did in fact reside in the particular loci damaged.

The moment we consider the more complex schemata, both the registering and the shaping of these "sets" require more territory; the evidence shows that minor injuries scattered over many localities, or toxic conditions affecting many cells to a slight degree, produce comparable disturbances. Schemata-building, history-making, effective imprinting and recall of relationships, flexible use of the past seem to require all the cerebral substance, and seem to be damaged by a wide variety of injuries that impair a sufficient number of the cells. The syndromes that we are here discussing illustrate the kind of qualitative descent we have in mind.

To use the schemata that have been formed in the past requires an equally complex schema-forming process in the present. Good traces, formed earlier, may be present as potential integrations and yet be unavailable for use because of the present shape of events now forming in the brain of the subject. When the present brain state has recovered, the old patterns also become available, and perhaps a few traces from the interval in which a continuous amnesia seemed to make any trace formation and storage impossible.

With good presentification there are shapes which summon other relevant (and resonant) shapes. With poor presentifying we are limited to those massive summations of many repetitions we call conditioning, or trial-and-error learning. The oft-repeated routines are available, but not complex schemata with meanings.

With the same cerebral cortex and the same set of old traces, even the normal person's capacity to insert his will effectively into a challenging field fluctuates widely; at times a man's present schemata will make him sensitive to remote consequences, dynamically in touch with a wide field; at other times he is restricted to an immediate present, under the dominance of some spontaneous but pressing motive, some external invitation or pressure.

These reversible functional changes mingle with the effects of irreversible organic changes in the amnestic syndrome and make the testing of the powers of the patient a difficult process. In addition there are "modes of approach to a problem" and ways of defining a situation, as we shall see in the section which follows, that determine whether a patient can perform, or not. Where an "abstract approach" (to use Goldstein's language) is required, the brain-injured seem especially handicapped, even though the part-responses seem to be intact.

LOSS OF THE ABSTRACT ATTITUDE

It is difficult to compress into a brief space all the meanings that Goldstein (1952) intends when he describes the brain-injured as tending to behave in concrete fashion, as lacking the capacity to perform abstractly. It is even more difficult to devise tests that will quantify this change, especially foolproof tests, for it is quite apparent that an observer must possess both insight and imagination that can quickly seize on the principle at work in a patient's performances.

This loss of the abstract (or categorical) attitude was especially apparent in the performance of those with frontal-lobe injuries, and at one phase in his work it seemed that he was about to propose a series of tests that would determine whether brain pathology was confined principally to the frontal lobe or not. As time has elapsed, this defect has been found in connection with Korsakoff's psychosis, general paresis, senile changes, chronic alcoholism, and tumors that also produce aphasia. It is also found in the feebleminded and in the uneducated, although in the latter case this product of poor training can be overcome. In those with extensive brain damage, the defect, Goldstein believes, is a capacity defect, irremediable and absolute.

It appears, therefore, that Goldstein is describing a lower form of brain functioning that may be expected, whatever the location or nature of the pathology, if the damage is extensive enough to produce a general impairment. Whether the loss of the abstract attitude also entails a general change in the personality is a question that has stirred a great deal of semantic dust. The reader can best decide this matter for himself when Goldstein's observations (and their interpretations) are laid before him.

In one place, Goldstein (1952, p. 248) attempted to compress his meaning into a concrete example, speaking first in parable and then attempting to abstract the principle:

"We act concretely when we enter a room in darkness and push the button for light. If, however, we reflect that by pushing the button we might awaken someone asleep in the room, and desist from pushing the button, then we are acting abstractively. We transcend the immediately given specific aspect of sense impressions; we detach ourselves from these impressions, consider the situation from a conceptual point of view, and react accordingly. Our actions are determined not so much by the objects before us as by the way we think about them: the individual thing becomes a mere accidental representative of a category to which it belongs."

Others have noted a similar quality of unthinking impulsiveness in the brain-injured. Watts and Freeman describe the patient (after lobotomy) who sees the sign in the hospital corridor and reacts almost reflexly. "Pull in case of fire" was not a signal for a discriminative choice reaction. The patient did not read the fine print, did not allow the impulse to elaborate; there was no kink in the reaction chain in which impulses could be elaborated before they released action. Others like to describe such action as automatic or stimulus-bound. The facts suggest that, in these patients, stimulating situations arouse immediate, unreflective actions instead of roundabout, deliberate, reflective action fitted to a wider field.

Goldstein evidently considers that "pause to reflect" to be an opportunity for logic to be applied, for the setting to be placed in its proper category (ideally *sub specie aeternitatis*), and for proper deductions to be made. The social creature, scenting criticism, uses the interval to search out an appropriate rationalization or justification (the new auto must be purchased for no selfish whim, but for the sake of the family's needs or the health of a wife). The "appeal to reason" seeks out a description that all right-thinking men can understand, or, let us say, all who share an ideology or a religious faith. For whatever reason the appeal to remote things is made and the second thought allowed to develop prior to action, this elaboration does not occur in impulsive children, in psychopaths, in the brain-injured, in those under the influence of alcohol or drugs. (Amusingly, we call the effects of some drugs "mind-expanding," whereas, in fact, the area of concern is restricted.) Speaking simply, bluntly, unmindful of host or guests present, the lobotomy patient shows a deficit that, Goldstein believes, arises from his need to act concretely, immediately, habitually, automatically, rigidly.

Developed into a philosophy of conduct he has expounded at length in many volumes (see Bibliography), Goldstein's meanings are most precisely indicated by the specific test performances that he and his pupils have described in detail. Like the brain-injured patient, we seem to want to know what happens, concretely, in these lower-order actions so common among all brain-injured patients. Out of a much longer list of "traits," Goldstein and Scheerer (1941) selected eight for testing. It will be noted that some of the trait names are provocative and ambitious, suggesting such knotty problems that testing itself must be "put to a test."

Eight Traits That Define the Loss

The patient fails to detach his ego from the outer world, or from his own private experience.

The statement of this trait implies an understanding of the development of attention in the child. Once upon a time, this view runs, we were all so fused with our environment that self and not-self were as yet undiscriminated. (The child's toe and the bars of his crib have an equal status at this point.) Even the adult can be imperfectly detached, as he shows when he projects. He knows the boundaries of his body; he can differentiate between his own stomachache and the effect of a blow that was aimed at his solar plexus from without; and he differentiates between the threatening object and his own anxiety (usually). But when he reads into the passive face of his interlocutor an aggressive intent that is actually rooted in his own hostility, it is apparent that the discrimination process is not working well. Social workers who use their own normal brains in dealing with clients in riot-torn areas of conflict have trouble keeping objective and subjective events apart, their own egos separate from the events which disturb them.

Goldstein and Scheerer are hitting at something more primitive, a much more pervasive defect. They describe a patient who cannot take a comb from the table and bring it to the examiner, on command, without pausing to comb her hair. (A comb? It is something you run through your hair. What to do? Pick it up and pass it through your hair. This is a concrete way of knowing, similar to a child's definition: e.g., a sword is what you stick into somebody.) Either she does not hear well, or cannot break up a concrete habit chain and redesign it for the present occasion. Stimulated by a part of a verbal-auditory stimulus pattern rather than by a reading of the experimenter's intention, she failed to trim away the adventitious parts of this agglutinated reaction. Such a cluttering-up of action with old routines corrupts the patient's behavior, mars the conversation of the senile (who begans his remark with "I always say ..." and is easily distracted from the topic being developed by his interlocutor), just as we sometimes see it mar the behavior of the normal.

Asked to repeat the sentence, "The snow is white," the patient does well enough, but he balks when asked to say, "The snow is black." This is senseless, contrary to the facts, and he is as unwilling to perform in this fashion as the person who cannot assume a certain role in a play (because that is just not the way a man should act). The patient finds it difficult to pretend, to merely imitate an action, such as drinking from a cup, when the action cannot be done concretely and completely (i.e., when the cup is empty, when he is just making a demonstration).

Piaget once noted a similar difficulty in some of the very young children he studied. He, too, describes an "egocentric" form of understanding. To the child who knows full well what a brother is (he has one) and what a son is (is this not the name his mother gives him?), it is nonetheless difficult when he is required to understand the usage when he is the brother of a brother and when others are also addressed as his mother's son: "I am not a brother, I am me; I am mother's son, not he." He has not arrived at the point of using an "outside map" of these relationships. He is not yet decentered, objective, viewing the family relationships from outside.

If the brain-injured return to this simpler form of understanding, it is not to be understood as a regression so much as a simplification, as a descent to a level that is still possible. Goldstein and Scheerer add the warning: it is not mere simplicity of an action, for many of the concrete performances of the brain-injured are complex enough. The old lawyer in Cozzens' *By Love Possessed,* who is at home and can function among legal technicalities that would stump a beginner, but is in other ways suspected of growing senile, could have been drawn from life. The tester must be on guard in planning test materials.

We might remind ourselves, also, that a decentering and recentering of life, such as the Communists aimed at in their brainwashing techniques, is not an easy matter for the well-socialized person. We can recall this stubborn concreteness, too, as we watch the deliberations of the Security Council on television. From kindergarten child to diplomat, the trail of the deficit can be followed. The brain-injured, we might note, are human, all too human, with slightly more of this trait than the normal shows.

The patient cannot assume a mental set voluntarily, consciously.

Acting out a command, imitating, pretending, demonstrating also require this "detachment of the ego." The patient can read the time from the face of the clock but is puzzled as to how to proceed when asked to set the hands so that they designate some arbitrary hour. He can count or write when he is set to work on these tasks by the examiner; assuming the counting attitude on command or in imitation of another is something else. He can name the months seriatim but is stumped by "What month comes before June?" He cannot search fore and aft on some internal calendar, so to speak. He does not scan his memories to pick out the relevant one that would fit the present scene, which needs to be analyzed according to many categories.

The patient cannot give an account of his acts to himself or to others.

Although the patient can act (when properly started on an action and fully supported by stimuli), he cannot represent an action, think about it, communicate an account of it to others. He would be a poor man to post as an observer. He reminds us, again, that to live through an experience and to make a history of it are two different actions; to repeat a conditioned response or run through an action learned by trial and error is different from the communicable understanding of what was done. Asked to throw balls into boxes placed at varying distances, the patient does well enough, but he cannot give an account of the spatial arrangement (or the sequence of his localizations). His actions are not converted into any describable time-space map. The patient's inability to put into words what he can do (mix paints, point to, knit, or whatever) makes him seem aphasic, but he has no difficulty in hearing or speaking, per se. Let him use the speech mechanism concretely and the absence of any articulation defect will be evident.

The patient cannot shift reflectively from one aspect of the situation to another.

The brain-injured patient behaves as though limited to a single "set" for each setting. He finds it difficult to shift gears, and is left behind as conversation shifts quickly to a new topic. He can keep two things in mind if they "go together" as parts of a familiar sequence, but a series of arbitrarily selected acts, particularly a series that includes conditional action, is too difficult (if A happens, do B, and if X happens, do C, but if Y happens, avoid doing either and do Z). Head devised such tests for his aphasics, some of whom could speak and hear, but could not obey when directed: "Put your hand over your mouth and close your eyes; put your right hand on your left ear." These are difficult for some brain-injured patients who have no other evidence of aphasia (unless we devise a special name for it: amnestic aphasia, a Goldstein-type aphasia).

The performance of the brain-injured, interrupted by some distraction, is not easily resumed. (He is like the board member who rambles in his discourse and then, suddenly, has to ask his neighbor, "Now, where was I?" Too many performances of this type and the board member will be suspected of advancing senility.)

Goldstein and Scheerer note that shifts in ambiguous figures (such as the vase figure of Rubin, which is also a pair of profiles) do not occur as in the normal. The teacher of experimental psychology will point out that in any class of thirty there are one or two who have difficulty in appreciating these alternating figures. Again, the stickiness and lack of flexibility in perceiving is a factor that has many degrees and affects the normal as well as the brain-injured. The observer may note that this factor is not quite like other cases in which a shift in set is "reflective" or "voluntary." It is as though certain reflex possibilities had been passed over and never exercised, and had remained concealed behind some use-and-wont facade of habits.

The patient cannot hold in mind simultaneously several aspects of a situation.

Simple reactions are managed; choice reactions are more difficult. On the other hand, where a task requires a fairly prolonged retention of a directing set, the patient may lose his way, either shifting to another task or stopping when his task is unfinished. Even more difficult is a task such as fitting a piece into a feature profile while watching to see that not only the shape, but the lines on the piece, fit the profile and its lines. Variations in the lines can throw the patient off, although he has been asked to disregard them and watch only the shape. Thus Goldstein and Scheerer seem to have found both hypertrophied and subnormal forms of rigidity-flexibility.

The patient cannot grasp the essential of a given whole, or break up a given whole into parts, or isolate the parts and then resynthesize them to fit a fresh insight.

Here again we are dealing with a level of organization that is difficult for the child, the uneducated, the person with subnormal intelligence. The patient hears the words of the story, and misses the point, even when he can retell it in a concrete fashion. He sees all parts of the cartoon, but it is somehow "over his head." Losing his way among details, his storage of experience is also defective.

In any act of serial synthesis, as when the pieces of a comic strip are exposed serially and have to be stored and fitted together before the "message" pops out, or as when the bits of a line drawing of a familiar object are seen separately and the subject is asked to name the object, the fusion is something more and other than the act of perceiving the parts. The *aha* moment as the Gestaltists call it, is a common experience, and striking. A subject, allowed to peer through a tube and to move the far end so that an aperture traces the outline of a familiar object, may learn to operate this visual maze with increasing facility. He learns his way about the figure. Even when he feels familiar enough with the sequence of turns to attempt to draw the outline, he may not tumble to the fact that he is drawing the outline of a wooden shoe until it is almost complete, so that he can see all parts simultaneously. Difficult enough for the normal adult, it is more so for the brain-injured. The latter can see many figures (e.g., the cartoon) with all parts in view and still miss the essence, the insight which gives meaning.

The patient cannot abstract common properties reflectively.

The patient may be asked to classify skeins of yarn of every color and tint, according to a sample, or according to a named category. Finding all the reds is a task that sets the patient on a search for skeins that are identical with the sample handed to him. He may give the colors that do not go together concrete names: strawberry rose, violet, jade mist, Egyptian gold, wood-moss, frosted honey. The more precise the comparison object, the more he is sure there is none other like it: his names isolate rather than unite with a row of similars.

This suggests that events are discrete in an unusual degree. Yet there are concrete ways in which objects go together: asked to group an assortment of objects, he will place a knife and a plug of chewing tobacco together, or a match and cigarette. He overlooks such categories as all wooden objects, all long objects, all metal objects. Shown one of these categories, he responds: "They just do not go together." What Goldstein calls the "categorical attitude" has a way of uniting most diverse objects, of suggesting "similars" that have never been seen or used together. Thus, instead of seeing many diverse possible essences, ways of classifying objects and of finding uses for unusual "means objects," the brain-injured are stuck in concrete usages.

Normal human beings with intact brains may also function far below their category-making potential. The tester must be wary lest he be misled by a performance due to special interests of the patient, a lack of discrimination training, or a cultural trap that has insisted on one way of diagnosing settings. Even the type of instruction makes a difference. Told merely to classify the skeins of colored wool, he may stand confused. But when he is instructed to "pick out all of the reds and put them there," or is given a sample of classifying to follow, he may continue. These brain-injured patients, like children, seem to prefer full instructions, outside regulation that is complete. Too free a design of testing gives them difficulties, and, besides confusion, they may experience suspicion as to the tester's intent. Like the intelligence tests for adult patients, which have to be standardized against performance of similar adults (for age, education, socioeconomic status, and so on), these tests of abstraction have to take into account the probable status of the patient before brain pathology developed.

The patient has difficulty in planning ahead.

As illustration Goldstein speaks of the patient who can easily find his way about the ward and into other rooms (and floors) of the hospital, but who carries no "inside map" of this field. He cannot draw the spatial design that would represent it; and if he is interrupted in the course of traveling from his ward down to the floor where occupational therapy goes on, he may become "lost." He is like the motorist who learns his way about a new territory by street signs but has no sense of direction, no cognitive map.

The ball-and-field test that Binet used gives these patients difficulty, as it sometimes does the child with a mental age of less than ten years. The difficulty is similar to the one the patient shows when he is asked to demonstrate how to use a key when there is no lock or door. (An earlier psychology would have spoken of a loss of motor images.)

In short, the mind of the patient does not rush ahead. He is the very opposite of the man with a "blown-up brush heap of the imagination" who never can take the situation before him at its first intention, but has to test a variety of hypotheses before moving. Sometimes the normal mind suffers from an excess of plans: he sees heroes and sunset deaths, knights and their Guineveres, spies and plotters, until not only are things not what they seem, but he cannot act simply and directly. We say, "Oh bosh! If these cloud-minded dreamers would only come down to earth and learn to react to things as they are, to the possible and the probable, they would be more effective." The brain-injured patient stands at the concrete end of this continuum. He is bound to a simpler and much more stable reality; in fact he may not be prepared for the variety and change that real existence offers, and so a hospital environment is required.

A Summary

Goldstein has made numerous attempts to compress all these behavioral facts into one statement that will symbolize their essence. One who cannot make such a last step sometimes feels a little like the "concrete-minded" patient, with a string of particular acts whose essence is not yet grasped. On one occasion he wrote of this group of patients:

"They are changed with respect to the most characteristic properties of the human being. They have lost initiative and the capacity to look forward to something and to make plans and decisions; they lack phantasy and inspiration; their perceptions, thoughts, and ideas are reduced; they have lost the capacity for real contact with others, and they are therefore incapable of real friendship, love, and social relations. One could say that they have no real ego and no real world. That they behave in an abnormally concrete way and that they are driven to get rid of tensions are only expressions of the same defect. . . . they are abnormally rigid, stereotyped, and compulsive, and abnormally bound to stimuli from without and within."

Again, to emphasize the generality of this "Goldstein syndrome," these changes have been identified in the thinking of schizophrenics and of patients suffering from alcoholism, hypoglycaemia, arteriosclerosis, general paresis, Pick's disease, concussion, carbon-monoxide poisoning, and diffuse cortical injuries. It has not been possible to present any statistical analyses of the extent of lesions or the locations of injuries. The test scores on the batteries of tests used by Goldstein and his pupils show the deficit varying along a continuum (with some "normal controls" also performing at the level of patients with known brain injuries). The mere statistical summary of scores, Goldstein feels, with the mere summary of successes and failures, is not as important as the analysis of the manner of solving problems, the quality of the behavior. Although it does injustice to the richness and the imaginative quality of Goldstein's thinking, it may help us to grasp his concept if we compress his major conclusions into a brief list.

1. Brain injuries produce four types of defect. The first type is "near effects," losses that depend on the location of the injury and produce negative symptoms. The patient may not hear, see, smell, taste, or make the movements expected. Such "near effects" may destroy the "instrumentalities of speech," as in motor or sensory aphasia, where the articulation of speech sounds or the perception of the spoken word is faulty.

2. In the second type he may suffer from what we might call "catastrophic behavior." This arises each time his task requires him to go beyond the level at which he can operate and while he still retains enough of his capacities to anticipate disaster.

3. In the third type he develops a variety of techniques for avoiding these disorganized states and of defending himself against demands with which he cannot cope, still struggling to make the most of his impaired equipment.

4. In the fourth type a complex set of changes appears which amounts to a personality change, a new method of approaching reality:

a. The patient tends to take each separate situation concretely, and in both spatial and temporal isolation. From the onlooker's point of view, he does not grasp the situation as a whole, for his approach excludes a great deal from this simplified grasp. Within this isolated concrete grasp he can operate successfully, even performing complicated concatenations of movement, finding his way about the hospital and performing skills that are well-learned.

b. The patient does not abstract from the totality "essences" which suggest a number of similars, nor does he make new organizations easily. The spatial schemata that the normal person constructs are replaced by what Tolman once called "strip maps." These strips are fragile and do not reach far ahead. He does not cumulate a pattern of actions just passed through, nor does he relocate himself when introduced into the middle of one of these strips. Like the child with rote memory of a poem, he has to go back to the beginning, once he gets lost. He is a creature, therefore, of the here and now.

c. The storage of traces, involved in any delayed responses and in any construction of a history of what he has lived through, is so difficult that he is forced to react to an immediately present and visible field. He does not project a distant future, and he has difficulty in representing his past (and in preventing it from intruding upon his present constructions, fusing with them). He can betray the effect of a past when he does not remember it as the normal person does.

d. He is highly distractible at times, and stubbornly persistent at others (when more flexibility is required). Where he is in the midst of a familiar routine, he clings to it stubbornly, almost as though it were a zone of safety.

e. He requires more of a supporting situation than the normal: he cannot demonstrate, act out, imitate (especially when the action is related to another, remote field). When he is able to live in a stable and simplified environment (with a capable "organizer" by his side), he functions best, and he remains placid and easy to manage under conditions that might bore a normal person. Sudden shifts in his surroundings fill him with anxiety and with a catastrophic sense of impending disorganization (a behavioral abyss), and make him irritable and emotional: he feels threatened.

f. Living in the present moment, he forgets absent ones. His way of "relating" to the latter may make him seem calloused and indifferent. Returned to the heart of his family, he behaves with normal responsiveness.

g. Immersed in his restricted field, he finds it all but impossible to take an objective look at himself or his situation. This "inability to separate the ego from an outer world or from its present needs" makes his activity an expression of "animal training" rather than a function of imagination and reasoning.

h. This immersion in the present moment also goes with an extreme egocentrism, and it creates difficulties in his relationship with and understanding of those about him. It also makes him quick to use all tension-reducing mechanisms; he is less able to tolerate frustrations in view of goals.

APHASIA

The clinical facts associated with the aphasias are difficult to classify. The location and extent of the lesions have a way of disregarding the aims of the theoretician. There are few studies that have had adequate anatomical studies at postmortem, and still fewer with normal control subjects studied in comparable fashion. Since Broca's identification of a region in the motor area (third frontal convolution in front of the fissure of Rolando, on the left side in the right-handed), published in 1861, our notions of brain functioning have changed; the localizationists have departed from the almost phrenological conceptions that ruled in the early part of the last century, and more than a century of neuroanatomical and behavioral studies has added a mass of evidence that makes the modern clinician wary of all certitude. Weisenberg and McBride (1935) confess: "even today, more than seventy years after the time of Broca, we are almost as far away from the solution of cerebral localization of aphasia."

A few clinicians have been inclined to look at some of the disturbances classified as aphasia as due to a disturbed functioning of the brain as a whole. They interpret the speech changes as the result of defective insight, a poor grasp of meanings, an inability to "propositionize." Others continue to look for defects in specific part-mechanisms located in specific portions of the brain, with specific connections for each phoneme received or each syllable stroke produced. While few of the holists have been ready to go as far as Karl Lashley, with his notion of an equipotential cortex, there is a tendency among these interpreters to look at the various types of speech disturbance as due to lesions of greater or lesser extent. Their classifications suggest a hierarchy of language disturbances, in which a semantic aphasia would be placed at the top. In this type there is a loss of the more complex meanings and a certain difficulty in the more complex ways of speaking; the lesions are believed to be slight and diffuse. At the bottom of the hierarchy, these holists would place the restricted losses of sensory and motor function which affect the "instrumentalities of language" and which spare the more complex forms of thinking and perceiving. (The specific motor losses are located in the forward portion of the brain, where Broca first discovered a motor center for speech, and the specific sensory losses are typically in the posterior brain.)

There is no possibility of our reviewing and critically evaluating the mass of literature bearing on this complex subject. One study will have to serve for the many, but it is one of the more careful ones and can serve as a model to show the nature of the problem.

The study of Weisenberg and McBride extended over a period of six years (1929-1935) and involved a detailed examination of 234 patients. A rather exhaustive battery of psychological tests was employed, some of which were devised especially for aphasic patients.[15] Sixty of those studied were clear-cut cases of aphasia, free from complications that might obscure the findings. Control nonaphasics were also tested. (The authors had discovered that some medical students, given Head's tests, performed as did aphasics.)

THE NATURE OF THE DISORDER

Weisenberg and McBride believe that the term *aphasia* should be used to designate "a variety of psychological changes occurring with a unilateral cerebral lesion and appearing chiefly but not altogether in language processes." The presence of nonlanguage changes should not lead to an unnecessary extension of the meaning of this term; the many nonlanguage phenomena that are found in any extended series of cases, including changes in general intelligence and in the capacity for abstract thinking, are not an essential part of the *aphasic* changes but simply flow from the fact that lesions which cause aphasia are often diffuse and extensive. At times the disturbance is sharply confined to language performances; within this area, the different spheres of reading, writing, speaking, and understanding do not undergo changes *en masse* but vary enormously from patient to patient, being sharply localized in some and more widespread in others. When any extended series of brain-injured cases is examined, there will be those whose loss seems to involve a change in general intelligence, with the simple and direct forms

---

[15]The tests are fully described in Weisenberg and McBride 1935. They include measures of speaking, naming, repeating words, understanding spoken language, reading, writing, arithmetic, controlled associations, sentence completion, absurdities, vocabulary, formboards, imitation, and drawing.

of expression and understanding of speech little changed. That such a change in general intelligence is not a universal accompaniment is shown by the fact that many of these patients are able to succeed as well as the normal group (of similar educational and socioeconomic background) in test performances that do not depend directly on language.

Weisenberg does not believe that it is fruitful to classify patients into groups according to the part-functions of reading, writing, speaking, hearing (as the localizationists and diagram-makers do). The *pure* types of defect are rarely found. In his own series he described four types: (1) those with predominantly expressive changes; (2) those with a predominately receptive impairment; (3) a mixed group of expressive-receptive changes; and (4) an amnesic type that comprised less than a tenth of his cases. The frequencies of the types show that the expressive deficit is the most common (43.3 per cent); it is followed by the receptive (28.3 per cent); the expressive-receptive impairment occurs in 20 per cent.

The Expressive Type

In his 60 cases, studied intensively, Weisenberg found none that was a *pure* case of expressive disorder. Some slight impairment in understanding usually appeared with careful testing: the substance of a statement might be repeated, with difficulty, but in such a way as to show a lack of understanding; the absurdities test would be missed or the significance of some verbal direction; or failures on the Stanford-Binet Vocabulary Test would show that the patient's ability to recognize words was involved. Performance in nonlanguage tests and in practical social behavior indicated that the deficiencies did not depend on changes in intelligence but were manifestations of the aphasic disorder.

The expressive group has some resemblance to the group originally described by Broca, with the defect primarily in articulation. In the more severe cases the patient is limited to a few words. The more emotionally charged expressions tend to persist, as well as the more highly automatized reactions (such as his own name and address). Counting, the days of the week, "Hello," "Goodbye," can be managed, and many speech responses appear when the appropriate setting calls for them, even though they cannot be produced on command, or when an action needs to be described.

Speech is slow, monotonous, lacking in normal accent and inflection, words are slurred, and frequent substitutions (Homus for Thomas, hasket for basket, jair for chair, brints for bridge) appear. Some patients show a tendency to use a single expression on all occasions. Commonly the patient recognizes his errors and attempts to correct them. He can spell the word aloud, at times, when he cannot say it. However, in the expressive series there are all degrees of recognition: sometimes it is spontaneous; sometimes a form can be selected from a series of alternatives presented; and occasionally there is no recognition at all. In the latter case a garbled form of expression nonetheless seems to carry a correct meaning for the subject. Oral reading is less affected.

Writing disturbances commonly parallel those in speaking, but they may also vary independently. Simplification in sentence structure is common, and omissions, halting speech, and a lapse into a "telegram style" are observable in the cases with more severe brain damage.

A test designed to reveal the aphasic's grasp of relations, such as the analogies test ("Rain is to summer as snow is to _____.") proves to be difficult, even though the patient seems to understand vaguely what is expected of him and can give the meaning of the separate words. Sentence completion also gives him difficulty. Word *patterns* (and the meaningful relationships they symbolize) are difficult to grasp; here the performance of the patient falls below his nonlanguage performance (which also sometimes suffers), as well as below the performance of a comparable group of normal subjects.

Weisenberg's expressive type resembles a *verbal* type of aphasia earlier identified by Head. As in Head's group there are some difficulties in the reception as well as in the production of speech, although the defect is more apparent on the expressive side, and the patient often recognizes his errors. Wide fluctuations in the patient's performance (as between emotional, automatic, reactive, and voluntary propositionizing) argue against the loss of specific sensorimotor speech movements or the loss of "images of words."

The Receptive Type

In this type the expressive function remains at or near normal level. The characteristic speech is rapid, often at a rate above normal. Difficulties in articulation do not retard their speaking, and, at a distance, the speech sounds normal, with natural inflection, rhythm, emphasis.

Writing disturbances parallel those in speaking, but are less severe. There are difficulties in word *order* (rather than in word *form*), and circumlocutions abound ("animal of the circus" for elephant). Sentence completion is called "sentences vacant of completeness." Grammatical confusion is common, word order is changed, and speech is full of neologisms: one patient is "actuated" (stimulated), and another is "refined to his bedroom." These slips are often allowed to pass as though unnoticed, as though the meaning had been communicated. There seems to be no close relation between the awareness of these defects and intelligence (or the severity of the disturbance).

Weisenberg lists typical phrases used by his "receptives":

The dinner was enjoyed by me;
I have trees of apples in my yard;
I drove up the long side of a car;
I think I must have done it over a little bit because I can't read
    this morning;
at the day in its morning;
I trust I am now learning to do my best to secure the ideas
    to put myself carefully to operate the item to me which was
    seemingly away when needed so much by me.

If we were to describe this as a regression in speech, it is obviously not a change toward any simpler childhood level. Tests of intelligence which involve language items reveal an impaired performance, but, unlike the expressive's halting responses, the receptive gives a response (possibly confused) or none at all. Perseveration is common, the answer to one question showing up in subsequent responses. The nonlanguage tests are superior to those involving language and vary independently of the disorder. The general social adjustment of this group was extremely varied, a few showing pronounced and persistent emotional disturbances, others making a satisfactory adjustment.

The Expressive-Receptive Type

This group shows a mixture of the two forms just described and appears to be more severely damaged in both expression and reception. Expression in writing, Weisenberg found, was superior to that in speaking, even in those patients who had not been skilled in writing before the disorder. This group also tended to show more general deterioration, affecting nonlanguage performances as well. The patients' everyday habits of eating, dressing, and so on seemed superior to what one would expect from some of their language and nonlanguage test performances. A few of these patients showed the labored and difficult speech of the expressive type, while others (seriously limited to a sentence or two of automatic character) would use their limited equipment with "ease and freedom."

The Amnesic Aphasic

A much more sharply delimited impairment appears in this relatively rare type of aphasia. The patient has difficulty in evoking names, whether for objects, persons, conditions, or qualities. His articulation is free enough and effortless, but his difficulty restricts the patient to the more automatic, colloquial, familiar, emotional expressions. Names which he cannot use in voluntary speech may appear in automatic series. While he can count, he cannot name the number of objects exposed before him, nor can he name the day of the week without resorting to the automatic naming, during which he can halt at the correct word. Thus his recognition outstrips his voluntary usage of words, his word *finding*. There is little grammatical confusion, and his understanding and reading comprehension are disturbed but little, if at all.

The name-finding difficulty appears in both speaking and writing, and there is difficulty in repeating sentences, for the names heard and understood are not well-retained. His appreciation of the meaning seems superior to his ability to retain or use the names in the phrases and sentences.

Language tests, such as the one which involves finding antonyms, are particularly difficult. Performance in the nonlanguage tests is less impaired. The person who has enjoyed the fruits of a good education, has had a good vocabulary, and is accustomed to use fluent speech will appear to be markedly damaged by this defect. His general behavior will show little disturbance.

His habits, other than the verbal ones, his interests, and his general social attitudes may remain relatively unchanged. Games and illustrated magazines are enjoyed.

WEISENBERG'S FINDINGS

It is apparent that new studies with new tools will continue to produce new classifications in the data and new theoretical emphases. Improvements in tests for aphasics give precision to the descriptions of individual cases, but do not always produce sharply defined categories that correspond to any behavioral or physiological theory. Weisenberg's findings are more in the tradition of Head and Hughlings Jackson than in that of the diagram-makers. His conclusions may be summarized briefly in the following seven points:

1. Aphasia is not simply a disorder in representing objects and actions verbally, or in understanding such verbal representations. There are defects in nonlanguage processes in some patients, and when test performance depends on word usage and understanding, there is a defect in measured intelligence. (A university professor could not tell what was wrong with the picture of a telephone with two receivers.)

2. There does not appear to be a single, fundamental, essential defect that is found in all the cases of any extended series. Diversity is the objective finding. One patient will have difficulties in all tests that involve verbalizing; another will show inability to think and act spatially; a third is amnesic (having difficulty with names); another can write much better than he can speak; another understands well but cannot articulate. Save for the fact that the deficits touch the language-communication area, our diagnostic term has little specific implication.

3. There is sometimes a change in social behavior, but not always, as some have urged. It does, of course, force new adjustments, but these vary with the nature and severity of the defect. The surprising fact is that a very limited change in the social personality can exist beside a marked aphasia.

4. While many of the changes seem regressive, the term is not very useful, for the defect in no wise carries the individual back to earlier and simpler levels of speech. The amnesic searching for a word is quite unlike the child who has not learned the word or the discriminative behavior it represents. Social attitudes and nonverbal skills do not regress correspondingly.

5. Similarly, the preservation of the automatic and emotional components can be overemphasized. Although in general, it is the older, simpler, more automatic, more highly charged (emotionally), more passive (reactive) that is preserved, while the voluntary, novel, and complex falter, there are too many exceptions to this general rule. Complex forms may be preserved; simpler and older forms may be damaged. Thus there are lines of cleavage in these disturbances which affect language more than nonlanguage responses and which skip over some of the recent and complex patterns to strike at early and automatic forms of speech.

6. The general defect in intelligence stressed by Goldstein, and the loss of such modes of thinking as abstract or categorical procedures, was not found

in many of the Weisenberg series. What intellectual loss occurs tends to affect specific performances in which language functions, but the language defects are specific: where it is a defect in articulation, the general intellectual change tends to be slightest; in the more severe expressive-receptive cases, the deficiency in intelligence is apt to be marked. It is possible that language usage has penetrated the structure of action more completely in some patients than in others, and in these instances the change in behavior is apt to be more marked. Weisenberg does not find, however, any clear-cut relationship between the gravity of language defect and the amount of intellectual loss. Weisenberg thus veers away from two extremes: the disorder is not limited to defects in language (in many cases); it may be so confined to the speech process (in others) that no general intellectual defect is discernible (by the tests).

7. Finally, the question of localization has to be dismissed, briefly, as a clinical opinion, for Weisenberg reports only three necropsies on his sixty cases studied intensively. Head's data also lacked the requisite postmortem examinations. We do not know precisely what has happened to these brains. Damage which *seems* to be local sometimes produces pervasive disorders, and damage known to be pervasive may also produce sharply defined losses. In one of Weisenberg's *amnesic* cases (the sharply defined form resembling Head's *nominal* aphasia) the damage was extensive (an astrocystoma that implicated almost half of the left cerebral hemisphere). Another case classified as receptive had a sharply localized scar over Broca's area.

In spite of the dearth of evidence, Weisenberg concludes that most lesions fall in the dominant hemisphere (the left cerebrum in right-handed persons), in the anterior portion in the cases classed as expressive, in the posterior portion in cases classed as receptive. Yet in the cases studied Weisenberg thinks it probable that both anterior and posterior portions were affected in some degree, the differences in behavior indicating the difference in degree to which each portion is involved. (Thus the Broca-Wernicke distinctions with which the study of aphasia started tend to persist, without benefit of adequate evidence.)

The advances in neurophysiology have done much to locate the damage responsible for losses in vision, hearing, smell, taste, and in the motor control of specific muscle masses, but the problem of where to locate the damage responsible for either the understanding or expression of speech remains obscure. There may be reason in the arguments of the holistically minded clinicians who think of these more complex "unities" as involving the brain as a whole, even if the involvement varies with the different clinical types. The emphasis of Jackson may also still be germane: it is the functioning of the structures which remain that accounts for the speech and understanding of the aphasic, not the locus damaged. The three-legged dog has a gait that is not simply that of a four-legged dog minus the missing sensorimotor pattern. Thus a local injury will have both local and general consequences, the latter offering greater problems to the tester.

EPILOG

Looking back at the opening paragraphs of this chapter in the light of the evidence we have reviewed, one might conclude that neither the localizationists nor those who believe in equipotentiality and vicarious functioning have been the victors. The notion of a psychophysical parallelism which has guided research is incompletely demonstrated: there are small injuries that produce massive effects and large lesions with negligible consequences. Enough has been achieved, however, to draw a tentative map of functions even if it must contain many silent areas and fail to locate some of the more complex functions.

Proceeding from small and precisely located lesions and continuing to the more pervasive and massive brain changes, we have, in effect, shown the truth in both views. Goldstein's "near effects" which alter what he calls the "instrumentalities of language," on the one hand, and his "loss of the categorical attitude" which does not seem to be associated with any precise lesion, offer examples. Modeste's parietal lesion and the amnestic syndrome indicate the two extreme types; the aphasic patient often shows both the "near effects" and the more widespread changes in mental functioning.

We have also discovered that the "near effects," the precise sensorimotor losses, are much more easily tested than those pervasive results of brain damage. Not only are the latter changes revealed in a change in *quality* of response, in the *manner* of approaching tasks, rather than in precise scores on very specific successes and failures, but they are found to overlap similar defects in controls who have no known injury: the schizophrenic, the uneducated, and the person of less than normal intelligence also behave in this so-called concrete fashion. We can understand what patient study and what an effort at standardizing these tests will be required, if they are to be used in appraisal of brain damage or in estimation of recovery from, say, carbon-monoxide poisoning.

In addition to the direct and immediate effects of brain damage, the clinician must consider the reaction of the person to his impairment; the evidence suggests that it is in helping the person reshape his reactions, in helping the family understand the nature of the defect, and in arranging conditions so that the person can function as well as possible, rather than in trying to restore damaged functions, that the clinician can help most. By and large the gains through reeducation and vicarious functioning which Lashley was able to produce in his experimental animals are not matched by human recoveries. Recoveries there are: the amnestic victim of alcoholism or of carbon-monoxide poisoning may surprise his physician and demonstrate that what the latter viewed as an irreversible change (destruction of cells) was a passing physiological state that damaged the functioning of the brain as a whole. When the brain resumes its normal functioning, the mental processes are restored.

The wide fluctuations in the performance of a single patient show that the damaged brain is in as much need of good hygiene, both mental and physical, as the normal, and perhaps more so, for any damage to this most complex twelve-billion-cell network reduces that margin where stress can be tolerated, and errors perceived and corrected.

We can learn much about human behavior from those with brain damage. Their behavior shocks us into a realization of the shortcomings of some of the thought models we have been using. A surprisingly large residue of automatic actions is left in a patient like Courbon's old lady or Brickner's Mr. A., yet they are "imitation people." Courbon's nondemented presbyophrenic knew her categories but identified no one, preserved an old social attitude but could not remember what had happened yesterday. Mr. A. still talked the language of the cotton exchange and pretended to be about to resume his profession, yet could neither project a real future nor act on it. The imaginative and purposive person who can plan possible actions suitable to his needs and then act upon them is, in effect, dead. The mechanical shell of automatisms can be as deceptive as the skillfully posed figures in a waxworks museum. Had our thought models been capable of reminding us of all that brain lesions could alter, perhaps we should not have been as willing to embark on psychosurgery. If more of our contemporaries were familiar with the nature of the ecstatic's aura (associated with epilepsy), there would be fewer who seek to escape from their limitations by using drugs which also produce sometimes a temporary and sometimes a permanent brain damage (along with psychedelic "trips").

Finally, the study of damaged brains has prepared us to look at two pervasive and sometimes chronic psychotic changes, and to examine the physiological-anatomical hypotheses which attempt to account for them.

Chapter 10 • The Affective Psychoses

There are depressions and elations that sweep the individual out of reach of ordinary help. The emotions are not merely more intense but have undergone qualitative changes; instead of being responses to the common frustrations and successes of everyday living, some of them are so inappropriate or unjustified that clinicians are apt to attribute them to endogenous causes, to changes within the tissues that are, to this day, obscure in locus and in nature.

These affective changes are accompanied by changes in perception and action, in thinking and belief, so that we are dealing with a total change in the functioning of the person. Rarely, he is deluded and hallucinated; occasionally he is suicidal; and sometimes he is so filled with "the power and the glory" that he seems to be playing God. Usually these patients have to be hospitalized to protect them and those about them from the consequences of their acts, and to save the family from scandal, embarrassment, and possible ruin. The "free-spending" manic can soon deplete his capital, and his uninhibited antics and obscenities can land him in court. The depressed patient, even as he is convincing his family and his physician that he is once more his own usual self, is a suicide risk and requires constant and vigilant supervision. If these affective changes resemble those which are found in the normal, and which become somewhat pathological in the neurotic, they have become radically different in quality by the time they reach the psychotic level.

MANIA

The clinical picture of mania, according to Dr. Henri Ey (1954, pp. 47-118), is so easily presented to beginners in psychiatry that it is the one most commonly used in teaching the nature of a psychosis. It is especially easy to identify in its most blatant form (agitated mania), but it is not easy to understand and explain; and there are milder forms of elation which lie near the normal (hypomanias and euphoria). The latter intrude themselves, sometimes, as "mountaintop experiences" in the lives of the normal, and sometimes are given a religious significance by those who undergo them, particularly when they are experienced in a religious setting. The rituals of the peyote cult and of the LSD enthusiasts can also produce these latter types of "elation," as well as their opposite forms ("bad trips"); some of this admixture of drug effects, susceptible subjects, and religious intentions have been accepted by a few of the devout as genuine mystic experiences, indistinguishable from those of "true" mystics (see H. Smith 1964).

The clinician finds that there are forms which include mixtures of anxiety, guilt, and rage. Moreover, mania and melancholia often alternate within the same patient, with transitions that are abrupt and dramatic. When the diagnostician-theorist has searched for the early infantile experiences that, in his theory, might account for the punitive superego of the melancholy patient who feels so guilty that suicide seems the appropriate way of ridding the earth of a useless clot of clay, he is puzzled to see the same person, a little later, gay and guiltless, as though superego, ego, and id had fused. He can now do no wrong: he is perfect, powerful, and ecstatic. Such a complete transformation of melancholia into mania can occur within the brief hour of recovery from the last of a series of electroshock treatments. As an example, let us consider a case from Jean Delay (1946).

A woman of 42 had suffered from three years of an agitated depression with Cotard's syndrome, delirious ideas of negation and anticipation of an unending suffering. At times prostrated, at times agitated, sleepless, pale, and perspiring, this woman complained of having no organs: no heart, no bladder, no kidneys, no intestines, no rectum—all had been obliterated, and nothing remained for her but to endure forever this unimaginable suffering.

With the beginning of electroshock treatment, regular sleep returned. At about the fifth session, her anxious emotionality (hyperthymia) gave way, and along with it her paroxysms of arterial hypertension disappeared. However, the delirious ideas persisted, and between the fifth and the eighth electroshock one witnessed the paradoxical spectacle of a patient who kept repeating her themes of negation and of immortality without the least emotion, as if it were a story about someone else or of some old fable.

These ideas whose mere enunciation had formerly been accompanied with sobbing and agitation seemed no longer to affect her. The tenth electroshock abruptly released a transitory manic state with euphoria, joviality, flight of ideas, wordplay *(coq à l'âne),* various facetious and indecent expressions, and the reappearance of insomnia. She boasted of her great beauty, her great capacity for love, her success with men, and the wonderful influence she wielded over all those she approached. She laughed and sang at the top of her voice. The twelfth electroshock brought a return to her normal equilibrium of temperament and a resumption of normal sleep patterns. She left the hospital a few days later, cured of her attack.

A COMPARISON WITH LOBOTOMY

Delay's concept of *humeur,* an affective disposition that normally drives and organizes our actions but which can become disorganized, covers the facts and implies that they are accounted for by some central neural process that can become ill, some cell group in the hypothalamus. The *humeur* is the essence of emotional and instinctive forces: it contributes an agreeable or unpleasant tone to mental states as it oscillates between the two poles of pleasure and pain. What the word "consciousness" accomplishes in grouping the whole range of *noetic* phenomena, *humeur* does for the instinctive-affective aspect of mental life. Normal *humeur* is an equilibrium of inhibitory and excitatory impulses, and when it is disorganized there may be an excess of one or the other.

The changes which Delay reports in the above case have a certain resemblance to those reported by Watts and Freeman (1941), who treated obsessions and involutional depressions by prefrontal lobotomy. The neurosurgeons operated as though with the intent of severing a connection between ideas (and the cortical circuits which carry them) and that hypothalamic center that the descending fibers would ordinarily arouse. When aroused, this center would produce patterns of emotional expression and, at the same time, send fresh neural charges upward to further intensify the concerns of the patient. Their patient Abby, who retained her delusion that she had contracted syphilis even after the operation, was no longer worried about it, and could discuss the matter with a bland indifference, as though her emotions were no longer aroused, now that the corticothalamic pathways had been severed. Delay's patient, too, retained her nihilistic delusions into that period when she could discuss them without concern. In the one case, the surgeon's knife had severed (Watts and Freeman believed) a specific corticothalamic tract leading to the "center" of emotional expression; in the other case, the diffuse patterns of electrical discharge involved in the treatment had accomplished a similar effect through changes that are still not understood.

The clinician who can repeatedly produce such mood changes by a physical therapy such as lobotomy or electroshock comes to believe in a material substrate for the *humeur,* since he can alter it directly. The holistic psychologist warns us to be on our guard, lest this view lead us to bypass the difficult task of studying the relations between mood changes and the more extensive dynamic changes within the self-system and between the self and its milieu. On the other hand, simplistic materialism invites us to join with those who see the manic-depressive psychosis as of an unquestioned genetic origin, a view which further tempts us to neglect possible rational (in contrast with physical, nonlogical, purely empirical) forms of therapy.

Attacks of mania (as well as attacks of "suicidal depression") insert themselves in the midst of lives that seem, to outside observers, to be running smoothly enough. They bring an abrupt change in emotional tone, in motivation, in feeling about the self and the surrounding world, and in capacity to attend, to control one's actions, and to persist in rational plans. Ideas and actions seem to spill forth, pell-mell, uninhibited and unregulated; or, as in melancholia, the patient seems to have frozen in a fear of life and of action or to have turned against his very self in savage, self-destructive guilt. The associates of James Forrestal (see Rogow 1963), who had known him through the years, could not believe that his illness was anything more than an operational fatigue, such as some good soldiers experience after too long exposure to combat. As Secretary of Defense he had endured a long bout of overwork during the war. He had been too vital, too strong, too tough; then one day he plunged from an eighth-story hospital window. The phrase *déreglement de l'humeur,* which Delay uses as the title for his discussion of manias and melancholias, is an apt one, but we need to remember that these surges of emotion are also accompanied by profound changes in every other dimension of the personality. Along with the positive and easily identifiable signs of the illness, there are negative changes in thinking, in attention, and in belief that are much more subtle but equally central to the change in behavior.

THE TOTAL CHANGE OF PERSONALITY

When we examine all the changes that make up the manic attack, we find that all three aspects of the classic triad, feeling, intellect, and will, are affected: the autonomic nervous system functions differently; the appetites are whetted (eating and drinking increase); the waking and sleeping rhythm is altered; and all sensations of fatigue disappear. Along with a mood of "God-almightyness" (with a quite unwarranted feeling of power and perfection), there is a flight of ideas, a deterioration of reasoning and of the forms of belief. Movements, gestures, and words multiply, while meaningful associations and high-level skills deteriorate. The elementary act replaces the highly developed one (a slipper is fired through a window on impulse, clothes are ripped off, and obscenities are shouted), and in this sense there is a regression in behavior (the return to infantile tantrums is also a descent in the level of performance). A hitherto "proper" housewife may be openly seductive or exhibitionistic, or she may masturbate openly. A reflex type of pleasure and pain is experienced in the place of the more complex emotions of joy and suffering, and unreflective belief (with frankly expressed delusions and hallucinations) replaces the reflective form of awareness.

Although mania is most commonly found, clinically, as one of the phases of the cyclic manic-depressive psychosis, it can exist (and recur) separately as an independent syndrome, or as an aspect of other types of disorders that have a most varied causation. There are hypomanic auras which warn the epileptic that another attack is coming. A manic syndrome has been reported in patients suffering from a tumor of the third ventricle, and surgeons have reported that direct manipulation of the hypothalamus (either manually or by electrical stimulation) in the course of a brain operation has produced manic symptoms.[1]

---

[1]This last fact is not clear-cut evidence of a necessary, sufficient, and localized center for the disturbances in mania. Grinker and Serota implanted electrodes in the upper posterior angle of the nasal septum in a waking human subject, under local anesthesia. When electric current was passed through this electrode, one subject reported profound anxiety; another went into protracted and uncontrollable sobbing; a third "felt his life pass before his eyes"; and a fourth felt the end of the world approaching (see Grinker 1939).

White (1940) has reported contrary evidence. He used direct stimulation of this same area when it was exposed in the course of an operation. In five patients tested, the stimulation raised blood pressure and increased heart rate with the electrode placed on one point, and caused a slowing at another point of contact, but "there were no psychic manifestations ... no emotional changes or alterations in the level of consciousness."

General Appearance, Attitude, Ideomotor Expressions

Talking, shouting, gesticulating, the manic patient expends his energies as though he possessed a boundless supply, yet these are disordered actions. Clifford Beers (1908, p. 95), who had just emerged from a depressive phase into mania, seemed possessed by a fury of writing.

"The supervisor gave me large sheets of manila wrapping paper. These I proceeded to cut into strips a foot wide...a real letter usually required several such strips pasted together...and on one occasion the accumulation of two or three days of excessive productivity, when spread upon the floor, reached from one end of the corridor to the other—a distance of about one hundred feet. My hourly output was something like twelve feet, with an average of one hundred and fifty words to the foot."

The mood of these patients is, for the most part, euphoric, but it is also fickle, rapidly swinging through the whole spectrum of passions: furious rage, panic, jubilation. The patient is a "good fellow," boisterous, teasing, growling, clowning, but also angry, erotic, obscene, destructive. In such a rapidly changing state, no well-organized and persistent engagement with the surrounding field develops. There is no persistent directive set that remains goal-oriented. Janet's Flore "makes the gesture of catching a fly, dancing a waltz, kissing her nurse, destroying a paper": the movements are kaleidoscopic, "fugacious," and are not unified by any inner core of meaning. Punning, shouting, smashing, shoe-hurling, the energy spurts out in jets of uninhibited action; we could call it "birdbrained," and — like the bird — the patient's bright eagerness shifts with each passing sight or sound. The responses thus cued are abundant, but of very little value. Unless sedated or otherwise controlled, he would disorganize the ward, smash the furniture, flood the bathroom, tear the sheets, and in a dozen ways add to the cost of hospital services, menacing the peace and safety of other patients and personnel. The tranquilizing drugs, such as chlorpromazine, seem made to order for the manic, who needs restraint of some sort (continuous baths, a strait jacket, or a room so padded that he cannot harm himself).

All the while, the observer can get all manner of responses from him. He is in contact with his surroundings, but it is a crude, insensitive, momentary, inaccurate, inattentive, and distorted contact. His world is a flitting, rapidly changing field; he has no end in view save the very nearest consequence of his action, and even this is scarcely "regulative."

More than seventy years ago, Magnan described such patients as jumping, turning somersaults, rolling on the floor, upsetting the furniture, singing, disrobing, tearing clothing. Never fatigued, the manic's strength seems multiplied. He is literally rest-less, and does not pause to sleep any length of time. There is scarcely any weight loss; appetite for food and drink has increased (see Ey 1954, p. 54).

Face and posture change, the manic's voice fills out to a full-throated laughter, a hearty tone, and speech has a special form: telegraphic, elliptical, full of puns and wordplay, sound runs away with sense. His verbal "expectorations" often miss any human target: he shatters language even as he rips the fabric of his clothing (see Lorenz and Cobb 1952).

The agitated manic is playful, dangerously playful, recklessly playful, and only half-aware of what he is doing. His euphoria is self-maintaining, as though he were reaping a huge profit from his foolish sallies. One more calm than others, merely euphoric, may sit writing letters to his generals: each contains a few simple "directives," and the series has less sensible structure than the moves of a boy playing Monopoly. Yet he has the poise and grandeur of a General De Gaulle in one of the latter's more euphoric moments: he believes he is commander-in-chief. The patient's feeling of success, so baseless, is a measure of his total lack of self-criticism. Yet in this same euphoric period, as though half-aware that it is all a joke, he takes his medicine from the nurse when ordered, and goes to bed at her direction. He pauses to explain that the visitors to the ward (who are physicians) are autograph seekers. But at other times his gay fantasy may surpass any world of make-believe: his letters are mailed to the highest political authorities; his "grandeur" may lead to quarrels with his superior officers; and his "playful" blow can prove lethal (see Janet 1928, pp. 384 ff).

There are moments in the experience of some manics when they believe that they have discovered the greatest secrets, received communications from divine sources, discovered wonderful knowledge. They believe that their "inner light" surrounds them physically. One manic, writing late at night and believing that his "illumination" might disturb the neighbors, wanted the curtains drawn so that the intense brilliance that surrounded him would not spread into the street. Recovered, the manic cannot put the content of his "revelations" in any communicable form (even though his certitude still holds), and some emerge from these experiences with a yearning to reexplore the world that was briefly revealed. The moment, they claim, was worth years of ordinary living. A religious person, like a few of the present-day LSD cultists, may be certain that he has experienced "union with God," that his was indeed a divine madness.

The Flight of Ideas and Unreflective (Asséritif) Belief

Listening to the speech of the manic and watching his fugacious behavior, we become keenly aware of the negative side of these changes: there is so much missing. Chief among the missing factors are two processes: (1) the regulative work of some central tendency that keeps thought and action persistently on target, and (2) the critical, validating, testing process that either converts simple impulses into justified, reflective actions or discards them as either not worth bothering about or as much to be abhorred.

A manic hospitalized in the Phipps Psychiatric Institute is described by Muncie (1948, pp. 301 ff):

"He told his story easily. For six years after securing his doctor of philosophy degree in chemistry, he had been in an industrial research laboratory. His relations with his chief were not good, he felt his work was not appreciated, and he had received no recognition. Two weeks before admission, when he saw one of his own products shelved, he cut official red tape, and negotiated a successful independent deal with a university for a test of his product. When he returned from his trip, he was changed. He talked continually and said, 'I've tasted tiger's blood. I am a success and I am the man for my chief's job.' He tipped a head waiter three dollars, bought an expensive gold pencil, left four woodcocks at the club for the vice-president of the firm, a man he barely knew, with a facetious cartoon and a note, 'I've gone the limit.' He talked to a salesman about buying an expensive car which he could not afford, discussed with one the possibility of buying his father-in-law's home, suddenly resolved to have his child christened and put it through in six hours, wired congratulations to a classmate he hadn't seen in eight years whose wife he heard was to have a baby in two months, decided on the spur of the moment to come to Baltimore, and brought the whole family along, driving recklessly and stopping only to send unnecessary telegrams in every direction."

Between the mild euphoria of the hypomanic (who is just a little "high") and the most agitated forms of mania, we could arrange a series of "exhibits" and show a gradually increasing disorganization, with more frenetic speech and action at the extreme.

The disorder in overt action is duplicated by digressions in the course of writing a letter, and in the wandering flight of ideas continually verbalized: the manic is apt to "lead with his larynx," vocalizing before thought and letting the speech mechanisms run themselves. His thought is almost pure "free association," free of all guidance or constraint. There is obviously no lack of "drive" (if we can use that term in the sense of an aimless push), and no lack of responsiveness to stimuli. It is the "set toward a distant goal in a field that is well-grasped" that is lacking. Action, speech, and thought all break up into partial, fragmentary, meandering, local, all-or-none reactions; the transitions from segment to segment involve sharp breaks, klang-determined changes in direction, mechanical associations, stimulus-bound diversions. Speech pours out in abundance, rapid, excited, endlessly flowing, but it is as aimless and erratic as the course of a stream of water from a hose held by an infant. (A rose is a rose o' my heart, my heartfelt admiration for the admiral, Paul Jones is a rose by another name, the Crying Shame of Flying Fame across the street from Schermerhorn, Schermerhorn of the rowing squad with the weak heart, dark heart of Conrad, heart of darkness, dark of the moon, high noon of Noonan's bar, the Schoonhoven crossing the bar, and so on.)

A Noetic Quality

To the manic his effusions are of immense value. They possess a noetic quality. Even his sensory impressions are saturated with a penetrating wisdom. A partially recovered manic patient (Custance 1952, p. 31), writing of his visual sensations, observed:

"The first thing I note is the peculiar appearance of the lights—the ordinary electric lights in the ward. They are not exactly brighter, but deeper, more intense, perhaps a trifle more ruddy than usual. Moreover, if I relax the focusing of my eyes, which I can do very much more easily than in normal circumstances, a bright starlike phenomenon emanates from the lights, ultimately forming a mass of iridescent patterns of all colours of the rainbow, which remind me vaguely of the Aurora Borealis.

"There are a good many people in the ward, and their faces make a peculiarly intense impression on me. I will not say that they have exactly a halo around them, though I have often had that impression in more acute phases of mania. At present it is rather that faces seem to glow with a sort of inner light which shows up the characteristic lines extremely vividly. Thus, although I am the most hopeless draughtsman as a rule, in this state I can draw quite recognizable likenesses. This phenomenon is not confined to faces; it applies to the human body as a whole, and to a rather lesser degree to other objects such as trees, clouds, flowers and so on. Colored objects make a particularly vivid impression, possibly in view of the associations they arouse.... and, curiously enough, so do large vehicles, particularly steamrollers, railway engines and trains. Perhaps the associations of childhood are involved here. Connected with these vivid impressions is a rather curious feeling behind the eyeballs, rather as though a vast electric motor were pulsing away there."

This sense of some "inner light" that also illuminates the surrounding world, this seeing into things, these brighter colors, this marvelous empathic relation with the universe, this appearance of forms as though they were raised (or embossed) designs on an actually plane surface, keep recurring in psychological literature. Vincent Van Gogh was striving to put down on canvas effects that he experienced. Separated over decades, these accounts of experience seem almost to be a succession of plagiarisms, so much do they repeat themselves.

"In a way," Custance adds (p. 47), "I had fallen in love, too, with the whole universe." When these manic states occur in the devoutly religious, the patient is prone to interpret them in terms of his beliefs, and in the mild euphoria of "beatitude" to believe that he has experienced either a "union with God" or a kind of elevation into divinity.

The New Quality of Belief and Action

What we have been saying could be put in other words: the manic loses his standards, his tests of truth and of decorum. While he continues to gloat in his "success," his actions seldom validate such a feeling. His power to see through things and his certitude are, in fact, neither noetic nor prophetic. He has also fallen into a childlike form of belief, in which the mere existence of thought or gesture makes the objects or actions symbolized real, true, possible, valuable. If his earlier development had managed to separate the ego, super-ego, and id into independent systems of opposing and mutually corrective forces, so that "I want" has to wait on "it is possible" and "it is good," the destructuring in the psychosis has melted them down into something, perhaps not infantile or primitive, as many psychoanalysts are inclined to say, but certainly something inchoate and unstructured, although it still contains elements from a lifetime's learning. Guillaume Monod's experienced divinity had a background of theological training to give it shape and content. Clifford Beers was acting out the role of "the great organizer of the mental-hygiene movement," for which the times were ripe. Others act out the role of fascinating woman, great tycoon, genius-inventor. Whichever direction his values point, the manic finds cues for an easy route to success. Self-realization? He is *it,* and there is no inner critic, no mocking commentator, no scolding censor, no sense of reality to say him nay. If others rise in his audience to object, they betray (to him) that they are dull and unappreciative, or, as Beers put it, simply cool minds, unprepared to receive the white-hot revelations that he can give them.

The Sources of the Manic's Energy

Restless, free-wheeling, indefatigable, boisterous, sleepless, the agitated manic seems to have an uncontrollable and boundless stream of energy. Objectively: digestion and appetite are improved; respiration is more rapid (and deeper); the pulse is speeded and blood pressure is increased; and a vasodilation with flushing and a slight rise of skin temperature adds an impression of ruddy health. Subjectively, there is a sense of power: everything goes easily; everything is a marvelous success.

Two possible sources of this surge of power suggest themselves. A surge from below could be sparked by some localized changes in those hypothalamic cells that regulate the vital processes. Was it not in another group of sick cells (such as those at the margin of a cortical scar) that Penfield identified the origin of the epileptic discharge? "Everything is easy," one of Janet's patients notes on the day prior to his epileptic attack. The whole day has been filled with successes. "Everything is easily done. I have a thousand times more force and intelligence." With the experience of such auras, some patients learn that the states are dangerous: if they do not watch out, their excitement will lead straight into a seizure. (See Janet 1928, pp. 380-448.)

There is a related view, suggested by Janet's analysis. The sudden surplus of energy could be viewed as a *gaspillage,* a sudden burst of free expenditure in simple actions that occurs because some of the other and more costly actions, which normally bind energies, have suddenly been canceled, or lost, or thrown aside, or shortcircuited by some as yet obscure shift in action (and in cortical functioning), for it is not merely a surge of affects, as the name *thymergasia* seems to imply, but also a loss of much of that power to delay, inhibit, and regulate action which makes a man human and rational.

Suppose, Janet suggests (1928, p. 408), you have drawn a large sum of money for a voyage. Spending carefully, during your travels you arrive at the point of the final purchase of the ticket home. You discover to your surprise that you have much more cash in your pocket than you need and that a dozen coveted articles can now be purchased. In all probability you will launch yourself on a little spending orgy, and with a free conscience. You may even make some rather foolish purchases. No matter, you had saved the money. It had been set aside for the trip. You earned it. So, whee! Such is *gaspillage.* The dread of running short has disappeared. There is no longer a possible mountain of things to do, places to see, bills to face. All the anticipated possibilities that you had carried, in the form of prudent anxiety, have been liquidated. Thus the lid (of concerns) is off.

If we could link the sudden fading of this fringe of rational concerns, this descent from the level where many costly future-making plans kept our energies bound up, to a lower level where short-term, elementary, fragmentary "pulses of movement" abound, we could account for the apparent spurt in energy by this transformation into cheaper currency. Mania would then be as much a *loss* of cortical power as a *surge* of hypothalamic energy.

We do, in fact, observe the drop in quality of action. The actions that fill the manic's hours are indeed the less difficult ones: they require less control; they do not have to be corrected; they are not constantly bounded by the vigilant tension that keeps them related to a more remote field. They are "expectorated," as though there were no critical audience and no tomorrow. One might compare such a shift with the one a schoolboy displays when, too long confined at lessons, he is released from discipline and joins in a mass of shoving, shouting peers who pour onto a playground.

MELANCHOLIA

Melancholia has a thousand faces. To the aging business and professional man, its appearance may coincide with the end of his power to dominate and compete: suddenly he begins to lose the initiative; and he recoils from conflict that he fears will be too much for him. To the artist it can come as a sudden emptiness, a failure in his creative gifts. To the woman who has capitalized on her personal and physical charms, it may enter along with the feeling that she is no longer attractive, that men have begun to turn away from her, that life is over. To Don Juan it comes with the realization that the game of sexual conquest is not worth the candle; indeed, the candle and the zest have gone out.

Melancholia comes in varying intensities and durations. It can be an extension of the pernicious inertia of neurasthenia, lasting only a few days, but carrying with it the sudden conviction that life is no longer possible and that the self is a worthless thing. It can take the form of a long series of recurrent chutes in the will to live, each interrupted by the return of lucid and active living. The individual may endure these interruptions as though they were caused by some underlying glandular weakness. In some it is felt as an actual chest-constricting *anguish* that squeezes the body and stops thought, possessing the sufferer as though an outer harness were crushing him. It can vary from a merely passive aboulia to an agitated, restless, crying, hand-wringing, "fulminating" form called agitated depression. Sometimes it seems to be precipitated by obvious outer events; when these serve to explain the mood, we speak of a *reactive* depression. Loss of love, failure in business, the discovery that one's pain arises from a malignancy, the shock of an operation (or the exhaustion that follows a difficult childbirth), a catastrophe—the list of possible exogenous sources is endless. In the depressed these occasions seem to have so depleted the powers of resistance that the will to live has stopped.

When it creeps up on a person insidiously, in late life, along with failing energies, lowered metabolic rates, and a diminished supply of pituitary and gonadal hormones, it is likely to be named *involutional* depression, because of the age-linked changes: cessation of menstruation and loss of sexual energy. When the onset is swift, and unrelated to visible outer events or identifiable physical changes, we tend to view it as of endogenous or genetic origin, even though the implied causes are still hypothetical. In this last form it may be followed by an opposite swing into mania, with recurrent attacks separated by lucid intervals. This form is called the *manic-depressive* psychosis.

When melancholia descends, the springs of life seem to dry up: the pinched expression and the drooping posture suggest the weeping willow. Matching this posture, both the inner visceral changes and the subjective withdrawal of all tentacles of hope and aspiration complete the picture of despair. Even the sluggish colon participates in this general nonfeasance.

Motivation is not only withdrawn, but thrown into reverse gear. Where the patient's values and hopes formerly lay, a sense of guilt and of failure emerges. The very best in him suddenly changes quality: the beckoner becomes the torturer, the former source of satisfaction a poison, the helper a hurtful goad. Where he could once give, defend, demand, compete, protect, collaborate, as occasions demanded, he now gives up in advance; if we once called the sum of these positive thrusts "the life instinct" (as Freud did), we are tempted to invent a "death instinct" to take command of his depressed retreat from life. "What's the use?" he asks, as he crushes every hope in advance, avoids every challenge. As though certain of but one thing, namely that every path leads to the grave, he does not even bother to adjust his shroud: even his clothing is disordered, his body allowed to remain unclean.

These twins, mania and melancholia, have one quality in common: the wide swings of mood are so exaggerated that they carry the individual beyond reason. The manic is not God, as he seems to believe, able to reach out and touch the stars, in tune with the infinite, irrepressible, indefatigable. He is in danger of exhaustion. The melancholy one, who, at the other extreme, feels he can do nothing, has nothing, hopes for nothing, deserves nothing, and *is* nothing, has in fact many good years of life ahead: his guilt is pardonable (and possibly insignificant); his resignation from life is premature; and his worth is still as great as he can make it on some later day when he has recovered.

Neither the melancholiac nor the manic has good judgment, although in our impatience we may feel that — for once — the depressed person is telling the truth about himself (a significant observation about ourselves, perhaps, comparable to a revealing phrase of Hazlitt that struck Secretary Forrestal forcibly: "I believe in the theoretical benevolence and the practical malignity of man"). It is tempting, as we interpret his sense of being persecuted as a projection of his own hostilities, to turn moralist and thus aid and abet the sick person's tormenters, as Job's counselors did. "Depression is aggression turned inward" is a frequently used formula; used by an incautious counselor, it might have a potent effect on a patient already filled with guilt, who might feel that it points the finger at his essential hatefulness. (Here we should remember that suicide is often an aggressive action, intended to wound those who are near and who should have loved the victim more. "They will be sorry," he mutters, as he plans to create trouble all around.)

The manic, as we have seen, is in poor contact with reality. "I can do anything you can do, better," he is *certain,* recognizing neither the outer difficulties nor his own inner limitations. "I shall fly to Rome, talk with the Pope, initiate changes in our beliefs about the Holy Virgin," one of Janet's patients announced while she was still confined to the Salpêtrière. She added, as she tried to show how light she had become, walking about the ward on tiptoes as if she were about to take off in winged flight, "Don't put me on your scales. They are not to be relied upon. I *know* I am getting light enough to fly." In his airborne certitude the manic has no need for authorities, advice, the newspapers: he is clairvoyant, powerful.

In mild dosage, such enthusiasm frees the hypomanic for action that his normal inhibitions had prevented. Clifford Beers came out of hospital, still slightly manic, raging against all institutions for the mentally ill, at their stupidity and callousness (and particularly at a certain resident physician who had tried to set him straight); he called on the president of Yale University (a trained psychologist) and sent out letters to leading psychiatrists and public figures, calling them together to found the National Society for Mental Hygiene, *and it happened!* (Perhaps some of his optimism is still ricocheting among social workers and clinical psychologists.)

Other manics have talked with God. Like Father Divine, or his French counterpart, Guillaume Monod, their certitude is so catching that faithful converts gather around them, providing a limited validation of their delusions until the individual becomes sure that he is either a god or the emissary of one.

The melancholiac, on the other hand, is nothing. If the manic's "I fear nothing!" is a genuine expression of his feeling, the melancholiac's fear of nothingness is also saturated with a *certitude* of impending disintegration: death haunts him like a "presence," either approaching him with a majestic and inevitable step or beckoning him (as the railing on the top of the Empire State Building summons the suicidal person to jump, until to save himself he must draw back). In a strange agony he struggles with an invisible tide that he can feel sweeping him toward the abyss. Even at the moment when the doctors have assented to his discharge, and his actions and words suggest that he has improved, a sudden *chute* back into depression will reinstate his suicidal intent and send him leaping from the eighth-story window or blowing out his brains with a shotgun. The calculated risk which the physician and family take becomes acute at precisely this point where everyone is ready to relax, believing that the worst is over.

If the melancholiac's view were true, if he were in fact subject to all the slings and arrows of an outrageous fortune, if he were in fact overwhelmed, beaten down, crushed, weighed down by disease, poverty, and impending death, and if those who had once loved him had abandoned him, we could then say, "I understand, and sympathize. Your view of life has turned dark because life itself has darkened."[2] But the problem of melancholia is not the actual burden of living, not the real injustice *which exists;* depressions will still occur after our war against poverty has been won and after massive efforts to rescue the many who find themselves in the midst of circumstances they cannot master have succeeded, for there is little correspondence between the pressures of existence and the melancholy mood of depression. We note the fact that, instead of instigating coping actions calculated to improve matters, the depressed person worsens his condition in thought and deed, loses motivation and all belief in himself, launches into positively self-destructive actions.

Because depression is an experience common to most of us, in some slight degree, we can empathize and sympathize with the mood. It is more difficult to see the psychotic form objectively as a normal outgrowth of a particular life-history. It is equally hard to identify any specific physiological process that makes it emerge in an otherwise "unjustified" fashion. The "attack," like the attack of anxiety that has no clearly defined object, can come unbidden, unjustified, unannounced; and when it recurs from youth to old age, with long interpersed intervals of lucidity and productivity, it takes on the quality of a recurrent disease-process that lies somewhere outside the self-system, something that rests on changes "down among the cells," something that wells up like an inky black cloud to stain the field of awareness (as though something had gone wrong in the hypothalamus).

PHYSIOLOGICAL CHANGES IN THE DEPRESSED

While the changes in thinking are studied by one group of clinicians, other groups have centered on physiological changes. Summarizing some of these, Cameron (1963) points out that depressed males, classified as *retarded depressions,* tend to be impotent, poor sleepers, poor eaters, constipated, and below their normal weight. Women who grow depressed tend to become frigid, and to have infrequent and irregular menses. In agitated depression there is more activity, handwringing, pacing to and from, picking at the body surface, rocking, and audible and visible "suffering."

The sympathetic branch of the autonomic nervous system contributes to the appetite loss, and if anorexia is not averted, the refusal of food can produce a central neuritis. Diethelm (1950, p. 210) comments on two patients who died from such a central neuritis: unwilling to live, refusing all food, vomiting up forced feedings. This roundabout path is a partially voluntary suicide, protracted and painful. In spite of a first-rate staff and well-planned efforts to prevent the outcome, a good clinic could not prevent it.

---

[2] If one accepts the story of the melancholiac, and if one follows out his complaints to check them, some 98 per cent of the patients will be found to have "good reasons": failure in exams, marriages on the rocks; financial and legal difficulties, pressure of work and responsibilities. But a similar series of "insults" existed before the depression, and exists in others who have never experienced a mental illness. The "abnormal state" goes beyond a realistic appraisal of one's difficulties and capacities, and is produced by "insufficient" causes.

Careful studies of the blood constituents have shown that the composition of the blood is within normal limits; the average cholesterol level is 10 per cent above normal, but it is as high in many normals who are not depressed (see Sperry 1954). There is a greater variability in blood constituents, enough to suggest that in depressives the homeostatic controls may not operate as rapidly or within as narrow limits as in the nondepressed. Some studies have reported abnormalities in sugar tolerance. A disordered metabolism, due to defects in the enzymes or in the cells of the diencephalon which regulate so many physiological changes, has been suggested as one of the root causes.

States of drowsiness with vasoconstriction of cerebral blood vessels, as well as states of cerebral hyperemia, have been produced experimentally with drugs. The fact that an excess of folliculin produces the latter change, and of bulbocapnine the former, has led the speculative theorist to consider the possibility that the body's tissues may actually produce "poisons of the will" that affect personality and mental processes (see Baruk 1958).

Kraines (1957), who looks on the diencephalon as the seat of the difficulty, sees the illness as a kind of temporary vital failure: the psychomotor retardation (in some), with fatigue, anorexia, weight loss, and sleep disturbances, points to the hypothalamus and associated reticular system, he believes. Since there are many factors that can disturb the functioning of these cells (endocrine changes, circulatory changes, nutritional inadequacy, metabolic instability, toxins), the search for causes of the depression has led to these multiple physiological sources.

Thus, while it is true that, when we search out the beginnings of an attack of melancholia, there are often clearly visible blows of fate that have served as precipitating agents, there are other occasions when the states seem to have no origin in the outer world and no clearly visible cause within, and in all of them there is a disproportion, an exaggeration, and a "going beyond" the limits of useful and adaptive responses. What is a pernicious inertia, a feeling of emptiness, or a nameless dread that we call "free-floating anxiety" in the neuroses, in the depressive psychosis becomes a state that engulfs or possesses the patient: it arrests the normal coping mechanisms, and assumes the quality of a global vital arrest, a complete loss of nerve and of the courage to face life. If the state contains an additional component of restless and agitated aggression, the latter is still of the destructive, self-accusatory type.

THINKING IN DEPRESSION

When depression strikes, how does thinking proceed? In an effort to present a systematic and well-documented answer to this question, Aaron Beck (Beck and Hurvich 1959; Beck *et al.* 1961) has summarized extensive data obtained from interviews with psychiatric patients undergoing therapy for depressions. The patients were seen over periods ranging from six months to six years. Handwritten notes made by the therapist at the time of the interviews, notes about their thoughts and feelings made by the patients in the interval between therapeutic sessions, contents of dreams and free associations produced in the course of analytic therapy were compared with similar data obtained from patients who were not depressed.

To the changes in the external world about them, the depressed tend to give a stereotyped form of response, often inappropriate and irrelevant. Whatever touches on their personal attributes reminds them of their inadequacy. Should a passerby smile or fail to smile or fail to greet them, their feeling of inferiority is immediately increased: "People pay no attention to me. They smile in derision. People are no longer friendly." The depressed woman who sees a mother with a child, or who hears another mother praised, is sure that she is a bad mother herself. The praise of others reminds her of her own inadequacy. Even in their free associations and private ruminations, long trains of thoughts "on the dark side" cloud their consciousness.

Low self-esteem, persistent downgrading of the self, in spite of actual roles and accomplishments, along with ideas of deprivation (lack of resources, lack of friends, lack of ways of coping with surroundings, lack of traits that make the average person lovable), all persist in the face of all evidence to the contrary (real opportunities, actual money in the bank, overt expressions of interest and affection and esteem). It is as though some "central affective state" (or some central nervous-system condition, in turn under the control of toxins, endocrine deficiencies, or enzyme abnormality) were acting as a chronic inhibitor to all evidence that would support a contrary (and valid) feeling tone. It is as though the normal corrective experiences were systematically arrested. When this state is in force, all the virtues seem to have flown, while all of the failures (and any real defects) are magnified, exaggerated.[3] Constantly comparing himself with others, the depressed patient feels that he is inferior: poor in spirit, a poor spouse (or son, or lover), a poor performer in his chosen social role. Such a patient is ever ready to assume the blame for whatever turns out badly (in the business, in the home, in interpersonal relations): "It is all my fault."

Interestingly enough, low self-evaluations were found to strike the areas which had been highly valued by the person prior to the onset of depression. A housewife who expected of herself a high degree of competence in the management of the household and in fulfilling her wifely duties blamed herself for not getting up to prepare her husband's breakfast, but she freely confessed to a sexual affair, with little evidence of guilt. Fidelity was not one of

---

[3]A curious effect can be produced by a too concerted (and clumsy) attempt at reassurance. The "count your blessings" theme can intensify the guilt of an already depressed person. Now he *knows* that he *ought* to feel as he does not. Even the minister or priest who comes to speak to him about a religious consolation that is available to him may discover he is adding to the patient's distress. Diethelm warns (1950, p. 216) "In religious scruples, the aid of a minister may be required, but one must keep in mind that the minister is a helper and not a healer, and that he should work in cooperation with the physician and under his supervision. Too many visits by a minister will tend to cause the patient to consider his illness as a religious problem." Sister M. William Kelley (1961) comments, in the course of reporting a survey of depressive psychoses in the members of religious communities, on the effect of religious practices in these communities (which include systematic self-denial and deliberate and controlled self-examination). Sometimes they operate insidiously to exaggerate larval forms of depression if they are not exercised wisely under expert direction.

the lines she carried; her affair gave her no sense of guilt. The persistent self-evaluation and self-accusation acts as any persistent set: it is easily triggered by whatever changes occurs. Thunder and lightning at the picnic, while not indicating God's wrath, seemed to accuse the depressed housewife: she had picked the wrong day and was to blame for the misfortunes and discomfort of her guests.

Overwhelming press would give us a shorthand symbol for the depressed person's feeling about his surroundings. Duties that demand more than he can give, that divide and disorganize him, and that loom like a gigantic, exhausting, overwhelming mass, impossible to fulfill, make him wish to withdraw, escape, resign, cut down, evade. Yet the nagging voice of conscience still holds him responsible. The superego, we might say — using Freud's language — is merciless. The patient may hear a voice, nagging, accusing, prodding him to do what he cannot or will not do. It pushes him in two opposite directions at once, insisting that he perform actions that are mutually exclusive. But these self-instructions never seem to get him anywhere, and do not release actions that liquidate his feelings of guilt and incompleteness. He gives the impression of avoiding action, of being in full flight from these very liquidating actions; the "impossibility" of doing opposite things almost serves as excuse for nonfeasance. It's "damned if you do and damned if you don't," so little or nothing is done. When this pressure to do exists in its mildest form, as it does in a very mild obsession, it can seem like a richness of possibilities, as a groundwork for productive actions, even when it is the beginning of disorganization. In more complete depression, this splatter of invocations to action has replaced action. Rather than accusing it of blocking action, let us say that action is blocked, and in its place there arises a more or less disorganized sense of overwhelming press.

From these impasses the patient can formulate no clear and realistic path of escape. Yet escape from the intolerable conflicts is a constant thought, and along with this "no exit" quality comes the thought of escape by suicide. An alternative to suicide would be to disappear, to duck out of responsibilities, to seek out some "desert island," some other city where in anonymity one could live among strangers who demand nothing at all. Usually the vigilant superego will not allow the depressed to escape. The conscience would hound him at every step. He cannot hide under the covers (though some patients try going to bed).

Beck stresses the systematic error in these self-evaluations. Like the experimental subject who, blindfolded, systematically points to the wristward of the point stimulated on the volar surface of his forearm, the depressed person misidentifies himself, mislocates himself on a kind of interpersonal map that he carries about with him. This "purgatory error" puts him at the bottom of the class, makes him the one least attractive, least responsible, least lovable. His inferences from the stimulating context about him show overgeneralizations, overinclusiveness, cognitive distortions, arbitrary interpretations, and all the errors are in one direction. A glance from the elevator operator means: "He thinks I'm a nobody." A depressed intern, questioned about a hospital procedure by the chief of the clinic, thinks, "He doesn't have any faith in my work." The alternate hypotheses simply do not occur; we can describe this thinking as *mood-constricted.*

This same mood constriction could also be called *selective abstraction,* for it emphasizes and exaggerates any small detail that is congruent with this depressive mood. Thus the depressive could be said to go out to meet (and construct) this world that seems so black to him. It is as though he were a resonator set to receive bad news, tuned to a depressive frequency; over this beam comes material to validate his distortions, immediately. It is not that all men are liars, and always so, but he is continually finding evidence to support the generalization, and the contrary evidence is tuned out. Going to extremes, magnifying and minimizing in a manner always congruent with this dark mood, he creates an unpleasant and hostile world that congeals around him, solidifying, closing him in. At the very moment when his active and outgoing forces grow weaker, the barriers to any action grow increasingly impenetrable. Soldered to his past (and all that he can recall is similarly mood-constricted) and enclosed in a snake pit, all that the depressive learns from experience reinforces his attitude.

One aspect of the change in thinking in depressions makes it necessary for the history-taker to be on guard when asking such a patient to recall his past, for this recall is as distorted as his current perception of himself and the world about him. It is even possible that a certain clinical stereotype of the prepsychotic personality of the depressed person may be attributable, in part, to such retrospective falsification of the patient's own life story. His earlier fears, his childhood, his relations with his wife, his sex practices will all suffer in the recall and in the telling from his chronic self-accusatory and world-denigrating tendency. Added to this is the need to rationalize and to explain, still as strong in the depressive as in the rest of us. He wants to know how he could possibly have become what he is, and in his search he may utilize the words of his physician (and the latter's efforts to give him insight), exaggerating them and incorporating them into his delusions. Like the priest who comes to pray with the patient and to bring him spiritual counsel and consolation and who discovers to his horror that what he has said has been interpreted as further proof of the patient's guilt, the physician may discover that he, too, can become involved in this type of distortion. Kraines (1957, p. 227) describes a patient who

"...recalled all the details of the psychopathology discussed with her analyst, enlarged, elaborated, and distorted all that had been told her. She felt that she was a 'monster' for hating her sister, that she was 'filthy' for having had incestuous desires, that she was 'awful' for competing with her mother, that she had no right 'to have children as sexual symbols'—all concepts learned during analysis."

Changes in the Dynamics of Thinking

If we look not so much at the content as at the ongoing process, there are certain changes which could be called *physiogenic.* This term, used by Kraines (1957, p. 258), suggests that the stream of impulses reaching the diencephalon and cortex is not sufficient to maintain the usual level of alertness. A general impairment of intellectual functioning results, a *functional* impairment that will persist as long as the depression is in force, and disappear with complete recovery. Kraines speaks of a student

"... who was in a depression, [and who] made such low grades in his first semester that his dean advised him that he was totally unfit for college work. The next semester [this student] in a mild manic swing, led the class scholastically. A comparable case is that of a draftsman who was discharged because he couldn't do his work; later at another place he was employed for the same work and was considered one of the best men in the firm."

The mind seems to function as though some "power factor" had been turned off. The mechanisms are there, the pieces of information, but they are not or cannot be used. If there is such a thing as a *poison de la volonté,* whether hormone or toxin or defective enzyme that operates on the diencephalon and cortex to slow down the associational processes, it introduces a feeling of confusion and unreality, hinders the "imprinting" process so that immediate recall functions poorly, weakens the power of concentration and the power of making decisions, slows down the rate of mental activity, and solders the individual to sections of his remote past, instead of permitting the fresh development of vital relations to the present, to the events just past, and to the nascent future.

We have met so many of these symptoms in describing the neuroses that we are tempted to look on this state of depression as containing all the symptoms we found in neurasthenia and in the obsessions, only in more intense degree. The *feeling of unreality* and the uncanny sense of having been here before (*déjà vu*) Janet had also described in his psychasthenics. Perhaps many of these same patients would be diagnosed as mild depressions today, and perhaps the basic fact is that there is no sharp borderline separating the neuroses from the psychoses and that the depressive, manic, and schizophrenic states are simply deeper levels of what we met in neurasthenia, anxiety states, neurocirculatory asthenia, and obsessive-compulsive states.

In this feeling of unreality, the patient describes something comparable to the experience of the tired student who reads the words of the assignment in a foreign language but can get no meaning from the passage. The patient sees the nurse move about the ward, but wonders, "Is she a real nurse, or just someone dressed up in the uniform?" This man, who looks like his brother, "Is he really my brother?" The facade of the hospital wing, just opposite, is as artificial as a stage setting made of cardboard. All these expressions seem to suggest a certain loosening of the grasp upon the real, the vital contact and sense of ownership. The world is distant, hollow, unreal. We could call this change in perception a projection of his own feeling of estrangement. It shows a certain incompleteness in the grasping and presentifying. Needless to say, significant interpersonal relations suffer under this alienation process: wives fall out of love with their "strange" husbands, a man looks with indifference on the job that had formerly aroused his full interest and attention. Perhaps the *déjà vu* illusion of "having been here before" is part and parcel of a poor perceiving process, a poor temporal structure to action: there is so little difference between a recalled memory and a present scene, so little accurate placing of memories, that present and past are blurred, confused. Although these patients are seldom disoriented for time and place, they are confused. Their minds move slowly. They focus on things imperfectly. Their feeling about what they see is dulled, weakened. They read but do not understand what they read. (Yet, curiously, they sometimes imprint the material well enough so that it arises, spontaneously, days later. In this sense they are like the student whose mind is a blank before the examination, but finds when he settles down to reading the questions that the answers arise). All these instances seem to add up to an imperfect grasping, attending, bringing into the focus of full awareness.

The defect in immediate memory seems to be more a matter of failure to perceive and attend in the first place, but when it is continuous, the person is certain that his memory is failing. He writes himself notes, comes to the clinic with a paper on which he has written down the symptoms, since he is sure he will forget to tell even the important things. He can no longer trust himself to drive his car in traffic: he might miss a traffic signal, forget to make a turn, fail to register what he is doing. The "registering" and "history-making" that proceed normally as our experience unrolls are here felt to be defective; and the records of the patient's behavior suggest that there is both a subjective distortion or exaggeration of the symptoms as well as efforts to compensate for the sensed loss.

The interminable hesitation, the inability to act decisively, the weakness of interest (or thrust of action), the inability to concentrate, to finish actions promptly, or to discharge action tendencies, the slowed associations, the paucity of speech add up to a loss of will, of moral force, of integrative strength or *action-force*. When this very general trait, which affects every phase of living, enters into relationship with the altered sex-drive that is characteristic of depressions, some interesting combinations occur. A man may center on his loss of potency as the primary factor, see his whole "virility" threatened, and seek extramarital affairs, unusual sexual stimulation, in an effort to recapture or prove his manhood. A wife grown frigid, and turning against sexuality, may lose interest in her husband, or use her frigidity as the central factor in her self-accusations: she was not meant for marriage, she has not been a good wife and mother, she does not deserve the husband she has. With its tendency to move the sexual factor into the foreground and to look on a libidinal history as the essential factor in understanding the psychosis, psychoanalysis assists the rationalizing tendency of the patient. All his difficulties lie here! When, following a series of electroshock treatments, the patient's potency returns, and with it some lifting of the other depressive phenomena, the full validation of the rationalization is completed. But it is also true that, with recovery from a depression (whether the physician or the patient has focused on the sexual factor or not), appetite returns to normal, thought processes speed up, attention and the power to decide resume their former vigor, sleep patterns return to normal, and normal sexual desire reappears, along with potency and orgasm.

There are two ways in which depression alters the temporal structure of action, in addition to the weakening of immediate memory. The first is that time seems to grind almost to a stop, the day drags, yesterday seems ages ago, but when there is work to be done, there is never enough time. The makeready for a job is interminable. It takes hours to dress. Things just do not get done. In the depth of a depression, behavior seems to grind to a full stop. When he looks and contemplates all that he must do, he cries, "Time must have a stop!" When he looks, as a voyeur, at the way the present drags by and at the remoteness of yesterday, he says, "It *has* stopped!"

The second is that he finds old events, long forgotten, now return to join up with the present field. He is "soldered" to this old past, and it is an unpleasant past, colored by his present depressive cast of mind. In part this crowding in of old memories may be due to their superior imprinting (as compared with the more recent ones), in part to their congruence with his present mood, and in part to the fact that he is not actively interested in an immediate future. There is no present plan to exclude them, no good grasp of current reality to preoccupy him. He is like the old gaffer who has retired from active life and now harks back to the good old days.

Dreaming

Since dreaming has occupied more and more attention of psychopathologists, and since psychoanalysis makes so much use of dreams and free associations, it is worth noting that in the depth of depression many dreams are reported by patients who insist that they had rarely dreamed before. The content of these dreams reflects the waking concerns of the depressed person, and they take on a nightmarish quality. They are so disturbing that they come to be one of the dominant concerns of the patient: they interrupt his sleep, intensify his misery, bring premonitions of disaster and death, revive some of the more horrible memories that, in health, had been successfully suppressed or kept out of mind, and suggest to the patient that he must be losing his mind.

If old anxieties, old conflicts, old "sins," arise in depression, may it not be that the dynamic trends they reveal are the causes underlying the depression? Has the man of 50 who had long forgotten his boyhood conflict over masturbation, but who now is preoccupied with it in depression and wondering if it had caused his present state, in fact hit upon the cause? What if he again forgets all about it when he recovers his potency and the depression has fled? It would seem the part of common sense not to look on dreams as the cause of sleep, or their nightmarish quality as the cause of depression. It would also seem that the revival of old conflicts, such as the one over boyhood masturbation, is also a part of a typical depressive pattern of thinking, not the cause of the depression.

Kraines (1957) thought he could see a relationship between the patient's illness and his dreaming, but unlike those who emphasize the importance of the "dream work," he hypothesized a biochemical process. Recent studies

(Snyder 1965) of depressed patients who also suffer from loss of sleep (and from dreams with a "masochistic" affect) show a marked reduction in REMS (the rapid eye movements that are observed in dreamers as their eyes "pursue" objects in their dreams). A recent report of a case undergoing two-day cycles of manic-depressive fluctuations has been made by Bunney, Hartmann, and Mason (1965). They report that wide shifts in mood and in waking thought content came with the regularity of the tides, and where these alternations are accompanied by physiological changes, there does not seem to be any good pyschodynamic explanation of the endocrine changes. These observers, like Kraines, view the physiological rhythm as the regulative factor.

Fatigue

Fatigue is another constant concern of many depressives, and it can be literally prostrating in its severity. Kraines observes (1957, p. 148) that in a series of 1,300 cases seen over a 15-year period, this complaint appears in 75 per cent of the cases. Common sense searches for the source of the exhaustion, for overwork, for excesses, yet when this symptom is viewed as part of the quartet of physical changes (psychosomatic changes, sleep difficulties, eating difficulties, psychomotor retardation and fatigue), and when, in addition, the fatigue emerges in a setting where activity has progressively declined and is now minimal, this natural interpretation fails. Even when the patient sleeps excessively (as he does in the beginning and terminal phases of depression), he awakens exhausted, too tired to get up. He sleeps but does not rest. He rests but is still tired. The fatigue seems to spring from some more basic physiological source.

These patients are not only tired, but fatigable. Action runs down rapidly. The effects of moderate exercise and an effort to resume activity produce such contrasting effects at different phases of the depressive cycle that clinical opinion is radically divided. One therapist will look on exercise as positively dangerous, and on any encouragement to effort as playing into the self-accusatory trends already too strong in the patient (he tends to take on too much anyway). Others insist that the lift to respiration and circulation, the fillip to the whole organism, is restorative in spite of the patient's disinclination, and these clinicians will use a "total push" therapy to move the retarded, apathetic patient into activity, hoping that, like a resistant motor that is finally started, the action will recharge the run-down batteries of the physiological system. The consensus seems to be that this type of therapy works best as prophylaxis, in the early phase of the illness, and again in the final recovery phase, but that in the deepest trough of the depression such a "total push" adds insult to injury.

Hypnagogic Images

One interesting side-effect associated with sleeping difficulties is the emergence of hypnagogic images. A patient who formerly, in health, plunged immediately into deep sleep, now reports that he sees all manner of shapes, and in "technicolor." Illusions may have the vividness of hallucination, yet be sensed for what they are, productions of his own imagination: he sees frightening animals, hears his name called. All these symptoms disappear on recovery from the depression.

Anorexia, Weight Loss, and Other Appetites

Anorexia and weight loss are common accompaniments of depression, but there are also swings from anorexia to bulimia. In the former there is simply no appetite, no desire for food (even when there is strenuous exercise). Food doesn't taste right, look good. It simply does not appeal. Neither does smoking seem as enjoyable. The swing into bulimia, in which the craving for food is excessive and the patient cannot eat enough, reminds us that depression is also a disorganization, a deregulation of behavior, that reaches down into the basic homeostatic mechanisms. There are similar flareups (particularly in the early or later phases of the depression) of excessive sexual desire, followed by complete loss of sexual appetite. The "visceral brain" seems to be disordered, now overactive, now underactive. Subjectively these are experienced as intense cravings: "It isn't carrots or cabbage or any other nonfattening thing I want. I want bread and butter and meat—the fatter the better. It's got to be highly seasoned, too, so that it burns a little as it goes down. I eat until I feel stuffed; but half an hour later I'm as hungry as if I hadn't had a bite." A corresponding emergence of nymphomania, voyeurism, exhibitionism, and the use of pornographic literature and other methods of increasing sexual excitation is reported in the literature of depression. In many instances the frank emergence of these patterns is a revival of old preoccupations, long mastered, but now uninhibited and uncontrolled. This depression phenomenon reminds us that the failure in the patient's action systems is not confined to diencephalic mechanisms: it is the "higher level" that is here defective. Perhaps we should consider the kinds of controls which existed prior to the illness. For the person for whom "sex is all," the need to demonstrate his virility may produce excesses, including perversions, in a desperate effort to demonstrate that his "value" can be preserved. For another, long struggling to achieve purity in thought and deed, the disappearance of sexual desire may be received as a blessing that compensates for some of the unhappy aspects of the illness.

Because this deregulation of sexuality seen in depressions may be the original occasion for abnormal practices, the person who treats sexual disorders should consider the possibility of this kind of origin. Kraines observes (1957, p. 292), "Sex is so basic a drive that its patterns, once grooved, like a gorge carved by a river, tend to pursue the original pathway despite changing circumstances." For this reason a depression in the adolescent years, before the sexual trends have taken firm shape, may have serious sequelae.

A Test for Depression

There is greater agreement among psychiatrists about the depth of the depression they see in the patients before them than in their interpretation of this depression, in the causes they assign, or in the diagnostic labels they apply, and what they see before them may be affected by their theoretical predilections, the therapies they like to use. In planning treatment, in evaluating the outcomes, and in estimating the course of events while the patient is under observation, it would be helpful, therefore, to have a relatively objective standard to use in the assessment of the patient's progress. Since these tests would have a certain foolproof quality, they could be administered by less qualified, less thoroughly trained, less "expensive" personnel; hospital administrators and chiefs of service would thus find them of value, particularly if they could be validated against the judgment of the most competent staff members.

These tests, or rating scales, require the subject to estimate his own condition. Some of them require, in addition, careful observation of the patient by the physician while he is being interviewed. A list of items, based on the literature of depressions, and phrased so that the significant aspects of a depressive illness can be canvassed in objective fashion, is then applied to patients who have been carefully evaluated. The items are scaled (so that the degrees of a trait or symptom can be recorded), the nondiscriminating items are discarded, and a final battery is tested against a patient population (both depressed and nondepressed) and against the judgment of the most competent staff members. Its reliability is also tested, although this offers some special difficulties. If the test is given again soon after a first testing, the patient may remember his earlier responses. If it is postponed, the illness may have actually changed so that low reliability can mean progress in cure. If the "split-half" method is used, the reliability may represent a halo effect (the spread from certain items, or symptoms, to others).

Wechsler, Grosser, and Busfield (1963) explored six areas: (1) physical functioning—sleep, appetite, elimination; (2) motor activity—retardation and agitation as manifested in energy level, character of speech, and motor behavior; (3) motivation or drive—interest in surroundings, plans for future; (4) mood and affect; (5) intellectual functioning; and (6) self-devaluation and guilt. In exploring these areas, they constructed some 34 test items, which, after some 37 psychiatrists had studied them and offered criticisms, were finally reduced to 28. With the scaling of each item a total maximum score of 131 for the most depressed, and of 28 for the least depressed, could be attained. The items which finally emerged included 14 which had to do with the patient's attitudes and feelings, 5 related to physiological functions, and 9 which called for observations by the interviewer. In the first group there were questions designed to draw forth the patient's comments about his ability to meet current situations, his past, his future, his memory, his interests, his suicidal preoccupations, his guilt feelings, his present mood, his initiative, his persistence in completing tasks, his fears or anxieties, his ability to concentrate, his concern about his present situation, and his self-esteem. In the second group he was asked about appetite disturbance, sleep disturbance, weight changes, changes in amount of energy, and disturbance of bodily functions. The third group called for the clinician's judgment of his motor activity, voice quality, pressure of speech, ideation, rapport with interviewer, personal appearance, ability to concentrate, degree of tenseness, and amount of energy. With three to six "levels" for each item, the structured interviews could be converted into numbers, and these numbers correlated with depth of depression as estimated by the most competent judges.

In the study of Wechsler and his associates, the reliability between raters (as determined when independent observers rated 158 patients) yielded an average coefficient of 0.67, ranging from 0.52, when the scales were filled out on the same day, to 0.78, when they were filled out a week later. (The experimenters suggest that the lower figure may represent actual diurnal fluctuations in the illness.) When the ratings were made by two interviewers who shared the same patient but asked questions taken from different portions of the test materials, and who could observe the patient as he answered (in any case), the reliability coefficient jumped to 0.88. When the scores of patients judged as nondepressed were averaged, they yielded values of 69 or lower in 80 per cent of the cases; the depressed group had scores of 70 or above in 80 per cent of the cases. Thus there was some overlapping, but not a great amount.

When four groups were constructed on the basis of the best clinical judgment (nondepressed, mildly depressed, moderately depressed, severely depressed), the mean scores were 46.7, 56.04, 76.53, 98.14. The ratings of improvement following therapy (the values here reported are all post-treatment values) are related to scores on the test for depression. Used at different hospitals, quite similar results were obtained, showing that, with changing staff members and changing validating personnel, the test continued to function in "foolproof" fashion. The value of such an instrument in measuring the success of various therapies (about which there is much controversy and a heavy investment of interest by proponents) is obvious.

Rough as this instrument is, it may serve a very useful purpose in the planning of treatment and the evaluation of therapeutic results. Since it emphasizes an aspect of the diagnostic process on which agreement is possible (the depth of the depression), it may facilitate in recentering treatment, especially where there is disagreement as to the diagnostic categories and where certain theoretical predilections may get in the way of both diagnosis and treatment. Wechsler notes that "theoretical conceptions of etiology held by different schools of psychiatry influence judgments of diagnosis and severity. Studies of consistency in application of diagnostic categories have disclosed a considerable proportion of diagnostic disagreements."

Beck *et al.* (1961) have constructed a similar inventory for measuring depression, have achieved similar (and slightly higher) reliabilities, and have demonstrated a similar consistency in the ratings by experienced psychiatrists of the depth of depression, and a similar inconsistency in the choice of the diagnostic categories.[4] Each of the categories used by Beck varied in the di-

---

[4]When two psychiatrists see the same patient and estimate the depth of the depression, and when they scale this depression in four steps, 97 per cent will fall either on the same steps or on adjacent steps. The consistency of diagnostic classifications is only 74 per cent.

rection of the group of traits as a whole. Split-half correlations averaged 0.86 (corrected for attenuation, 0.93) Beck also notes that the depth of depression may be as great in such a category as schizophrenia as in the manic-depressive group.

What the Tests Leave Undone

The tests for depression are based on the patient's answers to questions that deal chiefly with his present status. As deeply as a patient may be depressed at the nadir of his cycle, when he recovers he will give the kind of answers the nondepressed, "normal" person gives, or he may swing into hypomanic and manic euphoria. The emotional "weather" has changed. If there are three or four clearly identifiable steps down into the depth of depression, and a corresponding number of stages in the return to normality, and if these "levels" can be tested and validated by expert clinical judgment, a test might show where the patient is *at the moment.* When he has returned to normality, his scores will not vary from those of the person who has never had, and will never have, a depression.

When a highly valued and widely respected public servant like James Forrestal commits suicide, there is apt to be a cry: "Why didn't we do something to prevent it? Why do we not make periodic surveys of our men in key positions to forestall any such occurrence?" Considerations, both humane and practical, are advanced to support this demand. Forrestal's biographer, Rogow (1963, pp. 347-49), issues a call for serious consideration of the problem:

"If more is to be known about the mental and physical health of our political leaders, physicians and especially psychiatrists may have to reassess their traditional attitude toward the privacy of the doctor-patient relationship. At present, that attitude makes it difficult if not impossible to investigate in a systematic fashion the extent to which medical resources are involved in the complex interplay of politics, personality, and policy."

After noting the difficulties in constructing and administering a mental-health examination, Rogow cites "the battery of psychological tests 'to determine personality and motivation' given to the Mercury Astronauts."

In spite of the prestige of the Space Administration, and in spite of the authority invested in those psychologists whom the profession has accredited for assignments of this sort, even in these hands the tests do not have the *predictive* validity that we could hope for. In his prepsychotic period, the future manic-depressive patient does not express depressed thoughts, nor does he show a residue of them after he has recovered to a normal level of functioning.

One study of men under stress of semistarvation (Schiele and Brozek 1948), in which interviews and batteries of tests were used to detect those who would "break" under rigorous experimental procedures, found that, in spite of all precautions taken, there were some who underwent serious breakdowns.

Reviewing the performance of those who broke, and comparing it with those who came through successfully, no identifying scores could be found.

At the moment, with tests that have a very low predictive value, if any, with a psychiatric profession largely untrained in the construction, administration, and interpretation of test scores, and with the possibilities of misuse of authority, the time does not seem ripe for the establishment of any such thing as a Federal Board for the Review of the Mental Health of Public Officials. Even the prediction of recurrence of attacks of manic-depressive illness, once a record of a previous attack exists, is little more than a crude statistical probability. (Four out of five will have a second attack.) This bare fact has more predictive force than any of the tests or interview procedures can claim. It is a conditional prediction: it will hold, as a probability, if nothing is done to forestall a recurrence; if the kinds of pressures that were at work prior to the first attack continue; if no advance in insight into the way a self operates and no improvement in the general hygiene that governs the distribution of energies is made; if no supportive factors enter the field; and so on. Whatever genetic and constitutional factors may have existed prior to the first attack will continue to load the probabilities. But when one identical twin commits suicide, and the other does not, we seem to be justified in hoping that even an unfavorable constitutional loading can be overcome.

THE CONCEPT OF A MANIC-DEPRESSIVE PSYCHOSIS

There is a *concept* of a manic-depressive psychosis that is clearer than the recorded clinical facts. Like the historian's account of the reasons for the Franco-Prussian war, the *theory* of this psychosis is rigorous and permits a great economy in thinking. The facts themselves are "messy." In the clinic, diagnoses of the same patient vary (from physician to physician, and from time to time), and across the state borders the proportions of manic-depressives and schizophrenics found among first admissions differ. Thus manics can be "misdiagnosed" and, discharged as cured, return to hospital to be admitted as schizophrenics. When Sandifer discriminates a Type-A depression from a Type-B, he also notes an intermediate *mixed* group. The diagnosticians (and the clinical facts) do not behave in accord with logic-tight categories. The concept can be traced to Falret (1854), who identified an illness that he called *folie circulaire*. It was given a more precise form by Kraepelin in 1896, who set up criteria that would distinguish it from schizophrenia and from other affective disorders.

In this illness, mania and depression succeed one another in irregular fashion, with lucid intervals between attacks, and with a rhythm so independent of external circumstances (both as to duration and recurrence) that the course of the illness seems to be *internally* regulated.

Both the terms, *rhythmic* and *cyclic,* are misleading: either mania or melancholia may recur alone, in an individual case, or in irregular sequence; there are mixed forms that include facets of each extreme; the recurrence is so unpredictable that the pattern of succession can scarcely be called rhythmic; and, occasionally, the pathological state assumes a chronic form without interspersed lucid intervals. Typically the attacks reach a terminus, the patient improves with or without therapy, and in the lucid interval which follows, the normal functions which are restored show no measurable impairment. Thus it is a functional, reversible disorder, without persisting organic sequelae.

THE GENETIC FACTOR

The geneticist who studies the relatives of the patient adds a striking note to the description: if one member of a pair of identical twins is affected, there is a 90 per cent probability that the other member will be affected by the same type of psychotic process. From the mere identification and isolation of a cluster of symptoms that recurs in the clinic population, we have approached one kind of explanation of the facts. Add, still further, the speculation that this dominant gene probably controls some neurohormonal complex which periodically produces deficits or excesses of some substance that normally keeps man's emotional swings within safe bounds, and we have further refined our concept, even though we must admit that the nature of this protective-regulative substance and of the neurohormonal deficits is still obscure.

The genetic data and the speculations about neurohormonal regulators are advanced by Franz Kallmann (1954), among others; the most impressive of his supporting facts are the identical-twin data drawn from a sample of 206 siblings (27 monozygotic and 55 dizygotic twin pairs). In order to center on a precise target for investigation, Kallmann used cases that were hospitalized for psychosis, and excluded all depressions that began after age 50, all extreme mood changes associated with menopause or early senility, all reactive depressions in which a bad life-situation seemed to provide an adequate basis for personality disorganization, all psychoses in which there were hallucinatory episodes, and all instances of agitated depression with anxiety and hypertension. Thus a "pure" form (cyclic, rhythmic, acute, self-limited, middle-life) of attack emerged by this process of exclusion, a concept that contrasts with the varieties of affective psychoses which make up the clinic population. The endogenous-genetic concept fits the group formed by this diagnosis by exclusion.

In the Kallmann concept, it is possible for two pairs of identical twins to appear within the same family, one pair being both schizophrenic, the other pair manic-depressive; but it would not be possible for one identical twin to be manic-depressive while his twin is schizophrenic. In the raw data supplied by the clinics, however, there are individual cases diagnosed as manic-depressive on their first admission and later hospitalized and diagnosed as schizophrenia. Among the manic-depressives, who make up from 5 to 15 per cent of the first admissions to our mental hospitals, there will be many so diagnosed who also show hallucinations, come out of very bad life-situations, or show agitation, restlessness, and anxiety along with their depressions.

Some of these have experienced their first attack in late life. These other affective psychoses, which Kallmann would exclude from his study, also behave as his manic-depressives in one respect: they generally recover, without residual effects or signs of progressing deterioration, and experience recurrent episodes. (The group of senile depressions on an atherosclerotic base would be exceptions to this generalization about recovery.)

This disorder, which, in Kallmann's thinking, is determined by a single dominant gene, affects the offspring of manic-depressive parents (50 per cent of whose children have the psychosis) in a way unlike the excluded forms.[5] Kallmann believes, therefore, that some of those who have attacked the genetic hypothesis have probably failed to isolate the essential manic-depressive illness, as he has delimited it. Returning the attack, he invites his detractors to study twin pairs more intensively, since, here, in the monozygotics, the essential traits of a genetically determined illness are isolated by nature. "Improve your diagnostic skills here," he seems to say, "with the identical twins as your teacher."

There are other odds and ends which emerge in this genetic analysis of a "pure" type of manic-depressive psychosis. His evidence shows, Kallmann reports, that when the illness occurs in monozygotic twin pairs inclined to obesity, it is the more obese member of the pair who shows the widest mood swings. He and other observers[6] have noted that two out of three cases show the pyknic habitus, a body type that, in addition to the tendency toward obesity, has a greater susceptibility to cardiovascular disorders (and less than normal liability to tuberculosis). Within the monozygotic twinship, Kallmann found that one member of the pair could have a more pronounced trend toward the depressive end of the cycle while the other tended to show elation more frequently.

Those who conceive of self-regulation as a power that is slowly and painfully acquired through a social discipline will find Kallmann's concept of the manic-depressive psychosis somewhat puzzling, since he seems to posit a regulative mechanism whose presence or absence depends on a single neuro-humoral entity determined by a dominant gene. The slow process of learning to express and inhibit impulses in the light of personal goals and social consequences would require hundreds of thousands of conditionings (or as many efforts to formulate and strive toward objectives), according to the first view. According to Kallmann's view, we should be looking for a chemical packet, or some medication that can substitute for it, with much the same outlook as those who hopefully believe that administration of LSD-25 will solve such a complex disorder as alcoholism.

---

[5]The likelihood of finding a manic-depressive in any sample of the general population lies somewhere near four in one thousand. Kallmann's theory would prepare him to find one member of an identical twin pair affected with one of the excluded types of psychosis, without having to revise his concept.

[6]Slater, Hoffman, Lange, Ey, Luxenburger, and others support Kallmann in this emphasis on constitution and genetic makeup. See Chap. 2 above. See also Fuller and Thompson 1960.

This problem of the "regulation of behavior" is illustrated by the reaction of the parent who, starting out on a trip with children who are "problems" (i.e., are restless, difficult to control, excited, apt to become nauseated), decides to solve the whole problem by giving each of the children a small dose of bonamine (or some equally potent ataractic drug). What the drug does for the patient whom the psychiatrist finds difficult to restrain (and he is more likely to use thorazine, stelazine, or another of the new and potent tranquilizers), the milder bonamine does for the children; these drugs relieve both parent and psychiatrist from having to use other forms of restraint, or from carrying out the kind of habit training (or discipline) that might build other self-regulative devices (or powers) within the child or patient.

The Typological Approach

This problem of self-regulation, which becomes so patent in the manic-depressive psychosis, is handled in similar fashion by the typologists. Jean Delay (1946, pp. 1-5) appears to take this tack in his description of what he calls the schizothyme and cyclothyme makeups. In their extreme forms these constitutions (and body types) become manic-depressive and schizophrenic; in the milder versions that we count as within the normal range, both of these trends are present in varying but less extreme degrees; and in a series of individuals these constitutionally determined trends will produce all the varieties from the extreme introvert (schizoid, shut-in) to the most outgoing extrovert.[7] The latter is warm, in close contact with the persons around him, quick to respond and to catch and reflect a mood, empathizing easily, a sympathetic type, a likable character. The other is cold, withdrawn, out of touch with his surroundings, and so in need of an extended rational and interpretative framework that he remains inhibited when he does not have it. It is hard to get through to him unless one is fully in tune with that private, logical, schematic framework (i.e., unless one enters into his delusional system). We might call him a "constitutional Cartesian." Folk psychology links the extroverted personality with the Latin temperament, the introverted with the colder Scandinavian mentality. We could easily imagine the former to be predisposed to those ups and downs in moods without apparent cause that appear in the manic-depressive, and, in contrast, imagine that the schizoid is in danger of the apathy and withdrawal of the schizophrene or of that unreachable, autistic, and hallucinated state of the paranoid person.

Delay uses the terms *sympathique* and *apathique* for these types. The sense of the word "sympathique" is carried by the physical example of "sympathetic vibrations." Such a person strikes responsive chords in those around him, and he is welcomed as a "member of the club." The "apathique"

---

[7]Minkowski (1927, p. 80), who also accepts a typology of mental illness, describes the thought of the schizophrene as spatial, as though he were trying to reduce the normal action that occurs within psychological time to a mathematico-deductive geometry.

type neither stirs others nor gives the impression of being stirred himself. Decidedly, he does not "send us," and thus, to more than the usual degree, he remains an *outsider*. That this latter condition can be a passing dynamic state is amply documented in Janet's discussion (1928, pp. 216 ff) of the "morose inactive." These psychasthenics have a way of falling into and of rising out of this state of apathy, emptiness, and lack of rapport; in this state they feel the unreality, the uncanny quality, of persons and places around them. They do not empathize nor react fully; even a brother or a sister seems strange, as though some actor had been made up to play the part and had succeeded in producing a good imitation that was still something short of the real thing.

The fact that the manic-depressive psychosis is associated with the pyknic habitus in only two cases out of three should remind us that, even if trends can be demonstrated, the illness, body type, and life-style are not associated in any one-to-one fashion. However, the typologists insist: these are constitutional types, in no sense the outcome of life-experiences, but instead the determiners of the course and dynamic properties of these experiences. Odd that a bodily and psychological constitution should make one man prone to hyperrationality, in which his action is all "sicklied o'er" by a network of inhibitory considerations, a veritable thicket through which stimuli have to penetrate before practical action can occur; where an opposite type has the thinnest of protective shells and is prone, therefore, to show the widest swings in mood, to be the first to become "engaged" and the first to break off, deeply disappointed and disaffected. The latter would be the one carried away by the crowd, or by the enthusiastic salesman, and the first to feel overwhelmed by a sea of troubles. The difficulty of the schizoid lies, on the contrary, in an aloofness that, too often, permits him to react only after the opportunity is past, e.g., when he reads about it in the newspaper. Given to rumination and long, long thoughts, he is also likely to be filled with symbolic-autistic fantasies that are not validated and that mesh poorly with reality.

These two temperaments, or instinctive tonalities, are concepts that may have been derived, in the first place, from contact with patients who had been segregated into clinical categories. They become, in turn, the clinician's prejudgment, and influence his assessment of the probable prepsychotic personality. But they also create difficulty for the clinician who has on his hands a schizophrenic who had been diagnosed as a manic-depressive two years ago. Such a clinician might derive a little comfort from the observation of Kallmann: "Procedurally, it is one of the most difficult tasks of a psychiatric research unit to procure adequate evidence of past pathological mood swings in persons who are temporarily stabilized, and relate it to patients requiring no extended hospitalization." This same difficulty may lie at the root of the conflicting evidence which challenges this stereotyping, for the very area where valid evidence is difficult to come by is the area in which we build clinical stereotypes, pseudoscientific confabulations to bridge the gaps in our knowledge. Neither the person himself nor the family are very good witnesses, nor are they too interested in such discussions, or capable of taking an objective view of such matters, any more than the manic patient, who does not care to pause and discuss his earlier moods: he had *never* been depressed, he is now sure.

Whatever the final consensus may be about the existence of these "types" (in any but the conceptual realm) and their relationship to type of psychosis, both the constitutional concept of the cause and the current types of psychotherapy based on it raise as many problems as they solve. If it is a constitution that is illness-prone, we have yet to discover the specific cyclothymic mechanism. If the essential illness is a sickness in the hypothalamic cells, precisely how does the diffuse effect of electroconvulsive therapy produce changes in these cells, affecting a genetically caused weakness so as to shorten an average hospital stay of six months to an average of three? The answers are most confusing.

EXTRAGENETIC FACTORS

After we have assigned the disorder to "incontestable" genetic causes and have identified a biotype (body and personality type) that is well-rounded physically (pyknic) and extroverted psychologically (syntonic) and that has a labile emotional life (easily boosted into jubilation and ecstasy and as easily plunged into despair), we still have to note that one-third of the diagnosed manic-depressives do not fit into this latter category. Ey quotes the work of Mauz (1930) and Luxenburger (1942) as pointing to 64 per cent of the cases in the pyknic habitus defined by Kretschmer (1925). The existence of the "exceptions" forces us to consider other possible factors. Even if a biotype existed, even if it provided a basically low threshold so that ordinary stresses become pathogenic, we would have to consider those ordinary stresses. Faced with this question, Ey suggests that we consider the following possible extragenetic causes.

1. Cerebral lesions may disturb the integrative network. (These would include the effects of gunshot wounds, accidental traumata of varied origins, tumors, arteriosclerosis and the resultant changes in circulation, and changes produced by encephalitis and meningitis.) None of the studies of brain changes in manic-depressives has revealed clear evidence of a precisely localized histopathology or physiopathology whose existence is both necessary and sufficient.

A very large amount of research on both human beings and animals has been devoted to the identification of "centers of emotions." Electrodes implanted to excite specific points or to record cell changes within a precise area (by means of EEGs), and direct manipulation of third-ventricle cells (or stimulation of same) in human beings who can report conscious states while being operated upon, have produced a mass of contradictory evidence, and an even greater volume of interpretations that support a variety of opposing theories.

In the place of well-supported conclusions we have hypotheses and affirmations, such as:

a. There is a specific center for each major emotion.

b. Mania is the consequence of a primary and localized hyperactivity of cells in the hypothalamus.

c. Stimulation of the floor of the hypothalamus, manually or electrically, will (and also will not) produce identifiable emotions.

d. Excitation or excision of subcortical tissues (such as those on the floor of the hypothalamus) will alter motor, visceral, and glandular *expressions* of emotions, and change physiological processes, but will leave the emotional behavior relatively intact.

e. The sham rage produced by decortication is not true rage, and should be called a pseudaffective response.

Since the hypothalamus is normally in constant contact and interchange with the cortex, with a two-way stream of impulses (corticothalamic and thalamocortical) binding this autonomic center into a wide-reaching network of "controls," it can be a "center" for emotions only in a virtual sense. In turn the hypothalamus is continually bombarded with both excitatory and inhibitory impulses from the pituitary, from the reticular apparatus of the brain stem, and from viscera and skeletal muscles. Thus the gonads affect the pituitary and hypothalamus, just as the stimuli from distance receptors can arouse the reproductive system. When we think of this expanded network of connections, with the center "affected" by the periphery and the latter "under the control of" the center, it is difficult to place any perception, emotion, or action in any one spot: it is the system as a whole that is perturbed under pressure; it is the person who acts. When there are wide swings in mood, such as in the manic-depressive psychosis, we have no good logical ground for anticipating that the "sickness" will be localized in a particular group of cells: it is a dynamically interacting whole that is changed. In so insisting upon the complexity of the relationships, and in endeavoring to think in terms of a "dynamic imbalance," we need not discourage anyone who is looking for a specific factor that can throw the whole into its pathological phases. Rather, one should expect that many of these disturbers will be found. The single-gene notion does, however, seem to become less probable in such a holistic conception.

2. The endocrine products of thyroid, pituitary, ovaries, testes, and adrenals have all been suspected to be contributing causes of the mood swings and of the deregulation of action and thought. Again, though each may be contributory, none is essential and sufficient (witness the poor relationship found to exist between the involutional changes and late-life depressions).

3. Metabolic disorders, vitamin deficiencies, liver or kidney failure, lactic-acid production, blood sugar, blood cholesterol, protein metabolism, acid-base balances, and basal metabolism have all been suspected to be pathogenic agents.

4. Toxic agencies have been found to produce manic-like behavior (e.g., alcohol, hashish, cocaine, nitrous oxide, amphetamine, atabrine, nicotinic

acid). A variety of therapies has been suggested by clinicians operating with hypotheses suggested by these facts, but none of them has been particularly successful, although each has produced its "reported recovery or improvement" in the hands of some enthusiast. Bellak enumerates a list of fifty-odd agents which have been tried, including cobra venom, whiskey, dilantin, atropin, theelin, acetylcholine, histamine, decholin, liver extracts, methedrine, and nicotinic acid. Taken as a whole, such a list bears testimony to the deep conviction that something which can be taken by mouth will solve the cyclothymic's mood-swing problem, compensate for a deficit in regulatory *substances,* restore the balance in a system so that once more the "consequences of action in a perceived field" may play their normal role.

5. Traumatic emotional experiences—loss of love, failure in business or vocation, pressures of work, stress of combat—have been thought to produce these releases of emotion or provide the final straw that breaks the too weak tolerance for stress of these susceptible individuals. Summarizing the factors listed in the life-history of patients diagnosed as manic-depressive insanity, Travis (1933) found that there were 2 per cent who had no listed precipitating causes. The balance of the records included such factors as marital maladjustment (33 per cent), death in the family (17 per cent), childbirth (11 per cent), a physical condition (11 per cent), economic worries (10 per cent), antagonism to parents (8 per cent), and sickness in the family (8 per cent).

The greater the emphasis placed on such exogenous factors, the more the diagnostician is inclined to take the case out of the *"true* manic-depressive" category and to place it in another one called *"reactive* depression." The pure case that is "incontestably" produced by a genetic factor thus becomes a "thymergasia" with no known exogenous cause. One would expect that a clinician, sure of his genetic theory, would not look on anything but the most patent and extreme stress as a sufficient cause for psychotic depressions or elations; indeed, many stresses might be left out of consideration, since they are of the type that the ordinary person carries without breakdown. Where such exogenous causes are in fact important, the exclusion of these cases from consideration would certainly lead to confusion for the geneticist studying family records, since most of these items fall on one member and not on his relatives. Either the geneticists have been clever in selecting just the right patients for study, or their insistence that exogenous factors are of minor importance is correct, or the sufficient stress will appear, sooner or later, in any life with a sufficiently vulnerable system. For all of his eclecticism, Ey never reaches the point of questioning the primary role of the genes in this disorder.

What Ey finds worth emphasizing is the fact that an attack of mania or depression is not something like a mild toothache, something local and all but peripheral to the main structure of the self-system. Instead, it is something which alters the very essence of a self-in-action. It has to be conceived of as hitting the very *center* of selfhood, or of affecting the system as a whole.

Local or not, it alters thinking, reasoning, self-regulation, the sensible contact with reality, the action into the future; it changes valences of perceived objects, the liveliness and extent of the field that is lived in (vital space-time); it releases poorly conceived actions, lowers the powers of self-criticism, overwhelms the remaining organization of behavior, until reason is either destroyed or made to serve these nonlogical, affective tides.

SICK CELLS IN THE DIENCEPHALON?

If we could identify the precise nature and location of that illness in the cells which regulate our emotional life, say, for example, in some portion of the hypothalamus, in which so many autonomic functions center, or if we could accept as proved the theory that, somewhere in the lower third of the thalamus (or in some other precise area not too remote from the third ventricle), there were cells whose excitation with an electrode would produce genuine emotional experience or whose excision would reduce a person to a state of terror, guilt, and depression, or if we could find the precise chemical that had the affinity for a specific neurovegetative complex so that either mania or depression could be quickly canceled, we would have arrived at the goal that has been fantasied by many theories and therapies. The Vogts' discovery of hypothalamic lesions in their postmortem study of the brains of hebephrenics is evidence of one use of this notion of an illness in specific cell groups. They have also advanced (1951) the notion that manic-depressive insanity behaved as though governed by a recessive gene. Thus we would have to look on the sickness of the cells as an expression of a specific constitutional weakness. Perhaps the next step would be to look on hebephrenia as an extension of this same illness to a point of no return, with irreversible changes destroying the cells. (Such an extension of the sick-cell theory would not fit Kallmann's interpretations, in which the manic-depressive twin never has an identical, schizophrenic twin. Perhaps different loci for the two illnesses would then be urged.)

Kraines writes (1957, p. 508), "Assuming that the diencephalic-reticular systems constitute the site from which these symptoms arise, and remembering that psychic forces do not play an etiologic role in the typical manic-depressive patient, one must inquire into the nature of the pathologic process." He discusses the hereditary data, and argues that the hereditary susceptibility must lie in this same diencephalic-rhinencephalic area, and that the precipitating factors must lie elsewhere *in the body*. He discards diet from the list of probable causes, thinks circulatory changes (vasomotor spasms with resultant anoxia) might be involved, believes that endocrine changes should be placed high in the list of suspects, notes the frequency of the pyknic habitus, and believes that gonadal changes may prove to be the most fruitful type to study. He thus views the diencephalic-rhinencephalic-reticular systems as mediating mechanisms of the illness, and any other factor or combination of factors as the secondary or precipitating causes.

Jean Delay (1946) sees the problem as one of discovering the factors that disturb the balance between cortex and hypothalamus: a weakening of inhibitory functions or surges in the instinctive pulsions that arise in the hypothalamus may be responsible. Located at the crossroads between "body" and "mind," the hypothalamus becomes the focus of all the conflict between the socialized tendencies and the instinctive pulsions that rise from the tissues. It is both the animator and inhibitor of the cortex above; the latter, in turn, binds the more primitive regulator within a wider "life of relationships." Whether the upward flow of impulses from hypothalamus to the cortex is dynamogenic or inhibitory depends on an affective quality that is determined by a process within this group of cells which no one, at present, seems to be too clear about. The hypothalamus is the regulator of the ebb and flow of emotions, the vital center without whose support the ego can issue no commands, the wellspring of mental energy, and the source of those obscure rhythms in mood that become, in the manic-depressive patient, mania or melancholia. With this scheme in mind, Delay warns against crediting to a sudden increase in emotional charge what is due to a deficit in inhibitory power, or vice versa. The corticobasilar *equilibrium* is at fault in the psychoses.

Although Ey calls the manic-depressive psychosis the mental illness most clearly of genetic origin, the nature and location of the tissues which give way remain unknown. It would still hold, as in the fracture of a bone, that there are always external pressures as well as an internal weakness. Even if we could identify some factor in the adrenal-sympathetic system, some neurohormonal substance whose poor resynthesis produces toxic factors, some acute illness of the hypothalamic system that regulates the vegetative system (and emotional expressions), we would also need to relate the "breakdowns" to some press. Whatever the inner sources of the deregulation may turn out to be, they do not lead into irreversible or degenerative changes in this psychosis. Only the *actions and emotions* of the temporarily deranged mind (such as a suicide, or the attempt to cross Fifth Avenue while in a state of exaltation, or some public performance of manic quality, or some open confession of a real crime under the urgency of guilt and depression) can lead to irreversible effects. As for the patient's ecstasy or anguish while ill, these are easily forgotten on recovery and seem to leave no harmful traces. It is almost as though recovery had brought about a shift in gears, so that the normal memory systems can replace the ones of the psychotic period.

PSYCHOANALYTIC HYPOTHESES

One might argue that, by the very nature of its methods, psychoanalysis cannot produce anything but the most tentative of hypotheses. Its free-association method, its interpretation of dreams, its introspective and retrospective reconstruction of the earliest phases of infancy and childhood cannot claim any great accuracy, and when this highly subjective interpretation is carried on while the patient is in a depressed or maniacal state, all the data will be subject to the gravest distortion. Since the bulk of these attacks occur, for the first time, in the years between 20 and 40, the strain on the recall process is great indeed. The view of a prepsychotic self obtained from the mouth of a depressed person would certainly require the support of objective data, which is almost wholly lacking in the studies of busy psychoanalysts, whose efforts are concerned with the present mental condition of their patients.

Beginning with Freud (1917) and Karl Abraham (1927), psychoanalysts have linked melancholia with mourning, with the loss of love. Since there is not always an actual loss of a loved one in the cases of psychotic depression a clinician sees, it follows that whatever precipitated the change in the cases without such loss must have symbolized some earlier loss: some little "loss" in the present must reactivate a state of mind and a drama that was first enacted in infancy. It is true that some depressions are precipitated by the death of a parent, sibling, lover, or superior, but others are precipitated by a failure in some important relationship (with wife, husband, lover), or by a disappointment in some relationship with an institution, or by a professional failure, or—most curiously—by a sudden marked professional success. It is difficult to believe that the common element is indeed that "loss of love" that the psychoanalysts' theory posits.

It is only by projecting the current dynamic trends onto an earlier scene enacted in infancy that the psychoanalyst is able to make his theory work, and in so projecting the current conflicts onto a *myth of development,* he is able to wring from the current scene the meaning that interprets symptoms. At the same time he reveals his own view of the socialization process as it is enacted in the Western world.

For his purpose he utilizes a quartet of trends. In the beginning is the need for love: the child's helplessness, his incompleteness. His need for guidance and support creates a basic anxiety and a basic set of demands. These demands are answered more or less willingly and more or less completely in most homes. There is little evidence that the mothering of the manic-depressive patient is radically faulty, but even if it were perfect, there comes a time when the pressures that force a child to mature, to feed himself, to undertake a whole series of developmental tasks, thrust him from his little kingdom where he has ruled so completely. He learns that he must put forth effort, strive, discipline himself, give up, comply. If he has internalized the good mother and developed an appetite for her approval, he will also agree with her that some of his own impulses are bad. Yet he cannot help feeling resentment at parental authority, and at the same time feeling guilty for this welter of lethal hate that arises within him. There will be other forms of guilt: guilt as he feels himself unloved, for not having achieved as he should, for not having obeyed as he should, and for not having completely eliminated the impulses which still rise within him. He is guilty because he has lost the full love of that first significant other (and of that internalized other, the superego). So we have (1) the need for love, for more love than is easily obtained, for unconditional love, (2) the compensatory striving that requires compliance, denial, ascetic-masochistic maneuvers, (3) the resentment against the other and against the symbolized other that has been incorporated, and (4) the lethal hate, guilt, and anxiety that arise from it, and the self-hate that arises because the unregenerate portion of the self (and the nonfeasant self) is unloved and unlovely and undeserving of love.

This quartet represents an unstable equilibrium of trends which, instead of rapidly and permanently resolving itself, can sometimes generate an interlocking fixation (an arrest of development), and provide a groundwork for later regressions and return engagements. The more resentment accumulates (along with a hate and a sense of guilt), the more the individual must compensate, undo, suppress, and the more he is likely to deny his own feelings. The quartet of guilt, need for love, hate, and self-hate constitutes a vicious cycle that, laid away, lurks to spring into action when the going gets rough. In an infant all this groundwork may be laid down at the stage of toilet-training, when, though a runabout, he seems bent on remaining an infant and frustrating his mother, yet still is in need of her understanding love and skillful mothering. This early deadlock can be quickly laid aside: the battle of the sphincters is soon over for most of us; we do learn to control bladder and bowel needs. In some this is learned at a cost: the image of the other one that is stored away will be split, having been shattered during the conflict, and this fracture underlies a tendency toward ambivalence and coping mechanisms that are actually self-destructive.[8] The openness, the naive confidence of an infant, once so unalloyed, will never again be the same. This scarring in early infancy can be repeated and reinforced in the peer group, on a playground, where in their first year at school children learn the shape of a very imperfect "justice," at adolescence (when the craving for intimacy leads to the formation of twosomes, and, sometimes, to betrayals), and at every stage in which crises center around love, guidance, achievement, conformity, power, and that growth in the direction of shared ideals which produces the socialized man. It can emerge to alter the dynamics of all interpersonal transactions. (Are you for me or against me?)

This quartet will reveal itself in the kind of rapport a depressed patient can establish with his analyst, who is faced with the task of identifying their sources if these ghosts of an earlier period are to be laid. The *current* dynamics, which center around conflicts that are so common in our society that they seem at first incapable of generating any extreme and irreversible changes, are thus viewed as not the most important sources of mania and depressions. Rather, the analyst urges, these sources lie in those earlier and originally sensitizing transactions whose residues have persisted in the unconscious of the patient. Forward and backward, down into infancy and back up into the recent past, the analytic explorations (by means of free associations and dream analysis) will weave interpretations that can be given to the patient

---

[8]This "other one" becomes the censor, inside the individual. All parent figures take on its qualities. The ones in authority, the "image of the laws," the policeman, the teacher, the critic: all in turn arouse this unfinished ambivalence and make it difficult for the individual to learn with grace.

as explanations of his conflicts, as indicating the very roots of his feelings. These interpretations also point to the changes that he must undertake to unlock the fixations and undo the faulty ways that he has been using in coping with his impulses and with the others who now replace that first censor. The patient will have to learn that, in fact, he asks too much; that he does not know how to evoke the precise responses in others that he needs; that he is too preoccupied with pleasing and hurting "the other one" and does not consult his own heart; that he surrenders too much and in consequence hates too intensely; or that his loving is both aggressive and self-destructive because he is compulsively acting out an old drama and mis-identifying those around him as though they were characters in that earlier drama.

Why are the present precipitating factors, shared by so many others who do *not* become pathologically depressed, so pathogenic in this case? Why is he driven beyond the borders where emotions cease to be compensating and self-regulating reactions and instead serve to fixate mania or melancholia? The answers run:

1. Because there was an unusually traumatic period, back there.

2. Because this is an individual with a special constitution—witness the 25 to 1 probability of finding an affective psychosis in the near relatives.

3. Because this is an individual who is endowed with a stronger hating mechanism (death instinct) than the average.

4. Because this person had a higher degree of oral dependency, therefore made more excessive demands, and developed—when the environment failed to comply with them—greater resentment.

5. Because an accelerated growth and an overweening ambition, made compulsive by early imbalance between ego, superego, and id, has forced this individual into a taut self-regulative pattern that is highly vulnerable, setting in motion vicious cycles such as indicated in the above-named hypothetical quartet.

6. Because the loved one that was lost had been the target of great hostility, and, internalized in the form of superego, now directs hatred against the self, who in turn feels a murderous hate.

Each of these reasons has been emphasized by one or another of the analytic authorities as these have extended and elaborated the thesis Abraham first proposed. Melancholy, seen as an episode of grief, gave the clue and set the analysts looking for the lost love-object that was being mourned. If, as postulated, the patient regresses to an ambivalent, pregenital stage, the questions arise: "Does he regress, now, because of that earlier drama and its scars?" "Why has he waited so long?" "Is the descent caused by some present state of affairs that is now forcing him to act out trends that are more appropriate to a pregenital level (in the way that frustration brings an obscene vocabulary to the lips of the carpenter who has pounded his thumb)?" In simplest terms: does his difficulty date from an exceptional childhood, or is he simply an adult coping with his difficulties by descending to a childish level?

Much of the language of psychoanalysis is figurative and metaphoric. It has to be translated and given precision if it is to escape from the self-validating level of mythanalysis. When Freud points out that the mourning and melancholia refer to an internal loss, a lost person that has been incorporated, we might translate in this fashion: along with the mother's milk, the child incorporates her values; she comes to dwell within him symbolically, so that in thought her benediction is sought, unconsciously and automatically, as action is planned. The better she was as a mother, the more painful it will be to act in wayward fashion (until other satisfactions, other voices, other personalities serve to extinguish this primal Oedipus fixation). Normally the child begins to see the world the way the people next door see it too. His inner authority expands to include the gang on the playground, the teacher, the baseball hero, and so on.

The ambivalence directed against an incorporated love-object is a mixture of compliance and affection and resentment and guilt (it is multivalent and almost too complex for words) that develops as successful growth and multiple but conflicting loyalties find a more or less satisfactory resolution in firm and positive action. The analysts seem to imply that these conflicts are more acute in the manic-depressive, no matter how well he seems to resolve them when viewed from without. He is a conforming man, says Arieti (1959, I, 434), an outwardly successful and adapted man, but inwardly things are in confusion. "He is generally efficient, and people who do not know him too well have the impression that he is a well-adjusted, untroubled individual. On the contrary, he is not a happy man." Arieti chooses to call him outer-directed rather than other-directed. In fact, he has special difficulties with these "others."

All manner of ad hoc hypotheses have been developed by Abraham and those who follow him:

1. There is a constitutional and inherited oral eroticism.

2. There is a special fixation of libido at the oral level.

3. There is a severe injury to infantile narcissism (a disappointment in infantile love needs).

4. There is a repetition of the primary disappointment in later life.

Mania, which remains an essentially unexplained fusion of ego with superego, may depend on some biologically determined cycle like the fusion of ego with id that occurs every 24 hours as we fall into sleep and dream.

All of this, however, is more strategy than science. It reveals how an analyst looks on the symptoms that we all see, but these hypotheses (which could be elaborated indefinitely, so fertile has psychoanalysis been in inventing word puzzles) have not been supported by the type of longitudinal studies that alone could validate them. Since some of them refer to an inner dynamics that once existed in an infant (whose own mother could not see the relations at the time) and which cannot even be recalled by the patient himself, it may be that the very nature of these hypotheses precludes any possible evaluation.

Like many other theorists, Arieti attempts to sketch the prepsychotic personality of the manic-depressive patient, but, as has been the case so often, without validating longitudinal studies and without statistically impressive evidence. He suggests three patterns:

1. The rigid conformist, duty-bound, an imitative rather than creative man, a stable and incessant worker with a life-style not far from that sketched for the coronary cases seen by Jacob Arlow (1945).

2. A more immature and dependent type who still yearns for an unconditional bliss, who has not developed good work habits, but who, feeling guilty, has developed techniques for enlisting aid and for making others feel guilty, and usually has "elected" a particular person to be his leaning post.

3. A type who gives the appearance of hearty and outgoing friendliness but who is only superficially related to others, a shallow activist who escapes into reality yet never "grasps" it. This is the type that Pascal excoriated, ready to check meditation and any deep self-awareness by any and all kinds of diversion. They are pseudo-psychopaths who are forever trying to avoid the full realization of their unhappy condition, who laugh in order not to cry, but who fall into depressions from time to time nonetheless.

Arieti (1959, I, 430) confesses, "our knowledge of the psychodynamics of these cases is still fragmentary." Indeed, the whole attempt to study the adult depressive "from the inside" and to make such a self seem rational (when its essence is its irrationality) forces the analyst into the position of projecting what everyone can see onto the screen of an infancy which no one, as yet, knows much of anything about. It leads him to project into the individual's past a set of imputed psychodynamic relations now believed in operation. And we have already noted to what extent the thinking of the depressed person about himself, about his past, is distorted. Here and there an analyst has been led to affirm some special constitution or inherited endowment, to postulate a type of nursing experience (that has never been validated), or to invent some special dosage of the death instinct (to account for the violent suicides committed by these depressed patients, a suicide that is "hatred turned in"). Every dynamic trend that the analysts speak of (such as that resentment we feel when we have conformed and deprived ourselves to win approval) exists, no doubt, in the depressed person as in the normal individual. To the degree that the analyst's thinking has seen through that outer face of the ego which the manic shows to others, it has also suggested something about Everyman. But to make it helpful in the causal explanation of the manic-depressive psychosis, the conflicting trends have to be measured, or carefully estimated, so that they can be shown to be stronger in the prepsychotic personality of these patients. We do not know that much about them, and we do not have the measuring devices to estimate, in comparison groups of normals, the kind of balances implied.

The manic-depressive is "antinomic man," writes Henri Ey, repeating a judgment of Binzwanger. But this is simply taking the symptomatic facts over again, and reifying them into some essence within. To be sure, he is a creature of moods, of ups and downs without sufficient cause, of extremes, of love and hate, of black and white, and of an uneasy swing from one extreme to another, always passing through the balanced position and never staying long on a stable course. But we would have to formulate this "swinging from one extreme to another" (which sometimes passes the point of no return into psychotic fixations) in some "life-style schedule" that could be assessed before the fact, if we are to predict the course of the psychosis. As it is today, prediction is possible only after a depression has occurred in late life. Then, reports Rennie (1942), 79 per cent will have a second attack, 63.5 per cent a third, and 45 per cent a fourth. Yet these are "life-styles" that maintained a normal adjustment for forty years or more before the first attack struck. Perhaps an analysis of depressions that strike early, during adolescence and in the early twenties, and those which make their appearance late in life, would yield material for a revealing comparison with normals who have escaped the illness altogether. Since such studies have not been made, we are left with "postmortem" inferences and ad hoc hypotheses. We are left with mechanisms that resemble those of the normal and that can differ from the latter only quantitatively, and the grim genetic facts which testify to some (as yet unknown) susceptibility.

AGITATED DEPRESSIONS

Descriptively we can isolate from those depressions that are retarded, apathetic, difficult to move, another group that is agitated, restless, pacing to and fro, wringing the hands, seemingly unable to rest in one place for a moment, driven, anxious, full of plaints. Kraepelin, the classifier, after linking mania and depressions in a single cyclic disorder, was driven to look on this group as made up of "mixed cases" with both manic and depressive symptoms fused into a single combination. The mood of these patients is definitely depressive, however, and they are totally lacking in the euphoria the manic shows. Noyes and Kolb look on the agitation as simply an expression of a strong anxiety component, as though the patient anticipated some impending harm (or punishment) that was about to befall him. Kraines (1957, pp. 350-54), who would place this form along with the involutional melancholias, urges that the category be renamed, since the symptoms and treatment of both types are not demonstrably different from those in other depressions of the endogenous-genetic group, and since changing diagnostic fashions produced this artifact by attaching the diagnosis "involutional" when a first depression arrives in late life.

Bitterness, hostility, resentment seem more to the fore, but if we "explain" this by positing a stronger dose of the "death instinct" in these patients, we are simply reifying the phenomena. The patient demands that he be punished, and is at the same time fearful and resentful. "We assume," observes

Cameron (1963, p. 519), "that it is the superego that demands it." This combination of reification and tautology entraps us all as we invent categorizing words that "explain" what our science fails to clarify.

Cameron (1944, p. 883) makes a good suggestion about treatment of these cases that deserves to be applied more widely, in other diagnostic problems as well. He notes:

"Their need for simple occupation and encouragement is too easily overlooked because any directive effort on their part appears to the inexperienced to be entirely out of the question; but actually this is a group that in the long run is very likely to repay every effort at constructive therapy made on the occupational level."

Titley (1938) is persuaded that this disorder differs from the manic-depressive psychoses, since he found, when he reviewed the prepsychotic personality data for the two disorders, that the agitated-depression patients (descriptively identified by three aspects: "depression without retardation; psychomotor unrest; and anxiety relating either to self or to environment, even at times merging into anxious delusions") showed a characteristic prepsychotic personality that included the following features: "narrow interests, difficulty in making adjustments to change, asocial and unfriendly attitudes, intolerance and poor sexual adjustment, a rigid ethical code, proclivity for saving, extreme reticence, marked sensitivity and anxious trends, stubbornness, overconscientiousness, and meticulosity." In contrast, the manic-depressive patients studied did not depart from the normal in their prepsychotic makeup.

The group of patients diagnosed as involutional melancholia were found to have had the same type of prepsychotic personality as the agitated depressions when Titley applied the same method of analyzing case histories. His groups were small, and in spite of his own careful study of the life-histories, others may find that such personality data may prove to be of doubtful value in differentiating the disorders. The differences in present behavior are real. It is these symptom clusters, visible at the time the patients enter hospital, that lead the classifier to create a special category. The categories are dynamic, and may represent stages in an illness that is notoriously full of transitions. There are fluctuations in dynamics, mood changes, and shifts in the flow of energy, the perceptual grasp of the world, which cover the whole scale of moods, from anguish to ecstasy. Furthermore, the patient that today complains principally of fatigue, and appears to behave like a neurasthenic, may pass through an obsessive-compulsive stage in which there seems to be a heightening of the conflicts, a sharpening of the hostilities aimed at the ego, a loss of control of the part-processes. On the wide-ranging cyclic swings from mania to depression, with mixed states and transitional zones in which a pressure to act is combined with anxiety and intropunitive attitudes (as in the agitated depressions), there is a continuum of changing dynamic states. Although a deficient integrative power seems to be a common factor throughout the series, the series does not seem to rest on any fixed "anatomy of the personality" or on any known and irreversible organic lesion, for, after the cyclic changes, the same patient may rise to calm confidence, behave normally, resume productive living, and look back in disbelief on the behavior that he now hears described and has all but forgotten.

In the depths of his depression he shows, according to Farrar (1951), "an almost incredible concentration upon the single purpose of self-destruction. The formerly devoted husband or wife or parent, the business or professional man who has conscientiously fulfilled all his obligations as a good citizen and has observed the customary social, legal, and religious sanctions, now becomes totally oblivious of all of these relationships and of what are normally the most elementary duties. These matters are simply not in the patient's consciousness. What, for example, is to become of his family is not a problem for him to deal with because it does not present itself to his mind, or if it does it is as if it were of no concern to him in the presence of the one overwhelming impulse, the fixity, exclusiveness, and urgency of which is something that cannot be experienced and can hardly be appreciated by the normal mind. Recovered patients have tried to describe this state which to them also in retrospect seems scarcely to have been possible."

This "gunbarrel" mental vision, as Farrar calls it, is a dynamic thing, a change in the range and scope of presentification, in the mood, in the capacity for action, that arrives with the depression. He has not been this type of man. He will not be this type, later, when he recovers. When we describe the intropunitive hostility that turns against the very self as the work of a hypertrophied superego, it is well to observe that this is also a narrowed superego, a gunbarrel self-evaluation. It is quite different from the premorbid self-regulative process that existed in health.

To complicate the diagnostic problem, these dynamic changes do not respect the categories we set up: bits of schizophrenia may sometimes emerge, and when these "signs" are numerous, we begin to name another kind of "disease." We are gradually becoming less category-bound today, and are prepared to see bits of schizophrenia, obsessions, neurasthenia within the same patient. What a symptom cluster may become is not determined by the cluster present now. A dynamic state should not be mistaken for a permanent life-style. (Perhaps we should begin by an effort to dispel the illusion of the constancy of the human personality.)

These "shelves," or points of arrest, where for a period (of days or of months) a patient may rest, with certain predominant trends in thought, feeling, and action remaining relatively unchanged, are worth description; it is important, for therapeutic contacts, to understand the dynamic factors at work at the time; but they should not be reified. More importantly, we should not be trapped into looking for the unique determiner in the germ plasm (that makes an agitated depression different from an involutional depression, for example), nor expect to find some unique and irreversible change in some diencephalic nucleus for each of these patterns, for the fact is that they are reversible, whatever the underlying and contributory somatic factors in these behavioral trends may be. If the neurotic depression is self-limited, lasting but a few days (or weeks, at most), we should not be quick to set it aside as something totally different from a manic-depressive depression which endures for 18 months. It differs in degree, and in duration.

These considerations become important for treatment. Consider the single item of threat of suicide. Farrar makes this sage observation:

"... there is one point to be especially emphasized: the diagnosis of neurasthenia or of a neurosis is no guarantee that a serious or fatal suicidal act will not occur. Although there is evidence enough to bear out this statement, there has been a rather widely credited assumption, supported by medical authority too, that a patient who is merely 'nervous,' perhaps under private care at home, is not a suicidal risk. Depression is depression whether we call it neurasthenic or reactive or involutional or manic-depressive; and an attempt to differentiate a benign from a more serious mental state on the basis of an arbitrary psychiatric diagnosis is to incur an entirely unwarranted hazard."

It is possible that, as we devise tests that will give us a quantitative measure of the depth of a depression or of the amount of alienation and delusional quality in a schizophrenic pattern, we can describe the phenomena as they exist instead of warping them to fit a rather wooden and static classification scheme. We may grow to feel that the states are dynamic and transitional, capable of being modified in both a positive and a negative direction (down into schizophrenia or up into a normal level of anxiety). The search for definitive signs, for prepsychotic personalities, for specific infantile histories, for identifying interpersonal backgrounds, for specific lesions in the diencephalon, or for abnormalities in a specific chromosome represents the continuing influence of an older static conception of mental illness. Although such searches are intended to economize effort in therapy, they are a poor substitute for vigilance and the skills of the artist-healer.

MELANCHOLIA OF THE INVOLUTIONAL PERIOD

There are many ways of ordering the data of the clinical field. One could classify melancholias according to ages and emerge with melancholias of childhood, of adolescence, of early maturity, of late life, and so on. In the first group one could place those reactions of the infant to separation from the mother. In the melancholias of the climacterium, one could place all the depressions clinically grouped as involutional melancholias, no matter how loosely tied these seem to be to the glandular changes that occur in this period.[9]

---

[9] One study of 38 women diagnosed as involutional melancholia reports that, in 17 of the cases, the menopause occurred from one to eight years prior to the onset of the illness, and in one considerably after. (Malamud, Sands, and Malamud 1941). Wittson (1940) reported that 47 per cent of his cases occurred during the menopause; 16 per cent antedated these changes; 28 per cent followed by more than five years; and 8 per cent occurred more than ten years after. The selection of the climacteric as a causal factor to be used in naming the disorder of a patient is, of course, bound to affect such relations as these we have just reported. If we select all first admissions to mental hospitals diagnosed as involutional melancholia (see Bellak 1952), we find that the diagnosis begins to appear for ages 35-39, reaches a peak at ages 50-55, and continues to be applied at ages 65-75. The menopause itself is more sharply centered, occurring more frequently after 40, whereas the peaks for melancholia are reached earlier, between the ages of 30 and 40. The changes at the climacterium that are judged to be relevant to this disorder are broader than those immediately associated with cessation of menstruation. The changes in sexual desire, as well as in reproductive capacity, are also loosely coupled with this "change of life."

A classification system of this type would involve a great deal of repetition if each clinical grouping is to be completely described. There would be, for example, the anorexia of the separated infant, the anorexia nervosa of the adolescent girl at the threshold of reproductive life, the anorexia of the woman in the involutional period. Each of the depressive symptoms would recur; and in varying settings with varying conflicts and preoccupations, the observer would see different reactions to the symptoms and different ways of coping with conflicts. All this would tempt the patient to construct rationalizations and lead the physician to posit different dynamic explanations to account for the symptoms. The depressive symptoms at the entrance into adolescence are matched by similar symptoms at the climacterium. One physician may ascribe the adolescent girl's self-starvation to her oral fantasies of impregnation or to a sensed equivalence between being fat and looking pregnant. Another physician sees the anorexia of the woman at the climacteric as a revival of that early disappointment of the girl who discovers that she is not equipped with a penis. Since (so the psychoanalytic argument runs) having a child is a psychological equivalent of acquiring a penis, the woman at the climacteric is suffering from a revival of an old disappointment, for now she can no longer have a child. Whoever seeks a more general explanation may spot the change in status and outlook or the threat to one's status, and the deficiency and rigidity in the person's coping mechanisms as the important factors, rather than the single factor of presence or absence of a particular endocrine substance and the accompanying psychic states.

For all the repetitiousness, the task of working through the varieties of melancholia seems to be required if we are to arrive at some notion of the essential nature of the depressive reaction. In this way, perhaps, we may be able to penetrate beyond the surface structures and easy rationalizations that are so obvious. Some of our understandings of both adolescence and the climacterium are culturally defined and consensually agreed on. The question is whether these definitions affect the patient and hence *produce* the symptoms or, instead, confuse the patient and distract the physician from the search for scientifically more valid causes. A social definition (and explanation) can both help and mislead us. In any case, the sharp differences in the developmental tasks and the settings in which the symptoms arise can help us to break loose from some of our concrete preoccupations. Obviously, we are not going to explain the depression of the infant separated from its mother by referring to some glandular failure or to the cessation of a sexual relationship, factors so frequently on the lips of those who deal with the melancholias of the climacterium. Perhaps we shall come to a description, finally, that will include a few general factors common to all depressions, along with a variety of specific ones that are appropriate either to a particular period or to a particular person's life-situation. There are, of course, specific tasks that we expect each individual to accomplish at each developmental stage, and it will be helpful to identify some of the particular coping mechanisms that are used at the climacterium. Hopefully, one would also look for those most general relationships that occur with monotonous frequency at all ages and in all settings, for out of these we might fashion a "scientific" account of the depressive reaction.[10]

On the surface, no other form of melancholia offers a more obvious "endogenous" clue. The cessation of menstruation in women, the decline in sexual potency in men, express changes in the endocrine system. The loss of interests, the faltering memory, the introduction of "feelings of effort" and "feelings of pressure" in actions that had formerly been discharged with ease and efficiency, and the general sense of a loss in vital thrust that we see in many aging persons, all suggest a general vital decline, a slowing down of the energy system, a damping of the fires of spring; the physiologist can point to changes in basal metabolism that are related to the changing status of gonads, pituitary, adrenal, thyroid glands. It seems that a counselor might urge aging clients to undertake fewer new projects and to restrict their daily output, and to recognize the fact that they must live within their new and more restricted biological means.[11]

The involutional period is also one in which some individuals become unemployed and unemployable. With children grown and the nest empty, the concerns which have so long kept the aging woman occupied are now lacking, and the woman of few interests, for whom her children have been the main source of her sense of significance and worth, has a special problem of readjustment. The involutional period is also a period of "final evaluations." When youth faces pressures and defeats, it is always with the vague conviction that things will shortly take a turn and that radical improvements in the trend of things are possible, but for the aging male who is faced with enforced retirement and for whom "the facts are in," the climacterium opens up a vision of a future in which he sees more and more of less and less. His life-situation suddenly has "no exit": he feels he is in a trap. This closure of the field is based partly on the actual scarcity of new opportunities for the aging, but it is also due to a deficiency in the energies required if one is to embark on new ventures, risk failures, meet the demands that go with "getting started." New business ventures, new marriages, new loves, new interests, new homes, new families founded, new professions undertaken seem less and less possible as the years pass. If there are fewer opportunities, fewer invitations, there is also less plasticity, less flexibility, so that we can attribute some of the aging person's problems to the type of personality: narrowness of interests, or a chronic asceticism that has sacrificed almost everything in life for a single aim that is now blocked. To these factors we can add the impotence (or decline of sexual

---

[10]It is interesting that in two rather thorough treatments of depressions, by Ey (1954) and by Henderson and Gillespie (1956), the former devotes less than three pages to melancholy of the involutional period, the latter devote 23 pages. Kraines is of the opinion that the preponderance of evidence is against the retention of it as a separate entity. Some choose to describe it as an unrecognized variation of the manic-depressive psychosis.

[11]As if to dramatize this general vital failure, the children born to older mothers just on the threshold of the climacterium have a much greater likelihood of being mongolian idiots. For mothers over forty, the ratio runs as high as 125 mongolians to 1,000 births. Although these children are now recognized to be genetically different, there seems to be some relationship between aging and this kind of failure in genetic transmission.

desire) which puts an end to a particular form of the lust for life that, in some lives, has been expressed too narrowly.

The patients placed under this diagnosis can represent a selected group, if one excludes, as some clinicians recommend, all those who have shown depressions in an earlier period, all those whose present depression in the involutional period has been preceded by wide mood swings such as characterize the manic-depressive case, all those with paranoid and aggressive features (with projected hostility), and all those in which there is clear evidence of brain damage or early senile changes with cerebral arteriosclerosis (or other degenerative changes). Kraepelin helped to set the fashion in 1896, by separating such involutional depressions from the manic-depressive disorder. Thus, first admissions whose first mental disorder is a depression that occurs in the climacterium, and who have no record of the above excluded features, comprise a kind of diagnostic artefact. Kraepelin himself changed his opinion following the work of Dreyfus (1907), and restored these involutional melancholias to the manic-depressive group. If the agitated forms of the depression are excluded, the symptoms of involutional melancholia will be limited still further, although in this case the identification of the element of restless, agitated, aggressive behavior (and its exclusion) may not add much to our understanding of causes and outcomes.

It should be added that this syndrome is found in women three times as frequently as in men, and that clinicians in general do not follow the recommendations for exclusion given above. There will be, for example, among the reported cases, a woman of 68 who has had earlier and recurring depressions; there will be others that have had periods of elation; a few will have arrived at their present status after having experienced years of a more or less severe obsessive-compulsive neurosis. There will be a few for whom their present involutional depression marks a complete change from a former gay, outgoing, and extroverted pattern of actions and interests.

When diagnostic preferences fluctuate so from clinic to clinic, when the ages in the group vary from 30 to 70, when physical factors form one of the important criteria for one diagnostician (e.g., menopause) and while some diagnosticians are impressed by the life-style of the patient (retarded, submissive, intropunitive rather than hostile, agitated, resentful), one can see that communication from clinic to clinic will be poor: the psychological factors associated with the diagnosis will be varied, and outcomes and therapies diverse.

In spite of the rather confused state of the data, certain trends keep recurring. The involutional group seem to have fewer ancestors who had mental problems than the manic-depressives, from whom Kraepelin wanted to separate them (20-30 per cent of involutionals have such ancestors, as against almost twice as many manic-depressives).[12]

---

[12]Palmer and Jardon (1941), who reported these facts, had a small group of patients on which to base their judgment. (See also Palmer and Sherman 1938; Palmer 1942, 1946.) Henri Ey reports that his patients in this group do not differ from the manic-depressives in the number of antecedents with mental disorders (33 per cent as against 34 per cent). In view of the

In the matter of prognosis, opinions remain sharply divided. The earlier view tended to be pessimistic, looking on the process as one slow to develop and slow to respond to treatment. Henderson and Gillespie observe (1936, p. 187) tersely: "The course of the condition is apt to be very prolonged." Later studies, especially those making use of shock therapy and the newer drugs, tend to describe this particular depressive syndrome as the one most likely to react favorably to treatment. Noyes and Kolb note:

"Before the introduction of electric shock treatment, about 40 per cent of the patients with involutional melancholia recovered. Convalescence, however, was slow, and those who recovered were frequently ill for two or three years. With the use of electric shock, more than 50 per cent of the involutional melancholia patients show prompt recovery."

Others would set the recovery figures even higher, between 80 and 90 per cent. Before shock therapy, the average duration of the hospitalized involutional depression was from nine to twelve months, with a few cases remaining depressed into the third and fourth year. Convulsive therapy has shortened hospital stay and improved the outlook for recovery. It has also decreased the likelihood of suicide.[13]

Although many clinicians point to the endocrine failure as contributing to the onset of the depression, there has been little success in securing an amelioration of the mental state with hormone therapy. The older depressives, in general, are less responsive to all forms of therapy. Hoch and MacCurdy (1922) pointed out that as long as good emotional contact with the surroundings persists, the outlook is favorable, but that such symptoms as a "flatness of affect, autoerotic behavior, bizarre hypochondriacal delusions" make the outlook unfavorable. It has been suggested that there is a schizophrenic-like deteriorative form of involutional melancholia that proceeds slowly toward dementia.

DEPRESSION IN WOMEN

Common sense tells us that the ways in which women react to the change in their status at the climacterium are as various as the ways in which girls react to puberty, or the ways in which young mothers react to motherhood or to the loss of a child. Perhaps common sense is inclined to exaggerate the constancy of life styles, but it does not expect a fairly stable integration of needs, presses, and coping mechanisms to suddenly disintegrate or to undergo regressive changes. Although personality structures change through the years of

---

difficulties in making adequate search among the ancestors and relatives, and in view of the findings of Koller and Diem, who showed that nonpsychotic patients also have a high percentage of spotting in the ascendants (66.9 per cent as against 77 per cent among the ancestors of psychotics), it is apparent that it will take the most meticulous research design to validate the impression here at issue.

[13]According to one set of figures quoted by Kraines (1957, p. 456), 7 per cent of a group of manic-depressives not treated with electric shock were suicides, as compared with less than 1 per cent who had been so treated.

development and decline, there is a great deal of stability, even in the face of changes in life-situations; our safest assumption would seem to be that no drastic personality changes will occur in the lives of most women at this period. The menopause does not arrive suddenly, unannounced, creeping up to pounce suddenly upon the unsuspecting female. Gradual changes have been occurring over a period of years, and a mature woman has some knowledge of the nature of these changes and of what she must do; she cannot plead ignorance like some uninformed adolescent girl who is totally unprepared.[14]

Such an ardent champion of womanhood as Simone de Beauvoir (1949, II, 399-421) would have us believe that, next to puberty, women are called upon to face no greater readjustment than that to the menopause; whoever reads her analysis of the difficulties faced (and of the types of efforts to adjust that women develop in response to them) is invited to see the period as highly pathogenic. So many voices are raised in our time to point out that we are living in an age of anxiety and that it is increasingly difficult to get out of this world alive, that we need to be cautious lest these plaints sweep us into a neurotic view of life.

The objective signs of the approach of the menopause are unmistakable: menstruation first becomes irregular; the intervals between periods grow longer; the discharges are scantier; the ovarian hormones fail; and the discharge of ova ceases. There are "hot flashes" (vasomotor disturbances), dizziness, sweating, headaches, neuralgias, insomnias, anxiety states, which vary from individual to individual in variety and intensity; there are psychological accompaniments of irritability and depressive moods, which, in the rare case, ripen into the involutional psychosis. Some of these psychological signs have long accompanied the low-hormone premenstrual period in each cycle. The period of premenstrual tension, in which some women are irritable, restless, and self-critical, sometimes produces behavior similar to that of the rigid and compulsive type described by Hamilton and Mann (1954). They are driven to clean, scour, polish, set their houses in order, as though in an effort to expunge some unconscious feeling of guilt and uncleanness.[15] All these disturbances can be related directly or indirectly to disturbed endocrine functioning. Some of them are directly the consequence of the ovarian failure; others reflect a more

---

[14]To arrive at a firm estimate of the number of women who undergo serious physiological and emotional changes with neurotic or psychotic consequences would require a kind of record-keeping that our society does not possess. It would not be far from the mark to guess that between 10 and 15 per cent suffer changes that are serious enough to warrant professional assistance (medical, psychological, psychiatric), and perhaps 0.1 per cent will undergo the types of change we have been calling involutional depression. Since not all of the latter are hospitalized, and since these depressions are of every degree of severity, this latter estimate is not a firm one.

[15]The cupboard disease of the premenstrual period is matched by similar actions and speech in the depressed male, and the passage from devaluation (in which everything seems empty, worthless, indifferent) to pejoration (in which a positive loathing describes them as dirty, dangerous, obscene, disgusting, stinking) is characteristic of the descent into a deeper layer of depression. A patient of Janet (1928, pp. 302 ff) said, "This balcony is a good place for a public urinal.... If I fall in love with a woman she is sure to become a monstrous and soiled

general imbalance in the endocrine system as compensatory realignment of body chemistry follows; and some of them represent psychological reactions to these changes and to the change in general status and expectations.

A Chicago study (Allen 1939), reporting observations made on 1,000 women during their menopause, indicated that 85 per cent had experienced symptoms of such minor nature that no interruption of daily routine had been required. Only 15 per cent had shown marked symptoms. It is even more striking to discover that these changes, so directly traceable to endocrine changes, are not easily corrected by endocrine treatment, just as women suffering from an involutional depression do not improve under endocrine therapy; and anorexia nervosa in the postadolescent period, which often leads to cessation of menstruation and changes in the reproductive structures, is not corrected by the administration of hormones. Pratt, who reported a study in which control subjects were used (received placebos), found that there was little difference in the improvement of the groups. (Independent evaluations by another physician who did not know which patients had received the endocrine therapy eliminated any experimenter bias.) Both the mild and transient character of these symptoms and the effects of suggestion seem to be involved.

It thus seems we could well view the climacterium as merely one of a series of incidents, challenges that have to be met in the course of development: going to school, passing through puberty, choosing a vocation, getting a job, becoming engaged, marrying, giving birth to a child. At each of these "test points," the individual's assets and liabilities are measured. One child will experience separation anxiety (on entrance to school), while the rest of the class give little evidence of stress. One adolescent girl will experience anorexia nervosa; a hundred classmates will overeat a little and experience no more than the average amount of adolescent turmoil and confusion. Perhaps a third of the brides will experience some frigidity or inhibition about sexuality; two-thirds will enter the marriage relationship without qualms. At these transition zones, our coping mechanisms, our habits and beliefs, and our general emotional stability are tested. The vasomotor symptoms, the cessation of menstruation, the glandular-physiological readjustment, and the new "status" are taken in stride by most women, and are treated lightly by

---

thing that crushes me with her dead weight.... That man in whom I became interested for a moment has suddenly become a dirty porter reeking with alcohol. If I hear someone tell the age of a woman, this makes me think that the women are all getting older, that we are walking toward the grave, and then I become overwhelmed by the thought that I shall be buried alive."

What the analyst calls "anal-erotic" interests are mingled with dirt, disgust, death, soiling. Such linkages may indeed have their roots in associations formed in early toilet-training, but the movement of these linkages into the foreground of the depressive's thought is another matter. Searching for the words to express his "transvaluation of all values," including his changed self-value, where in this world can he find the metaphors if not in "shit, piss, and corruption"? Death, disease, excreta enter the thoughts and language of the depressed, summoned by a present state that is caused by current conditions. The state makes use of ancient associations, even when the state itself is not caused by those old linkages, for the latter are universal, available to all.

most physicians. The normally integrated personality finds ways of meeting the endocrine-paced changes, and if there are new types of deficit, new emotional needs, the individual who possesses the glands also possesses the means of solving the new tasks.

This kind of cautious and conservative common sense seems needed when we read such judgments as Benedek's (1952, pp. 353, 356):

"There is no other period in life—except puberty—when internal changes of the organism put the individual's capacity to master those changes to such a test. And while puberty may be difficult for many girls, even greater is the number of women who at the time of their climacteric show signs of stress, strain, and emotional disturbances of variable severity. . . . Much of the exaggerated fear of menopause appears to be culturally determined. It is an expression of the expectation— in woman and in man alike—that the abating sexual function will be experienced as an irreparable blow to the ego."

In her analysis of one of her cases, Benedek implies that a hormonal decline "mobilized a regression of the ego's integrative capacity." Because the woman did not produce enough "libido" to meet the demands of living and to accomplish what she herself felt was fitting and right, and because her ego was impaired, she felt frustrated, grew panicky, and went into a psychotic episode.

Consider these judgments of Deutsch (1945, II, 462, 463, 472):

"It is indeed a critical period, and whatever influence the changes in hormonal activity may exert upon the whole psychosomatic picture, there is no doubt that the mastering of the psychologic reactions to the organic decline is one of the most difficult tasks of a woman's life. . . . The climacterium is known as the 'dangerous age,' and a certain type of aging woman has become a comical theatrical type. . . . The suggestibility of women in this life period increases markedly, their judgment fails, and they readily fall victim to evil counselors. . . . The climacterium not only has a tendency to repeat the neurotic and psychotic states of puberty, using analogous defense mechanisms; in addition, neurotic features that previously appeared as character traits become intensified, just as in puberty."

Try as we will to go beyond such statements of opinion about the severity of this challenge of the climacterium, either in trying to arrive at the precise ways in which women do meet the challenge or in trying to describe those personality organizations most apt to succumb under this test, we find ourselves confronted with a paucity of data, with a variety of contrasting literary, impressionistic sketches. The perception of the signs of aging, of the loss of physical attractiveness, will send one woman to the beauty shop and initiate all manner of compensatory efforts to enhance her charm through clothes, hairdo, jewelry. In her fear of being devalued, she may undertake new work, new studies, reviving a career once begun and then abandoned, or she may draw, dance, paint, take up philosophy to fill that emptiness in her "interior castle." She may even compensate in seeking new romantic adventures, as though compelled to prove that she *is* desirable, to someone. She may seek a kind of symbolic or substitute expression by endeavoring to promote young men of talent, or by drawing the successful into her orbit, by setting a table, by entertaining, by conducting a salon where the "doers" of her society shed some of their glory on an older woman who fears that she is "finished."

But what she does, precisely, will not be a simple function of either the endocrine failure or her aging. The bulk of her age peers finds ways of "solving this problem": they discover new challenges to meet and a variety of ways of maintaining their sense of worth. Life does not suddenly stop. It is conceivable that there is a character type that has depended too exclusively on a coy and seductive way of coping with life and who now will fear a total collapse of her coping mechanisms. This would better explain that "drowned ego" of Benedek's patient than some simple withdrawal of the biochemical substances secreted by a gland. Titley, Hamilton, Mann, Noyes, Kolb, Malamud, Sands may have a point when they stress the rigidity in make-up, the narrowness of interests, the general lack of plasticity, in their cases of involutional depression, for this type finds it difficult to change, and many of the alternate courses of action have been allowed to atrophy. There is little doubt that the changes of this period announce in unmistakable terms that life is a one-way street, with a very certain and not to be desired terminus not far away. Although this fact has existed throughout life, it now becomes more apparent each day and living can become, suddenly, a dying. Those who have never come to terms with the fact of death, or who have never settled a long-standing quarrel with someone who has gone ahead into the shadows, or who have never and cannot now bring themselves to make investments that will endure beyond the tomb, are now seriously threatened. When the sexual-affectional adjustment has always been marginal, focusing on a rather tenuous relationship with a sex partner, the difficulties will now be intensified.

When, however, as in the pages of Helene Deutsch and Simone de Beauvoir, woman at the climacteric is made to appear inactive and morose, or depressed, agitated, and slightly paranoid, or as hysterical and suggestible as an adolescent, or a rather silly and stupid person in danger of falling prey to gigolos and Hindu swamis, one is moved to discount the observations on the ground that these observers are unacquainted with average women and mothers, that they have seen too many neurotic or psychotic women in their busy practice (or in that milieu de Beauvoir so cleverly describes in *The Mandarins*), for their descriptions strike one as drawn from a group of bored, hysterical, anxious, depressed women who are trying to face the problems of the involutional period with character structures that are weak, immature, rigid, distorted. They tell us much about the exceptional woman, but little about the involutional period per se. Psychology has much to learn from psychiatry, but its judgments of the normal should not be obscured by this taint of the pathological. Even the clinician seems to suffer from an educated disability.

Perhaps the sensible thing to do when we speak of melancholia in the involutional period is to recognize the special problems of making a good life at this period, to observe the physiological changes that go with aging and take them into account in formulating an adequate dynamic picture of an illness of this period, but at the same time to free ourselves from the notion that any of these changes has any inevitable or even any statistically significant relation with psychopathology. Each of the seven ages of man provides an interesting backdrop against which to view all deviations, but we should be sure that we are constructing a true and factual account of this backdrop.

Deutsch's Account of the Involutional Woman

Because of the nature of his techniques, a psychoanalyst cannot collect impressive statistical samples, even when his entire lifetime of practice is included. Given five new patients a year, and analyses running up to 70 months (with a median duration of 17 months), his case histories can be rich in detail, but, in toto, they cannot be statistically impressive, and because the women studied are suffering serious psychological disorganization, they are obviously not a representative sample of aging womankind. When, therefore, a psychoanalyst sets out to write about women in general, or women in the climacteric, on the basis of his very limited experience, his every impression should be accepted with serious reservations. Even if we were to take the total population of all the psychoanalytically oriented clinics in the Western world, there would be a professional bias and a class bias in the data (for only the well-to-do can afford such treatment), and most of the analysts follow rather slavishly the original dicta of Freud, many of which were written before the turn of the century. Deutsch's views are nonetheless worth our reflection, not merely because they reveal the analyst's biases about this involutional period, but also because they are offered by a woman. Not all female psychoanalysts have accepted some of Freud's sometimes crude and typically masculine observations about womankind. His strictures represent a kind of Central European conception that was finally caricatured by Nazi writers, and perhaps they have a kind of bitter truth about them, epitomizing something that a hundred feminist writers today are trying to counter as they create a new "feminine mystique." The "truth," in short, can be a kind of social truth, a comic truth, a delusional truth which is actually accepted by some of the women who suffer, most of all, because of it.

Deutsch begins her description by calling the climacteric a "narcissistic mortification," a wound to self-love. The involutional woman, who had received from nature a gift that had guaranteed for her a biological significance, at puberty, now finds that Nature is an Indian giver, taking it all away. If the entrance into sexual maturity and all of its "rights and privileges" (not to mention responsibilities) brought her joy, how can she be expected to feel as she is retired, put on the shelf? She now knows that she will not be as attractive, sexually, as she has been; she can no longer bear children. Her children, each one of whom compensated for that earlier insult when she discovered that, unlike her brothers, she had no penis, are now fully grown, preoccupied with children of their own. They no longer need her.

If she fails to realize and readjust to the fact that her old reasons for existence are gone, she will be in danger of rapidly becoming a meddlesome grandmother, an unwanted and interfering mother-in-law, a person who does not "know her place."

The beauty and charm of a budding femininity that once made her so attractive at sweet sixteen have been fading, gradually, for years, and now a series of "insults" (deposits of fatty tissue, hirsutism, varicose veins on the legs and thighs) announces something that, if not catastrophic, is very unpleasant. She is forcibly reminded that she is not immortal. One of the most important themes which served as an organizer of her actions and which brought rewarding and satisfying experiences suddenly threatens to leave her entirely.

Not every woman accepts this drift in affairs. Some will read with interest the remark of Princess Metternich, which Deutsch quotes (1945, II, 471) in support of her own observations that sexual excitability long outlasts the cessation of reproductive capacity. Asked, "When does a woman cease being capable of sexual love?" the Princess replied, "You must ask someone else, I am only sixty." As if this discovery that their sexual life is not wholly over arouses a false hope of an eternal youth, and a compensatory overdrive (in a person who has long overvalued sexuality), a few of these aging women will seek to prove that they are still lively. Like an older man, who boasts that he can still play a good game of tennis (or who boasts of his newest intrigues), the involutional woman may seek to draw around her young men, attractive lovers, proofs of her youth and charm; her efforts to use cosmetics, dress, and every seductive wile can carry her beyond anything her normal efforts to be attractive had produced in young maturity. These excesses may lead to inevitable dangers and disappointments. Without girlish inhibitions, and with the fear of pregnancy gone, she can be more abandoned in her search for something, something *beyond the ordinary,* something to fill her emptiness (that is, if she is actually empty and bored, and in one of those psychasthenic states Janet described so well). If the interest of her husband (or her interest in her husband) has waned, or if he has grown absorbed in business and professional preoccupations (or golf, or fishing), she may feel robbed, cheated, abandoned. The Emma Bovarys who entered marriage with all of the romantic illusions that a convent education and much novel-reading had fostered may try anew to seek that fulfillment their marriage has denied.

This can also be a period when compensating interests outside the home are pursued with an almost feverish intensity in an effort to fill this new void. If her interests have been too narrow, if she had sacrificed some of them while she was building a home, this can call for a second period of growth; on the other hand, if her pursuits are too narrow, too egoistic, too narcissistic, she can become absurd. The aging coquette is at first amusing and exploitable; then she becomes a bore, and even downright annoying. If her new interests, which she works at so sedulously, give her a new spate of opinions (on painting, international relations, mental health, Oriental rugs), her borrowed and superficial conversation pieces may fail to make her the personality she fantasied she might become. Narcissistic wounds lead to narcissistic compensations in a narcissistic personality, and self-centered efforts directed toward the defense of a threatened ego do not make egotism any more attractive. The new capacities for affectionate, realistic, and productive relations with her world, which must be found if her significance and worth are to achieve real validation, require another sort of outgoing interest and another kind of learning.

Comical, pathetic, even tragic, this "puberty in reverse" revives old conflicts, and the new "wound" revives old compensatory strivings, some of them childish. One kind of woman begins a diary (as she did in puberty), suddenly feels too important for her home (as she did then), craves the challenges of a new sort of life, a new love, and new responsibilities: something to replace the deadly round of unpunctuated living that threatens to make her dull. New clothes (a few on the outlandish side to help make her "colorful," interesting), distracting the onlooker from the telltale signs, will hide the fact announced by her mirror. Even if the admiration has to come from men whom she would have spurned when younger, it soothes her wounded ego and supports the desired illusion. Her husband, poor fellow, does not quite know what to make of all this, nor is he quite aware of this void which has to be filled, nor is he capable of filling it. He is too familiar: like an old shoe, he is comfortable, but not very exciting. Negative adaptation has long ago set in, and old quarrels, old awkwardnesses, old scars, have dulled the sparkle of what was once a crystalline thing. In short, he can no longer "emotionize" her. Something new, strange, exotic, exciting, is required.

Without the market created by these involutional women, the culture-mongers, the "improve your personality" experts, and the professional guides and counselors would suffer. (Note, it is a woman who makes these observations.) "The suggestibility of women in this life-period increases markedly, their judgment fails, and they readily fall victim to evil counselors." Perhaps we should note that physicians, priests, pastors, psychologists, and psychiatrists are included in this group of professional guides. The involutional woman is visibly present in the Sunday morning church audiences. Some of these women will grow preoccupied with religious matters, seek mystic experiences, become ascetic in their manner of living, seek some kind of philanthropic self-sacrificing test. One thinks of the *gray ladies*. Deutsch quotes an old German proverb: "Young harlot, old nun." The mildest reaction of this type is found in the woman who finds the involutional changes bring a blessed release: she feels freed from "the curse," and can now forget the whole problem of sex, returning to those other pursuits she has always considered more important. A complete denial of all sexual expression serves a few who are in search of a self-purification, now easier to accomplish than in youth.

One can understand a certain jealous attitude among some involutional women, particularly among those who have not found fulfillment in a normal sex life. For these women, the actions of youth appear "disgusting" and "foolish." This form of Mrs. Grundyism is hypersensitive and punitive where anything suggesting erotic pleasure is concerned. (Of course, many of these reactions occur among involutional males as well.) The revival of sexual interests, and the foolish effort to compensate for aging, can carry a few involutional women into a new version of old repressed, or latent, homosexuality, bringing into play an element that has silently colored many of their friendships with women.

In some measure age is entitled to a slightly depressed outlook on life. Its losses are real. Many things are over for the aging, in fact. The end which looms ahead is not to be denied: one cannot get out of this world alive. Failing energies and a weariness of the flesh make the discharge of responsibilities increasingly difficult. Since these aging women are now in competition with younger, more energetic "strivers and strainers," whether it is a matter of affection, power, or some test of skill, they are threatened with failure. If the individual is one of those tightly organized (and very productive) beings whose superego has never been too tolerant of nonfeasance, she will likely find the decline in output intolerable. On the other hand, the one who has succeeded through charm (and woman's wiles) is now forced to realize another kind of narrow margin on which her successes depend. Her charm will have to assume a different form: a maturing is called for, new ways of giving and new ways of meriting that human love we all need.

Therese Benedek has hinted at the changes in motivation which accompany the menstrual cycle. Others have agreed that in the premenstrual portion of the cycle, when both estrogen and progestin secretions are at their low ebb, a woman's mood is not at its best. Altmann, Knowles, and Bull (1941) reported "an outburst of physical and mental activity before the onset of menstruation, coupled with high tension and irritability and preceded or accompanied by depressions. Housework, classwork, organizing of research, redecorating furniture, or remodeling clothes were undertaken in addition to all routine doings on such days. In fact, one of these subjects was the first to direct our attention toward that phenomenon which was jokingly called 'cupboard disease.' " Added to all of this compulsive activity, there is an increase in the critical feelings toward the self and toward others.[16] There is a certain analogy between this premenstrual "burst of feeling" and the changes in the involutional period, when the glandular support for action is permanently lowered.

Deutsch also believes there is a marked increase in the fantasy life: fantasies of new romances, of rape, of seduction, of prostitution. As neurosis in general

---

[16]This relationship with the "superego" that we call self-criticism is more or less constant in some personalities. They have an unforgiving conscience, we say, and are the products of an unhappy relationship between a child and its parents. It is rather striking to note that this relationship between the ego and superego fluctuates with "the time of the month." Thus to the observation of Durkheim, who was prone to remind us that the guilty of this world are the punished ones, we could add a footnote to the effect that the conscience-ridden self may be suffering from low hormone output.

revives the conflicts and repressions of infancy, the climacteric revives old problems of puberty. As a symbol of this return to puberty, Deutsch (1945, II, 470) quotes a Dr. Wiesel: "I am struck by the case of a patient who formed a thick strand of snow white hair during puberty; this strand later disappeared, but reappeared in the climacterium at the same spot and with the same dimensions." Such a striking example is well-calculated to impress the credulous (involutional women, perhaps), and its implied overtone could be summed up as: the repetition of pubertal changes is complete, biologically, psychologically, as witness this instance of a structural change based on a glandular condition. "I wanted to show," Dr. Wiesel concluded, "to what extent the symptomatology of puberty can be likened to the events of the climacterium." Deutsch adds: "Wiesel's conclusion as to the organic symptomatology is true to an even greater extent of the psychic." This sort of "physioanalogy" and "psychoanalogy" may be worth preserving for posterity as demonstrating how the human mind works as it carves out relationships in an area not yet thoroughly studied by scientific methods. What factual basis it has must be limited to some such meaning as that the hysterical patients Deutsch has seen bear many resemblances to hysterical adolescent girls. Since a psychiatrist seldom works out a full-length portrait of normal women, the real underlying meaning may be simply that hystericals resemble one another, whether young or old.

A second generalization of similar import also needs a qualification: "All these modes of behavior in which we can find similarities as between puberty and the climacterium may be intensified into psychosis if there is a disposition to it—into puberal psychoses in young girls and into climacterical psychoses in aging women." Statistical studies do not reveal any burst of mental illness at either age period.

One factual item is laconically reported by Kinsey et al. (1953, p. 736). Tabulating "total sexual outlet" for a sample of 173 involutional women according to ages (see Table 11), Kinsey notes that this very gradual decline parallels very closely the decline in his much larger sample of this same age period (when the data are collected without any consideration of the menopause). Some of the decline may be due to the hormonal changes, some to the readiness with which some women seize on these changes as an excuse for discontinuing a relationship in which they were never particularly interested, and some of it a declining interest on the part of males. In isolated cases there are contrary trends (as when the disappearance of the fear of pregnancy actually releases a greater frequency of outlet).

Among the statements we cannot evaluate is Deutsch's impression that "almost every woman in the climacterium goes through a shorter or longer phase of depression" (p. 473). Or, consider the following (p. 474):

"It is my impression that feminine-loving women have a milder climacterium than masculine-aggressive ones.... Apparently these women (the artists in love) possess a psychic cosmetic in a certain form of narcissism, a cosmetic that other, less resourceful women try to replace by rouge, massages, and youthful dress. The

TABLE 11. *Total Sexual Outlet for 173 Involutional Women.* (After Kinsey *et al.* 1953, p. 736.)

Age	Frequency per Week
1-2 years prior to menopause	1.5
During menopause	1.0
1-2 years after	0.7
3-4 years after	0.6
10 years after	0.4
20 years after	0.4

former remain young for a long time, the latter maintain that they feel young.... Feminine erotic women, experienced in love, accept the inevitable with greater dignity and calm than the spinsterish, frigid, even frustrated ones.... Beautiful narcissistic women whose beauty seems to be the center of their existence, often make one wonder: 'What will they do in the climacterium?'... Before they are surprised by the disaster, they avert it by gradually turning to an occupation that later will supply them with a gratifying substitute."

Since these generalizations are, as yet, unsupported by a validating study of normal women, they serve only to symbolize Deutsch's beliefs. In this type of "projection test," Deutsch's theme seems to run: "Those who have been successful, as women, in maturity, tend to be successful, as women, in the climacterium." To the strong, as usual, many things are possible, including the power to adapt to change, to enjoy life in the climacterium.

Realistic and practical in her advice to aging women (learn to enjoy what you can enjoy and invest your energies where they are productive of real satisfactions and triumphs; resign yourselves in the face of the changing reality), Deutsch adds many perceptive comments about grandmothers, mothers, mothers-in-law, and those others who have "missed the boat." About those who are so anxious to hurry the emancipation of women from the traditional womanly roles (calling their sisters out of the kitchen and nursery to stand in the production line and to work at the jobs men dislike at wages slightly below those paid to males), she notes: the emancipation will benefit women only if it includes ample opportunity for them to develop their femininity and motherliness.

To the depressed involutional woman, whose sexual adjustment had never succeeded too well, Deutsch's chapter would make troublesome reading, adding to all the other forms of self-accusation the hint that she has somehow failed to be sufficiently loving and womanly. In a very real sense, the depressed woman feels this already, and now the sanction of authority (the woman in the white coat) adds a final blow.

The Prepsychotic Personality of the Involutional Depressive, Male and Female

In spite of the confusion about diagnosis (and this confusion must affect the composition of the group), there has grown up among clinicians a general impression of the kind of personality which existed before the patient entered a depression at the involutional period. In retrospect, reviewing the case history, one often gets the impression that the patient was headed this way for some time. Since there are three women for every man in this category, it is not surprising that Noyes and Kolb (1963), in presenting their impression of this prepsychotic personality, use the pronoun "she" in referring to the person. Their brief sketch of these patients is worth quoting as a clinical impression. It may be that this impression is affected by the present status of the patients; it is also possible that a knowledge of the patient's life-history may influence the selection of the cases to place in this loosely defined category.

"In a significant number of cases of the involutional depressive reaction, there is found a certain general type of personality makeup and of habits of life. Usually the patient was an anxious child with a background of early fundamental insecurity. A review of the patient's previous personality and temperament often shows that she has been a compulsive, inhibited type of individual with a tendency to be quiet, unobtrusive, serious, chronically worrisome, intolerant, reticent, sensitive, scrupulously honest, frugal, and even penurious. Usually, too, she has been of exacting and inflexible standards, lacking in humor, overconscientious, and given to self-punishment. Such persons have been mild, submissive, and sensitive to the moods and feelings of others. They have never been boastful but have depreciated their own worth, which often has actually been high. Not rarely they have been exploited by the selfish. The prepsychotic personality has been marked by a rigidity that represented a neurotic defense, and the patient has been perfectionistic, prudish, and prone to feelings of guilt. The personality has been superego dominated. Many involutional patients have been self-effacing and self-sacrificing and have had an exaggerated need for, and dependency upon, the approval of others.

"Undoubtedly involutional depression evolves out of a masked neurosis of earlier life. In some instances, hostile and aggressive impulses have been repressed with difficulty. Many psychiatrists consider, in fact, that the prepsychotic personality of the involutional depressive type has been developed as a reaction-formation against aggressions. Often the patient's sex life has been suppressed or unsatisfactory. Her interests have been narrow and her habits stereotyped; she has cared little for recreation, has not sought pleasure, and has had but few close friends. Frequently the patient has been a loyal subordinate, meticulous as to detail rather than an aggressive, confident leader. Many have been fidgety, fretful, apprehensive persons. Others have been characterized by caution or indecision."

The Hamilton-Mann Study

That the Noyes-Kolb stereotype applies to men as well as women, and that other clinicians have found data which support a similar view, is made clear by Hamilton and Mann's study (1954) of patients admitted at the Westchester Division of the New York Hospital over a 30-year period

(1920-1950) and diagnosed as involutional psychoses (169 women and 150 men provided the case histories that were reviewed in this study).

The average age at admission for the women was 52, for the men 57, with ranges of 38 to 72 and 45 to 71, respectively. Above average in intelligence, with an educational and socioeconomic history that would locate them in the middle or upper social strata, they are described as responsible, productive, and with a good capacity to organize their own activities. Their ability to delegate responsibilities or to work easily with others was notably lacking, and they were short on capacity to appreciate the feelings or viewpoints of others. This made them: "hard, uncompromising drivers when in executive positions, but they were known for getting results. One half of the men were in positions where they were directly handling money. The personality traits most frequently mentioned were: conscientiousness, meticulousness, narrow interests, and adherence to a rigid routine. However, reticence, prudishness, stubbornness, oversensitiveness, and penuriousness were descriptive adjectives that could be commonly applied to both sexes." Looking at the records of their patients as children, Hamilton and Mann found that they had been healthy and well-socialized: they were notably neat, conscientious, and helpful. Closely attached to their mothers (or some mother-surrogate) who were usually the dominant parents (the fathers tended to be the subordinate figures in the homes), the type of relationship was one well-calculated to develop strong superegos. The weaker fathers (found in three-fifths of the cases) contained an unusual number of alcoholics. Others had died while the patient was young, and some had been divorced.

When these patients were young adults, they tended to shoulder responsibility early, and they adjusted to a triad of duty, obligation, and "doing the right thing." They also gave evidence of a certain resentment against the very role that they assumed so well. They were conscientious, but they also felt "hard done by."

Hamilton and Mann stress the rigidity in these personalities: they seemed lacking in imagination and sense of humor; they had very narrow interests; they did everything according to schedule;[17] they were stubborn in resisting change. Serious, full of good works, they did not take time to play.

Sometimes these well-socialized adults carried their "good deeds" to the point where their actions not only went beyond the line of duty but seemed calculated to make everyone around uncomfortable. The housewives were overconcerned about their homes, overdirective and oversolicitous to their children, until their compulsive actions made the home anything but a place for relaxation. The men prided themselves on overtime, worked without vacation, and looked down on the "jokers" and "morons" who wasted time on movies, spectacles, sports. As though they had actually been compensating for some deficit in integrative force, they seem to have had to tread gingerly through life, to constrict the range of their interests. They act as though, with their small capital, they could not afford to waste a bit of it and hence missed many of the joys and "celebrations" that balance the living of others who are less constrained. These are signs of what Janet called low psychological tension.

Lacking spontaneity, acting under careful and preplanned control, humorless, and a bit on the prudish side, these patients were respected but not well-liked. The

---

[17]The wife of one male patient observed: "He did everything according to a rigid schedule. I got kissed three times every morning and twice every night. We had sexual relations at 10 P.M. on Saturday nights."

physicians who studied their histories described them as showing a "notable lack of personal charm." (Transfer and countertransfer are tenuous.) Neat, orderly, conscientious, rigid, tense, serious, responsible, perfectionist, self-critical, this group may have suffered from a long-standing "neurosis" prior to being hospitalized, but it would have to be called a character neurosis, and it had enabled them to do more than "get by." They were productive and responsible citizens.

It was not easy to obtain a sexual history, for they were secretive, reserved, and aloof. Good rapport required long and patient effort. Almost all the men, and 75 per cent of the women, had married. Only half the women had children. When they did finally unburden themselves, they reported enough masturbation, extra-marital affairs, induced abortions, and strong erotic feelings with guilt to make the physicians who studied them conclude that they had entered adulthood with a normally strong sexual drive. When sex hormones were used with some of the patients, the resulting increase of sex tension seemd to aggravate their condition. (Suicide attempts were more frequent in this group.) An increase in sex tension that is sometimes associated with the climacteric also was found in some of these men and women, and they reacted with shame and guilt.

These tightly organized personalities had not only adjusted, but, by all middle-class criteria, had adjusted well (save in those personal qualities that make for charm, ease of interpersonal relations, and a flexibility and spontaneity that make life more enjoyable). When they arrived at the climacterium with its failing energies, with opportunities to demonstrate worth curtailed, with forced retirement, with children no longer a preoccupation, they behaved as though their life-styles had grown brittle in the tautness of their self-control; the additional blows initiated the depressive phase. Financial insecurity, sickness and death in the family, conflict over emancipation of children, physical illness of the patient, and visible signs of some failure so great that the patient and his family and friends were conscious of his "loss of face," found them without the reserves or the flexibility to rise above these blows. Loss of appetite, difficulties in sleeping, bodily concerns (especially about elimination), loss of sexual desire, difficulty in remembering, inability to do the "extra work" that had so long boosted their sense of worth, fatigue, neuro-circulatory symptoms finally brought them to a full stop.

Now that such patients are treated earlier and both chemical and electroshock therapies are available, three-quarters of these cases will respond with distinct improvement, in contrast with the former, more advanced groups that were treated largely by psychotherapy, encouragement, hydrotherapy, and occupational therapy (thirty years ago, when only 40 per cent recovered).[18]

Hamilton and Mann interpret the strong work-drive in these patients as a compensation for a strong but unrecognized passive-dependent need. They quote one of the patients, deserted by his father in infancy and shortly after by his mother, as saying: "When I took on extra jobs, I see now I was proud of my ability to do more than anyone else. It made me feel better than others who had more advantages in their early life. Yet I realize now, when my illness was starting, I began to block getting to my work and finishing it, and was irritable to my wife for not helping me more, and it ended by my wife's having to stay up at night to push me into finishing."

---

[18]These patients resemble those whom Wittkower, Rodger, and Wilson (1941) studied in their search for a common personality pattern in patients with neurocirculatory asthenia. Another common personality type found in this latter illness was also a sober, reliable, trustworthy perfectionist type with a keen sense of duty.

Hamilton and Mann speak about the patients' unsatisfactory identification with their fathers, pointing out that many had lost a father early. Others, the son of very busy and very successful fathers, had received very little attention and less affection from them. This same complex was identified by Jacob Arlow (1945), in his study of patients suffering from the anginal syndrome, as an ascetic-masochistic element behind hard-driving behavior that never seemed to bring any personal satisfaction. The origin of both their inner insecurity and their continued need to "go beyond," to do better than their superiors, was attributed to an unsatisfactory identification with the father, one founded on fear rather than on admiration.

The fact that this pattern keeps cropping up in widely diverse illnesses may have some significance. Does it mean that these taut, unpunctuated, and unrelieved lives have pushed capacity to its limit, so that a life-style becomes brittle? Does one more straw break the backs of these camels? Never having developed flexibility, never having found it easy to depend on or collaborate with others always sure that "I can do anything you can do better" and having traded affection for respect, do these systems now "break" (with a coronary, with neurocirculatory asthenia, with an involutional depression)?

Or is this sensitivity to a life-style a medical preoccupation? Are the psychiatrists who treat these patients merely reflecting what is all too generally felt by those who do not carry "the white man's burden" too well? Are the Chinese and the citizens of undeveloped African countries less filled with high expectations, more content with a humble lot, more flexible and able to bend with the forces that beset them rather than break in stubborn opposition? It it the dandipratted ego Western socialization develops that is to blame?

Should we pinpoint the superego, and in accounting for the overbearing concience with which these patients seem to be plagued, study the relations between infant and parents at that point where the first conditionings laid down the basic dynamism underlying all regulative efforts? Or should we, following the tradition of Janet and his more recent successors, look on the integrative forces of the individual, that mixture of assets and liabilities which includes everything from decayed teeth to membership in the Elks, as a rising and falling power to adjust that has no single cause and that cannot be corrected, completely by any single therapy? In such an eclectic view, whatever makes a difference can serve as cause, or, corrected, can lift the integrative powers and health *in some degree.*

Exceptions to the Stereotypes

The search for a "coronary personality," a "gastric personality," a "neurocirculatory-asthenia personality" warned us that there is not a unique personality structure responsible for each "breakthrough" which damages a particular organ. The unusually severe spasms of small blood vessels and the symptoms of Raynaud's syndrome are not the specific outgrowth of a particular personality constellation. There is good reason, therefore, to be suspicious of the present clinical consensus, even though there may be a truth in the general impression that a certain type of rigid, conscientious, highly socialized person who has suppressed and contained his aggressions is also brittle, frangible, and vulnerable to the stresses of aging.

This note of caution is supported by the findings of Malamud, Sands, and Malamud (1941). In their group of 47 cases, they identify such outstanding traits as: introverted (15), extroverted or outgoing (15), sensitive (15), timid (12), pleasant (10), conscientious or pedantic (9), hypochondriacal (8), underactive (7), prudish (7), work-interested only (7), very religious (5), stubborn (5), dependent (4), anxious (3), shiftless (3), frugal (3), aggressive (3), autistic (2). The frequencies with which these traits were mentioned as outstanding features of a personality warn us that quite varied combinations can be expected.

There is the timid and dependent person, worrisome and hypochondriacal, who leans on one person through the years. This deep attachment might be that of a daughter for a mother who was originally overprotective and oversolicitous, and who literally absorbed the daughter who in turn finally became the mother's only support; having completely restricted her own social life, the daughter finds herself, at the death of the mother, without the power of facing and coping with life on her own. Entering into a deep depression, terminated by suicide in her late forties, this passive-dependent person is in strong contrast to the next case of suicide a physician meets.

In such a series there are the outgoing and pleasant individuals who are also militant prohibitionists, pedantic sticklers for details, chronic worriers. The concomitant features make these extroverts close to the constricted type of Noyes and Kolb and of Hamilton and Mann.

But the three who were characterized as shiftless suggest it is not merely the taut and rigid system with narrow interests that is frangible. Some persons can be immature, weak, never well-organized, never autonomous or responsible, carried along by family and friends as a sweet but ineffectual member of the group until, late in life, they are unprepared for the challenges that, mastered earlier, would have toughened and matured them.

There is also the alcoholic-depressive who has learned to use alcohol as a sedative and as a means of escape from "insoluble problems." Kraines describes a case, aged 32, consuming on the average a quart of whiskey daily.

"In giving his history, he related how he had been 'well' until the age of 18. 'Then I suddenly got attacks of heart palpitation. The doctors couldn't find anything wrong with my heart, but I felt that I was dying. I couldn't sleep, couldn't work, and the only thing that would give me any relief was whiskey. I'd take half a glassful at a time to quiet down.' His cardiac neurosis, which was the presenting symptom of a depressive attack, disappeared after six months; but by that time, he had become a chronic alcoholic."

There is no firm date at which a cardiac symptom must make its appearance, and the pattern that emerged in this case at age 32 can emerge in the involutional period. We have already seen that those who have sought a precise personality pattern underlying neurocirculatory asthenia have found some very diverse types, including the rigid and constricted pattern.

Grouping the constellations of traits which seemed to favor a poor prognosis, Malamud, Sands, and Malamud noted that limited interests, timidity, sensitiveness, hypochondria, and "pleasant" traits were associated with poor prognosis, while the underactive, introverted, anxious, religious, shiftless, autistic, conscientious, and prudish traits were weighted in favor of recovery or improvement. It is obvious that none of these traits exists in isolation; it is a dynamic constellation within a single personality that undergoes the type of disorganization we call a depression. Each of the traits can function in constellations that provide other corrective or compensatory features. A dash of conscience can "season" a generally shiftless and poorly organized personality, and a "pleasant outgoing" can temper an otherwise underactive and religious personality. We cannot arrive at prognosis by chopping up the person into isolated traits.

These reflections on the varieties of prepsychotic personality should remind us that a depression is a dynamic state of affairs: a withdrawal from action, a drastic change in the view of the self and of the world, a disruption of the normal rhythms of eating and sleeping, a loss of desire and hope. It can occur in widely divergent personality settings and when it appears *the person is not like himself.* What Federn (1952, p. 274) said about the manic-depressive psychosis, in which these bouts of depression alternate with manic, excited phases, is equally true of these depressions of the involutional period:

"The symptoms of manic-depressive psychosis are typical and well-known, and but little dependent on the prepsychotic individuality. At the peak of either phase the gap between the genius and average person, wise man and fool, is leveled, and difference in background and education is erased. Before this kind of psychosis, human values fade away as before death itself. Just as organic matter is coagulated by freezing and by boiling, so are all the features of normal mental life blotted out by depression and by mania. And, in analogy with temperature and organic life, only in the middle layers of emotion can a prosperous mental life develop."

The conclusion that emerges resembles the one of Cohen and White (1951) as they reviewed the causes of neurocirculatory asthenia. Although the vulnerability of these patients is often related to their personality structure, there is no single structure that has a title to this kind of weakness. There are quiet and resilient, patient and long-suffering, cheerfully submissive souls that weather great stress without breaking. There are boldly aggressive, successfully demanding, outwardly forceful patterns that suddenly crack and go into alcoholic or suicidal phases. It will be recalled that the clinicians who interviewed, tested, and studied the group of subjects in the Minnesota semistarvation experiment could not predict those who would break under the conditions imposed upon them, nor could they, on reviewing the evidence (once the breaks had occurred), locate in the original protocol signs of that weakness which made the difference.

In addition to this aspect of the problem, these personalities do not have the fixity of Gibraltar: some wax stronger, some wane. Rising and falling, with assets increasing or liabilities growing, they are altered by internal changes and external press. Coping mechanisms develop to make them stronger; traumata and fixations scar and weaken them. Brain tumors, infections, arteriosclerosis, surgery, and other changes attack the very substructure of the action systems. Consider the triad, therefore, rather than one-factor causes: personal history and personality pattern, physiological state and constitution, external pressures and competing demands. The dynamic product that emerges in a specific symptom cluster, such as we find in depression, is not something easily predicted by those who center on any one of the three sets of variables.

ELECTROSHOCK THERAPY FOR THE DEPRESSIONS

ECT, or electroconvulsive therapy, is referred to as a purely empirical therapy, for the very simple reason that its efficacy remains unexplained in spite of serious efforts to rationalize it, to experiment with the procedures, to study neurophysiological changes, and to fit it into the generally accepted theories of mental illness. It deserves the most serious attention, if for no other reason than the reported remission or improvement it produces in some 70 to 80 per cent of manic-depressives (in the depressed phase) and an even higher percentage of involutional melancholias.

Olmansi and Impastato summarized the results obtained by the application of various forms of convulsive therapy (particularly electroshock) following its introduction in the late 1930's. Although their report was published as early as 1942 (Cerletti and Bini had published their work with electroshock just four years previously), they found studies involving some 2,152 cases in the literature. Scattered through four diagnostic groups, these cases responded to electroshock as shown in Table 12.

The figures for schizophrenia in Table 12 are the least impressive; later studies have confirmed this first, unfavorable impression, and some have shown that, of patients treated by psychotherapy and without electroshock, comparable percentages are discharged as recovered or improved. The percentages for involutional melancholia and manic-depressive psychoses have continued to remain high in subsequent reports; Noyes and Kolb (1963, p. 541) report 80 per cent full or social recovery for all patients treated. In spite of certain risks involved, this form of therapy continues to find widespread acceptance.

The risks are as follows. After treatment there is a dulling of all mental faculties, but the changes gradually disappear (for the most part). A temporary retrograde amnesia, an occasional amnestic syndrome that persists, a period of confusion that gradually clears seem to be the principal findings; where extensive psychological tests of memory, perception, and discrimination learning are carried out on patients six months after treatment, all but a few cases show no measurable residual losses. Kraines (1957, pp. 469 ff) goes so far as to insist that, even with repeated series of shock treatments, there is no increase in these residual losses so long as the treatments are spaced so as to allow recovery from one series before another is begun. Fatalities are

TABLE 12. *The Results of Electroshock.* (Based on charts by Olmansi and Impastato on display at the New York Academy of Medicine Graduate Fortnight, Oct. 1942.)

Diagnostic Category	Number of Cases	Remissions	Improved	Unimproved
Involutional melancholia	158	69.0%	20.2%	10.8%
Manic-depressive	596	59.5	27.8	12.7
Schizophrenia	1,184	28.7	34.1	37.2
Unclassified	214	39.7	31.3	29.0

rare (1 in 6,000). There have been repeated warnings from physiologists, supported by experimental evidence obtained from careful study of the brains of animals similarly shocked, and by postmortem studies of a few patients who have died during ECT, that there are "frequent multiple perivascular and meningeal hemorrhages, shrinkage of the cytoplasm, nuclear changes and marked glial proliferation, subarachnoid hemorrhages, perivascular gliosis" (Rennie 1943, pp. 134-35). We may consider them one more example of "brain damage without residual personality changes."

The majority opinion among psychiatrists has ruled against giving too great a weight to these risks involved in ECT. They urge that: (1) no other treatment brings as rapid a relief; (2) it shortens a costly hospitalization from six to eighteen months down to two or three weeks, and some patients can be treated as ambulatory patients in a general office practice, remaining at home the while; and (3) although depressions are usually self-limited (eventually), there is always the danger of suicide. A follow-up of manic-depressive patients (half treated by ECT, half untreated) showed that, with shock, 1 per cent of the ECT patients committed suicide, whereas 7 per cent of the untreated patients did so (Huston and Locher 1948).

Arguments For and Against ECT

Weighing the pros and cons, Noyes and Kolb (1963, p. 541) reach the conclusion (which is widely shared) that:

"In the depressions of involutional melancholia and of manic-depressive psychosis, the improvement following electroconvulsive shock therapy is striking. In 80 per cent or more of these disorders, five to ten treatments are followed by full or social recovery. *Prior to the treatment of involutional melancholia by electric shock therapy, protracted depression, sometimes lasting for years, was the rule.* Early treatment of this disorder and of the depressions of manic-depressive psychosis by shock therapy will save many patients who would otherwise commit suicide" (my italics).

According to numerous studies (e.g., Ey, Bernard, and Brisset 1963, pp. 227-28; Noyes and Kolb 1963, p. 541), this therapy in no wise guards against a recurrence of depressions. ECT, by itself, does not bring the patient any insight into the nature of his problems or his symptoms. If one were to assume, contrary to the genetic bias of Kallmann, that psychogenic or situational factors help to precipitate the illness and are worthy of the status of *causes,* these are apt to remain unaltered (along with the prevailing lifestyle). The patient who recovers returns to his former selfhood, save for the fact that he now carries the scar created by his memories of the depression and its treatment, and by having passed beyond that point of no return where his emotions no longer served to regulate productive action but became instead a source of deregulation.[19]

It will be true that many patients will prefer this kind of "no nonsense" therapy. It does not pry into their private lives. It treats their symptoms as though the latter were indeed "mechanisms," something that a good biological engineer could correct, and something that the individual himself need take little effort to correct. Many patients do not have the capacity or the inclination to enter into a long and searching personality study, nor do they have any desire to "negotiate" a new approach to life with the help of a counselor. Many therapists who resemble plumbers and engineers more than they do spiritual guides or artist-healers not only find it easier to handle cases in this efficient and impersonal fashion, but look on their critics as "faith healers," swamis. In the matter of efficiency, there is no question: a well-organized clinic can process a large number of electroshock treatments in a morning with a limited staff, and the cost of the electric current is small.

The work of the artist-healer forces him to empathize, cajole, persuade, seduce, emotionize, arouse, frighten, *motivate the patient.* The task of awakening hope in the depressed and of restoring the appropriate brakes on the manic, the demonstration of a warm and human concern that cares enough to discipline and guide a patient, are replaced—in these simple shock treatments—by a scientific and impersonal efficiency.

Some clinicians who use shock therapy look on it as:

1. A most potent form of suggestion. The expert who manipulates the electrodes says, in the potent language of action and gesture, "The trouble is in your brain. These electrodes will be fastened to the sides of your head. The shock will produce changes in your mood, in your consciousness, including a

---

[19]One patient, whose treatment proved ultimately to be a failure, resented the procedures of electroshock bitterly. Ernest Hemingway confided to his friend Hotchner (1966, pp. 279-80):

"What these shock doctors don't know is about writers and such things as remorse and contrition and what they do to them. They should make all psychiatrists take a course in creative writing so they'd know about writers."

"Have they stopped the treatments?"

"Well, what is the sense of ruining my head and erasing my memory, which is my capital, and putting me out of business? It was a brilliant cure but we lost the patient. It's a bum turn, Hotch, terrible. I called the local authorities to turn myself in but they didn't know about the rap."

This last statement reveals that Hemingway's delusion of being wanted by the F.B.I. was still in effect, a delusion he had carefully concealed from his physicians in his determination to get out of hospital.

brief period of coma and confusion." (See, for an excellent example, Kraines 1957, p. 408.)

2. As an occasion around which to develop psychotherapy, some of which can be introduced in the period before the shock; the review of personality trends, situational pressures, ways of coping with difficulties can be continued in the more receptive period that follows shock (in the more successful cases).

3. As an occasion for desensitizing the patient to his own symptoms through an explanation of psychosomatic relationships, and as a part of the "explanation" of how the shock therapy is supposed to work.

4. As an occasion for introducing a thorough plan for rehabilitation in the post-shock period, and for a continuing follow-up that will provide support for that patient's effort to make a renewed and improved attack upon his life-situation.

When all of these psychotherapeutic adjuncts are utilized to the fullest it will be difficult to assess precisely the proportion of the results that is due to the ECT itself. Those who insist that this form of therapy is able to produce only a symptomatic cure argue that it must always be used in conjunction with psychotherapy. Perhaps figures for the "pure" electroshock can be obtained from institutions (public hospitals) where individual psychotherapy is all but impossible, or from those therapists treating outpatients who cannot afford the more costly and time-consuming forms of counseling.

There seems to be a general agreement that the patient just launched in one of the manic-depressive cycles is less responsive to ECT. Kraines is of the opinion that these patients recover, untreated, in any case, and in as short a time as the patients shocked at the very beginning of their illness. He is ready to admit that several shocks per diem may reduce an excited manic to a state of quiet confusion and thus reduce the risk of exhaustion of both patient and staff, which fact suggests that electrical restraint should be added to others that have been used (continuous tepid baths, straitjackets, tranquilizers), and adds a certain sadistic aura to the treatment that the more squeamish among the staff will dislike.

The results that are reported for very mild depressions, particularly when the shocks are applied in the final or recovery phase of a long depression, show the highest rates of recovery and improvement. On the other hand, at the very nadir of depression, or in the early phases, a brief improvement is apt to be followed by a return of the depression, as though there were some endogenous process that required a certain period to complete itself, and that could not be hurried by such an extraneous agency. (See Kraines 1957, p. 458; Diethelm 1950, p. 151.) All the studies of the therapeutic use of ECT have shown that some patients do not improve. A few are actually in worse shape following the shocks. This is not surprising considering that patients vary in age, in the severity of their illness, and in the number of preceding attacks. Diagnosis is not yet such a precise affair that it will exclude all who should be spared this therapy.

How Does ECT Work?

We are left with an empirical "cure" and a number of unanswered questions:

1. What accounts for the 20 per cent of failures (patients who persist in their depression or go on to more serious deterioration) even when we limit treatment to the depressions or the depressive phase of the manic-depressive psychosis?

2. What proportion of the cures reported are actually cases of neurasthenia or psychasthenic depressions (which have normally yielded to all manner of therapies, with a success ranging from 60 to 80 per cent, or to the mere passage of time)?

3. What proportion of the recovered and improved cases are in the fifth and sixth stages of a depressive cycle (as Kraines describes it) and would therefore recover, shortly, in any case?

4. What weight should we assign to suggestion, to the fogging up of consciousness, to the loss of alertness and of memories which keep alive hatred, resentment, depression? How much is to be attributed to hospitalization and bed rest, to being accepted as an "organic" case by a "regular physician" who does not probe into the inner recesses of one's mind.

5. What accounts for the endorsement of this "cure" and for its extension to the treatment of psychoneurotics, if not the fact that there are many psychiatrists who are not equipped to do psychotherapy and many patients who either cannot or are unwilling to collaborate in such a venture (which is inevitably costly, demanding, and time-consuming)?

Some of the speculations offered as rationalization for the cure's success are neither impressive nor likely to stimulate hypotheses that can be tested. There are psychiatrists who have linked the treatment with the ducking stool, beating with brooms, and other harsh treatments dealt out to witches in a former day. St. Theresa's "firm measures" that she recommended to her Mothers Superior, faced with nuns who fell into states of *sécheresse,* were not as grave a threat as this scientifically refined procedure, yet both St. Theresa's methods and electroshock fit the beliefs and needs of some patients who feel guilty. Like insulin, which also tests the very limits of the patient's vital capacity, this insult to the physiological system arouses a reaction, a compensation, and following the shock, the sluggish sympathetic nervous system "fights back." If this new level of arousal is maintained and the reticular-hypothalamic centers now facilitate the awareness of and reaction to challenges and opportunities, replacing the low-grade parasympathetic vagus-mediated retreat and withdrawal by a more normal reaction to stress, this "fillip" to the patient's physiology may be the important aspect of therapy for which we can discover better substitutes with fewer hazards.

The precise manner in which electroshock alters mood and action and thinking is, at present, unknown. The physicist points out that much of the current actually passes over the surface of the cranium, especially when subconvulsive shocks are used. Some of it induces: (1) a depression of cortical activity,

(2) a wave of vasoconstriction responsible for some local blood clots and consequent cellular damage, and (3) a massive cortical discharge that produces tonic contractions of the musculature followed by clonic contractions similar to those seen in an epileptic seizure. When subconvulsive shocks are employed, the therapeutic gain is reported to be less or nil (see Kraines 1957, p. 465); it is generally agreed (among those who use shock therapy) that whatever good comes from the therapy must take place at this point where the convulsion occurs. Kraines is of the opinion that the pituitary is somehow involved, and if this gland (which is situated so near the hypothalamus) is also the "master gland" that arouses other endocrines to action via its hormonal substances, some of the effect of the shock may very well be biochemical, in which case a more direct and precise route may be discovered (as a skilled repairman can discover better ways of repairing a radio set than banging on the cabinet or giving the circuits a massive dose of alternating current). The general change in the action of the sympathetic nervous system is also followed by new corticothalamic balances, in all probability, but the precise nature of these changes has yet to be identified, so that speculation amounts to little more than a reification of the observed changes in thinking and action.

Noyes and Kolb (1963, p. 542) leave us with this terse statement of the puzzle:

"The use of electroconvulsive shock is entirely empirical. Many theories, both psychogenic and physiogenic, have been suggested as explanations for its therapeutic action, but no one has offered a satisfactory explanation for the results obtained either by electroconvulsive or by insulin therapy. Some investigators suggest that cerebral anoxia, a result common to all shock therapies, may somehow be the basis for the mental improvement. In both hypoglycemic and convulsive shock therapies, the brain is deprived of energy and oxidative metabolism to a degree that renders it inadequate to support cerebral function. The mechanisms producing these conditions are different, however. With hypoglycemia the brain is deprived of glucose and the cerebral metabolic rate is depressed. With electroshock, brain activity is raised to such a high pitch that cerebral function cannot be sustained by the oxygen and glucose coming to the brain in the blood."

Reviewing the various suggested explanations of treatment, Rennie (1943) finds such a wide range of "theories" (which have scarcely changed in the last 25 years) that one is led to wonder whether we have, in fact, gone beyond the ancient ducking stool (and other attempts to drive out the spirits). One is reminded of Pareto, who repeatedly called our attention to the fact that, in the history of civilization, the reasons for our actions change, but the central core of performance remains surprisingly constant.

Rennie reports various authors suggesting:

1. It frightens the patient out of his depression and delusion by forcing him to fight for his existence. Looking back at the treatment employed in the last quarter of the eighteenth century, Diethelm (1941) had this to say, "The curative effect was taken on its face value and there was no need to under-

stand the psychological factors involved. In many therapeutic procedures fear was the unrecognized dynamic factor which caused the patient to lose hysterical symptoms, to break through a catatonic stupor, or to control himself in his manic excitement or in states of anxious agitation. This lack of psychological analysis is to be expected in even the greatest physicians of these centuries."

2. It weakens the tyranny of the superego.

3. It breaks up rut-formations, checks vicious cycles, stops the faulty ways of coping with reality.

4. The amnesia and confusion prepare the way for new integrations.

5. The escape from death ("electrocution") brings a joy of rebirth and a willingness to reevaluate life.

6. It prepares the patient for intensive psychotherapy and facilitates transfer.

7. It strengthens the forces of control.

8. It stimulates appetite, inciting tremendous oral craving and equally strong satisfaction in eating (a guiltless fulfillment).

9. It provides a sedation effect, better sleep, improved appetite, weight gain, interruption of preoccupations, and better rapport.

The contradictory and rather superficial character of these "rationalizations" shows quite clearly the slender basis of certitude on which this rather radical but wholly empirical therapy is carried on.

All report amnesia present in some degree. The memory loss is greatest for the period immediately preceding shock, and it extends as the series of shocks grows longer. It is accompanied by a general dulling of consciousness and by confusion. After reviewing all the biochemical theories (including the concept of cortical anoxemia), Rennie concludes: "The actual reasons for its effectiveness are not known and may be primarily in the psychological realm."[20]

Like Kraines, Diethelm (1950, pp. 150 ff) sees the treatment as ineffective in stopping a depression in its earliest phases, and he notes that, with the increasing popularity of this treatment, the number of patients who enter hospital after having been unsuccessfully treated by electroshock has increased. "There are no publications which present conclusive, or even likely, evidence that acute depressive episodes which cleared up after a few convulsions would have had a prolonged course without the treatment." He also frowns on the treatment of ambulatory patients in a physician's office.

Wortis (1962), reviewing the journal literature for 1961, raises the question "Is electroconvulsive therapy obsolete?" He points out that after an initial burst of enthusiasm following the original report of Cerletti and Bini in 1938, the mid-1940's saw the beginning of a growing skepticism as to any permanent value of the treatment, and with the introduction of the new drugs

---

[20] A revealing observation of Arieti (1959, I, 449) suggests that what goes on in the minds of the patient and the psychiatrist is not always put down in the protocol: "It is advisable that electroshock therapy and psychotherapy be administered by different therapists. One of the fantasies of the patient (probably to a certain extent connected with the manifest recovery from the attack after shock treatment) consists in the feeling of having received enough punishment and, as a consequence, of being redeemed. The psychotherapist should not be seen as the punishing agent."

TABLE 13. *Death Rates for Suicides (1940)*.

Age	Rate (Per 100,000 in Age Group)
Under 15	0.1
15 to 24	6.1
25 to 34	13.5
35 to 44	19.4
45 to 54	27.7
55 to 64	34.4
65 to 74	33.2
75 to 84	34.4
85 and over	26.6

in the 1950's, this trend away from electroshock grew more pronounced. Physicians were more certain, apparently, that whatever "damage" the drug therapy might produce was most apt to be reversible. Increasing attention has been given to combinations of preparations which sedate, activate, raise mood levels, support cortical activity, depress muscular tension, alter circulation, suppress the hypothalamus, activate the pituitary, check tremor, facilitate sleep, allay tension, produce a mild euphoria, and so on. Increasingly, with the development of these synthetic compounds, the therapist has worked on the organism: the patient's mind is viewed as the body's mind, and the art of psychotherapy is replaced by the science of biochemistry. If this seems an exaggeration, we can at least note the rising consumption of the new psychopharmacopoeia, reaching 200 million dollars annually (according to Shaw *et al.,* 1959). A new set of iatrogenic effects has emerged: the "thalidomide babies" are simply one of many striking examples. Other side effects reported during the past five years include: agranulocytosis, thrombosis, thrombophlebitis, suicidal depressions, hepatitis, red-green blindness, addiction to meprobamate, optic atrophy, fetal damage, jaundice, dermatitis, seizures, manic excitement, and pigmentary retinopathy. (See also Wortis 1963, 1964.)

THE PROBLEM OF SUICIDE

No discussion of depression would be complete without some consideration of the problem of suicide, for every deeply depressed patient has to be regarded as a potential suicide, even in the final phases of his recovery (and perhaps especially then, when the vigilance of a staff or family is relaxed). Early release from hospital (where he has been closely supervised) is always a calculated risk.

Kraines (1957, p. 209) reports that "practically every patient 'thinks of' suicide, particularly during the depths of the depression," and that in his case records about 8 per cent made some sort of suicidal gesture. Other mental disorders also contribute suicidal attempts, some of which are carried out under delusional beliefs and in response to "voices" that command them. The suicidal risk mounts with increasing age, to judge by the vital statistics for the United States as a whole (see Table 13).

When, in round numbers, there are 150,000 first admissions to mental hospitals in the United States per year, there will be about 19,500 within this group who will be diagnosed as manic-depressive psychosis or involutional depression. This group, and a group of approximately the same size who are not hospitalized (and who never appear on any statistical table) but who are equally ill, form a pool in which the "suicide potential" is very great. Dublin (1963) puts the annual rate of *recorded* suicides at 19,000, the number of *actual* suicides at about 25,000, and estimates the number of those who *attempt* it but fail at between 175,000 and 200,000.

Where careful studies of cases of suicide have been made, the evidence is clear that in about half of them there is some form of mental illness prior to the attempt (see Stearns 1924). It is possible, of course, that some of those who are not thought to be mentally ill may be suffering from a mental depression of abrupt onset and great intensity at the moment of suicide. Aggression turned inward is the common characteristic of suicidal mental patients, according to Farberow, who reports: "All of them showed greater hostility than did a control group, but those who actually attempted suicide tended to direct their hostility inward. . . ."

Some would agree with Esquirol (1838, I, 335, 639), who asserted: "Suicide offers all of the characteristics of mental alienation. . . . Men do not cut short their days unless they are in delirium and all suicides are alienated." Such a complete rejection of the possibility of a rational suicide is close to the view of the Catholic Church, which is *absolutely* opposed to suicide on any count, but it overlooks such ritual suicides as were once practiced among Hindus (in which the widow was expected to join her husband), or the suicide of honor that was considered a mark of nobility in old Japan, or the voluntary drinking of poison by the members of the court at Ur (who intended to join their dead ruler in that new Kingdom in The Beyond). It also overlooks the long list of variables (other than mental illness) that are positively related to suicide rates.

The French sociologists Durkheim and Halbwachs, who made extensive studies of suicide rates in different populations, tend to discount the mental-illness factor and to look at the behavior as a symptom of social disorganization, of loosening bonds between the individual and his society, or as a symptom of disorganization in the group life. Others have shown mounting rates of suicide in times of depression, when unemployment increases and boxcar loadings go down; and such correlations suggest causal relationships. Yet it is the disorganization and the *anomie* that are critical, Halbwachs insists, for the same increase in the rates also occurs in periods of rapid industrialization and expansion (when people are uprooted from their old community ties). The high rates that followed the defeat of Japan and the breakup of the old regime (including the changes in family life and in the "respect for the elders") can be fitted into this disorganization-anomie thesis.

The choice of the social and impersonal factors rather than those within the individual biosocial history, and the preference for gross material changes rather than the conscious reasonings of the individual, seem to represent a kind of occupational bias. When we look more closely at the kind of bond between the social change and the decision of the individual to end it all, we are moved to emphasize its very tenuous nature. When we look more closely at the figures, we find that the high suicide rates affect from 25 to 35 per 100,000. In the United States, where the rates varied from 10 to 17 per 100,000 over the years from 1900 to 1960 (with low points in the postwar years 1920 and 1945, and a very high point at the peak of the great depression, 1933), the rates mean that for every 1,000 children born, 16 white men and 5 white women end their lives in suicide. (The rates for the nonwhite population are *lower*: 7.2 males and 2.0 females of all ages in the year 1960.)

Statistical studies have linked suicide rates to race, religion, age, sex, marital status, urban neighborhood, season of the year, wars, depressions, and types of legal or societal punishment directed against the act. All the linkages are slight. One gets the impression, as one studies each of these "bonds," that somewhere on the sociological map there is a man who is aged, Oriental, Buddhist, male, widowed, who is living in a postwar period in poverty, facing chronic illness, growing more and more depressed on Christmas Eve. Summing up all of the positively linked indices, one might arrive at a suicide "loading" (or potential) that would make him one of the most suicide-prone persons in the world. Yet the rates warn us that it is the ninety-ninth one, and the hundredth, of all who die who take this exit. The surprising fact to keep in mind is that the rates are so low. Normally we do take arms against the sea of troubles, cling to life, hope, endure, and most societies have codes of conduct and belief which support such decisions for life. Esquirol's judgment is one expression of our own code. Society frowns on suicide, for it needs soldiers and citizens; families frown on it and feel disgraced, let down, when it occurs within their household; the vast majority condemn it as a cowardly act. We imply, in our collective judgment, that this life is a socially and not an individually owned thing. This act was not something for the individual alone to decide. And it is simply "out of the question."

Yet there have always been a few to defend "the rational suicide." Dublin (1963, pp. 8-9) cites the instance of the Nobel Prize winner, Bridgman, the Harvard physicist:

"At the age of 79 he was suffering from the terminal stages of cancer when he shot himself. A colleague quoted him as saying, 'I would like to take advantage of the situation in which I find myself to establish a general principle; namely, that when the ultimate end is as inevitable as it now appears to be, the individual has a right to ask his doctor to end it for him.' He also left a note declaring: 'It is not decent for Society to make a man do this to himself. Probably, this is the last day I will be able to do it myself. P. W. B.' His colleague stated that the day after Bridgman's death Harvard University Press received from him the index for the forthcoming seven-volume collection of his complete scientific papers."

Another one of those for whom chronic ill health provided the reason was George Eastman:

"At 77, he had been suffering for some time from a serious and painful sickness. Rather than become a burden to himself or his friends, he shot himself. He left a note reading, 'To my friends: My work is done. Why wait?' His intimates were confident that at the time of his demise, Eastman, one of the great benefactors of his generation, was as rational as ever."

"I have thought the matter over carefully," the rational suicide might say, "and my judgment after full reflection is that I should bring my life to a close." Such a decision may have much to recommend it, but when we remember the delusional character of the depressed person's thinking, the way in which the negative side of a set of memories tends to become dominant in one of these "times of trouble," the tendency toward self-accusation, the distorted perceptions of the surrounding field, the loss of hope, the certitude that there is no one who can help, the feeling of alienation, guilt, and loneliness, it is quite apparent that only the exceptional person has any right to be sure that his careful survey of all the facts is not depression-tainted. It also seems that the board of competent judges who might be called in to validate such a conclusion will enter upon their deliberations with a heavily weighted prejudice against the act.

Looked at from a distance, the suicidal act is one of those mixtures of rational and voluntary choices with unconcious, physiological, and impersonal factors that push us into actions for reasons we do not know. The reasons assigned are legion: mental illness, depression, chronic physical illness, loneliness, failure, rejection by family and friends, hate (and the desire to injure someone), poverty, hopelessness of one's condition, addictions that cannot be mastered (or accepted), family discord, loss of love, hypochondriacal worries, fear of losing one's mind, guilt, or the need for self-punishment. Like the hari-kiri on the doorstep of an enemy, a suicide can be *against* someone. In most general terms, it is a failure of ego-strength, of that integrative force which at other times has been able to rise above difficulties and to persist in the face of misfortunes.

Looked at in such general terms, the *cause* of a suicide is anything that has made a difference, that has weakened this integrative power, that adds to the burden of difficulties. Since the rescue teams which have been formed in all our major cities are able to dissuade many of those who call them by showing their concern and providing even a small dose of "tender, loving care," one is tempted to see the predicament of the one who attempts suicide in terms of a deficit in this same department.

On the other hand, there is abundant evidence to show that weak egos can emerge from hothouse environments, where solicitude and overprotection have created dependent, infantile, demanding selves that are ill-suited for this world. The judgment of James (1896, p. 47), which is also the judgment of Toynbee, when applied to history, points to another side of the truth:

"Sufferings and hardships do not, as a rule, abate the love of life; they seem, on the contrary, usually to give it a keener zest. The sovereign source of melancholy is repletion. Need and struggle are what excite and inspire us; our hour of triumph is what brings the void. Not the Jews of the captivity, but those of the days of Solomon's glory are those from whom the pessimistic utterances in our Bible come."

Again, looking at suicide in the large, the rational element decreases, and the reasons assigned for the action grow increasingly trivial, as we enter the territory of mental illness. A patient may claim that God has commanded him. A girl suffered from sexual impulses that were making her lose her mind. A paranoid patient threatened to commit suicide unless he were released, and then, when released, jumped from the Washington Monument. A 56-year-old woman committed suicide because Nixon lost the election. The observation of groups ranging from the normal (where a rational suicide is possible) through the neuroses, and finally to the psychoses, would yield a series of "reasons" less and less adequate.

This emphasis on the lack of adequacy in the reasoning, however, misses the essential fact about most suicides. Suicidal impulses, with whatever motivation, are apt to occur in those catastrophic moments when the individual has been pushed just beyond his limit for organized behavior. A young man who has been studying nights in order to prepare himself for an examination which would open up a career for him (and exhausted by long effort and prodded by an ambitious family who want to see him "get somewhere") may be swept into one of these catastrophic moments when he reads the examination and finds that he cannot answer any of the problems. A lonely youth, shy with women, greeted with an amused smile and a flat refusal, may—before the night is out—attempt to cut his wrists. The parents of an adolescent may find that their refusal to let him use the family car was "the last straw." The number and variety of these crisis-points are infinite, for they simply represent ways in which the pressures on a system with limited integrative forces mount until this "point of no return" is reached. Some suicidal acts should be called "gestures": they are appeals for help, the methods are patently ineffectual, and they are made at some place where others are bound to discover the attempt before it is too late. But these "hysterical" and histrionic forms also contain some of the irrational, delusional, disorganized quality that we associate with neuroses and psychoses. Unfortunately, some of these "phony" attempts succeed, and all who work with such persons are agreed that the folklore to the effect that "those who talk about it never carry it out" is incorrect. Years of productive and satisfying living can be cut short when one of these "gestures" proves irreversible (whatever epithet we chose to describe them: phony, infantile, hysterical, irrational).

Although this discussion of suicide occurs at the close of the chapter on depressions, other mental disorders contribute to the annual table. Table 14

TABLE 14. *Suicides among Patients with Mental Disease.* (From Dublin 1963, p. 171.) *

Mental Disorder	Number	Per Cent	Average Annual Rate of Suicide per 100,000 Resident Patients
Cerebral arteriosclerosis	6	9.7	31.9
Involutional psychosis	7	11.3	80.4
Manic-depressive	5	8.1	87.4
Dementia praecox	31	50.0	30.1
Other	13	21.0	46.1
Total	62	100.0	34.0

*Patients in New York Civil State Hospitals, Apr. 1957 to Mar. 1959.

shows the suicides among patients with mental illness when allocated among five classifications.

EPILOG

A child can become "high-strung." His interactions with his environment will then lead to raised voices, tears, punishment, resentment, further excitement, and further tension. On the base of this mounting curve of tension, further episodes of wild anger can break out, with a blind disobedience. On the other hand a progressive withdrawal may end in an impenetrable posture of sulking and resentment which excludes all negotiation. States which have a certain resemblance to that state of frustration which Maier (1949) described as "behavior without a goal" supervene, and while they endure, behavior takes on a spontaneous, unmotivated, nonadjustive, unregulated form. Like an experimental animal that wildly attacks the learning apparatus or recoils in a corner, the child who has reached this point can no longer profit from his errors or improve in discrimination. Like a psychotic, he is "unreachable." These efforts of parents and therapists can meet a stubborn barrier.

Behavior, so fixated, tempts us to posit some self-defeating end, some masochistic appetite for punishment, some will to fail (or to fall ill), since these states produce, in fact, such ends (see Stephen 1960, Menninger 1938, Reik 1925). Sulkiness can have an almost suicidal quality, since the child refuses to participate in or take advantage of the opportunities that are opened to him, and blind rage can be more destructive of the self and its true purposes than the punishment of those who are its targets and who are apt to respond in kind. The hand of forgiveness is bitten, counteraggression is provoked (whether intended or not), and any progressive reintegration with the group becomes impossible. (For a successful therapist's views of such cases, see Aichorn 1925.) In thus going beyond the point where negotiations, discriminations, and corrective experiences are possible, these end-states tend to provoke drastic countermeasures in those who surround the child (or the psychotic), and these in turn reinforce any paranoid or masochistic beliefs on the part of the individual himself.

No longer reasonable, and no longer in charge of his own actions, such an individual seems to be *asking* for a padded cell, or shock treatment, or a ducking, or blows, or a straitjacket, or chemical restraint, or, if he is the child of "progressive parents," for more imaginative measures. Chlorpromazine is one of the first thoughts which enter the mind of the physician who deals with a difficult-to-manage manic patient. For, since words, gestures, reasoning, and reasonable treatment (including just punishment and earned rewards) fail to produce the desired actions, all that remains seems to be some nonlogical *force* that will alter the "mechanisms" directly. The clinician who treats the manic, or the depressed person, dreams of affecting the hypothalamus, through which emotional expressions are finally integrated and distributed to the tissues. The therapist who confines the autistic child to a room where Skinner-box levers permit him to discover the consequences of his manipulation of the levers intends to *force* him into a renewed cathexis with his environment by thus confining him so that the relentless laws of learning can operate.

Over the centuries, various methods have been tried by the physicians who have had to deal with psychotics: the blow of electroshock, the ducking stool, the drastic purge, the bloodletting, the chemical that blots out the undesired actions. The newest ataractic drugs, the shock therapies, the lobotomies, the stimulators (such as meprobamate, or aventyl HCl, or dexamyl) that rouse the apathetic or depressed patient are simply the most recent psychiatric tools to perform this continuing function.

Where this type of treatment seems to work best (in the involutional depressions, where 79 to 90 per cent are reported as improved following electroshock, for example), the effects are notoriously symptomatic, that is to say, good for the current attack only; and they give no guarantee of permanent improvement in behavior or of any change in susceptibility to further attacks when later rounds of mounting tension begin. In the manic-depressives so treated, recurring bouts of mania or depression are the rule, even though the therapist cannot predict the time of their arrival or their gravity or duration. The "cured" person remains as vulnerable as ever. These methods that force a change in behavior do not improve the individual's ability to discriminate, to profit from experience, nor do they alter any organic or constitutional susceptibility which, if it exists, must require improved ways of dealing with frustrations and burdens.

Since therapeutic skill is now, as earlier, in short supply, and since the patience of adults responsible for the management of incorrigible children is limited, and since there is seldom available any lay counselor who can give the requisite amount of concern and affection (or who possesses the understanding and skill required by an annual crop of first admissions of several thousands of manic-depressives), and since hospitals are crowded and good institutional homes are limited in number, and since their own homes, to which such children or patients must inevitably be returned, are apt to remain unaltered, these quick and forced changes in the patient (even when managed by experts) are not likely to improve matters radically, powerful though the steady pressure to employ them may be.

These irrational states represent a fracture in the normal self-containing, self-regulative system. They may be caused by some constitutional weakness or susceptibility; simple immaturity or a failure in earlier discipline and affection; some current endogenous change that radically alters the level of arousal and lowers frustration tolerance; or some current failure in the coping powers that leads to a depression, and a disorganization of the perceptive-regulative process. The problem, it would seem, consists in finding some method of strengthening whatever residue of self-regulation still exists, and some way of increasing this power. We need to restore the balance of tensions within an integrative system so that it can begin coping again, instead of responding spontaneously, reflexly, mechanically. The therapist must find a mode of entrance into such defensively closed systems. When we rely solely on physical therapies to force change, we dodge the more difficult task, and seem to deny the existence of any more rational course. Our actions communicate to the patient: "It is not possible to reason with you. You need *outside* help. You cannot manage, poor thing. You have to be treated in a special way (as a set of mechanisms). You have no inside power. There is nothing 'in there' to be exercised, strengthened. I do not count on you to do much of anything. You can let yourself go now. Our treatment will do all that can be done. I do not have a great deal of respect for you." We communicate a similar belief in the essential weakness of the person when, with bad news to communicate to him, we pave the way with a proffered "good, stiff drink" or a tranquilizer. Mrs. X, we read in the newspaper, was informed of her husband's accident and is now under sedation.

The bonamine pill that converts the transatlantic traveler into a "body transported overseas" as well as "a body impervious to motion sickness" also bypasses any effort on the part of the traveler to find his sea legs. Only the captain and the crew are expected to remain vigilant. Whether one chooses to stay interested in the life on shipboard or to become a transported body is the question, along with the option to take a calculated risk of motion sickness as a step in learning to control it. In life, unfortunately, most of us do not have a captain and a crew who will ferry us over to the other side whether we remain vigilant or not. The child who starts out life with a protective family around him might wish that, sooner or later, the family would also hold themselves responsible for making him into an autonomous member of the crew, not simply a dependent "institutional case" for whom someone else must assume responsibility.

The religious will try to accomplish some of this by appeals to divine guidance. In some ways the humanist has a more difficult task; he is forced to adopt a rather hard doctrine. That is, he knows that life is short and that it can be a good one only if he makes it so. He has no divine providence to watch over him, no disciplined crew to look out for his comfort. And he knows by now that premature medication or forced therapies can only weaken his chance of becoming autonomous.

Chapter 11 • Flights from Reality: The So-Called Schizophrenias

Those who approach the schizophrenic armed with the common-sense categories of causality, identity, and contradiction often come away perplexed. These minds do not operate according to "the laws." They do not even obey the laws of operant conditioning, or of pleasure-seeking and pain-avoidance, or of simple reinforcement theory that does so much to reduce the performance of the laboratory rat to order. The reasonable and lawful expectations which work when we endeavor to predict and control the actions of the normal man are violated. Pleasure is seen on the face of the patient when disgust or pain should be there. He makes and persists in false generalizations that would be promptly extinguished by a normal person, who undergoes the corrective experiences that establish the outlines of a shared reality: he persists in error. Even Freud, who had developed a quasi-systematic account that made a place for irrational conduct, a "system" so loose and flexible that it could be warped to fit the wildest examples of action and belief, recoiled from the thought of trying to bring his kind of insight to such patients: even the rationale of irrationality could not be understood by these minds, and to interpret their conduct to them seemed futile, adding an even more complex task to the simpler ones they cannot master.

The schizophrenic has a way of engulfing therapists and their theories, sweeping both into the surreal life of his delusions. The analyst's effort to develop rapport, instead of culminating in a therapeutic transference, may aggravate the psychotic who is already troubled by any form of closeness. He may perceive his counselor as seductive, as sexually aggressive. To resort to hypnosis may intensify such a patient's feeling of being influenced, for the schizophrenic often complains of having thoughts put into his head, of being robbed of his thoughts, of feeling electrical (or magnetic) influences pass through his body. Even a simple offer of medication can be interpreted as one more of a long series of attempts to poison him that have had to be fought off. Needless to say, the shock treatments can be experienced by these patients as attempts at electrocution. Thus the theorist and therapist are moved to look for some way of altering the patient's behavior in spite of these elaborate defenses and misinterpretations, by some direct means that will break through and alter some essential neurophysiological process that is not functioning properly, a breakdown reflected in that behavior.

Sometimes the patient sits, apathetic, so deteriorated and so indifferent to all that goes on around him that he makes another human being feel like some impersonal factor, a thing. The therapist's speech may evoke an impersonal echolalia in which the patient parrots the words spoken (in a tone and rhythm that betray the lack of comprehension); or his words fall, like the sounds of the street traffic that come in the window, on ears that record but do not initiate meaningful perceptions of the sounds.

Perhaps it is not altogether true to say that therapists have learned as much about themselves, and about the nature of everyday rationality (which the patient has lost), as they have about the patients. Nor is it true that their words always fall on deaf ears: the mute catatonic who seems to be unhearing and unseeing will repeat one day something his therapist said two weeks before, showing that the latter did, in fact, get through. The total push of a hospital staff that is working together intensively to change the course of the disorder can reduce the number of patients who drift into a deteriorated delirium or apathy to a sixth of those admitted, instead of the 30 or 40 per cent that commonly end in irreversible psychosis when a hospital is a mere custodial institution without the staff or the interest to attempt the more difficult task.

The schizophrenic's deficits bring into sharp contrast the powers of ordinary folk, even of persons who are far below the intellectual level of the patients; and many of the latter show islands of rationality and skill, use an extensive vocabulary and exercise gifted imaginations: some who have aesthetic sensibilities and creative talents lack the simpler integrative power that is required to make a life outside of hospital and to keep in vital touch with a shared reality. One can write poetry that is acceptable to the editors of little avant-garde magazines; another produces a play off Broadway while still under treatment; and a third produces abstract paintings that a curator with a flair for modern art might be glad to hang in his exhibitions. One of the three "Christs" that Rokeach studied at Ypsilanti was able to bring a sensible book review to a group-therapy session, yet he stubbornly clung to the absurd notion that he was God. Another patient, who believed that she had been nominated "woman athlete of the year," kept a spurious file of letters, typed "copies" of clippings (about others), and photos that she had collected and woven into her private fantasy. Another, who regularly read the *New Republic* with interest, was sure that it was actually a propaganda source managed by the Vatican; as proof she pointed to the yellowish tint of its pages. Arrested on various "shelves" in their progression toward a more deteriorated terminal state, these minds can show a surprising residue of intelligence, subtlety of expression, skill in penetrating the motives of therapists, even while their islands of sanity are surrounded by a sea of delusion and many of the simple distinctions between fact and fantasy cannot be managed. The tugboats on the river are sending signals about him. The Catholics are opening her mail on the railway mail coaches.

Viewed against the backdrop of dereistic nonsense that composes the delirium of schizophrenics, the soundness of normal thought and action even at a very humble level stands out with striking clarity. Whereas the patients cannot make even a simple life for themselves (or are dangerous, or scandalous, or reduced to a helpless apathy), the nonpatient characteristically learns from his mistakes, foresees his needs, manages to keep in reasonably good contact with those around him.

BORDERLINES OF NORMAL BELIEF AND ACTION

There have been many who have sensed that schizophrenia is a "reality disease." Minkowski described it as a loss of vital contact with reality. The term "dereistic," which both Bleuler and Minkowski have used, means, literally, "away from the real." A diagnostician confronted with a borderline or incipient case of schizophrenia will have his own sense of reality tested as he tries to discriminate an illness from a slight exaggeration of the beliefs that are shared by a culture. Like a magnet, there are certain "fringe areas" that seem to draw the schizoid personality. Where the normal may enter and leave at will this "lunatic fringe" of telepathy, clairvoyance, spiritualism, the potential schizophrenic remains "in communication," withdrawn in "meditation," or "acts out" what the normal is content to imagine. Just beyond any reflective or objective validation, just outside the real, these realms may further contribute to a schizophrenic's disorganization.

Janet's Achille, who came from the Midi and grew up in a village where traffic with spirits was not regarded as too unusual, was helped into a delusional interpretation of what was going on within him by what we might call the mass delusions that circulated among the community, folk beliefs that for the most part no one paid much attention to, but which were believed in, nonetheless, and were ever available to the "odd one" who became alienated. So surrounded, the normal process of consensual validation, which should pull the individual back to more matter-of-fact beliefs, allows him to drift toward pathology, and even reinforces his hallucinatory experiences with corroborating tales.

THE HALF-DELUSIONAL WORLD WE LIVE IN

These delusion-supporting folk beliefs are, however, usually no more than latent possibilities, forms of thought whose full potential is rarely used. The normal individual does not find too much use for them, employs other routes to his practical goals, corrects his expectations as he finds himself acting too often in terms of this *au delà*. Flournoy noted how some members of the Geneva spiritualist circle remained strong in their belief for a while, then grew disaffected, and finally came to laugh at their former credulity as they moved outside the circle; others stayed longer, and a few became more deeply involved so that their whole life became wrapped up in "communications with the beyond."

Similar transitions in and out of believing groups are reported as common in present-day Ghana, where some, newly educated in Western culture, mingle with fellow tribemen steeped in the lore of witchcraft. The old spirit beliefs are still solidly entrenched, and the elaborate rituals of a very skillful group of practitioners help give them a kind of validation. Most of the tribesmen do not resort to witch-doctors in their everyday business, and it is the exceptional one who becomes possessed, or believes that he is in fact a witch. Common-sense practices govern most of the actions of the tribesmen.

When one of our own tribe develops notions about the blinking lights of the aircraft which fly overhead each day, believing firmly that they are signaling to him, we promptly identify the dereistic quality. When someone voices the notion that the liquor in the liquor store would be poisonous unless someone else bought it for him (the proprietor would slip the poison into the bottle were he to recognize that the patient is the purchaser), it is obvious to us that his suspicions have become paranoid. When some humble citizen, a minor employee in a bank, is suddenly sure that the F.B.I. is after him and that they have turned up evidence about his secret life, we are apt to suspect that he has lost his reason. When each of these men has started out life with the experiences that we share in common, when each has possessed at one time the common sense that protects men from absurdities, we ask, "What is the nature of that underlying (or inside) process that cuts short the normal validating process, or makes it suddenly unnecessary? Why has his belief fallen to this primitive (or infantile) level?" Some theorists have speculated about a "process schizophrenia" in which some neural, chemical, endocrine, enzyme, or toxic change has muddied the stream of thought and altered the course of action and belief, for it stretches our belief, and even threatens us, to view such a change as simply the cumulative effect of little things, small errors, minor wishful distortions (or fearful thoughts). How does "What if they are influencing me too much?" become "I am being brainwashed; I feel electrical influences that are changing my insides; my brain is being electronically polarized"? Uttered with all of the bland poise of a person who is conveying simple matter-of-fact information, the words of these patients betray that what may have begun as a normal give-and-take with the environment has undergone a qualitative change *at some point*. The theorist seeks the good and sufficient reason for such a change.

We know well enough that misunderstandings between perfectly normal people can develop to an almost delusional level from small beginnings, especially if the corrective transactions are cut off; but to be carried to extremes, the little mistake has to be compounded, the error validated by some fact, or some complementary error committed by the party of the second part. Ordinarily, we call this a comedy of errors, and, while the mutually compounding series of interactions can reach a climax of absurdity, we are optimistic about the conclusion: it will collapse of its own weight when one small grain of fact intrudes to blast the structure. However, farce can turn into tragedy as deeds begin to validate and produce errors. In our own time we have seen a not too bright ex-corporal turn a highly developed Western power into a machine capable of committing genocide. A pair of potential young lovers can gradually grow apart as each interprets the shyness of the other as coolness and each determines to wait for "proof" from the other or tries to test him by minor rebuffs. In a continuing dialogue with the world about him, and with those others who both give and validate his identity, the individual can move into a half-real, half-delusional private world. To the half-deluded, his pseudoreality is *out there,* as firm as a mountain of granite, as vast as the sea, and it seems to him that it will be there when he is gone, whether he turns his head away or not. He is sure that it is independent of his wishes and cannot be altered or willed away; indeed, he may be ready to defend it to the death. When the clouds of suspicion increase at the same time that the means of correcting them decrease, judgment can become so confused that practical necessities cannot be managed. At this "point of no return," the private world becomes delusion. The act that reveals how far this process has gone can be committed, finally, with an *absolute* conviction.

A SOMATOPSYCHIC CHANGE OR ERROR COMPOUNDED?

The growth of a progressively delusional system in such cases can be so stubborn, so resistant to correction, that we are tempted to imply some underlying motivational system, some primary process (neurobiochemical) that alters learning and robs the individual of his normal corrective powers. We ask, "Is there some unconscious complex that continuously distorts perceptions until they cumulate to this catastrophic level?" Or, we speculate, "Can it be some biochemical factor that alters perceptions, as the psychotomimetic drugs do, so that action is founded upon a wildly distorted private world and the normal process of extinction fails to reduce errors?"

Hesnard (1949) described the case of a hairdresser whom he had observed:

Living in a small village, this man gradually became more and more suspicious of his physician, an elderly man of good will with a somewhat authoritarian manner. Month after month, the hairdresser became more and more certain that this physician took a more than ordinary interest in him. At first the feeling was vague, the evidence slender, but his certitude that there was a malevolent intent increased, and his feeling became so insistent that he had to work out some explanation. Vigilant, he found signs. The clues were small: a strange glance, an accidental touch, a failure to greet him. These "mere nothings" crystallized around his original vague premonition to give it a "fact"-supported structure of belief; the residue of reason told him that this crazy quilt of "accidents" could not be shared with any other. In his fantasy life the kind of suggestion that the normal mind would have discarded became an affirmation: "He is going to make me the subject of some of his criminal experiments, probably of a sexual nature." (He explained all this to a psychiatrist, later.)

A fantasy system of this sort can be a sort of inner play, for a while. We smile at the child making mudpies. We even enter into the game and pretend to taste them, expressing our admiration for the fine baker he has become. The child knows it is a game. We would become alarmed if he were to begin to act out his game, requiring us to eat and swallow the pies. But this stepping-out onto the cloudbank of fantasy, as though it were firm rock, is precisely what the schizophrenic does.

Hesnard's hairdresser openly complained, one morning, that the doctor had entered his room, at night, in order to practice on him acts that were contrary to nature (after he had been put to sleep). When the hairdresser was asked to give some kind of substantiation, or proof, of these accusations, he could offer little that was convincing: a bruise, his own rectal pain (which, unfortunately, no one could share or observe, conjointly). Multiplied by a thousand, such circumstantial proofs can accumulate until the sheer proliferated mass does what reflective verification does for the sane: a core of meaning is formed that will draw each new event into its orbit. The daily newspaper will give proof, the radio broadcast, the pastor's sermon.

One evening, at dusk, after years of struggle against his persecutor, the hairdresser lay in wait for the unsuspecting physician, and shot him as he rounded a corner. Later he declared to the prosecuting judge, "One of us had to be destroyed. I have rendered an immense service to society in ridding it of such a hidden human monster."[1]

In like fashion, an episode of love can develop between a schoolgirl and her teacher, between a callow youth and that movie actress whose lovely smile "communicates" to him as she looks down so lovingly and reassuringly from the screen. Ruminating in secret, returning to the theater to look on that face, writing to her studio (finally) and receiving in return the photo distributed by her public-relations staff (to all "fans" who write in), he carries on a spurious private dialogue, to the point where some overt act finally reveals to those around him that it has passed the boundary of common sense.

When such a psychotic arises to testify in prayer meeting (or revival) about God's grace, about the efficacy of prayer (and his own long dialogue with divinity), he may not be spotted, at once, for what he is, for in his action he is expressing a belief sanctioned by an ancient and honorable tradition. The witchcraft beliefs in Ghana also support the woman who announces that she is possessed (or under the influence of some evil spell cast by some yet to be named witch).

THE FINAL TRANSITION TO PSYCHOSIS

We call the private world of the schizophrenic autistic and dereistic. We conceive of it as mushrooming in some dark subcellar, where the validating sunlight of facts cannot correct its growth, or within an action system

---

[1] With processes of this sort developing in weak and distorted minds, no public official is safe; the more prominent the "star of attraction," the greater the probability that he will draw upon himself the attention of some paranoid person.

that for some reason is operating below the normal level of perceiving, learning, conditioning, or, as some believe, in a mind beneath whose surface some old infantile trauma or fixation continues to work steadily to distort the course of growth. Sometimes the outbreak of the illness into an overt form that all can see comes suddenly, dramatically, and with outside "precipitating causes" in abundance (as often happens with the manic-depressive psychosis). Sometimes it arrives very early, as in infantile autism or childhood schizophrenia. Sometimes it develops so gradually and insidiously that even those who surround him are hard put to name the transition point: he has simply become more and more queer, eccentric, self-absorbed. Whatever its history, the transition point in the dialogue and the ultimate content of the delirium, even when all the inside story is laid out in as complete a phenomenological description as can be managed, may not reveal the nature of the *causes*. The religious *contents* of the various drug experiences are not the causes of the drug's action, any more than sleep is caused by dreams.

Process and dialogue, loss in reality testing and increase in fantasy life, exogenous precipitating factors and endogenous processes of some nonlogical impersonal sort, conscious reasoning and the work of unconscious factors, are so combined in this psychosis that the hundred years that have elapsed since Morel first identified his *dementia praecox* (1860), with a central core of symptoms that place it in the midst of the severe schizophrenias, have not produced a simple, clear, and concise explanation for the illness.

Borderline "Schizoid" Cases

The diagnosis "schizophrenia" is a serious one, and at present there is a danger that it will be used too often and on too slight evidence. There is, for example, a wide band of pathological forms of conduct in which behavior resembles now one aspect, now another of this protean disorder. There are manias with schizophrenic features, obsessives who are preschizophrenics and who, before they fall into more serious pathology, tend to be dismissed as neurotics and seem almost to be protected from anything more serious by their elaborate defensive rituals. There are hysterical patients, sometimes diagnosed as "pseudoneurotic schizophrenia," who show many of the features of the full-blown disorder but who are almost magically cured by therapies that are ordinarily applied to neuroses. Clinicians have come to speak of ambulatory schizophrenia, an illness that has some of the components of the more serious disorder, yet is not incapacitating and does not require hospitalization. A well-to-do family can maintain a brother or a daughter in an artificial environment (even hiring paid companions to provide a kind of imitation of life); ensconced in a room of his own, the schizoid self can loaf, dream, engage in a kind of "work" (on the occult, on some grand design for politics, or sexuality, or some electronic gadget) that never comes to anything.

Some of these near-schizophrenics are found among the perennial students who haunt the universities but never take a degree, the artists who move in and out of ateliers but never hang a picture, the cultists who are the first to be drawn to new religions, new drugs, new therapies. So closely do these persons simulate the true innovators, who are the lifeblood of any growing society, that they test our own discriminative powers. We have to examine their fantasies and probe for the negative signs in their behavior before we can separate the authentic from the near-schizophrenic. Some of these near-schizophrenics compose the band of narcotics addicts, drifters, dipsomaniacs, criminals, and deviates who clog the courts and keep alive the question: "Are these men and women sick, or just weak, or do they have essentially simple character problems; are they undisciplined selves whose families have failed to socialize them?"

In addition to this zone where a chronic deviance has stabilized itself at a near-schizophrenic level, neither improving nor progressing to a deeply psychotic end-state, there are cases in which *attacks* of an openly psychotic nature that invite the serious diagnosis are followed by a return to normal, in response to either therapy or a compensatory self-regulation that is as obscure as the original "loss of control." This single attack can be followed by a long history of normality that is as completely recovered as any careful series of examinations can demonstrate (see Sullivan 1931; but cf. Bleuler 1911, p. 255). Others experience a series of such episodes with lucid intervals of normality between "attacks"; this undulating process can continue for three or four years before it becomes clear that the fateful dénouement has finally come to stay. At this point, what had been a borderline case (or, as some are calling such cases today, "nonprocess schizophrenia") has become a genuine instance of "process schizophrenia."

The wide band of borderline and transitory forms that resemble the core cases (which, diagnosed as schizophrenia, make up the enduring body of long-term residents in mental hospitals and occupy half of all mental-hospital beds) has created confusion and controversy among those who describe, treat, explain this disorder. The very concept of the disorder is unstable, with vague borders that can shift toward an overinclusive fuzziness, covering all who have broken with our reality, or toward excluding all but the 16 (or 36) per cent whose symptoms have endured so long that the diagnosis can now be made after the fact, when one is almost certain that the normal self is dead and that the patient will never return to normal.

CONFLICTING GENERALIZATIONS

Whoever reviews the literature on schizophrenia, now a library in its own right, will discover that, in the hundred years since Morel first identified dementia praecox, this group of disorders have been viewed as:

1. Organically based, with a probable specific neuropathology underlying the symptoms, and with a fateful and irreversible course that moves to an end-state of deterioration and dementia.

2. A functional disorder that (even after the pathology has advanced to the point where hallucinations, deepening apathy, or stubborn delusions enclose the self completely from all vital contact with reality) can reverse its course;

after successful therapy the patient can be described as a complete recovery. There is no irreversible, organic, neural lesion.

3. An illness that has no fixed course and outcome, that represents merely the pathological extreme of a long series that reaches from neurasthenia through manias and depressions to schizophreniform processes. There is no specific cause that is both necessary and sufficient. Since it has no single cause, anything that makes a difference in human adjustment can serve as cause or cure.

4. A group of illnesses that are too often sloppily diagnosed. As with manias and depressions, where such work as that by Kallmann, Lewis, and Piotrowski seems to indicate a failure on the part of many clinics to establish clear concepts of etiology and therapy and to make proper diagnostic discriminations, there are those who believe that our present confusions and contradictions about schizophrenia are similarly rooted. When there are claims that cases of chronic and advanced schizophrenia are cured by some new type of "direct analysis" (or by chlorpromazine, or by insulin or electric shock), critics can often point to carelessness in the selection and diagnosis of patients; we want to know how many of the "magical" cures were actually instances of borderline cases, pseudoneurotic schizophrenia, or improperly diagnosed cases of manic-depressive psychosis, or first attacks and "beginning" cases, which are known to yield a higher rate of recovery, or in fact mild forms of neurasthenia (or psychasthenia), which yield to a wide variety of therapeutic efforts.

5. A way of life upon which we pass a social evaluation when we say "It is schizophrenic." Such social evaluations may be required to make a culture go, to permit the rest of us to feel safe, to save the life of the individual, but we should realize that this is a police matter, a "judgment of one's peers" (i.e., something *between* the patient and his society). Such a reaction to the problem of diagnosis reminds us that the revered shaman or witch-doctor of one culture may be confined as a schizophrenic in our own society, or that within the little in-group of deviates there is a firm agreement that the ruling morality is sick.

The above generalizations show that there is confusion about the concept, and about what constitutes the area to which it can safely be applied. It is therefore important to identify the standard which the most experienced group in our society use. Experienced psychiatrists share a strong conviction that there is a core group of cases which will have to be hospitalized for years and which will contain few recoveries. It is to this group that the theorist turns when he wishes to study a schizophrenic process at work.

PROCESS AND NONPROCESS SCHIZOPHRENIA

Since the days when Bleuler first summed up his extensive experience with schizophrenia, clinicians have been trying to differentiate among these illnesses. It is argued: "There must be more than one type. There are not only different types of behavior, but the courses and outcomes, the responses to therapy, are different." A recent attempt to classify schizophrenias studied among the patients at Johns Hopkins Hospital suggested that we might need some 22 categories.

Bleuler was aware of the problem (quoted from Freyhan 1958):

"By the term 'dementia praecox' or 'schizophrenia' we designate a group of psychoses whose course is at times chronic, at times marked by intermittent attacks, and which can stop or retrograde at any stage, but does not permit full *restitutio ad integrum*. The disease is characterized by a specific type of alteration of thinking, feeling, and relation to the external world which appears nowhere else in this particular fashion.... One comes closest to reality if one makes it clear that merely the general direction of the course of this disease is toward a schizophrenic deterioration, but that in each individual case the disease may take a course which is both qualitatively and temporally rather irregular. Constant advances, halts, recrudescences, or remissions are possible at any time.... We do not speak of a cure but of far-reaching improvements.... Definitive or transitory improvements occur spontaneously, or in connection with psychic influences or factors such as transfer to another place, a release, a visitor.... These improvements occur significantly less frequently in the chronic conditions than in the acute, but are not completely absent from the former." (For further clarification of Bleuler's views, see M. Bleuler 1931.)

Both Bleuler and Kraepelin, who helped set the fashion for more than half a century of psychiatric treatment of these illnesses, believed in an underlying trend toward schizophrenic deterioration, in some constitutional and endogenous causes which underlie the changes, and in the likelihood that "apparent recoveries" would be followed by a resumption of the course of the illness or, if the course were merely arrested, would show on closer examination that the recovery was not complete. Yet the trend over this half-century seems to have been away from their convictions; and with the willingness to expect a wide variety of outcomes has come a readiness to extend the diagnosis to borderland forms, in which most of the "brilliant" cures have occurred.

What the studies of the half-century since Bleuler have added, in the way of careful follow-up studies of those admitted to hospital as schizophrenics, is a healthy agnosticism about the existence of that universally present, underlying *process* whose trend is always toward dilapidation of the personality, deterioration, and fixity in delusion, for by every criterion that can be applied, a sizable fraction of the hospitalized group (10 to 25 per cent) fully recover from their attack (or attacks), never have a recurrence (at least not a psychotic one over a period of ten to twenty years), and lead productive lives that are as well-adjusted as those of many nonschizoid normals. If anything, our therapies have grown more eclectic, perhaps inevitably: given a psychosis of unknown origin, we are willing to try everything, and in a kind of total push, we hopefully accept "whatever will make a difference in the life of the patient" as therapy.

In the meantime, the diagnosis has tended to be applied somewhat indiscriminately to a wider and wider range of the borderland phenomena. We identify schizophrenic features in cases of manic-depressive psychosis, in obsessions, in hysterias, and in immature personalities. Such broadening of the concept intensifies the problem presented by the very real differences in the outcomes. Stephens and Astrup (1963), with the hindsight that comes from having made an extensive follow-up of some 178 inpatients treated for schizophrenia in the Henry Phipps Psychiatric Clinic at Baltimore, believe that they can identify two groups that differ so much they deserve to be treated as radically different types of schizophrenia; they offer *process* schizophrenia and *nonprocess* schizophrenia as sufficiently noncommittal terms for the present stages of research (where the causes of either type are unknown). Life-histories before the illness, behavior on admission, course of the illness in hospital, predictions of the staff upon discharge, and finally the subsequent history of the patients during a follow-up period of five to thirteen years after discharge, all went into the differentiation of the two types. With all this data and the longer view of the patients' illnesses, these investigators believe that in the future differentiating criteria can be applied to any new group of first admissions. Thus physicians will be able to predict outcomes and adjust therapies to the actual differences in the illnesses.

What has sometimes been referred to as a "hard-core" group, the process schizophrenias, emerged at the time of discharge from hospital, when only 7 per cent were described as recovered, 38 per cent as improved, and 55 per cent as unimproved. The comparable figures for the nonprocess group (possibly a lighter form of the same illness) were 19 per cent recovered, 54 per cent improved, and 27 per cent unimproved. (It is evident that if a clinic wishes to compare the therapies in use, or the skills of staff members, the indiscriminate assignment of these two types of patients to the various experimental and control groups could vitiate all findings.) At the end of the follow-up period, the nonprocess group contained 38 per cent recovered and only 3 per cent unimproved, the process group 10 per cent recovered and 49 per cent unimproved. Over this period of study, the nonprocess group behaved as though suffering from a mild, self-limited form of illness, whereas the process group contained a large portion of cases who continued to progress to deeper levels of illness and who did not respond to therapy.

In their process group Stephens and Astrup note that:

1. Introverted, schizoid personalities ("cold," withdrawn, preoccupied with an inner life) abounded. Described as a biotype by Kretschmer, these personalities are often identified as the typical prepsychotic form of character development. They are described as inhibited, meditative, "terrible metaphysicians," dreamers, obstinate, withdrawn, "hypersensitive," isolated, with occasional bursts of impulsive and poorly adapted behavior. However, although the type has been identified by Bleuler, Kretschmer, and Harry Stack Sullivan, this prepsychotic form of character makeup is actually not found in more than half of the patients hospitalized and diagnosed as schizophrenic (Ey, Bernard, and Brisset 1963, p. 468). A normal or extroverted (cyclothymic) personality is counted by Stephens and Astrup as more characteristic of the nonprocess group. Sullivan and Bellak also list this latter pre-illness life-style as one of the more hopeful signs.

2. Chronic schizophrenia was generally found in their near relatives, to the following extents: 5 to 10 per cent of parents; 10 to 14 per cent of siblings; 10 to 16 per cent of children; and 75 to 86 per cent of identical twins (the expectation for schizophrenia in the general population is only 1.6 per cent). Relatives of nonprocess schizophrenics, if mentally ill, tend to suffer from some psychosis other than schizophrenia. These facts are worth bearing in mind when we try to evaluate the genetic studies, especially since the diagnosis of schizophrenia has been made to cover many diverse illnesses. Furthermore, some patients thought to be nonprocess schizophrenics when first discharged from hospital later develop into obvious process cases.

3. They tended to have histories of poor social, vocational, and sexual adjustments. Adolf Meyer, and Terry and Rennie (1938), have stressed this point in earlier studies of Phipps' patients. They had been poor in schoolwork; their work-history was spotty, with frequent change in jobs and high-flown ambitions poorly suited either to talents or opportunities; their sex training had been premature, or inhibitory, or abnormally excitatory, and sometimes disorganizing. Vague, dreamy, abstract, impractical, they had adjusted poorly to work that required collaboration, steady effort, and alertness.

4. The onset of the illness was insidious.

5. Symptoms tended to endure.

6. Precipitating factors were minimal or absent.

7. Symptoms bore little relation to past conflicts. These seven items so far seem to describe an illness that arrives early, develops insidiously, has prevented the individual from ever establishing a good adjustment, has some inner (endogenous, genetic, or neurophysiological) basis, and is not directly linked with life-experiences or learnings. The nonprocess group, in contrast, had not shown any gradual personality changes, and had formed a good work, social, and sexual adjustment to life. The onset of illness in the latter group was frequently linked to clear and present external stresses, and the psychotic symptoms shown were easily understandable (and meaningful) when related to the precipitating factors and past history. Instead of an insidious onset, the beginning phases tended to be stormy, anxious, excited, elated, or depressed, and with marked expression of self-blame.

8. The patients could not give any clear or reasonable account of their psychosis. They were without "insight." In contrast, the nonprocess group could discuss their symptoms, giving vivid expression to their sense of the distressful events which they believed to be responsible for their illness.

9. Marked affective blunting characterized the process group. The nonprocess patients showed considerable emotion, were nearer to the manic-depressive group, were disturbed about their symptoms, wished for a return of their old selfhood.

10. Delusions were fantastic and bizarre, little related to each other, with paranoid features, sometimes (as when related to their bodies) so grotesquely described that the physician could not empathize with the patient. They included massive feelings of passivity, of being influenced, while fully awake.

The nonprocess group realized that their feelings of depersonalization were delusional and were more likely to be plagued by delusions of inferiority, guilt, or a general hypochrondiasis.

11. Auditory hallucinations (voices, hearing his own thoughts broadcast), tactile hallucinations (sometimes involving the sexual organs), visual hallucinations of mass scenes of murder and torture were common. The non-process patients lacked paranoid features, and both the delusional and the hallucinatory experiences seemed to be more related to a confusion, a clouding of consciousness.

12. Movements were often stereotyped, automatic, grotesque, and bizarre. Silly giggling and senseless behavior and posturing often made communication impossible. The nonprocess group, if hyperkinetic, showed natural and undistorted movements.

13. Mental processes showed disturbed associations, neologisms, perseveration, telescoping, disturbed symbolization, and a marked departure from the ethical and social feelings that had been present in the prepsychotic personality.

These two groups of patients differ in their behavior; the nonprocess group is much more approachable, seems to have symptoms that arise out of meaningful difficulties, permits a relationship that facilitates psychotherapy, and yields a much greater number of fully recovered and improved cases than the other. In spite of all advantages in such a separation of patients into these two groups, there are certain warnings that we ought to heed:

1. Recoveries do emerge from the process group, and there are nonprocess cases that move into a state of delusion and chronic deterioration. In the course of studying the two groups, these investigators found that there was a considerable "crossover" in the placement of the cases. The "signs" may differ at different phases of the disease. Patients wholly outside the psychotic category may "fall into it" (yesterday's obsessive or hysterical turning up today as a full-blown case of schizophrenia).

2. The dichotomy is not a sharp one, but represents two overlapping ranges on a continuum. Using a scale that expresses the saturation of process items in a given case, one might speak of a patient's "schizophrenic score." But although prediction might be improved, incorrect forecasts would still sometimes be made.

3. For all the improvement in our power to predict outcomes, we can be duly grateful: there are all too few firm generalizations in this field. Should such a discrimination as is here proposed also be used in redirecting therapeutic efforts, it might deepen the contrast between the groups, diverting effort away from the seriously ill and using staff time for those patients who are easier to empathize with, and who are more likely to improve. Thus the successes in psychotherapy would go up, while the residue of "core cases" would be left to be treated by those who use the less time-consuming and more impersonal forms of therapy (lobotomy, electroshock, insulin shock, chlorpromazine), or to mere custodial care.

Looking at the matter from the physician's viewpoint, we sense another danger. Adolf Meyer (Winters 1951, p. 457) noted it:

"The comfort of working under the cover of fatalistic and analyzed conceptions of heredity, degeneracy, and mysterious brain diseases—and from the relief from responsibility concerning a real understanding of the conditions at hand, and concerning the avoidance of preventable developments—is a powerful and unconsciously cherished protection, very rudely disturbed by these conceptions which make the physician partly responsible for the plain and manageable facts. I deny that fatalism is inevitable, without admitting that my conception should imply unwarrantable optimism."

Meyer made these observations when he was trying to establish the notion that schizophrenia was a cumulative habit disorder, a compounding of errors that need not have drifted to its psychotic conclusion, an illness that can be interfered with, a form of action that must always be viewed against the background of immediate causes and in the light of the purposes of the individual. In short, he viewed the symptoms as meaningful. Therapy required, therefore, a persistent though often painful effort to ferret out these meanings, so that common-sense measures might be taken to correct them. He made his residents unhappy by his criticisms when they brought him, not the concrete facts in a case, but classifications, mechanisms, imputed processes. His reasoning made him distrust Freudian formulations, and would have given him an equally potent reason for rejecting the "process" concept that has emerged in recent years in the clinic where he once taught.

These "dangers" are underscored when Stephens and Astrup report that within the process group the patients who went on to deterioration *could not be discriminated from those who improved*. If we call the process group the *real* schizophrenics, as Langfeldt (1937) does, and then add that prognosis is poor in this group, it is a small step to withdraw an intensive effort from them. Then we can count those who improve as schizophreniform illnesses, or as pseudoschizophrenias, but not as *true* schizophrenias, and we are back at the original, rather hopeless prognosis of Kraepelin.

THE CLASSIFICATION INTO FOUR GROUPS

From Kraepelin's day to the present, it has been the practice of clinicians to separate schizophrenic patients into four groups. This grouping provides a kind of descriptive economy, and familiar stereotypes can sharpen perceptions. They also invite the research worker to identify different types of causation, and they lead the clinician to anticipate certain characteristic outcomes. At this point such grouping does not seem to have served particularly well. Some are of the opinion that, since the consideration of greatest importance is the individual patient (whose life-situation must be understood and whose unique assets and liabilities must be appraised), effort should be placed on communication and understanding: a taxonomic enthusiasm can replace more productive effort. The predictions made on the basis of "type" are not only uncertain and full of exceptions, but could conceivably lead to either indifference ("this type is hopeless") or unwarranted enthusiasm (if a type should be judged as merely episodic and likely to be followed by prompt recovery).

Not only does the typing have limited predictive value, but the cases that are followed over the years are found to shift from one form of the disorder to another. Like the races of man, who resemble one another in their essential humanity, these different forms of schizophrenia also share in certain common qualities to which therapy must ultimately be directed. The illness mocks the categories by producing many mixed types which straddle the boundaries: the pure type is thus only a convenient "reference point." It is presented here simply as a step in getting acquainted with the disorder.

Some suspect that, in addition to being merely a dynamic stage in the development of a disorder, the type may be related to the way in which a staff (or a family) has handled a patient. A conflict between staff members, a type of discipline of the patients, may produce an increase in catatonic symptoms. Arrested at the moment on one or another of these "shelves," a patient may progress to join the residual core of institutional cases that are more difficult to differentiate in their common state of dilapidation and regressive changes.

In the eyes of Harry Stack Sullivan (1964, II, 27), our taxonomic enthusiasm is a form of logical obscurantism and leads only to increasing the distance between physician and patient, already made so great by the difficulties in communication. "It does not make one bit of difference, per se, whether a patient be labeled manic-depressive, hypothyroid, or sexually neurasthenic; the life-situation is what distinguishes him completely from any other patient, and places him almost entirely beyond useful statistical inquiry." Sullivan also believed that a physician's skill in modifying the course of the disorder depended on his ability to enter into and modify this "life-situation."

CATATONIC SCHIZOPHRENIA

The disorganization of the catatonic's movements makes this class of illness the most visible of all. It is also more likely to (1) have an abrupt onset, and (2) be related to identifiable conflicts and pressures. In view of the signs which Stephens and Astrup used to differentiate process from nonprocess schizophrenia, it is not surprising to find clinicians giving this class of patients a more favorable prognosis.[2]

The stuporous catatonic sits or stands, motionless. He shows no emotion, answers no questions, does not flinch from a feinted blow. He may have to be fed, dressed, and taken to the toilet (which latter procedure he so often circumvents that his soiling seems purposive). His motionless stance may make feet and ankles turgid, and if his purpose is to shut out the world, it is almost completely realized in this complete cessation of active give-and-take.

The excited catatonic strikes out in an unorganized and unmotivated aggression that hits whatever is near, purposeless though it seems to be. Unpredict-

---

[2]Henri Ey would enter an exception here. In his opinion the hebephrenic-catatonic mixture, identified by Kahlbaum in 1874 and described in much the same terms as used here, is one of the more serious forms of the illness. (See Ey, Bernard, and Brisset 1963, p. 502.)

able, full of mannerisms, his autistic-dereistic actions and postures express in motor terms what the silly verbigeration of the hebephrenic does verbally. Nude, attitudinizing, sleepless, hearing voices, he is explosive and disorganized in movement. His vegetative system also participates in the "attacks" of salivating, sweating, and muscular hypertonus.

Both positive and negative suggestibility are present in extreme forms: (1) automatic mimicry, echolalia, and compliant, waxy flexibility that outdoes the hysterical, on the one hand; and (2) mute, stubborn, resistant negativism (doing the opposite of what is requested) that outdoes the obsessive-compulsive. What the catatonic cannot produce is an action that is voluntary, purposive, rational, sustained.

Although the prognosis for this group is generally more favorable, some catatonics progress to the hebephrenic form and undergo rapid deterioration, or to the paranoid form and remain in an arrested stage, neither recovered nor deteriorated.

Although it is admittedly exceptional, the following study reported by Robert Knight (1946) deserves a place here, if only to set the record straight and restore the balance that is distorted by too inclusive generalizations.

Knight's patient was barely 17. As he stood by his bedside in hospital, mute, resistant, refusing food, neglecting his bladder and bowel needs, his ankles gradually swelled. He had to be forced to sit or lie down. Some 387 hours of psychotherapy and 30 months of hospital care had passed before he was ready to attempt a trip home. Patient, persistent, one-way conversations had probed his defenses until at long last he had talked.

After his final discharge, he completed two years of college, joined the Navy after V-J day, and served for eighteen months with an excellent service record. He then returned to finish college. A "schizophrenic episode" had interrupted an earlier growth and development that had been remarkable only in its extremely normal course.

As Knight probed to construct a history of his patient's prepsychotic development, he found little in the family that could be called *schizophrenogenic*. The youth had made a good school record, played football, achieved Eagle Scout status, participated in youth groups in the church, and had given no evidence of conflict or concern in adolescence. If he was unusual, it was in a sort of early maturity that made him the one at the picnic who helped clean up afterward, the one at the dance who looked out for the girls who otherwise might not have danced. His father, described as a "pal," had encouraged him to carry papers, save money, achieve an early sense of responsibility. The family was above the general socioeconomic level of the town and owned a home that set them apart; theirs was a family with some culture, and they were friendly and without pretensions. Two older sisters had preceded the boy through the school system; one had married before the patient's illness began.

The onset of the illness was fairly rapid. "During his senior year of high school he stayed away from the football games in which he could not play because of a recent operation (appendectomy) and listened to them on the radio. He did not participate much in the camaraderie of the boys and, although he did not betray it at the time, he was disturbed by their rather outspoken sexual talk and attitude toward girls. He himself had a very few platonic dates, mainly with less favored girls. However, in spite of a certain reserve and aloofness, he was very popular and the margins of his high-school annual were filled with penned good wishes and predictions of high success from his classmates. He had decided to take a year in military school before going to college, and at once a number of boys who had been undecided what to do made their decision to go to the same place.

In a garage and filling station where he worked in the summer vacation following graduation, he seemed excessively slow at his work, and the proprietor had to let him go. He spent an unusual amount of time sitting by himself in the yard, or on the curb with his chin in his hands. When he disappeared from a dinner party and went off to walk by himself, his father sought him out, tried to get some explanation, but only evoked apologies. More and more the youth sat alone, staring into space. He seemed slow at everything he undertook. His eating almost stopped. He did not want to enter the house when he thought his unmarried sister's boy friend was there. He spent hours in the bathroom with the door locked. On the advice of a psychiatrist he was brought, finally, to a hospital.

As Knight describes his efforts to establish rapport with this youth, it is apparent just how persistent he had to be. The youth did not want to talk to anyone. The physician seemed to talk through an impenetrable wall, and the patient gave, at first, not a flicker of understanding or gratitude. Returning, day after day, asking permission to talk to him, showing by his persistent interest the nature of his purposes, he intruded to interrupt whatever the inhibiting process may have been. He tried to answer questions that may have been on the youth's mind, even though the questions were not raised, and to restore his interest in his family, his mail, the outside world. When contact was finally established and a conversation begun, a question would sometimes emerge that had been touched on weeks earlier, when the physician had thought he was not getting through at all. It was virtually a "laying on of hands," an insistent forcing of the patient to focus on what was being said, a persistent interest that finally broke the spell. Or should we say that, finally, a self-limited process passed?

HEBEPHRENIC SCHIZOPHRENIA

Almost as visible as the catatonic form, the silly, giggling hebephrenic, with his false jocularity and decorated costume or outlandish hairdo, may have arrived at his status at admission after a long series of insidious changes. His prognosis is not good: he tends to grow increasingly autistic and self-contained; his actions become disorganized; and his personal habits of cleanliness and good social behavior are replaced by soiling, wetting, gorging himself as he eats, neglecting his dress. His moods are varied and shallow. Speech and action are bizarre, incongruous. Fantasy and delusions (not well-systematized) show his limited critical powers and tend to center upon his body. Often hypochondriacal in the prepsychotic period, he now complains that his heart is on the wrong side, his bowels have been removed (or lost), his brain melted.

This caricature of a jocular fellow or a lively adolescent (or a hippie), at first amusing in his disregard of social values and customs, becomes a sore trial to the staff as the disorder progresses, hard to contain, impossible to discipline, until he curls up in fetal position and soils himself as an infant would.

Hebephrenia with Hypothalamic Lesion

Among the students of the adult forms of schizophrenia there have always been a few who were convinced that some underlying brain change must exist to explain these extreme changes in behavior. For the most part, their postmortem studies of those who have died in the course of an illness have not revealed clear-cut and consistent types of damage. The neurological hypothesis has remained one of those deep-seated convictions that persist without support. As Rimland has done for infantile autism, here and there theorists have presented evidence which suggests that at least in a few cases neural lesions may be involved.

Hebephrenia is a form of schizophrenia that tends to occur at an earlier age than either the catatonic or the paranoid form. Emotional "attacks" of wild excitement alternating with tearfulness and depression, and with marked incoherence in thought, mark this vivid and "senseless" pattern of behavior. A pattern of silly, impulsive, shallow, and otherwise inappropriate behavior, with inadequate underlying motivation and with interspersed ideas of being influenced and watched, leads gradually into a deterioration of the personality that one observer refers to as a "molecular disintegration": the pieces of action no longer are bound together by an ego with plans. Bizarre delusions accompany hallucinations of sight and hearing that make waking behavior like that of a person in a disordered dream. (For more descriptive data see Henderson and Gillespie 1936, pp. 210-11.)

Guiraud (1950) is of the opinion that, if we select the forms which appear early and pass rapidly to an acute terminal dementia, the illness can be correctly described as a *diencephalic degenerative change.* There are many autonomic symptoms that accompany the disorder, and these would fit in with this hypothesis. Epidemic encephalitis, and illnesses which selectively affect the midbrain and the posterior part of the hypothalamus, often produce symptoms like those of hebephrenia and catatonia.

What Guiraud calls *athymhormie* (the emotional-motivational deficit so prominent in this disorder) can also be interpreted, he believes, in terms of the generally accepted role of the hypothalamus in motivation and emotion; he includes in this concept the lack of interest, the poverty and inappropriateness of emotion, the loss of vital relationship with the environment. He cites nine cases, reported by Vogt and Vogt (1948), in each of which there was an uncomplicated hebephrenia with deterioration and death; in each case anatomical studies at postmortem showed lesions of the diencephalon.

In such a view as this, the somatic changes are primary. Because of their location within the neural apparatus, they produce changes in instinctive-affective behavior. Such a disorder should therefore be called *somatopsychic* rather than psychogenic or psychosomatic. The precise nature of the hypothalamic changes is left unspecified: it might be of genetic origin, or the result of trauma or of the invasion of microorganisms or of some toxin that attacks these cells selectively.

Guiraud, like some other theorists, tends to generalize: "there is *always* a systematic illness of the vegetative centres in the encephalon" (my italics). In his opinion, to apply psychoanalytic or behavioristic analyses to the personal histories of these patients, and to arouse pain and guilt in parents by a probing that inevitably implies that they have been at fault, would be a wicked waste.

PARANOID SCHIZOPHRENIA

In this form the delusions are more systematic, but the disregard for facts and the patent contradictions betray the impenetrable psychotic process. With considerable intelligence preserved and with disorganization arrested, the paranoid may be discharged as a social recovery, even though a schizoid quality remains: he is likely to remain suspicious, withdrawn, bitter, and his actions keep others at a distance. Indeed, many have shown these same qualities in their prepsychotic personality and have never really adjusted socially, even to a small circle of friends.

Typically changeable and shallow, his delusions are nonetheless occasionally acted on, and when these are of a persecutory nature and charged with counter-hostility, his impulses may be homicidal, his upsurges of violent feelings felt as "uncontrollable." The idea of being influenced, so common among schizophrenics, here assumes bizarre and elaborate forms. His delusions are far more systematic than those found among the hebephrenics. In an educated paranoid, his delusions can issue in a book (which he peddles from publisher to publisher, each of whom hesitates to handle it) in which he gives an elaborate account of a world plot of the Catholics (or Jews, or Masons) with detailed descriptions of the operation of an international network and of the way in which "agents" have interfered with the patient's daily life, caused deaths in his family, thrust messages under his front door, robbed his mailbox. In America (according to Arieti 1959, I, 455 ff) his delusions are more likely to be persecutory, whereas in Europe they take the grandiose form.

As he leaves the hospital, that institution and its staff, including his psychiatrist are apt to have a special place on his private "world map." Most clever of all deceivers, his counselor is now seen to have used devious and seductive approaches; with his a strong appeal, he was the most dangerous of all. The paranoid thus includes and neutralizes the very means used to bring about his recovery.

SIMPLE SCHIZOPHRENIA

The least visible of all four forms of the disorder in its early stages, this one (first labeled *dementia praecox*) seems to be more of a "withering on the vine," a slowing down of development to a full stop, a slow decrease in all vital contact with reality, a loss of all interest and effort. The "What's the use?" attitude of the psychasthenic has reached its acme. Prognosis is poor. Although the patient's arrested growth may be related to some obscure factor in his life-situation, this factor is difficult for an outsider to see, and the patient

is not interested in changing anything, in registering any complant, or in helping the psychiatrist ferret out the source of his difficulties.

Although he may make a good start in life, show promise as a student in
the grades, seem normal enough in the play group, the vital thrust that should
fire him with ambition and carry him through the disciplines of apprentice-
ship or professional training at the threshold of adulthood runs down. No
psychedelic cultist needs to urge him to become one of life's dropouts. He
cannot, in fact, be instigated, cajoled, aroused to action. Instead he sinks
gradually into apathy, indifference, withdrawal. His development has stopped
at the threshold of life, as though down among the genes there had been
lacking that lust for life that normally organizes and activates all striving.

At first unnoticed, showing no hallucinations or delusions, less visible than
the three types we have described, his behavior grows more and more inappropriate: his feelings are too shallow; small things are too inhibiting; his
indolence is terrifying to the family that has hopes for him. His pecularities
may be intensified by the efforts of those around him to exert maximum
pressure. (Perhaps it is in this interplay that the motivation for that one-room
existence away from the family originates, as Hare's study seems to indicate.)
What he is able to carry out under prodding and complete direction, he will
fail to do on his own. Freed from pressure, he drifts still further into a do-
nothing state; he is in danger of gravitating into the company of hoboes,
prostitutes, and irresponsible delinquents, or into a "life at the fringe," living
as an eccentric hermit, a collector of junk, a harmless one who stirs the
charitable to do something.

As in other forms of this disorder, communication grows increasingly difficult. Once he slips out of the normal interpersonal orbits, or is segregated
in an asylum (that cares for his body only), he is likely to progress into a
more or less permanent and irreversible deteriorated state, the acme of morose
and empty inaction. Dilapidated, changed irreversibly, he becomes a true
dement.

CHANGES IN MENTAL PROCESSES

There are a number of changes in mental functioning that keep recurring
in the published case reports. While none of these gives a clear indication of
the essential nature of any underlying psychobiological core process, their
sum indicates something about the dynamics of the illness and makes clear the
difficulties confronting the therapist, especially the therapist who approaches
the patient "with his bare hands," relying on ordinary means of communication.
The "talking cures" are necessarily difficult when words fall on the deaf ears
of the deteriorated schizophrenic or the stuporous catatonic, and the therapist's
efforts to communicate can be dangerously distorted when they are taken up
into the dereistic thinking of the paranoid patient. The ordinary procedures
used in motivating a patient are less and less effectual as he drifts out of
reach and down into the apathy and morose inaction of simple schizophrenia.
One can sympathize with the therapist who searches for some drug, some shock

treatment, some form of neurosurgery, that will penetrate these psychotic minds.

DISTURBANCES OF THE COURSE OF THOUGHT

Sometimes speech is well preserved, and even the sentence structure is intact, yet the residual intelligence implied by this fact is not used. Closer analysis of the verbal productions shows that whatever it is that cements our thought into one whole (and keeps it in close relation to transactions with reality) is missing. The familiar sounds are there, and even some of the familiar patterning, but the sense is lacking, the thread of meaning repeatedly broken. Ideas are therefore "flighty," and there are abrupt turns that leave the hearer nonplussed. From an almost intelligible discourse to a mere automatic naming of objects or to an elliptical and telegraphic style, from a highly elaborate complaint of persecution down to a jargon aphasia that is more a mouthing of sounds than true communication, the constriction and dilapidation of thought can proceed until only unintelligible bits remain, a kind of parrot speech (echolalia) or an impenetrable muteness.[3]

Examples of Disordered Communications

The three "Christs" whom the hospital at Ypsilanti, Michigan, assigned to a single room, so that they could be studied as they interacted, resented the experience and reacted to it as to a new form of mental torture. One of them "read between the lines" and realized that

"... those people who bring patients together to have one abuse the other through depressing—is not sound psychological reasoning deduction. Meaning a person who is set in his way, there is nobody on earth.... God cannot change a person, either, because God Almighty respects free will; therefore, this man is so-and-so and I'm so-and-so, and on those merits to try to brainwash, what they call it, organic cosmics through the meeting of patients one against the other—that is not sound psychological deduction also."

The *therapy* thus became "mental torture," "electronic dumping," "brainwashing": the patients could interpret as well as the research therapist, and their paranoid delusions stood like a rock against the suggestions, interpretations, arguments, and blandishments of their interlocutor. As Redlich (1952, pp. 33-34) suggested, the therapeutic interviews with an established schizophrenic tell the therapist more about the nature of the patient's deficits than about any way to cause changes in the illness.

Almost communicating something to his counselor, one of the three patients that were studied by Rokeach (1964, pp. 5-12, 55, 68, 74, 83), a tall, lean,

---

[3]The stages of speech development that Allport (1924) sketched pointed to (1) a reflex babbling, (2) a conditioned imitation (echolalia), and finally (3) a selection and fixation of useful (reinforced) verbal pointings. The final, voluntary stage of true communication is both the more complex and the more vulnerable; we can see a regression to the more primitive mouthings of sound in the schizophrenic.

soberly earnest "Christ," stood with both hands before him, one resting gently on the other, both palms up, as he explained that his name (Leon) was a "dupe" name.

"Sir, it so happens that my birth certificate says that I am Dr. Domino Dominorum et Rex Resarum, Simplis Christianus Pueris Mentalis Doktor ... It also states on my birth certificate that I am the reincarnation of Jesus Christ of Nazareth, and I also salute, and I want to add this. I do salute the manliness in Jesus Christ also, because the vine is Jesus and the rock is Christ, pertaining to the penis and testicles; and it so happens that I was railroaded into this place because of prejudice and jealousy and duping that started before I was born, and that is the main issue why I am here. I want to be myself. I do not consent to their misuse of the frequency of my life [by] those unsound individuals who practice electronic imposition and duping. I am working for my redemption. ... I don't want this electronic imposition and duping to abuse me and misuse me, make a robot out of me. I don't care for it."

Once when he sat holding his head, his counselor asked him if he was suffering from headache.

"No, I don't, sir, I was 'shaking it off,' sir. Cosmic energy, refreshing my brain. When I grab cosmic energy from the bottom of my feet to my brain, it refreshes my brain. The doctor told me that's the way I'm feeling, and that is the proper attitude. Oh! Pertaining to the question that you asked these two gentlemen ["Why do you think you were brought together?"], each one is a little institution and a house—a little world in which some stand in a clockwise direction and some in a counterclockwise, and I believe in a clockwise rotation."

Leon had evidently taken in and reformulated other bits of wisdom his physician had imparted to him, or which he had read in some popular exposition of psychoanalysis.

"The human has two squelch chambers. Some people have four. It depends. It's their privilege if they want one in the subconscious region of their brain. It's a little bit beyond the center point—about one and a half inches from the top of the skull—and it is an aid to the person. For example, if the squelch chamber is charged positively [Leon had served in radar reconnaissance in World War II], it will counteract negative engrams—grind them up—by grinding up I mean the faculties of the squelch chamber are such wherein sound is amplified into itself and the interamplification of the sound or engrams as such are squelched; that is, transformed through amplification that is so great that it is transformed into light, organic light as a secondary outlet that refreshes the brain to a certain degree."

Leon almost communicates. Most of his sentences hold together: they could be diagrammed, with subject, verb, object, and properly placed dependent clauses, but the meanings elude us. Do the "electronic duping" and the "cosmic energy" mean that Leon, like so many schizophrenics, and some spiritualists, believes he is under constant outer influences, that these forces or persons are either sending him great strength or robbing him of his thoughts, his identity (as his own forces fluctuate up and down the scale of psychological tension)? Has he tried to incorporate some popular neurology (with the hypothalamus just an inch and a half below the top of the skull)? Or some account of those experiments on animal memory in which the engram-bearing tissues were ground up and fed to another animal in order that the effects of training could be transported in the still-organized nuclear bits ingested by the second animal? Or is he acting out a bit of folklore about masturbation? The truth is that it is the *hearer* who is trying to organize a consistent meaning, to make something of Leon's "message."

And Leon misses communicating, because his speech is neither adjusted to his hearer, nor disciplined by an outside shared reality. It has moved toward mere *expression* and away from *communication*: it is an autistic wordplay, rather than language that is well-designed to make something happen within a hearer.

Consider the following letter from a student, written while in hospital for treatment of a schizophrenic episode, and addressed to her former teacher and counselor. After an almost stilted introduction and a perfectly normal salutation, she launched into:

"What is the purpose of trying to square the circle, unless you are a square in a social circle. Anyone want to shoot pool? Who's Pool? Why shoot Pool, poor fellow? Or on the other hand what is shoot? Why shoot? Possibly shoot is gun fire. Or shoot is a spring flower when young. Someone has given us one word for two things. If you run into a real dull faculty meeting try this: Shall we use shoot for gun or for spring flower? Faculty meeting now breaks up into factions, shoot against shoot, and you roller coaster down the chute-the-chute. Just kidding.... The situation is nevertheless pregnant with possibilities, if you will permit the use of an abused word such as pregnant, which, according to GB Shaw, equals baby withorwithout wedding ring."

The counselor is puzzled: Is she trying to tell him that her difficulties began with a pregnancy and a need for an abortion, and that she is the spring flower who has been shot (i.e., deflowered) too young? Or is this just an example of the flight of ideas, of a mind operating at a low level of psychological tension, of the random firing of associations with no central directing tendency (posture, intent, purpose to communicate)?

A still greater fragmentation is observable in the letter cited by Manfred Bleuler (1931):

"Dear Mother:

"I write on paper. The pen which I use is from a factory named Perry and Company. I imagine this. Above the name, Perry and Company, there is written on the pen, City of London. But not the city. The City of London is located in England. I learned this in school. I always liked geography there...."

Writing from his room in a mental hospital, this youth is reduced to a mere naming of what is before him, to a mechanical sequence of associations that pop into his mind, one thought dragging the next by its heels. It is not the missive organized and directed upon the mother who is waiting to hear from him.

In the next sample, although the shell of sentence structure remains, the words seem not only to wander but to be cluttered up with contaminating and irrelevant meanings. We can scarcely call the thought *symbolic* (unless we do the work of imagining the meanings intended), for the patient is not capable of speaking in riddles, intentionally. He cannot even lie, that is, keep a clear eye on the meaning intended while saying something that will produce a quite different expectation about his actions in the mind of a hearer.

"It is right painful and causes it to be right sorrowful and right undigestive matters. There practically was no digestive—no living—than, any more than borning in life. In that case we feel right close to stock and we look upon that stock of food—well, I have lost my worries—we look upon that stock as though feeling it wanted to feed us. That horse was a well-digestive horse and a fine animal. He had a way of dropping lights down the throat—some kind of a man had been very brutal to this animal—he had been lashed unbeknownst to us, and it went to his throat some way or other and hurt him, but he gave me this light to understand how he hurt. I hadn't quite finished dropping the light."

Dr. Muncie (1939, p. 154), trained in Adolf Meyer's clinic to look for meaningful interpretations behind all symptoms (by projecting the present act against the total course of a life and the actual surrounding situation, making the one the numerator and the larger whole the denominator of a meaning-producing "fraction"), asked the patient, who seemed to have made a mishmash out of gastroscopy and his own experiences as a farm hand for veterinarians, "And how did all this affect you?" He was told,

"It simply dried me all up in a ball—when I went to walk, was told to do things. Of course, I was blind most of the time and so blind I would bump into things. It was a matter of birth—bumping to travel. And when I was in bed it was a matter of birth beds—three doctors and nearly got a spark of life to attract attention to give me life."

From a vaguely intelligible yet disquieting form of communication (he seems to be telling something), the schizophrenic's communication can descend to a flighty, disjointed form, or to a kind of "word salad" in which understandable phrases are tossed together with neologisms and "symbolic" and irrelevant phrases. Even the pseudogrammatical forms become lost; the style is so condensed and private that it can scarcely serve the function of a secret language (i.e., to direct the future thought and actions of the subject himself). Words become play objects, verbal mudpies that are mouthed (or shouted) for their "sound effect" rather than for any communication. Sometimes they are mere echoes of an interlocutor's question.

Abstract and Concrete

"Why did he kill?" we ask, when a sudden and murderous action occurs, out of character for the murderer, an action without reasonable motive yet at least briefly premeditated. A homicidal schizophrenic might answer, "His tie was red." When Bleuler asked his patient, "Why are you crying?" the latter replied, "Because you are dressed in black." In both of these instances thought and action have run off the track, making an abrupt change of direction, confusing symbol and fact, flying outside the boundaries of a limiting common sense.

"Read this passage to me," Hanfmann (1939) urged her usually compliant patient, but the girl refused, complaining, "But it is not raining outside!" The test passage had read, "It is raining." The patient could not, would not perform in this fashion. On the other hand, when she was asked to read, "When the train passes you will hear the whistle blow," she not only complied, but added, "Yes, I do hear the whistle blow at night; do you?"

It is apparent that what the experimenter easily structures as a test situation (in which a patient is asked to read a sample of prose) is reacted to as a "real setting." The patient does not seem to be able to take the "as if" stance, to *demonstrate* the kinds of things she can do, to consider the possibility of some hypothesis, and to be clear about the distinction between a merely representational and a final action. Her structures are simpler, all or none. They exist. If she thinks "black," she promptly adds mourning, and someone is dead. If the line of print says, "It is raining," she must either put up her umbrella in the consulting room or object to the passage, refuse to participate in something that is not right.

The deeply deluded schizophrenic cannot lie, Janet noted (1926, pp. 248-53), for a genuine lie is a much more complex stance in life than he can manage. Like the problem of malingering in the hysterical, this question of the sincerity of the deluded, the firmness of the delirium, has caused considerable argument and created much confusion, especially in the beginning of his illness, when the patient seems merely to be playing with his fantasies, pretending to be what he knows he is not, and cautions his physician not to tell his family about them (knowing how he would be laughed at). When a very positive clinician orders "the commander-in-chief" to go to bed, or when he abruptly stops the flagrant and open effort by his female patient to seduce him, he is moved to say, "See, the whole delirium is a game. The patient himself does not believe it."

When, however, the patient is quite open about his obscenities (seeming to have lost all inhibitions) and has settled into the full-blown form of delirium, the latter has become a bloody truth, the very foundation of his life. He will die for it. He acts out his convictions without any regard for the very real consequences (as firmly convinced as the LSD-drugged patient who blandly prepares to step out of the eighth-floor window, certain he will float away into space).

Negative Aspects of Schizophrenic Thinking

Let us sum up some of the negative aspects of the schizophrenic patient's thinking:

1. His speech often expresses but does not communicate.
2. His words are often used in ways that are so unusual we suspect them of being symbols. However, our work to interpret them is something that

goes on in us: he seems to operate far below the level of one who tries to communicate with symbolic speech. Some of the "metaphors" represent the vagueness or looseness of his directive tendencies: his speech splatters about its target, producing near-misses that would be hilarious in another setting.

3. As the thinking deteriorates, its form drops from the level of well-ordered configurations to a broken, disjointed, contaminated, fragmented form, telegraphic, elliptical, with unexplained changes in direction, and without regard for a hearer.

4. The clear distinction between fantasy (or mere hypothesis, or merely spoken phrases) and a reality-ordered action is gradually blurred, until inner speech is no longer good self-direction. It becomes private, unrealistic, autistic, incomprehensible.

5. Test situations cannot be apprehended as such, and when they are interpreted by the patient, they become a part of the bloody reality (electronic duping, false directions, harmful agencies).

6. The evidence from the tests shows that what a normal subject can do easily (put these blocks into groupings that belong together) is difficult for the patient: he may fail altogether, or use methods that do not produce good categories. ("These go together because they are all Chinamen!" To the yellows of the test blocks, he adds the pencil in the examiner's hand, failing to put a boundary around the test setting. Or he excludes every block save one that is identical. Or he adds a blue: "This is a Chinaman dressed in blue denim.") This inability to use the categorical attitude has been called a *primary thought disorder* by Kasanin. Because this deficit also appears in "organic cases" (lobectomies, brain tumors, senile dementias), some have suggested that the patient's performance, being similar to that of the brain-injured, should be counted a sign of some underlying neurological process that is also the cause of schizophrenia. (See Kasanin and Hanfmann 1938b, Hanfmann 1939, and Parfitt 1956.)

7. This loss of the abstract attitude, as Goldstein called it, carries with it a lack of flexibility. Once the yellow blocks are grouped as Chinamen, they remain Orientals to the end of the test period. "I think of them that way, therefore they are," the patient could insist, caricaturing Descartes. They may also be large or small, tall or flat, angular or curved, heavy or light, soft or hard. They remain, for all that, Chinamen, once they have been so named. When this type of patient is asked how he likes it in hospital, he may reply: "I don't like it. The rooms are too large." This is the way they strike him. It is not that he has fallen into a clairvoyant grasping of reality as it truly is, or that he sees the *Ding an sich* (as some of those who experiment with psychotomimetic drugs seem to think they can do), but that his categories are both simple and fixed. As a result, he does not grasp his true identity, perceive his real predicament, understand what it means to be a patient in a mental hospital, or understand what mental illness is, what the therapist is about.

Not only is he stuck with his categories, but they tend to be rather simple. They do not fit the reality he is in. He cannot understand a test as a test, or therapy as therapy, or a physician-patient relationship as such. Some of his productions suggest possibilities that the patient may be playing with, at first, knowing that they are only half-real, but when the disorder progresses, the patient falls into a bloody certainty. At first plays of fantasy, then muddled half-truths, finally the delusions pass into a certitude where all the normal reality-testing powers no longer can correct them. Nor does he feel the need of any validation. The signs that the patient offers when asked for the causes of his behavior are trivial. How does he know that Miss Threadway loves him? Because there is a thread in his soup.

8. The lack of a normal energizing and directing agency permits a mass of irrelevancies, overinclusions, and sharp turns in direction, sentences that trail off unfinished, and an abrupt and complete blockage of thought. (Subjectively this gives substance and meaning to the patient's complaint: "I am being robbed of my thoughts!")

Parfitt's Observation of Sexual Delusions

Some of these points just summarized are illustrated by the observations reported by Parfitt (1962) from his study of a group of 61 patients. Eighteen women in this group experienced fantasied love affairs (usually based on very slight "signs" from their amours). Four had chosen doctors, three priests: Parfitt describes these as "safe" love objects, as though the patients had been counting on these targets to keep them within the bounds of ordinance. "I had the impression," he notes (in describing two instances in which women patients made frank overtures to him), "that the possibility of any active response on my part was not included in their train of thought." The flood of easy sex talk and uninhibited expression he took to be an expression of a general loosening of repressions. In the lighter cases the obscenities may appear to be compulsive, as though the words expressed themselves in spite of guilt (or fear, or hostility). Most of the patients, he thought, were casual, their expressions offhand, even when they carried such content as: "I want to be castrated to free me from the Freudian drive." Two women moved from job to job because they imagined their genitals were being interfered with. The relatives of two of Parfitt's cases wanted him to arrange ways of helping the patients sexually. In the more deeply involved cases, the patients were sure that their bodies had changed, that their sexual organs had become diseased, decayed, or shrunken. The ease with which the sexual impulse rises to the surface in this destructuring process leads Parfitt to observe that Freudian psychology is particularly suited to describe these patients. As the mind loses its other powers, a luxuriant growth of sex can occur.

The Dereistic Quality

Bleuler (1927) insisted on the dereistic quality in the schizophrenic's thought and action, and the term caught on. Minkowski (1927), who confessed his debt to his teacher, was echoing Bleuler when he defined schizophrenia as *a loss of vital contact with the real.* Since wishful thinking and distorted perceptions also occur among the normal, this loss must represent a difference in degree rather than a clear-cut or absolute difference. If the rational man is the norm, the schizophrenic is simply farther from the standard than most of the rest of us.

The concept of a psychosis as a *reality illness* strikes the modern ear as a surprising sort of working definition, but it points to the fact that the psychotic cannot grasp, communicate, adjust to, or collaborate in the work of managing and changing a shared reality. We must hospitalize him because he is dependent, or dangerous, or scandalous, a "social dropout," in need of "treatment." When he is hallucinated, and hears and sees what we cannot, his behavior becomes uncanny, unpredictable, even alarming; we seek to restore him to a vital contact with us and with the world around us.

Once grasped, this notion seems simple and clear, a workable formula on which we can agree. It merely states the obvious. But it also forces us to confront the baffling nature of *reality* itself. The very word, reality, seems at first to refer to something that is out there, something tangible that is easily verified, validated, something hard and fixed, something that will not go away or change while we turn our heads for a moment. But if we talk to the villager in Chan Kom, as Redfield did, we find that the "evil winds" are a very real thing (as evil and as real as the disease which takes the life of a villager's child). All the elders agree as to their potency. Everyone knows about the man who defied them, and died of it. Delusion or not, it is shared and it is reinforced in the course of the training of each child (until he escapes to the seacoast town of Merida); so long as this culture remains intact, we can predict, the reality of these poisonous, evil, disease-bearing winds will remain as hard as flint. We begin to wonder if the concept of "schizophrenia of the culture" might not be applicable here.

Madame Nijinsky, who became worried about her husband the dancer (who finally became a chronic schizophrenic), was advised—while his illness was still in its early phases—to consult the world-renowned Dr. Bleuler. When, after a long diagnostic interview, Bleuler emerged to speak to the wife, he said, "Madame, if your husband were not a Russian, I would say that he is schizophrenic. As it is..." As he spoke, looking across cultural barriers, he seemed to be saying, in effect, "Perhaps our own reality may appear a little distorted to those, over there." The oddities that one notes in an incipient case of schizophrenia are not wholly unlike those we sense in strange people who have other gods, who perform rituals unlike our own, and who seem to move and live in the presence of unseen witnesses and unseen forces we do not believe in. They, too, base their actions on a foundation of belief that seems to us to be unreal, vague, cloudlike, and full of fantasy.

There are other occasions when each of us moves away from hard and fast waking reality, and loses the stance from which all normal persons launch their projects. When, for example, we drift into a private revery, and more noticeably when we cross from the waking state into dreaming, we seem to release our grasp of something that we have taken for granted, of something that makes us behave logically, realistically, and with a sound sense of what is practical. We lose our grasp of the consequences of action. We are inclined to say: "The logic of feelings has taken over. The law of contradiction no longer holds. Opposites lie down side by side. We are free to do what would violate our waking judgment, or what would disgust us normally." Whether we can properly speak of "a logic of feelings" or not, it is clear that some different kind of "regulation" has taken over. Belief is suddenly too easy, unreflective. Our usual sense of what-follows-what is not in force. Our thoughts, impulses, actions, and *feelings* have begun to operate in undisciplined fashion. If we call them autistic, we are pointing to a certain spontaneous, uncorrected, automatic quality. Janet used the word *automatism* to describe the behavior of Achille, and this is one of the meanings of Bleuler's word *autistic*.

Sometimes this type of thinking is called childlike since, in childhood, wishes almost rule. But in addition to wishes we have to remember fears: do we not waken, sweating, from an anguish-filled dream, saying "Thank God, it was only a dream"? What shall we say of that other sensitive soul, whose *waking* hours are filled with anxiety, and who almost wills to escape it? For he wakens in the morning from his night of dreaming to say, as he gets out of bed and as his dawning consciousness begins to grapple with reality and to assume, once more, its leaden burden of concern, "What a dank and odorous swamp of pestilential *reality* this is. I have been floundering in it for so long." Evidently his reality is something far from that of the happy fellow who wakens with a bounce, eager to plunge into the day of exciting adventure. The one wishes he could go on dreaming; the other is impatient when anything deflects him from the reality which, alone, is truly rewarding.

Where shall we place the Mohammeds and the Mahatmas who build a new social order? We are not always certain whether to call them "dream merchants" or successful "*creators of reality.*" Mohammed had been depressed during that month of Ramadan in which Gabriel had appeared to him in a dream full of promise. On his return from his mountain cave, he was faced with the problem of convincing his wife, Kadijah, and all the rest of his household, of the *reality* of all that he had experienced, for he had believed in his visitor with a message. He might well have found himself in serious trouble had he clung to his belief and its *sacred* quality, while all those around him drew back, clinging to their convictions so long rooted in the tough and practical reality then common throughout the Arabian world. But Mohammed succeeded, and today some 430 million believers share *his* reality.

There is another point to be made. We speak as though dreams were wish-fulfillments, childlike, egocentric, autistic. We smile at Mohammed's description of Heaven, with its sensuous delights to reward the faithful, especially those warriors who might die in defending Allah and the true prophet. But besides this wish-fulfilling quality, in revery and dreams there are also mechanical couplings, contiguity associations, klang similarities that shift the course of this brand of autistic thought. As the waking self with a purpose geared into reality grows weaker, another mechanical process utilizes the associations: we can speak of *a lack of normal egoism* as a part of autism. The parts of the integrative apparatus have their own trends, tendencies, mechanisms that go nowhere in particular without some ego, some proper stance to guide them.

Finally, while we are smiling at Mohammed's Heaven, we have to remember Dante's *Inferno.* "Why," we ask, "should anyone free to choose the course of his dreams become bogged down in an Inferno? Only an abnormally sensitive person, or one who is depressed, would drift in that direction." Here an unregulated, unsound, uncommonsensical drift leads into that which is horrifying, terrifying. If all of this is the work of the id, as Freud would say, then the id and its unconscious is delightful, sentimental, horrifying, lusty, terrible, and *mechanical.* It seems to lead in all directions save toward that normal, productive, reality-bound form we count desirable. The trends we find in autism and dereistic thinking are many-sided, and not very disciplined.

These considerations serve to remind us that the word *dereistic* describes a quality that pervades a great deal of thinking outside of what we see in the schizophrenic. We spot this dereistic element in the adolescent's daydreams: he imagines great accomplishments, scenes in which he will return to strut in gold-braided elegance or white-coated wisdom before those who laugh at him now. Though we accept his daydreams as normal, healthy, on the positive side, we can also see that they are autistic, immature, for they neglect all the hard discipline that will be required in the years ahead. These dream accomplishments are easy! There are also bad daydreams, of defeat, of ostracism, of death (as anyone who is easily depressed can testify); these dreams, too, can possess us, operate in an autistic and dereistic fashion. Possessed by them, we are defeated in advance of all trying, and even the actual powers we own are sealed off by this semiautomatic defeatism. Even in the half-disciplined adult, there is a certain amount of this dereistic factor, operating just offstage at the fringe of our awareness. Perhaps our doting mothers and sweethearts have helped the trend along, as did those treasured folktales that filled our heads as children with dreams of accomplishment, adventure, and glorious and heroic deeds (like those that have made others immortal). Is it not really remarkable that most of us "simmer down" to the point of expecting the probable (and so become able to endure the actual)? We reserve for dreaming, for novel-reading, for self-indulgent fantasy *which we treat as such,* these wild flights "out of bounds," these creations of the "fool in our house." The long development that took us through this thicket of fantasy was slow, with a few breakthroughs and many grinding and punishing retreats; we literally had to hack our way through a jungle of fantasies in order to arrive at a sober, workaday view of the world. Easter Rabbits, Santa Claus, Aladdin's lamp, giants and headless horsemen, Alice in Wonderland and Rumpelstilskin—what a rich stream of dereistic consciousness courses through little heads, and to that provided by our culture, we add the inventions each of us makes on his own. The race has kept a social surplus of fantasies that still delight adults in their moments of leisure, some of it invented by odd fellows like Hans Christian Andersen or Lewis Carroll. Some of our private compensatory fantasies were set spinning when, stirred to an intense pitch by some frustration, rejection, or unjust punishment, we reacted to a crushing reality by our private version of that famous phrase of MacArthur, "I shall return!"

As in Chan Kom, where the elders set the pattern that shapes the private (and shaped) world of belief, so in any society there are always collectives and congregations to aid and abet this reality-shaping process: congregations where the elders pray for rain or for a healing; tribal gatherings where, like those in which the Zuñi children wait for the coming of the kachinas, we give a flesh-and-blood form to fantasies; cults like those of the enthusiasts who are sure LSD will expand our minds to a superior reality. How difficult for the developing member of the tribe to keep alert when all these dereistic invitations help to deepen an addiction to fantasy. In the schizophrenic the fantasy-correction process begins to fail altogether.

It is worth emphasizing that the released autisms can be of the most varied sorts. There are forms that are terrifying and self-accusatory, as though in a spasm of hate, as we let go of reality, our thought world was transformed, reflexly, into punishing forms that everywhere menaced us. There is the form of autism that is all but mute, damped down as though no surplus of organizing energy remained to activate dreams or fears: in this state of emptiness there is little left but the echoes of voices around us; the sounds stir echoes within us, like those of voices in an empty auditorium, but the sound is not converted into sense. In the terminology of an earlier day: The sensory experiences are intact but no perceptions form; there is no guiding apperceptive mass.

Autisms Stripped of Meaning (Autisme Pauvre)

A subtype of autism deserves the name Minkowski gave it, for it represents not only a detachment of all striving from the real, but a running down of all striving, the gradual decay of all motivation. The real that once took on an uncanny quality has become uninviting; it has lost its punch. Everything produces boredom and restlessness, and, finally, a state of emptiness descends. Thinking vanishes altogether, and the world ends, as Eliot once suggested, not with a bang, but a whimper.

Sometimes this *autisme pauvre* consists in a residue of mechanisms that have the outer forms of thought: composed of fragments, mechanically tied together, there is little sense or dramatic unity. No story is told. The fragments accomplish no important communication, not even good self-communication. Aggregates of symbols, mere word-play, the sounds are manipulated for the sake of manipulation. Here and there a clot of meaning will come to the surface, suggesting that some value might be found in that kind of analysis both Bleuler and Adolf Meyer suggested, an analysis that would not only gratify the observer's need for some coherent explanation, but might lead to the discovery of significant factors that would assist in returning the patient to a better relationship with his environment. Many of these residues point to earlier needs long since expired. Consider one of the cases of dementia praecox described by Jung (1907; also in Minkowski 1927, p. 103), the case of the shoemaker's sweetheart.

For years this woman had lived in the asylum, demented, deteriorated. She had outlived a director, all the nurses, and generations of young residents. No one knew anything of her past. No one came to visit her. Nor could she offer any information about her past. The living, vital, memory function that can turn back to survey the past and link it with the living present and the hoped-for future had gone. With this loss of memory and all vital structuring of action, anything resembling a normal present had also disappeared. In this *autisme pauvre* the most conspicuous pattern that remained was a stereotyped and continuing motion of her hands. She rubbed her palms against each other in this gesture until the surfaces were as leathery and tough as the heel of a barefoot boy. Like some automaton she sat there, always at the same place, always making the same stereotyped movements. One of the oldest nurses could recall that formerly it had been a gesture of greater extent and more specific form. Then, so long ago the nurse could barely recall it, the movements had reminded everyone of a cobbler sewing the leather surfaces together on his last. As a matter of fact, the nurses had a name for her, among themselves: "the patient who sews the shoes."

One day the patient died. An elderly cousin appeared to participate in her last rites. Jung asked him if he recalled the occasion when his cousin had fallen ill, and the old man searched his memories: "Ah, yes, I remember! The illness began at the time of a disappointment in love; she had a sweetheart who abandoned her." "And who was this friend?" asked Jung. "He was a shoemaker."

"Many persons," wrote Jung, "commit peculiar complicated acts which at the basis are nothing but complex-symbols. I knew a young lady who, when taking a walk, always wished to take along a baby carriage. The reason for this, as she blushingly admitted, was because she desired to be looked upon as married. Elderly unmarried women are wont to use dogs and cats as complex-symbols."

We can see that Jung looks on the complex as the source of the form of the action. But something must be added: playing the mother game so openly, as the young lady did, suggests a corresponding loss of the critical power of seeing herself as others see her. The very openness of her action suggests that the world of the others is, in some degree, lost. In the deteriorated dementia-praecox patient described above, it is lost altogether.

Jung developed his notion further:

"As shown by these examples, thought and action, both in general and particular, are constantly disturbed and peculiarly distorted by a strong complex. The ego-complex is, so to say, no longer the whole personality, as side by side with it there exists another being, living its own way and therefore inhibiting and disturbing the development and progress of the ego-complex through symptomatic actions which very frequently take up time and exertion at the expense of the ego-complex. We can readily imagine how the psyche is influenced when the complex increases in intensity. The most lucid examples are always furnished by the sexual complexes. Let us take for instance the classical state of *being in love. The lover is obsessed by his complex.* All his interests hang only on this complex and everything belonging to it. Every word, every object, recalls to him his sweetheart (experimentally even apparently indifferent word stimuli excite the complex). The most insignificant objects are guarded like priceless jewels, insofar as their value to the complex is concerned. The whole environment is looked upon *sub specie amoris.* Whatever does not suit the complex glides by: all other interests sink to nothing; hence there results a standstill and a temporary reduction of the personality."

In the case discussed above, this arrest of motion, this fixation on a wisp of movement that symbolized the one who, in going away, took away her life and her power to make a vital engagement with her surroundings, has reduced her mental life to a fragment that barely symbolizes what was once so vital.

This fragment of a gesture, this wisp of a memory, had persisted in spite of her loss of contact with the environment, as though somewhere, deep within some cerebral crevasse, there was an engram, with the neural impulses going round and round, the last surviving vestige of a once all-absorbing thought. While her life persisted, the deeply entrenched roots of a once vital relationship still functioned, now entirely cut off from the world of the hospital or the real world beyond. It must have taken shape at the time of that earlier refusal, when she ceased to participate in the life of the community. The "arrest" was half-compulsive (reflexive), half-conscious (voluntary). The gradual atrophy of all desires to redintegrate old social relationships has completed and fixated an introversive withdrawal; a gradual destructuring of action has proceeded, until only a core fragment of the once symbolic action is left. Such a movement fragment is not a true action: it points to no future; it has no tomorrow. If it is to be called a memory, it is a second-class form of recall, a kind of repetition-compulsion, a self-firing pattern, a "lesson once learned" that is repeatedly redintegrated (but not used) by the person who bears it. A lively memory would have remained oriented to a particular "going away." It would have had to change each day with the developing circumstances of an ongoing life and the increasing distance from that earlier time. True remembering had stopped, just as "vital time" had ceased. The pointless gesture, similar to some fragment of imitative magic striving to bring the whole man back, fails to undergo the normal extinction process of nonreinforced actions. So pointless, so arrested and fixated, it is not even a good *symbol* of anything in reality (least of all of that lover who left her). As outside observers, we might agree: "She died, spiritually, on that day of his departure; she never gave up yearning for his return." But so stubborn is this fixation that it does not atrophy: she stopped learning, growing, as a mother sometimes stops going ahead when a much-loved son dies; his image remains with her, unchanged, still the boy she knew. So this patient revived her lover, hour after hour, by a mechanism that grew so autistic, so out of contact with any possible world, so useless as a "thought plan," and so lacking in true communication, that it had degenerated to a wisp of hand-rubbing, a mere stereotyped motion, a private gesture that had lost its function as language. The callouses on her hands will be regarded, by the sentimental, as the living evidence of her devotion, and by her physician as evidence of her lack of recuperative power. They are the outward evidence of those "rut-formations" that the neurologist sometimes imagines as he tries to picture the reverberatory circuits he intends to interrupt by insulin-shock therapy or lobotomy. Like the marble toe of the statue of the saint, worn away by the kisses of the devout, the callouses are evidence of the persistence of a *ritual*. But the lively grasp of reality, charged with feeling, seems to have long ago abandoned this body. This kind of autism is a type of death-in-life, a conversion of a once vital relationship into a mere mechanism, a transformation downward. The fact that such mechanisms dwell in living tissues does not spare them from being mechanisms, any more than it spares church members from sometimes being the repositories of rituals that are no longer kindled by a lively faith, that have lost their once vibrant meaning.

It would be possible to develop a psychogenic theory of the origin of a psychosis from such examples: a failure in love-life, a crushing disappointment, an arrest of growth, a withdrawal from life, a gradual and progressive disengagement, a destructuring, a letting go, and a final dilapidation and deterioration. This case, in fact, symbolizes sequences of events some schizophrenics have lived through: a progressive loss of interest and of lively meanings, a *dérèglement* of thought and action, and with this letting go, a gradual substitution of dereistic thought and of autistic *movements* for life-attached, vital, growing, future-making thought and *action*. Such an interpretation of the end-states is understandable. To the psychasthenic himself, who places the highest value on love and who regards loss of love as the gravest defeat, it is not only understandable, but correct. To the psychiatrist who has developed an impersonal theory of the disorder that stresses some neurological or biochemical change as the primary process, this "love-history" will seem superficial, more dramatic than convincing; if he has worked out a plan for insulin shock, or daily dosage of three grams of niacin, as the corrective for this *dérèglement,* he will view the lived-through experiences as expressions of a basic biological disorder. Common sense is on his side, to a degree: we know that other girls have been abandoned, other widows left behind, without such disastrous regressions into extreme introversion and detachment. We also know of instances (in psychasthenics and obsessives, especially, where the love relationship is a precarious thing from the start), where both the abandonment and the detachment have been engineered. "I will reduce my life to a zero," Flaubert thought, as he tried to shake off the influence of Louise Colet. He plunged into artistic creation, eager to get back to this first love, where something more real and more perfect than life itself could be brought into being. Such a withdrawal is a *maneuver*.

We do not know much about the young woman who had been deserted by her shoemaker-lover, only that the "other possibilities" which other deserted women have developed did not develop in her after the arrest (for whatever reasons) of the love affair. If she arrested the relationship, it was not to convert the energies (and her suffering) into a work of art or a philosophy of religion (as Kierkegaard did). It was a much more complete arrest, and it is possible that the "turning away from life" we call introversion had begun earlier, even furnishing warning signs to her lover and sending him away because he could not find the responsiveness he looked for.

Dereistic Thinking Reexamined

Bleuler, who thought it important for the therapist to work through all the meanings of the symptomatic acts and complexes of the patient *in order to establish a vital contact* with these withdrawn and dereistic minds, never placed great weight on the theory that the illness was complex-determined. The complex may afford an avenue of communication, and a psychotherapist who aims at restoring a former vital relationship with life may use is as leverage, as a doorway. "All therapy with schizophrenics is psychotherapy," he said, repeatedly. But this is far from assuming that the complex is schizophrenogenic. A love affair whose rupture lay at that fork in the road where a psychosis began may have been (1) symptomatic and expressive, or (2) one factor among many others whose cumulative effects led into autism and withdrawal. Bleuler, like Kraepelin, assumed that there were constitutional, biological, factors at the root of the disorder.

Many have compared the schizophrenic's delusions to the dream experiences of the normal, and have tried to show how close delusional thinking lies to an instinctive core of motivation. But even when the "wishful" character of fantasy is transparent, we have to remember that, as in the dream, there is the other side of the matter. It is the lack of contact with a shared reality which makes both the dream and the dereistic thinking of the schizophrenic possible, and which gives to the word *dereistic* the meaning "without reason, without reflection, without practical worth, without the regulation of an active stance in reality"; something has been lost.

Our examples force us to summarize this approach to schizophrenic thinking as follows: Dereistic thinking may be instigated by cues from the world about the person, but, like dreams or revery, the thinking of the schizophrenic is not regulated by practical concerns, by reflectively validated beliefs, by respect for the possibilities. Rather, it regulates itself, either by the inner mechanical connections which join one thought with its successor, by superficial similarities (irrelevant to real tasks), or by complex-tainted and emotionally charged clusters of meaning which constantly irrupt to keep the round of thought within a narrow set of personal concerns. In some patients, the dramatic content seems to be high and there is a certain inner coherence to thought and action (even if it is autistic); in others the content descends to the level of a free-association chain, and the proliferation of thought may *express* much even when it *communicates* very little or nothing at all to the hearer (or reader); in some the content has descended to that level of Jung's patient who shows only the wisp of a sewing gesture, and a mechanical fragment of a symbol is all that remains (like the potsherd found in the refuse heap of a buried village).[4]

It was in their mastery of this technique of imputing meanings that Freud and Jung excelled; perhaps of all the founding fathers of psychoanalysis, it is Jung who deserves the appellation, "the poet of mental illness." The radical differences between these founding fathers reveal the looseness of the technique, but they were alike in a certain incurable romanticism. In their freedom from the inhibitions that are usually established by scientific training, and in their constant efforts to describe the illness *sub specie amoris,* their theories take on a certain dereistic quality themselves. Since their romantic "truths" are also widely cherished in our culture, it may be that— as Bleuler felt—they have a certain value for the therapist who would restore "vital contact." Such usefulness should not blind the theorist in his search for scientific explanations.

On such a continuum as we have suggested, the range of autistic thinking, the well-structured delusion of the paranoid patient will be near the top, while the patient with only fragments of old complexes, wisps of mechanisms (echolalia, stereotyped mannerisms), will be in that class called *autisme pauvre* (in the deteriorated patients), very near the bottom of the scale, the absolute zero of psychological tension.

At the top of the scale of autistic thinking, we might even place these products that have long raised the discussions of a relationship between genius and insanity. Even the imagination of the scientist can express some of this autism. His personal dream of the great crucial experiment includes a draft of his conclusive report that, like a penetrating intellectual bullet, will richohet around the world ("I shall disturb the slumbers of this world," Freud thought). Insofar as certain hard, experimental realities are absent from this scientific imagining (it is enormously economical), it is autistic, and in actualizing his idea he will have to come to terms with many inhibitors and reinforcers. If his whole plan is unduly bound up in a framework of thinking to which his earlier research and publications have committed him, in its exclusions of other work and other views it is also autistic. Absent are all the hours of drudgery, the tables of statistics which will have to be compiled, fed to a computer, organized, interpreted; absent are the negative instances, the times when the apparatus will not work; absent, for the moment, are the sharp criticisms of his colleagues who will promptly call his attention to the "controls" he is now neglecting. If his thinking is hasty, impatient, superficial, and ever so much easier and more swiftly satisfying than that slow and costly real operation, it has the characteristic autistic touch. It is all so satisfying except in one respect: the scientific daydream bakes no bread, proves nothing,

---

[4]"Reconstruct the civilization from a potsherd?" an anthropologist's student assistant might ask. "Reconstruct the dynamics of a living person from the fragment preserved in a deteriorated schizophrenic?" the young resident might ask his psychoanalytic mentor. "Precisely," Jung seems to suggest, "if your *understanding* of the illness is to be complete." "It is the best route to follow in re-establishing communication," Bleuler would add.

advances no secure basis for the next formulation, enhances no reputation, provides no basis for a new technology.

Thus autism can be found in that all-but-reasonable work of the imagination that will improve reality as it is applied, as well as in the clotted, mechanical, affect-laden, and fear-distorted complex-symbols, and, further, in the fragmented residues that persist, mechanically, in spite of the loss of any true semantic charge. At the end of the series lie the callouses on the palms of the shoemaker's sweetheart, which represent a transformation of meaning into tissue changes, into mechanisms.

Somewhere on this continuum we may also place some of our most cherished myths, whose symbols have illuminated our matter-of-fact world, shedding the light of meaning and at the same time screening away some of the reality that we must live with. For these myths are mixtures, too, clotted with much dereistic thinking, infused with a drama that differs from the ones in reality. We are sometimes prone to consider them "more real than reality," in the same sense that Proust thought of his novellas as superior to the experiences from which they were distilled. Many of the grand myths of our culture express something that appeals to old childlike and adolescent yearnings which have persisted in spite of our efforts to mature. They move us, appeal to us, flatter us, keep hope alive in us. (Is there anything more supremely egotistic, asked William James, than the Christian's confidence that he can both send and receive messages to and from the Most High, or his assurance that the latter is directly concerned about the fate of the little petitioner, and about his projects?) Are we not all half-dereistic, half-rational? Are not the best of our actions mixtures that contain affect-laden, complex-clotted, klang-associated curds of autism? Our very cognitive maps that we steer by are warped in their main coordinates, warped away from reality, as though some affect charged magnetic pole had altered our latitude and longitude, *on the map,* by its powerful attraction.

Bleuler's definition of the two categories of thinking is useful; it warns us to test both the thinking of the patient and the thinking about the patient, including that thinking which passes as most realistic in our society. But he has stated a problem, rather than discovered the explanation of why this form of thinking is so central a feature in the schizophrenic process. His statement does not explain why a person who has had all the advantages of a modern scientific education should drift into this pattern, with its affect-laden complexes, its mechanism-clotted irruptions, its abrupt turnings and aimlessness, its failure to communicate. Even when parts of it seem obviously to be wish-fulfillment or fear-fulfillment, and of a special value to a particular person, this does not explain why wishes and fears and autistic realization of needs should have suddenly taken over in these minds a function they are not allowed to enjoy normally.

When Bleuler notes that "the contents and aims of such unbridled mental activities always represent strivings which most deeply touch our innermost nature,...it is therefore quite obvious that dereistic aims are valued much higher than the real advantages, which they replace," he seems to add confusion to an already overworked teleology, for both dereistic and realistic forms of thought are "the outgrowth of strivings that deeply touch our innermost nature." The difference lies, in part, in the fact that one of the two forms is disciplined by reality, the other less so. Perhaps the world of the *real*, that tough core of what must be, will leave us unsatisfied and even deeply frustrated, at the very last, hopeful though we may have been all along. But it will be what it will be, like it or not. Perhaps the pressures to achieve the dereistic form of victory will be greater in those who find it difficult or impossible to win satisfactions in the shared matter-of-fact world. In those who find the contrast between the real possibilities and an inflated and childish type of aim (the narcissistic goals of the overprotected and "spoiled") too deeply disappointing and deflating, dereistic thinking will undoubtedly have a special motivation, and its consolations will be all the more dangerous.[5] In the individual with limited organizing powers, with limited energies for persistent striving, and with limited tolerance for the inevitable frustrations of living, the dereistic form will be an ever-present temptation. Since all these limiting "weaknesses" are common to the human lot, and since their opposite virtues are relatively rare, we may speak of a steady and almost universal pressure toward dereistic thinking as one of the natural aspects of human life. The point at which this pressure becomes overwhelming is difficult, if not impossible, to determine in advance. We have names for the weaknesses, but not measures; worse, since there is no science of the future, even a measuring scale would not predict the pattern of stresses that lies ahead. This crucial point of breakdown is not unlike the one at which the subject in a fatigue experiment gives up and says, "I can go no further." But unlike the fatigue experiment, where the subject is alerted in advance of the coming "giving-up point" (and may try to stave it off, or conclude that there is no point in trying too hard), the entrance into a psychosis is usually more insidious (and less a matter of decision). With little or no insight into the nature of the process (or even of its existence), the patient simply feels a change within himself, in his way of existing in the world, in the world around him. The psychotic does not stand aside from his psychosis and watch its progress. He *is* the process, and *in* the process. He evaluates his world, as always, but from a moving center and with decreasing powers. He does not evaluate his evaluation. That last self-critical level is lost.[6]

We can thus describe the normal maturing of an individual as a gradual

---

[5] We use a similar logic when we say that alcohol or drugs are not as important to those who can make a full and satisfactory life without them.

[6] Although they were self-critical to an extreme, Janet called many of his psychasthenics "terrible metaphysicians," for they were forever trying to get back of behind of beyond. Their ruminations, while expressing a weakness in decision-making, represented a kind of resting point, halfway between doubt and certitude. We are almost tempted to say that their rumination saved them from psychosis, that is, until the day when they fell through into schizophrenic certitude.

liberation of the mind from the bondage of dereistic thinking, and as a disciplined growth in reality-structured planning, until rational thinking displaces and dominates these fantastic and autistic flights. Would a man of the twentieth century wish to go back to that spirit-ridden period when the world of witchcraft was an acceptable way of accounting for ill health and misfortune? Would we substitute for the work of the weather bureau the old rainmaking ceremony? Animism, autism, dereistic thinking: we have been fettered by these internal weaknesses, and by our ignorance. One external barrier after another has fallen as man has rid himself of these autisms. Yet where autisms prevail, they show a surprising tenacity. The newly educated class in Ghana, as though taking no chances, often return to the old medicine. Whenever difficulties mount, in such a "mixed" climate of two cultures, the truth-bringer, who knows his limitations and sticks pretty close to what he knows, is an unwelcome (and not too impressive) figure. Of course, to those who own the healing shrines, and to others who have organized their hopes around some dereistic form of mystification, the new truths will be unwelcome. Not everyone is prepared to endure the trials, or the insights, that more realistic views of life call for.

In summary, then, we can say that a person tends to drift into dereistic thinking when:

1. His knowledge and skill run out.

2. His strength, fortitude, and integrative powers run down.

3. His needs grow so intense that his coping powers cannot gratify them in any realistic fashion, and when he is beyond the help of his peers.

4. That which is possible is far removed from that which he has been trained to expect and to hope for.

5. He is still undisciplined in assimilating reality. (The protected, who are nurtured in hothouse environments, and who have not developed either a tolerance for reality or coping skills, are prone to depend upon the exercise of personal charm or the employment of dereistic rituals.)

6. He is surrounded by a cultural frame that emphasizes and illustrates (with living examples) the dereistic powers.

7. His vital relationship with reality, particularly with social reality, has long been tenuous and narrow, so fragile that small insults break the bond.

8. States of fatigue and exhaustion, sleep, intoxication, sudden shock, failure, or loss of love reduce the functioning of the integrative network and narrow the field of awareness. To this type of cause we might add: drug states, toxic conditions within the organism, and, especially, the so-called psychedelic or mind-expanding drugs.

DEGRADATION OF THE EMOTIONAL LIFE

A mere listing, or classification, of the changes in emotional expression (shallowness, apathy, panic) apart from the living contexts in which these changes occur might miss their essential quality. There are, however, certain recurrent relationships that have long struck the observers who have tried to catch the essence of schizophrenic behavior. We shall describe them, here, illustrating them and commenting briefly. There is often noted, in these descriptions, a discordance or an inappropriateness of affect, a lack of harmony between the emotions expressed and the real-life setting in which they occur, or between what the patient says (and the implied experiences) and the silly giggle or expressionless physiognomy that accompanies his account. This is one type of "splitting" that helps give the meaning to this name of the disorder, *schizo*phrenia.

Sometimes we are tempted to reify the fact of emotional poverty into a cause, for it almost seems that the person acts as if he had systematically tried to quash every feeling, but, in the beginning stages in particular, the patient is apt to complain merely that he feels empty, that he wishes someone would emotionize him, that he is sinking into nothingness through no intent of his own. Then he experiences it as an automatic process whose end-state will surely be "nothingness." In the paranoid patient who is frantically apprehensive because he is about to be dismembered, or raped, or poisoned, the emotions mount to the ultimate in intensity, and he believes that he must fight for his very life.

These changes in emotional and motivational outlook can convert the warmly affectionate bonds within a family into indifference, or into intense hatred and total war. They may become a part of some bizarre set of principles, a geometry of action that he has adopted, and since the family cannot appreciate or adapt to his schema, they become disrupters, enemies. He moves away from them, or against them, or shuts them out with a tight-lipped and stubborn wall of silence. The extremes of murder and incest can come to the surface, in fantasies of seduction or of counterattacks, or in an actual living-out that forces the family to hospitalize what they cannot contain. Physician, brother, mother (whoever is near and close), can find themselves transformed into monsters, murderers, seducers, embezzlers, and the emotions appropriate to these inappropriate roles are the visible outer forms of the inner changes.

Emotional *expressions* can persist, as all but empty mechanisms, the mere husks of what may have once been vital feelings, and even though they have a cold and mechanical quality, these expressive acts tempt the observer to rationalize and justify them in terms of the history and circumstances of the patient, even when it is obvious, in the advanced forms of schizophrenia, that the original motivation has long since departed. (Mere expressions, they are no longer symbols to the patient himself.)

Impulses that are normally contained within a framework of vital relations (other affective "engagements") behave as though freed, as though a regulative self had abdicated or had suddenly been fractured into these bits of impulse. Out of all relationship with consequences, impervious to those whom they affect, having no tomorrow, the actions become "pure acts" or rather mere *movements*. They caricature the real thing or they resemble more childish or adolescent forms once tolerated at an early stage. Included among these are "extremes of instinct" (smearing or eating excrement, open masturbation or self-mutilation, erotic assaults on physicians and nurses, butting the head against the wall as though bent on self-destruction, complete refusal of food or gluttonous bulimia). When these are accompanied by the assumption of a fetus-like posture, they tempt us to use the term *regression,* as though the patient had gone back to that point of origin of some primary process that had caused all of the difficulty, an original affective fixation.[7]

Out of harmony with their surroundings (and with their own prepsychotic lives), they display both a coldness and a ferocity in their discordant and bizarre emotions. The homosexual caricature of love is common, and there are pieces of instinctual life that are more mechanical than vital. Where one patient shows instinct in excess, the next shows indifference and apathy. Collectively, the babbling, sulkiness, excitement, apathy, greed, stubbornness, masturbation, self-starvation, self-castration, frigidity, and eroticism present us with a mass of impulses that touch all extremes: only the via media of a regulated and vital contact with life is lacking.

It would be a mistake to look on these emotional expressions in isolation: they are aspects of a total intellectual-affective-volitional disorganization. Along with the primary thought disorders, there is also a primary affective-motivational disorganization, and perhaps neither fact should be made into the reason for the rest of the phenomena. The wide range of odd mannerisms, extremes of uninhibited emotional expression (from apathy to frenzy), the blunting and disorganization of feelings, the anxieties of some and the unfeeling inaccessibility of others, should warn us against looking for a "standard schizophrenic man."

Even when we try to gather these expressions into a single typical life-history, as Meyer did in the following (Winters 1951, p. 429), showing how the emotional changes are a part of a cumulating and compounding growth of poor ways of dealing with reality, we should be forewarned that there are many pathways into this psychosis.

"In cases of dementia praecox we find over and over an account of frequently exemplary childhood, but a gradual change in the period of emancipation. Close investigation shows, however, often that the exemplary child was exemplary under a rather inadequate ideal, an example of goodness and meekness rather than of strength and determination, with a tendency to keep good in order to avoid frights and struggles. Later, religious interest may become very vivid, but also largely in form; a certain disconnection of thought, unaccountable whims make their appearance, and deficient control in matters of ethics and judgment; at home irritability shows itself, often wrapped up in moralizing about the easy-going life of brothers and sisters; sensitiveness to allusions of pleasure, health, etc., drive the patient into seclusion. Headaches, freaky appetite, general malaise, hypochondriacal complaints about the heart, etc., unsteadiness of occupation and inefficiency, day dreaming, and utterly immature philosophizing, and above all, loss of directive energy and ini-

---

[7]Behavior that includes equally disorganized and regressive actions has been reported as a part of psychotic phenomena induced by the ingestion of morning-glory seeds. One patient showed catatonic excitement, became assaultive and unmanageable, lost control of bowels and bladder, and displayed religious delusions. (See Fink, Goldman, and Lyons 1966.)

tiative without obvious cause, such as well-founded preoccupations, except the inefficient application to actuality. All these traits may be transient, but are usually not mere 'neurasthenia,' but the beginning of a deterioration, more and more marked by indifference in emotional life and ambitions, and a peculiar fragmentary type of attention, with all the transitions to the apathetic state of terminal dementia."

Another excellent "composite portrait" is offered by Noyes and Kolb (1963, p. 334), in connection with their description of ambulatory schizophrenia. Since this description deals with a marginal form of the disorder, it, too, shows one of the pathways into the more severe forms.

"In that group of schizophrenics now designated as 'ambulatory,' these indications of social withdrawal are less evident. Their dubious relationship to life is expressed in doubts as to their aims, difficulties in making decisions as to their future, the means to get on or to find a central interest. Although at times they may appear to be driving and busy, their actions are performed to prove themselves. The adolescent may date to 'prove' that he can gain the attention of others as his peers do. Marriage becomes a means of 'proving' that one is a man or woman or that one can 'love.' The relationship with children is a means of establishing the fact that one can be a mother. All activity is representative of an autistic dramatization without full affective contact with the realities of life, as though there is a continuous screen between the inner person and those with whom he relates. The existence has an 'as if' quality; it is split from reality."

It is odd to find the authors identifying as schizoid what certainly is a universal human trait: the schizophrenic is like us, only more so. Does not man in general encode the stimuli that flow in via the sense organs (and the reticular-hypothalamic apparatus), so that a screen (or a kink in the sensorimotor system) always intervenes between the physical stimulus and the movement? In the schizophrenic the screen is a bit bizarre, an odd, weakened, and distorted one that does not enable him to deliver effective action into the field, to bind his anxieties, to develop and preserve good adaptations, or to continually organize and reorganize his efforts to fit a flowing and changing reality. As his "lack of fit" progresses, a point is reached where withdrawal, a blunting of affect, a distortion of perceptions and feelings occur: a precipitating event (a loss of a friend, being sent home from school, the discipline of a job, a venereal infection, or a spoonful of morning-glory seeds) can push him into frank psychosis.

In any attempt to describe the range of affective distortions, we bring together into one category the apathy or poverty, the disharmony between feelings and the discordance with real-life settings, and the exaggerated forms of lust, panic, self-hate, thereby setting up a problem that is full of contradictions. It is difficult to identify a single cause for this multiverse of affective changes.

One affective transformation is worth special note. The schizophrenic often begins his pathological course by reacting to his emotions themselves directly, by trying to manipulate them out of their natural context, with elaborate systems of self-control: Yoga, psychedelic drugs, systems of meditation and relaxation, systematic autoerotic practices. These can end in one of three *culs de sac*: (1) loneliness, apathy, withdrawal from life; (2) distortions and autisms that arise out of his "principles"; and (3) exaggerated pseudaffective responses that, even in frenzy, have a phony, cold, and mechanical quality (like the performance of sexual athletes who try to see how many orgasms they can achieve in rapid succession). Even in frenzy, these pseudaffective reactions lack depth and focus. All three of these paths progress, in the schizophrenic, to an emotional disengagement, a kind of autism. We say, of such a person, that he needs "emotionizing"; the patient himself makes use of this same expression: "I need someone to emotionize me, to arouse me, to love me, to make me feel and see. Otherwise I shall drift into emptiness. I feel that there is a wall between me and reality." Whether this wall was first constructed as an active defense against a too pressing reality, or represents instead the projected counterpart of a primary inner failure in emotionality, or represents a combination of the two that developed with no one intending the outcome, is the question that the therapist must face as he tries to reconstruct the development of this affective disorganization.

Sensorimotor Disturbances

The task of describing the symptoms of schizophrenia is, at the same time, an effort to identify the *essential* changes that can give us a clue to the nature of the disorder. Thus Hanfmann (1939) concludes her study of the thinking disorder with this note:

"The reduction or loss of the categorical attitude is to be considered not as a change within the intellectual sphere alone but as *a basic disturbance in the functioning of the total organism*. The intellectual and the emotional disturbances are probably only two manifestations of the one basic change. Furthermore, *the cause of this change* cannot be ultimately clarified by means of a psychologic analysis like that just made. The striking resemblance of the patient's behavior to that of a patient with a cerebral injury, while it appears to lend support to the theory of organic origin of the schizophrenic disturbance, is actually not a proof thereof" (my italics).

Others (for example, Parfitt 1956), after reviewing and classifying the principal thought disturbances, conclude that a lesion (or impairment of the functioning) of the frontal lobe is the most probable explanation of the schizophrenic's failures (1) in organizing his thoughts, (2) in planning, (3) in separating past thoughts from past events, (4) in recognizing absurdities, and (5) in insight into his own illness and his real-life situation. When such inferences are combined with the genetic data (of the type offered by Kallmann), we emerge with a disorder with difficulties in thinking, and in the affective and volitional spheres, traceable to a genetically determined weakness in the frontal-lobe functions.

Catatonic symptoms can also be made to point to a root-cause of a quite different order. This group of symptoms, first identified by Kahlbaum (1874) and described as a "tension insanity," has become, in present-day descriptions of schizophrenia, one of the subtypes of the disorder. Like Kahlbaum, many modern research workers look on the changes in motility as expressions of altered brain states; thirty years of study of forms of experimental catatonia, produced either by experimental lesions or by drug injections in animal subjects, have led them to focus on brain stem, hypothalamus, and the periventricular gray matter beneath the cortex. These investigators have produced behavioral changes so closely analogous to the symptoms of human patients (diagnosed as catatonic forms of schizophrenia) that there is now some basis in fact for what was speculation in Kahlbaum's time. What is now required, in addition, is some identifiable substance or process (1) that (unlike a neural lesion or some of the experimental neuroleptic agents that are not found in the living human body) is present in more than normal amount in the schizophrenic, (2) whose presence and absence parallel the appearance of and recovery from catatonic symptoms, and (3) whose production or elimination can be fitted into identifiable precipitating or therapeutic agencies.

There are two markedly different states that have been placed under this single catatonic category. The patient who is in *catatonic stupor* has a masklike face, does not communicate, is immobile. He may stand all day at his bedside until feet and ankles are red and swollen, or sit, motionless, on the edge of his chair, staring, or curl up, resistant to every effort to draw him out, get him to dress, eat, clean up. He is likely to retain saliva, urine, feces, although when he believes no one is watching, his soiling can be so aimed (with feces deposited in the exact center of a clean sheet) that it is easy to suspect a hidden stream of awareness (and hostility) behind the blank facade. In the same way he may eat greedily when he thinks no one is noticing. Catalepsy (with waxy flexibility), automatic obedience (put out your tongue so that I may prick it), insensitivity to pain, echolalia, and posturing are all present, with both extremes of suggestibility (negativism and automatic compliance).

In spite of the all but complete lack of communication and the apparent poverty of ideas and feelings, such a patient may emerge from his catatonia to give reports of statements that had been made to him in his mute period, ideas that were in his mind, reasons for his refusals. Noyes and Kolb compare it to the stupor that sometimes follows some great shock or bereavement, a kind of psychological death dramatized by this type of withdrawal, a "freezing" not wholly unlike the immobility of the bird in death feint. In some patients there are cosmic delusions hidden beneath this exterior; the patient may believe that he is acting to save the world, or that he is striving to avoid his own extinction in the holocaust that is about to arrive.

Catatonic excitement is a violent, aggressive, unorganized, purposeless, and unpredictable outbreak which may alternate, in some cases, with the stuporous form. In others it is the state that announces the onset of the illness; as it gradually wanes, the stuporous form emerges, with simple dementia. He may break windows, tear off his clothes, shout out his defiance (or his sense of power, or his mystical identity), and his restless agitation and sleeplessness (which resemble mania) carry with them the threat of exhaustion. Fused with homosexual delusions, the excitement may take the form of a flight in panic from an attack or of a vehement denial of accusations (hallucinated voices), or assume the form of an active and aggressive homosexual attack upon those near.

In some patients these catatonic phases recur in cycles; there are identifiable and parallel changes in excretion of nitrogen, water, and NaCl. Gjessing (1953) advanced the hypothesis that, at the turning point in nitrogen balance, a toxic substance altered the functioning of cells in the hypothalamus. The observable changes in heart rate, blood pressure, body temperature, metabolic rate, viscous saliva, and sleep reduction were interpreted as consequences of this center's actions. Fasting blood-sugar and glucose-tolerance curves are also higher during the excited phase. "The magnitude and direction of these changes leave little doubt that the mental disturbance is associated with increased sympathetic and diminished parasympathetic discharges." Gellhorn and Loofbarrow (1963) add that the metabolic changes suggest a thyroid deficiency, and that cortisone or thyroid therapy has sometimes alleviated the symptoms in the inactive phase (akinetic stupor).

The parallelism between the physiological and the behavioral data in the recurrent forms of catatonia should not lead to too hasty a conclusion. On remission the psychological and autonomic changes disappear first, the restoration of normal nitrogen-water-salt excretion follows. Gjessing also noted that emotional disturbances often antedated and accelerated the autonomic changes and served to signal the approaching excitatory phase. If, as some believe, the hypothalamic changes are responsible for the release of antidiuretic and thyrotropic substances, these affective-hypothalamic changes then become the crucial factors.

The hypothalamus, an intimate part of all emotional expressions, may have a disturbed function (1) because of direct chemical excitation, (2) because of a loss of normal cortical hegemony over its functions, and (3) because its upward-coursing excitations may be improperly encoded, interpreted, and distributed into appropriate action patterns. The bits of physiological evidence may need to be pieced together into a more holistic account. They represent the physiologist's contribution to the understanding of the observed breakup of the self in action: the glandular-visceral-motor changes signal the disintegration. The breakdown of normal homeostatic controls that regulate the balance of pituitary and thyroid is also involved.

Catatonic symptoms have been produced experimentally by brain-stem lesions, by follicular hormones, colibacillus, ACTH, bulbocapnine, eserine, acetylcholine, and DFP (di-isopropylfluorophosphonate). The last-named substance was injected directly via canula into the ventricle of a cat's brain and produced a three-stage series of changes beginning with itching, passing through tremor and increased skeletal muscle tone, to a final stupor and catatonia (with an inferred change in awareness). Placed in unusual and awkward positions, the cat remained immobile. The same substance, used in the treatment of myasthenia gravis, was found to produce nightmares, mental confusion, and hallucinations in human subjects. Feldberg (1958) suggests that when similar symptoms appear in the schizophrenic (without DFP), they may also be due to some impairment in the functioning of periventricular gray matter, analogous to that which the experimental injections in this area produced directly.

To the physiologist who can produce the analogs of catatonic symptoms in experimental animals by the injection of chemical substances (or by bilateral hypothalamic lesions), the temptation to look for analogous substances produced within the human body (but normally in amounts too small to produce pathology) or for analogous "physiological lesions" (failures in function which may represent constitutional weaknesses in the neural structures) is very strong. And he is prone to consider such changes as the primary and essential process.[8]

Autism as a Quality in Overt Action

The human spirit that becomes disordered, in schizophrenia, assumes a new attitude toward reality: there is . . . "a very peculiar relation between the patient's inner life and the external world. The inner life assumes pathological predominance" (Bleuler 1950, p. 63). Does not the inner life predominate, too, in realistic action? What is the difference? Minkowski (1927, p. 119) once tried to describe the contrast with a concrete example:

"Whoever takes up a task in the real world about him, whoever enters into a vital relationship to reach a goal that is significant to him, has given hostages to fate, in one sense; for if he deeply desires his goal he will have to submit to the tuition that every condition, every means to that end, imposes upon his action."

Even the simplest task requires vigilance. For example, driving a nail into the wall with a hammer forces me to take into account and adjust to the grain of the wood, the nature of the plaster, the underlying joist, the weight of the hammer, the length of the handle, the placement of my fingers. I must fuse all this, neglecting nothing, disciplining each move by corrective reactions that are related to that stance toward a goal which I steadily maintain. Concentrating on the action in hand, some of the more remote portion of the field I normally carry about with me drops away (I forget the stock market, the war in Viet Nam, and even my neighbor's cat that kept me awake last night). I am a nail-driver. But nail-driving is an action bound up within a series of concentric fields, in a vital and fluid relationship with them, and I can forget too much. If I forget that the nail is being driven in order that I may hang a picture, I may not slant it correctly, and if I hammer away, completely disregarding the announcement that the picture has evidently been broken in transit, or that the hammering is waking the baby, or that the nail is coming through the other side of the thin wall, and, absorbed in the act, stubbornly insist on finishing what I had started without regard for consequences and without regard for the larger setting which gave it meaning, I would be illustrating a sort of

---

[8]Gjessing's work on nitrogen balance has not been corroborated by other workers, and there are reports (see D. Jackson 1960, p. 5) of swings in nitrogen balance that are related to general nutrition and independent of changes in rhythm of pathological mental states. Pfeiffer and Jenney (1957) reported improvement in catatonic schizophrenics as a result of acetylcholinelike agents with effects analogous to Feldberg's DFP. Studies designed to show the influence of the cerebrospinal fluid of schizophrenics on the web-spinning of spiders succeeded with samples drawn from catatonics, but not with samples from other subtypes of the illness (see Bercel 1960).

overt autism. I have not retreated into an inner world, as the introvert does. Rather I have buried myself in action, uncritical action, action for its own sake, automatic action. Overt it may be, but it has lost its vital relation with that ever-changing reality which surrounds each of us. Action, dissociated from the whole that should regulate it, becomes mechanical, meaningless, autistic: it descends to mere movement. It reminds us of the action of the bureaucrat who has long forgotten the reasons for his regulations. It is the action of a schizoid personality who has lost interest in collaboration or in so shaping his actions and communications that they can function in the collective.

Minkowski (1927, p. 115) offers a second example to make his point:

"In a little apartment, modestly furnished, the family of a working man lives in rather straitened circumstances. The income of the father scarcely suffices for current needs. One day the mother announces that she wants a piano in order to make it possible for the children to resume the music lessons that they had begun some time ago when the family's situation had been better. The father tries to dissuade her; he advances serious considerations; the budget simply does not permit them to dream of such a thing. All in vain. She wants a piano and will have one. She knows how to sew. She finds work. Night after night she works, losing sleep. She no longer speaks of her desire. But one day the father, returning from the office, finds to his surprise, a beautiful new piano installed in the little apartment. There it is. It clashes with the rest of the furniture and with the whole life of the household. It is like a stranger, like some dead thing without a tomorrow. It was to serve primarily for the elder son, who had just gone through a schizophrenic episode, who is not a bad musician—to be sure—but who now seems to want to play late at night and thus manages to provoke complaints from the neighbors."

Minkowski directs our attention to two points: (1) the lack of a vital relationship between the act and the family situation, and (2) an autism that is not an introversive flight from reality. The mother could have imagined that she had a piano, or that she was playing it before distinguished guests. But no imaginary solution would do: she had to have the piano, even if it proved a nuisance or was completely discordant with the rest of her life. She is like the nail-driver intent on finishing the act he had started, perhaps at all costs, perhaps without considering any of the costs, or perhaps with a foolish overvaluation of only one of the possible consequences.

It is possible for actions of this type to be motivated by some former dream (e.g., the adolescent dream of a girl who wanted to be a musician, a dream her marriage had cut short, a dream that she hoped to see realized in her son). It could represent a woman's revolt against the stifling life of the wife of a petty bureaucrat. It is even possible that her action represents a hope that, through music, she could draw her son back into contact with the life around him, a contact he was daily losing as he moped away his hours in the little apartment. The closer her action comes to a workable relationship with the living reality, and the more constantly the action is regulated and changed in accordance with its consequences in the light of her goals, the less schizoid it appears. We, too, can be schizoid in evaluating a patient's action if we do not penetrate to that ever-changing inner relationship with a developing field. Since this relationship is fluid and changing (as the field changes and as new purposes emerge), and since the field itself consists in a series of concentric relationships (so that an act can be poor for the near effects, but good in the long run), the task is not a simple one.

Such an approach to autism is a wholesome reminder of the fact that we are all afflicted with a touch of this trait. Brand, the fiery priest whose heaven-bound thoughts carried his family into disaster, in Ibsen's play; Edison, whose stubborn certitude in the face of ridicule and indifference (and with complete disregard of simple tissue claims) carried him to success; the saint's retirement into the wilderness to get away from all entangling alliances and to free himself from the insistent claims of the realities of this world (while some rather pressing realities are neglected), all could be classified as examples of action with a schizoid quality. Whereas one schizoid person works out the maneuver in some interior castle between his own cloudy aspirations and an equally clouded vision of Heaven, seeking an otherworldly beatitude, the next person will make his schizoid maneuver in the open, driving his nail into the wall with complete disregard of consequences, buying his piano even though the action has no tomorrow. An "activist" can be schizoid.

This quality of the action without a future is revealed in a pathetic form in another of Minkowski's illustrations (p. 117):

"A young engineer, just out of the École Centrale, lost his position because he had made errors in his computations and in his designs. After a few vain efforts to secure work of the same type, he found a position as a simple secretary of an insurance company. Here, too, the same result followed; he made errors in fixing the claims for whose adjustment he was responsible. He then returned to his parents' home. There he underwent a rapid and profound deterioration.

"He became completely inactive, and wholly without interests. His parents were greatly disturbed and urged him to look for work. [And] he wrote out, in a single day, a hundred and fifty applications for work and sent them to various addresses, without seeming to feel any concern as to whether the effort had the least chance of succeeding.

"The next day he left, without saying anything to his parents, setting out for Paris, to look for work; he travelled, on foot, the ninety kilometers that separated his home from the capital; and in two days he arrived there in a piteous state. He was promptly arrested for vagrancy (since he could not give a sufficiently coherent and rational explanation of his condition) and he passed several days in prison before the matter could be fully explained."

Again we can see that *autism* can be quite overt. Action and idea are still partially geared into the milieu, but neither is realistic, productive, plastic, adapted to the changing circumstances. There is energy enough, in crude form. This process is quite unlike that in other schizophrenics, where there is a more or less complete withdrawal, a preoccupation with private fantasy. Overt or introverted, both forms of autism show a similar loss of vital relationship with the milieu: the essence of autism is found *between* the individual and his milieu, *between* the thought and the action, *between* the action and its field. Some autistic action is passive, covert, confined within the organism that sits virtually motionless. Some of it consists of wisps or fragments of what once was vital and closely related to a living present, but is now degenerated to a mechanical symbol of its former self, a symbol that has ceased to function as symbol *even to the patient*. Some of it is as overt and dramatic as mania, as when the paranoid patient acts out her belief that she is about to be raped by the physician. Although some of it is complex-clotted and obviously dramatizes important emotionally charged complexes, there is no certainty that these complexes have been causal; the notion that some primary biochemical (or neural) change underlies the whole descent into autism must remain a live hypothesis. Hanfmann and Kasanin are correct: the resemblance between the rather primitive and regressed forms of schizophrenic thought and those found in the brain-injured is so great that the objective approach is worthy of all our consideration.[9]

When a previously normal person descends gradually through the stages we call neurosis (e.g., obsessive-compulsive behavior) into delirium and into that *autism pauvre* in which nothing but wisps of meaning remain, losing, progressively, all vital contact with his milieu, we demand to know what causes the descent. In the richer and more active form, when he is like a waking dreamer and his autism is clotted with complexes, have we any more right to speak of the complexes causing the delirium (or of the repression that produced the complexes as cause) than we have of speaking of sleep as caused by our dreams? Shall we look on the descent as a failure in vital energies, a basically constitutional affair, the same kind of failure in growth that makes one seed produce a plant that withers as it matures, while another seed produces the fertile and viable kind? Or must we retrace the steps of the schizophrenic's development, watching the transactions which cumulatively developed into that final loss of vital relationship, seeking to discover within the dialogue itself the "laws of schizophrenic development"?

In order to act and remain alive we have to organize, carve out, structure a world about us. We *make* such actions and *appropriate* that world: it is ours; we have invented it; we assume consequences as we act; and the world we create is internalized so that it regulates our actions. Not only have we shaped a segment of reality and entered into vital relationship with it, but in the shape of expectancies and schemata, it now exists within us, represented. The sculptor intent on revealing the imagined form that is within the marble, absorbed in his work, could be described as fused with the block of stone, his tools. He is a part of them; they exist within him. If something approximate to the form he dreamed of appears, it is because hands, marble, chisel, hammer, muscles have been forged into a unity. Only a well-disciplined sculptor can see the possibilities in the stone and find the means to actualize one of them. He cannot choose a form inappropriate to the shape or grain of the stone, or make a blow without regard to what the chisel impinges on, nor can he disengage his atten-

---

[9]For the sake of accuracy, I must note that Minkowski is anxious to "scotch" all premature and oversimplified forms of materialistic theorizing: "The notion of a vital contact with reality...has nothing to do with physiology."

tion from his task and let hand and tool run themselves. Schizophrenic action suffers from just such breaks in the process of interaction: between the dream and its execution, between the movement and its objective, between the action and the surrounding field. If its essence lies in these "breaks" or "descents," then schizophrenia is most completely portrayed in that end-state, in *autisme pauvre*; the richer, complex-clotted constructions still reveal residues of normality, a kind of desperate constructive process still releases secondary compensations for all that is lost. It is this descent we focus upon when we search for the causes of schizophrenia. It will not be enough to say that autism is easier, or that it satisfies instinctive needs, long repressed, or that it provides pleasures and satisfactions, or an esthesiogenic "boost" to the person with lowered psychological tension. Teleologies of this sort will not do: they are as completely "after the fact" as the shaman's explanation of death as due to the departure of the spirit. If holism were to lead to such empty teleologies, we would have to join with Hoffer and others who attack them as nonscience, a form of nonsense that blocks scientific analysis.

Autistic Action in the Man of Principle

The nail-driver who forgets the plaster, the crying baby, and the people in the next apartment seems to have lost the whole circumambient world. He has descended to a hammerer with a nail. The woman who wanted a piano got it, but when it stood there in her poor apartment, it was an obvious misfit, and if she had ever entertained a dream of helping her schizophrenic son, his use of the instrument soon proved to be as much cut off from apartment-house living as her action in buying the instrument had been out of touch with the real situation of the family.

In other illustrations Bleuler shows schizophrenics producing actions that are internally well-structured and show a preservation of intelligence, but are simply devoid of any proper sense of social consequences. He describes a well-educated woman who sings at a concert, but who cannot stop; even when the audience whistles and hoots, she sings blithely on. He describes another woman, also of some culture, whose illness could pass unnoticed as she converses in a social group, but who cannot understand the reactions of her friends when she suddenly moves her bowels in the midst of a social gathering. Darr and Worden (1951) have described a young woman who had been followed from infancy, where she first gave signs of early infantile autism; she had been in and out of special schools, provided with special tutors, surrounded by paid companions, yet had never quite achieved those social sensitivities that most of us take for granted. Hiking in a mixed group of young people, and feeling a bit too warm, she stripped to the waist and could not understand why her companions insisted that she put the blouse back on.

These instances emphasize the loss of a social factor in ordinary judgment. Autism is a curious sort of self-ism in which the outer world is shucked off. If there is a predominance of the inner world, it is obviously a curious sort of inner world that is revealed in these particular examples. "What can they be thinking of?" we ask, as if schizophrenics are also "persons with a plan," a rational scheme into which their action can fit. The fact seems to be that this is an overt form of autism, with a *poverty of inner life,* with a defective schema or plan. Thus we have (1) a rich autism, with a proliferating but delusional inner framework into which absurd actions fit, (2) an *autisme pauvre* with only the wisp of formerly meaningful actions left in the form of stereotyped movements and without much in the way of inner planning or inner meaning, and (3) this third form, the overt autism in which the action itself is well-preserved but in which the vital relationship with a surrounding social field is lost.

The "man of principle" illustrates a similar autism. His case is just close enough to the philosopher's ideal of the well-examined life, or to our notion of a truth reflectively arrived at, to startle us into an awareness we might otherwise miss, certain as we are that our own "principles" are good ones. We know that a principle is often the last refuge of a scoundrel, that rationalizations are easy to come by after the fact, but we often assume that a life founded on good principles is, by definition, good. One of Minkowski's cases (1927, pp. 81 ff) gives us a caricature of ourselves that illuminates one aspect of schizophrenia, and shows that a principle is often very "economical," since it can substitute for a more active and realistic form of thinking, and it can save us the pain of acting with feeling.

Minkowski's Young Instructor

He was 32 years old when he came to consult Minkowski. He complained of a kind of "physiological decomposition" and a painful emptiness in his head, which latter symptom he blamed on excessive salivation. His voice had changed: its dead quality gave it an uncanny, graveyard sound. He was regressing, pulled back to his fifteenth year, to the time when he had been given his first instructions as a substitute teacher. There were no reported hallucinations, nor was there any note-worthy sign of a weakening of intellectual functions. The vague sense of something morbid was pronounced, however, and as the interviews progressed, he was diagnosed as a case of schizophrenia, already advanced.

His trouble had begun in a prisoner-of-war camp in Germany. He had experienced a "moment of truth," a "revelation" that had seemed to him to be a sign of a moral regeneration, and he began to detach himself from the life around him, to live by principles. He became interested in philosophic problems and wrote down a mass of his reflections, taking great care not to read any of the philosophers, hoping thereby to ensure that his reflections would not be distorted, that his creations would be original. He avoided people for the same reason: he needed time to reflect, freedom from distractions, time to perfect his plans. Since any Grand Plan ought to be based on solid experimentation, he decided to apply a single principle each week: justice this week (somewhat harsh, and military in form), temperance next week (followed by a program of complete indulgence), and then silence. When he was discharged from prison and returned to his job as a teacher, his application of his "Logicodeductive Method" to classroom teaching did not seem to work out so well. A martinet one week, and an indulgent and permissive friend the next, his supervisor felt that the young instructor needed a great deal of guidance. The instructor, on his part, complained of the suffocating influences, the demands of the routine requirements, the harness imposed upon him; he grew restive, "explosive," difficult. Even the resumption of work had been premature: his parents had urged him, and though they were kind enough in their insistence, they had betrayed him, destroyed his personal initiative.

In a task that requires a man to cajole, obey, command, deny, assert, submit, approach, avoid, construct, destroy, this was a one-principle man, a "Johnny one-note" who changed his tune each week, according to an inner geometry and not at all in accordance with the flowing and changing human world about him. Changed by the clock, his few categories operated mechanically; and, automatically scheduled, they required few if any decisions. Life was much simpler that way: there is a tremendous economy in a "standard operating procedure," as any bureaucrat knows.

He felt, now, that both his parents and his supervisor had done violence to his speech. They accounted for its graveyard quality, its lack of manly resonance. Yet this speech of his seemed, sometimes, to lead him into saying things in the classroom that were not his own, as though he were tricked by the sound of his voice, led into false thoughts and statements by his larynx. Both parents and supervisors were fine persons: he respected their wisdom; but they had destroyed his autonomy; they had seduced and coerced him.

Minkowski heard his young patient's story with the tolerant disbelief of a physician who knows that schizophrenia is due to a process that the individual does not create, a process whose true nature he does not recognize. For all the patient's superiority feeling, he was a schizophrenic, and for all of his dream of a complete mastery of life, he was moving progressively into worsening relations with reality. Adjustment, closeness, strength, vitality, plasticity were disappearing; perfection, wisdom, rationality, an examined life, an ordered plan, and perfect freedom were the inner illusions that hid from him his deepening impotence. We are not quite ready to believe Minkowski when he wrote: "He had no delusions."

As a maker of configurations, as a self that exists in close relationship with a world that he constructs and tries to come to terms with, the young instructor was moving through rigidly structured schemata, and his real actions were deteriorating. The good life calls for a great deal of self-regulation, to be sure, but the young instructor has something we could call a *mania for regulation*: his self-control has hypertrophied at the same time that the actual field of the possible has been stripped of everything that does not fit the narrow schemata. He has become all regulation, all principle. The little wisps of reality that seep through the mesh of his schemata have to be interpreted in terms of the subjective network that is regnant at the time, and he is therefore either impervious to, or in struggle against, or forced to distort his interpretation of, much of the reality that flows about him.

The obsessive and the schizophrenic could be called "antinomic" men. The opposites that all of us have to fuse and harmonize if we are to act (flexors *and* extensors, affection *and* firmness, authority *and* friendship, submission *and* self-assertion) these psychasthenics try to split apart, put into separate compartments: it is much easier to rotate the principles than to make them function side by side in harmony.

It is sometimes a shock to those who come within the orbit of these selves to discover how the schizophrenic is affected by their presence (on *his* cognitive map they are *demonstrations of a principle*). Warped into his cognitive map of the week, the persons around him form a kind of pseudo-community, and if one is not for him, one must be against him (if not this week, then next, when the military discipline goes into effect). The smallest decisions, for such a geometer living a logicodeductive life, are made under the Great Principle of the Week, and they become *demonstrations*. Thus a lively world becomes a geometrical design (if not a wasteland), and the vital sap is squeezed out of ordinary human relationships.

Such a schizoid personality makes a peculiar kind of history as he goes. He will have his blue period, his military period, his Goethe period, his monkish period. Looked on in retrospect, the path has had many abrupt turnings; one excess replaced its predecessor. What some schizophrenics show within an hour, in their flight of ideas, these geometers show in their series of designs for living; so extreme is each one of them that the actions could be described as a series of manias. He is a pact-maker who undertakes compensations and penances. He develops ultraprecise plans for his days and builds complicated defenses and precautions against impulses or contingencies, and he seeks perfection in simple things (sometimes in a bodily function, such as bowel movements), which can become such a source of preoccupation that we conclude he can no longer trust his own body to execute its simple reflex functions. As in the interpersonal sphere, where he deranges human relations, so in his physiology he sometimes produces chronic constipation, diarrhea, colitis, skin irritations. His perpetual analysis of simple personal relationships tends to kill all spontaneity. Even his sexual life becomes incorporated into a system of bookkeeping. (He will be able to supply the data for any future Dr. Kinsey.) To use the familiar cliché, he does not seem to know how to do what comes naturally.

In the place of the normal flexibility required by a lively and changing world of persons, this type of schizoid self tries to develop something more predictable, more geometrical, and in the process he squeezes out all life. What Minkowski calls a *"géométrisme morbide"* had some of the qualities of a machine, a nonliving logical system, and it avoids all of the confusions of an "indigestible," unpredictable, troublesome, frustrating reality. Villiers de L'Isle Adam wrote a fictional account of a young man who appealed to Edison for help when his love affair with a beautiful actress fell apart. He could love no other. He planned to kill himself. Edison promised, in this tale, to build him a mechanical sweetheart, so perfectly constructed that even her dog would be deceived, and geared (with inner Edison recordings) to speak and move precisely in the manner the youth wanted. If this model sweetheart did not say the correct phrases, it would be because the inventor had not been given the precise directions. A truly schizoid plan: pushing a button would release whatever the youth desired. Love would become a simple thing. One would not even need a handbook.

Minkowski tells us that as a boy his young instructor had been obsessed with the question of the stability of buildings, of the architectural problem of distributing stress, with the question of symmetry. He even felt compelled to walk in the middle of the street. A physician's medication could not be started save in the middle of the month, or the middle of the year. He worried about the balanced distribution of articles in his pockets; he placed his limbs in parallel or symmetrical positions; and his breathing was managed so as to fit into the symmetry of his movements. These obsessions flourished within him, altering his actions then as his Great Principles were to do later. This sort of schizophrenic thought has a great similarity to that of the obsessive-compulsive, and like the obsessive, many schizophrenics feel possessed, or they complain that someone outside is influencing them.

Once, when walking down the street, the young instructor felt too much impressed by the sight of a woman walking. He had to go back to his house, "seat himself upon a chair, cross his arms, take a position that was as symmetrical as possible, and set about reflecting. He had to resolve the problem: why should the body of a woman produce such a special impression upon a man. And he sincerely hoped that all this could be handled by mathematics, both the medical and psychological aspects of sexual impressionability." Thus the geometer must encode, reduce to principles, handle in the abstract, conquer by analysis. "Does not beauty of the highest and purest type consist in symmetrical relations? Is not the sphere the perfect form? And will not the body of man reduce itself to geometry when we can understand it?"

We sense the youth's difficulties: the ground beneath him and the world within tremble too much. If only it could be reduced to a kind of frozen, spatial pattern, an eternal sameness, then it would be ordered, safe, easy to handle. Even his past ought to be worked over, and it has a special attraction for him, since in recapturing it and ordering it, a unique perfection can be achieved: the action is over, finished, complete; only the analysis remains. The present, on the contrary, is so confusing, so open-ended!

This summary and analysis of Minkowski's case of the young instructor provides us with certain contrasts between this type of schizophrenic and the normal. What the normal accepts as life, and can enjoy, this type sees as a confusing scene that needs a plan. Life is a confusing chaos, a jungle, until something is made of it, something logical, rational, ordered. What the normal accepts instinctively, with a natural feeling (or evaluation) and deals with intuitively, this kind of schizophrenic must approach cautiously: it will require a "brainy" plan. In the place of feeling, he uses the idea; instead of depending on a simple affective reaction, he has to turn to principles of symmetry, balance, order (to geometry), or to justice, freedom, permissiveness. Instead of a direct empathy with persons, instead of allowing a social reality to penetrate and flow about him, he must stand at a distance, analyze it, find a principle that will order and explain it. Without this elaboration of the in-between process, he cannot deal with reality, and in his analysis persons tend to become objects, actions become skilled movements, and the whole is frozen in a geometrical design.

If manias and depressions warn us against too implicit a trust in emotions, the fate of the young geometer warns us to give the life of feelings its due. Unless we are to be as schizoid as he, using one principle one week and the other on the next, we shall have to find a way of fusing them. In the process of living that shatters multifaceted reality into "opposites" were to be described as typical of persons whose psychological tension runs low, we might actually see in these facts a way of fusing the descriptions of Janet, Minkowski, and Bleuler.

We begin to perceive the other side of the "trust your emotions" argument. Warm, outgoing, vital, leading with his emotions, one man makes his decisions in his hips before the message has reached his head. He is all heart, all feeling. He approaches life, as a lover (or with a whip), as his mood dictates. To be sure, he gets slapped, but the backwash from his vital thrusts also instructs him. His brother, all thought, always reasonable, cannot act until he sees the road ahead precisely ordered and completely anticipated. He does not like playing by ear: one gets caught unprepared that way. Since each action arouses so many unforeseen consequences, he can take small bites only, then, like the hypochondriac who "Fletcherizes" his food, chewing each morsel thirty times before swallowing, he must ruminate over it, digest and assimilate the tiny bit of experience, relate it to his past and his future. Although each bit is mulled over and enriched, his powers of digestion are strictly limited. Even though his principles make things easy, too much is excluded.

One can see how both extremes, the hysterical and the obsessive-compulsive, could profit from a psychotherapy which can produce a wholesome balance between the two extremes. Whereas the one needs to develop second thoughts and to introduce some order into a scatterbrained "trust your emotions" type of blind living, the other needs to have his inhibitions examined, his powers of action released, his ability to extemporize and to tolerate imperfection strengthened. As a teacher, the one makes overly copious notes, forcing himself to anticipate every ramification of a theory, every possible criticism. The other extemporizes too much and, for all his liveliness, creates a scatterbrained impression, full of witticisms and brilliant phrases, charged with feelings but disorganized.

Minkowski senses the *weakness* in his young hyperrationalist, his man of principle. It is obviously a weak sort of rationalism, as incapable of tolerating and including the welter of conflicting events as the overtly autistic nail-driver who could not include the picture, the crying baby, the neighbor on the other side of the wall. This is "rationalism by exclusion," and it illustrates a facet of repression that Janet understood and that the Freudians have largely missed.

ETIOLOGY AND THERAPY

For every theory there is a therapy. Since some of our therapies (e.g., ECT) are almost wholly empirical in the beginning, perhaps we should reverse the relationship and add, for every therapy a theory will be developed to rationalize it sooner or later. Sometimes the theory runs very thin: the convulsive neuromuscular "explosion" produced by electroshock or insulin shock, it was argued, will break up the rut-formations, the bad-habit fixations, the distorted rumination of the schizophrenic. The numbness and confusion that followed such convulsions seemed to prove the interpretation, and when, coming out of an insulin coma, a deluded schizophrenic hitherto wrapped up in his autistic world suddenly spoke forthrightly and with complete lucidity, some therapists concluded that this sweeping away of the debris of fantasy had enabled the true self to reassume full charge once more. Even though the patient lapses, again, into his delusions or emptiness, the clinician has seen and heard the person speak with clarity, and so he *knows* that behind the mask of insanity there remains the possibility of another kind of awareness and action. In a similar fashion the member of the drug cult can return from one of his "trips" full of certitude: he *knows* that there are other forms of consciousness (whatever value the waking self may finally put on these "expanded" forms).

Conditioning therapies have been successful in effecting limited changes in the behavior of hospitalized schizophrenics. For example, Ayllon (1963) has used food reinforcement to improve patients' eating and speaking habits. Even the most ardent behaviorists concede, however, that their techniques thus far have accomplished little with schizophrenics beyond making them somewhat easier to manage in the hospital.

KRAEPELIN'S LEAD

The ability to "do something to the self with a chemical" adds a very heavy weight to one kind of clinical opinion that has persisted since Kraepelin's time. He had gathered four groups of symptoms (paranoid, hebephrenic, catatonic, and simple dementia praecox) under the one head, believing that each type progressed to one common and fateful end, and he was positive that he was dealing with a somatic illness that had psychological manifestations. These "signs" depended on a faulty functioning of the brain that, in turn, might be rooted in some metabolic, nutritional, or even endocrine malfunction, or in some tissue-produced toxin which poisons the brain and produces a flattening of emotional life, a loss of will and interest in life, and a release of automatisms that are normally held within a taut intrapsychic system of regulative tensions.

The Neuroanatomist's Contribution

Throughout the three-quarters of a century that have elapsed since Kraepelin set up this category, there have been other "engineers of human behavior" who have sought the causes in neural changes. The neuroanatomists have looked at brain specimens of patients brought to postmortem: palpation, chemical analysis, microscopic examination, all manner of tests for the presence of hypothetical toxins have been made. Some of the foremost names in neurology have suggested as causes cellular changes in: the choroid plexus, the third layer of the cortex, the hypothalamus, the basal ganglion cells, glia cells (Spielmeyer, Nissl, Alzheimer, von Monakow). Every claim was backed by good evidence, but: controls were often lacking; the same changes were later found in the brains of nonschizophrenic patients; seriously deteriorated schizophrenics failed to show them; and some of them were undoubtedly due to secondary conditions (dietary deficiency, aging, liver dysfunction) not related to the disorder itself. In short, no brain condition has been discovered in seventy years of anatomical research that is essential, that is always present when the disorder is present, always absent when the disorder is absent. This is not to say that, in some schizophrenics, brain changes complicate and contribute to the deterioration. It is also not to deny in advance the possibility that some further advance in the technique of neurophysiology will enable research workers to identify a specific and invariable accompaniment of the disorder. We do not now have the evidence at hand, and if we were to define dementia praecox as an arrest of development with regressive changes in feeling, thinking, and in motivation, depending on brain changes that in turn rest upon metabolic disorders, we would be repeating what Kraeplin said. (See Benjamin 1958.)[10]

The Search for a Substance in the Blood

The organicist who looks for some impersonal cause of the disorder has not been easily dismayed. As one of them pointed out, the brains of animals brought to death through convulsions (anoxia, blood-sugar changes, insulin shock) may show no change in the nerve cells. It may be the same with the functional and sometimes reversible changes of dementia praecox: the guilty metabolic factor carried by the bloodstream to the cortex and producing what is virtually a chemical decortication may not be revealed by the postmortem examination. The villain has departed, or, if it is still present, it eludes the tests used.

The Taraxein Hypothesis

For seventy years organicists have studied the blood of the schizophrenic. Watching the numbed and incommunicative state of the frozen cataleptic, one is already half-convinced that some "inhibitor" is at work. As though to strengthen his hand, the organicist's discovery of the close resemblance between the disease symptoms and those produced by the psychotomimetic drugs has led him to a renewed confidence that he can find the culprit which robs cortical cells of their necessary oxygen, or calcium, or iron, or copper, or sodium, or whatever it is that is lacking in these patients whose "awayness" must be secondary to their own organism's self-dosage with the destructive chemical.

Remembering that the fatigued dog's blood can be transported to the circulatory system of the resting animal, there to produce the typical changes of fatigue, some investigators have carried out an analogous operation on human beings, transporting the blood of schizophrenics into the veins of normal volunteers. To make a long story short, the evidence is confusing and contradictory; there are both positive and negative indications. We need much better control of procedures and more certainty that no placebo effect (or suggestion) is at work. None of the behavioral changes produced in this manner has endured for any length of time, yet in a review of some 130 titles,

---

[10]Dunlap (1924), who placed his microscopic slides of schizophrenics' brains in a random order among slides of his "controls," found that two of his dementia-praecox slides were judged to be as good as those of one of his best "controls." The crudity of some of the anatomic studies was illustrated, in the course of the discussion of Spielmeyer's paper (1931), by an anecdote about the psychiatrist Southard, who was asked to discriminate between two brains, one of a feebleminded epileptic girl, the other that of a Harvard professor of bacteriology. He chose that of the girl as the sound one, and added that the brain of a distinguished associate professor of psychology had measurements within the ranges assigned to microcephaly. Gross anatomy certainly offers a poor clue.

McGeer and McGeer (1959) offered encouragement to the organicists: there is enough to show that "something is there"; "a spirit of optimism should prevail."

Heath *et al.* (1957) described a *taraxein psychosis*, taraxein being the name given to a blood extract distilled from the blood of the schizophrenic patient and injected into nonschizophrenic volunteers.

"The characteristic general change is evidence of impairment of the central integrative process resulting in a variety of symptoms. There is a marked blocking with disorganization and fragmentation of thought. There is impairment of concentration. Each subject has described this in his own words: some saying merely, 'I can't think,' 'my thoughts break off'; others, 'I have a thought but I lose it before I can tell you anything about it,' etc. 'My mind is a blank' is another common expression. It becomes impossible to express a complete thought. Often they will state only a part of a sentence. They appear generally dazed and out of contact with a rather blank look in their eyes. They become autistic, displaying a lessening of animation in facial expression. Subjective complaints of depersonalization are frequent. Attention span is markedly shortened with increase in reaction time. The symptoms often produce apprehension in the patients. The commonest verbalization of their concern is 'I never felt like this in my life before.' "

Heath's enthusiasm is marred by the vagueness of the signs, the absence of quantitative tests, and the absence of controls to rule out suggestion effects. Mesmer, who produced convulsions and tremors in patients by his "animal magnetism," and the witch-doctors who produced confessions of rides on broomsticks did as well or better to "prove" their cases. When Heath's data are placed beside those of Hicklin *et al.* (1959), who used a crosstransfusion technique, replacing or exchanging some 6.8 liters in the course of six hours, and who found that no apparent clinical changes occurred, either in the patient (who might be expected to improve) or in the volunteer (who might be expected to show beginning signs of the patient's toxic condition), the "taraxein hypothesis" is weakened. The patient continued to show visual hallucinations, the volunteer none, nor were there any signs of catatonia, delusions, ideas of reference or influence. Instead, about four hours after the crosstransfusion had been discontinued, the patient became more catatonic and more paranoid than before. The volunteer, oddly enough, showed (in a follow-up study) that he had improved his interpersonal relationships, gave signs of enhanced self-esteem, got married, and felt quite set up by what he had done (schizophrenic metabolite or no). A failure to prove the presence of the hypothetical agency does not, of course, prove its absence. Although, as Siegel *et al.* (1959) suggested, "taraxein is a hypothetical substance which explains some unique observations in the Tulane laboratories," we are probably safe in assuming that the taraxein hypothesis is still alive, and that the enthusiasms of the organicists will continue.

Changes in the electrically recorded effects of direct excitation of the cortical fibers have been reported by research workers who have used the rat's brain as an indicator of the presence of this x-substance in the blood of schizophrenics. German (1963) found that, with the patient's serum bathing these tissues, the measured aftereffects of stimulation rose steadily over a period of 40 minutes. An increase was also present when the serum of controls was used (patients diagnosed as manic-depressives, hysteria, obsessive-compulsive neurosis, Pick's disease, diabetes, alcoholism with depression, along with controls who had no illness whatsoever), but in the controls the rise lasted only five minutes. This physiological effect, in short, respected the diagnostic categories.

It is of course a far cry from the generalization, the overinclusion, the resistance to extinction, and the inability to screen out irrelevant and meaningless stimuli that the schizophrenic shows, to these recorded changes in the rat's brain when bathed with the serum of schizophrenic patients. The experimenters succeed in linking this measured effect with that produced by psychotomimetic drugs (atropine in toxic doses, which also produces hallucinations in human subjects, increases the amplitude and duration of aftereffects of the rat's brain in concentrations of one in 5,000). We can accept this recent evidence as an indication, a straw of fact in a gale of organicist convictions. For example, LSD produces no changes; O-methyl-bufotaine produces increases; mescaline reduces them. Rovetta (1956) has found that intravenous injections of schizophrenic serum produce decreases in the amplitude of visual responses. The x-factor in the serum of the schizophrenic patients remains unknown. Whether it can be isolated in future experiments, whether it is a concomitant which is not essential to the disease, and what its precise identity is remain to be seen.

The convictions of the organicist are strong. His logic sometimes leads us around the bush:

1. Schizophrenia is a behavioral change.
2. It arises from some disorder of metabolism.
3. Changes in metabolism may be induced by stress.
4. Schizophrenia is a thinking disorder induced by stress.
5. There are disorders in the schizophrenic's thinking.
6. Hallucinogenic drugs also produce changes in thinking.
7. Both metabolic disorders (and their x-toxins) and the hallucinogenic drugs affect cortical activity.
8. Thinking is a form of behavior that involves the cerebral cortex.
9. When we understand the action of hallucinogenic drugs (which produce a temporary psychosis), and identify the x-factor produced by the faulty metabolism of the patient, we shall have all the explanation required for the development of schizophrenia and can direct a chemotherapy to rectify the pathological changes.

Perhaps the research worker will find that his hypotheses have been tainted by the faulty logic that is typical of this illness.

Adrenochrome: A Promising Lead

Organicism is not dead, however. Witness the lively battle over adrenochrome, adrenolutin, and niacin during the last decade. Hoffer, Osmond, and

Smythies (1954) have made the account of their experiments, often told before meetings of psychiatrists, a dramatic one. It seems that there was a bit of serendipity arising from a frustrating experience in wartime when a medical officer could not get *good* adrenaline, only a deteriorated "pink adrenaline" with unwanted side-effects. There were also the exciting new "psychotomimetic" drugs that could be synthesized, whose formulas were known, whose dosages could be controlled, so that in living subjects something like a "model psychosis" could be produced experimentally. There was also a search for an "M" substance, a mescaline-like chemical that—unlike other psychotomimetic substances, which were produced by plants—arose in human tissues. The similarity between the chemical structure of the drugs and that of adrenaline finally produced the insight which made the "pink adrenaline" experience relevant. Searching the literature, they found that others had identified an adrenochrome and an adrenolutin, both breakdown products of adrenaline. There remained the problem of testing the effect of these compounds on human subjects, of tracing out their effects on tissues, and of relating the whole sequence of changes, from the stress that releases adrenaline to the metabolic changes (and failures) that produce the "M" substance involved in psychotic symptoms. Their work could have resulted, if successful, in emptying half the beds in our mental hospitals, for they would have had in their hands, ultimately, a chemical antischizophrenogenic drug. They had the example of Stockings (1940) before them, and his thesis demonstrating that mescaline could produce a controlled form of schizophrenia had earned him the Bronze Medal of the Royal Medico-Psychological Association.

They also had the example of Hoffman, who had prepared LSD-25 and, in 1943, had decided to test it on himself, taking what he believed to be an insignificant dose (250 micrograms). To his dismay he noted that his

"...environment was undergoing progressive change. Everything seemed strange and I had the greatest difficulty expressing myself. My visual fields wavered and everything appeared deformed as in a faulty mirror. I was overcome by a fear that I was going crazy, the worst part of it being that I was clearly aware of my condition. The mind and power of observation were apparently unimpaired." (See Unger 1964.)

When Osmond, Hoffer, and Smythies had obtained their sample of adrenochrome, they proceeded to make daring tests on their subjects and on themselves, when the effect of this substance, the strength of the dosage, the permanence of psychotic symptoms (if any) were all unknown. Their first subjects obliged them by reporting abnormal mental states. These varied from the classic signs of psychasthenia (which Janet had described in detail) to a depression that lasted for four days.[11]

---

[11]The wide range of signs, all familiar to those who have read the clinical and experimental literature, was diverse enough to make the drug appear nonspecific. In the case of the depression, which occurred when the wife of one of the research team was given the injection, a convenient ad hoc hypothesis was offered when her husband recalled that she had suffered an attack of infectious hepatitis a few years previously, an illness which may have sensitized her to that particular form of response.

The Niacin Hypothesis

An expanding stream of clinical and biochemical studies, tracing out the adrenaline-adrenolutin hypothesis, has followed. Multiple hypotheses linking the stress-produced adrenaline to the ultimate psychotic signs through a chain of intervening variables have been advanced, the details of which are too voluminous even to summarize here, and the end of this long road is not yet in sight. One of the latest events has been the published claims of Hoffer, announcing the cure of 13 out of 17 cases of schizophrenia by the administration of three grams of niacin daily, a substance he believed might have the power of neutralizing adrenochrome and adrenolutin.

Hoffer's paper, read before a group assembled to hear discussions of "Enzymes in Mental Health," had scarcely had time to be assimilated when a report of a similar trial at Rockland State Hospital, N.Y., was read in Chicago. Without proper controls, Hoffer had reported an improvement in his patients during the period when NAD (nicotinamide adenine dinucleotide) was administered, and a relapse when it was discontinued. Kline, who tried to replicate the therapy, used a sugar-pill placebo on half of his group of 20 patients, and found that the sugar pill and the NAD had effects so similar that no discrimination between the groups could be made.

We are forced to ask, "What else did Dr. Hoffer do?" Was it his enthusiasm, and the suggestibility of his patients, that resulted in a "lift" from their schizophrenic torpor? If so, the data would make an ironic coda to the decade of work of an organicist. Kline, interviewed by the inquiring reporter, made no suggestions as to what the possible difference in results might be due to, while admitting that he shared the organicist's central credo that some metabolic disorder was the underlying factor in the illness.

Benjamin (1958), reviewing the history of the adrenochrome hypothesis, notes:

"Adrenochrome, which had long been known chemically but had never been found *in vivo*, . . . was suggested as a possible candidate (among other causes of schizophrenia). Given intravenously, they reported that it produced, along with other psychological effects, hallucinations, including colored ones, thereby qualifying along with many other compounds as an hallucinogen. Apart from the fact that this finding is itself unconfirmed, both for adrenochrome and its close relative adrenolutin, there is no evidence whatsoever for the *in vivo* occurrence of these substances either in schizophrenics or in nonschizophrenics."

Conceived in haste, carried out in haste, charged with great enthusiasm, the procedures of Hoffer, Osmond, and Smythies, have, from the start, lacked both caution and the usual scientific controls. From the first administration of adrenochrome in their laboratory on Jillings, their willing subject, their work has been haunted by the possibility of a "placebo effect," a possibility that is greater in the midst of the infectious excitement that surrounds any miraculous cure, whether by Mesmer, or at the Grotto at Lourdes, or in the white-coated shrine of modern science. The extent of this suggestion factor is unknown, in any new setting. In an experimental setting only roughly comparable to that of the Hoffer-Osmond clinic, and in a situation where no such life-and-death issues were in the balance, Knowles and Lucas (1950) found that two-thirds of 59 subjects reported one or more effects which they believed to be caused by a "drug" being administered, when in fact a harmless placebo was used. Their experiences included such states as fatigue, confused thinking, blurred vision, relaxation, calm, aches and pains, gay feelings, relief from fatigue, greater energy, feelings of strangeness and unreality. The effects also had a high correlation with other measures of neuroticism, a fact we should bear in mind, always, when studying "volunteers for a study of drug effects" rather than some "total population" selected on other bases or random samples of normal subjects.

When a drug, such as LSD-25, of known and generally accepted potency, is used (instead of adrenochrome, a drug of uncertain potency and unknown to the average subject), the influence of the setting is again visible. Administered by a Freudian, the subject may report revived childhood experiences; one clinician, a Jungian, reported that his patient went through "archetypal experiences;" and in a religious setting, "mystic experiences" have been reported. In an impersonal and hostile setting, a subject may have experiences filled with horror and terror. So variable are the reported effects (a cure of alcoholism, the precipitation of a schizophrenic psychosis, the ultimate experience of "union with God," a complete clarification of one's identity, the total loss of interest in practical concerns connected with study for a career) that the core of biochemical change and its "pure" consequences is very difficult to estimate. One clinician will report that his patients never want to enter the drugged state again; the next finds himself besieged to repeat the pleasant experience; and some clinicians imply, in their reports of success with alcoholics, that their purpose was to "scare the hell out of the patient with a *tremendous experience.*"

Where so many purposes are served by a drug, and when it can be fitted into so many divergent settings, its effects will not be simple. This fact is one of the reasons why the organicists have produced such confusing data. Their conception of a human patient as a kind of walking test tube in which effects could be studied with complete disregard of psychological factors has made them unusually susceptible to error.

Hoffer and his associates have been violently opposed to any "organismic eclecticism," such as that which characterized the Phipps clinic when Meyer was the chief of the service. The reviews of life-histories which came from his clinic showed that all manner of bodily complaints had figured in these lives, and possibly weakened their integrative powers: early difficulties in nursing, night terrors, late maturation, infections, retarded development, enuresis, tantrums, fire-setting, weaning difficulties, convulsions, fainting, stuttering. Furthermore, these difficulties had occurred in persons with menstrual, gastrointestinal, cardiovascular, and other homeostatic disorders, such as fluctuations in temperature, susceptibility to infections, and skin abnormalities (see Terry and Rennie 1938).

When such a psychobiological potpourri is allowed to develop in a person who is in constant interaction with an environment and who is constructing holistic interpretations of what is taking place, the task of unraveling this web of relations (should the outcome be schizophrenia) is not likely to yield anything in the way of clear and simple causes and effects. On the one hand, almost any event may have made a difference, and so the second-guesser is not absolutely wrong. On the other hand, no clear-cut cause is likely to prove essential (i.e., present in every case). This leaves the therapist pretty much to his own devices. Anything that he can do to interpret, ameliorate, discipline, reeducate, encourage, restructure such a "holistic mess" will be therapeutic, but the artist-physician will have to approach the next case with a completely open mind, experiment with a new pattern of variables, grapple with a new pattern of resistance, and no simple handbook of procedures can emerge from that. Hoffer and his associates seem to want an *essential* factor, a *manipulable* one (if not a single one, then a clearly grasped and conceptually related set of variables) that can be shown to be present or not, right or wrong, and that will be so objective and manageable that the patient's behavior can be controlled.

BLEULER'S LEAD

There is a second school of thought that has always found Kraepelin's views uncongenial. Many of these workers claim to follow Bleuler's classic account of dementia praecox, and, more particularly, to respect the spirit of Burghölzli clinic. In a sympathetic description of his father's work, Manfred Bleuler (1931) has identified four therapeutic principles which indicate that in his practice, whatever his theory, Bleuler shared the kind of holistic assessment of the therapeutic problem that Adolf Meyer was suggesting to his colleagues in America. Bleuler urged:

1. A struggle against the patient's tendencies to autism. He may wish intensely that you would leave him to his own inner world. Tight-lipped, uncommunicative, withdrawn, he must nonetheless be reached.

2. Study him, in order to get in touch with him. Bring him back into vital relationship with those around him. Whatever his complexes, remember that a man does not live by them. Though he has regressed to the point of soiling himself and lies curled up in fetal posture, one does not have to leave him to himself, nor should the therapist put diapers on him and then join him on the floor, in order to enter his fantasy world and talk to him. Though one's theory implies that the patient is "living at the early oral phase," one does not have to feed him with a bottle or give him scraped apple. Touch the man in him, or the woman, not the arrested infant, *and the person is there,* behind the autism and behind the mask of regressive behavior.

3. Just as occupational therapy is designed, not merely to strengthen specific muscle groups, but to give the patient something interesting and significant to do, it should also be managed in such a way as to bring him into vital relationship with the hospital community. Forget the compulsion to analyze

the symptoms, forget the theory that explains fixation and regression, and focus on the actions that lead to a restoration of healthy relationships. Even assuming that the psychoanalytic interpretations (which Jung had urged on him) are true, dwelling on archetypal meanings is not a therapeutic type of communication, nor will it strengthen the weakened ego, nor affect that underlying primary process (the basic disorder, the constitutional weakness, whose existence he believed in as much as did Kraepelin).

4. Sometimes the discharge of a patient, his restoration to real life, in which he must face emergencies, will reveal powers of adaptation that remain hidden under the protective conditions of the hospital. It is well to assume that a patient has greater resources than he is currently showing. A certain amount of risk is worth taking. (Bleuler used the illustration of the physician Klaesi, who gave a very untidy and violent patient his handkerchief. The action shocked her into a sudden contact with cultivated human beings, to the point where she suddenly abandoned her delusional ideas.)

To a clinician who, like Bleuler in Zurich, or Meyer in Baltimore, approaches the schizophrenic with his wit, his common sense, and his "bare hands," every aspect of the patient's life in hospital becomes a possible therapeutic force. Holism leads to eclecticism, to a "total push" in which anything which makes a difference has therapeutic possibilities. All therapy with schizophrenics is psychotherapy, Bleuler often repeated, and it must be aimed (by whatever roundabout way) at that basic thinking difficulty, and used, not as one would mechanically administer a drug, but rather as one person would strive to reach out and touch another, in order to move that self that is still there (at least as a latent possibility).

PSYCHOANALYSIS AND ITS DERIVATIVES

Another group of therapies, also "barehanded" (making use of no drugs) but operating under the over-all conceptions of Freud rather than with the simpler framework of common sense of Bleuler and Meyer, have carried analytic practice into the territory once expressly forbidden to Freud's disciples. Forbidden or not, they *had* to try. Like the Matterhorn, schizophrenia was there. Believing in the essential truth of his insights, Freud's disciples have shown their faith by doing precisely what his own caution and prudence countermanded in advance.

Active Therapy

Some of these disciples have produced what their more cautious colleagues have called "wild psychoanalysis." Ferenczi, Rosen, Sechehaye, Azima, all share the belief that schizophrenia begins in bad mothering, in the *poisons* of rejection, seduction, overindulgence, or cold and impersonal disciplines that lay down the structure of the primary process which finally breaks through into one of the full-blown forms of schizophrenia. Determined to make up for what the schizophrenogenic mother (or father) had done, they hug, rock, pat, feed, bathe the patient. They clean him when he soils himself, take him to the bathroom and seat him on the toilet. Or they provide him with plasticine, or cocoa-colored clay and vegetable dyes so that he may smear, squeeze, mold, or otherwise symbolically deal with feces and thus extrude from his system the tendencies which, still arrested within him, produce the bizarre fixations that constitute his symptomatology. Thus they hope to free impulses for a going forward, and seek to release once more the full attentive powers of the patient for more adult forms of analytic work, and for living.

Some of these forms of therapy require the analyst to spend hours with a single patient, living with him, interpreting his every act, matching obscenity with obscenity, breaking through the patient's defensive barriers, and forcing the patient to acknowledge his presence, and to learn new ways with the analyst's "good mothering" to guide him. Michael Balint, one of Ferenczi's most trusted disciples and his literary executor, epitomizes one of the wilder forms of such efforts to restore a vital contact with reality: "It consists of hugging and kissing the patient and using four-letter Anglo-Saxon words."

An example of Rosen's interpretations is given in his own words (1959, p. 57, my translation):

"I was intrigued especially by the fact that the catatonic did not manifest anxiety in any outward form as long as he remained seated. But as soon as he got up he promptly showed signs of panic. He seemed to be looking for something. He looked about the room, emptied his pockets, pulling his handkerchief with every evidence of mounting anxiety. My own interpretations were in the direction of making him understand that he thought himself to be castrated and that he was looking everywhere for the missing penis. But my interpretations had no effect.

"And so my paranoiac patient came to my rescue with the solution to the enigma. He told me: 'He never asks whether he has a penis or not as long as he is seated, for in this position he is a girl. The girls do it in this position (he referred to micturition). But when he gets up he does it like the boys, and since he is not really sure that he is male he is trying to get an answer to this question.'

"If this interpretation was the right one, my problem from this point on was to convince my patient of his virility, and of the fact that he had a penis. And so, on our next session, when the patient arose I told him to put his hand upon his penis, and I even helped him to do it. From the moment that he felt his penis, he was reassured, and the anxiety was sharply diminished. He stopped looking around and left the room with me with an expression of relief. The symptom did not return."

Forced Regression

A few therapists have used what they call a forced regression, employing the sensory-deprivation techniques in order to intensify the patient's dependence, to exaggerate the therapist's power, and to enable the latter to enter into contact with the patient at a regressed level, feeding him and caring for him as one would an infant. All this is done with a view to restoring the damaged ego to an integrity at the level where its development went wrong:

before he can walk (to speak metaphorically), he must creep and crawl, and only after he has again traveled through the phases of development can an analyst approach him on the adult level with procedures appropriate to that level.

Bold in his claims, Rosen shocked his colleagues by his methods, yet so impressive were his reported results that even the conservative voice of Frieda Fromm-Reichmann was raised in association meeting to explain how this "wild analysis" could get results (and to caution her colleagues against its dangers). Boisterous, dangerous, tough as they were, she believed that his methods constituted too grave a threat for many schizophrenics (who fear, above all things, any invasion of that private world into which they have withdrawn). To quote her words, Fromm-Reichmann (1952) thought that

"...many of his interpretations are arbitrary, if not incorrect. Yet they work.... I am in accord with Eissler, who says that Rosen's patients emerge from their 'states of acute psychotic disturbance' because of the convincing, consistent intentness of purpose, attitude, speech and tone of voice with which he relates himself to them. His shocking random interpretations are one of his effective emotional tools. They are effective, irrespective of their truth or faultiness. However, what Rosen does with this method is not to cure schizophrenics, but to help them to emerge quickly from acute psychotic episodes."

Fromm-Reichmann's Principles of Therapy

Although she admits that her methods may not bring the patient out of his disturbed state as rapidly as Rosen's, Fromm-Reichmann would like to see:

1. The relationship between physician and patient kept on an adult level, strictly professional, with an appeal to that which is mature within the patient.

2. No efforts to "be a friend" or a mother, or to seduce, cajole, or otherwise invade the privacy of the patient.

3. Therapists realize the acutely dangerous aspects of any effort at love, friendship, or closeness with the paranoid, the homosexual, or those who already overvalue what they imagine a perfect love would bring.

4. Analysts resist the temptation to step out of their true role, remembering always that therapy may be serving their own needs rather than those of the patient.

5. An acceptance of the patient, an effort to reassure him and to reduce his anxiety, but at an adult level that is both realistic and humane.

6. Analysts remember that schizophrenics are threatened by any untoward offer of warmth. These patients are already having difficulties with *boundaries*, and undue closeness intensifies this difficulty.

7. Analysts remember that the schizophrenic is acutely aware of any insincerity, any feigned emotion, and unusually sensitive to either excessive warmth and sweetness or hidden rejection, and to turn the patient over to another who can do sincerely what the rejecting analyst must feign.

8. Analysts remember that schizophrenics have, already, great difficulty in handling their own hostilities. Anything that intensifies this problem or

invites retaliation may increase rather than lessen the patient's reasons for his loss of vital contact with reality.

A Follow-Up of Rosen's Patients

While Fromm-Reichmann was explaining Rosen's results and cautioning her colleagues, a follow-up study of Rosen's cases was being carried out at the New York Psychiatric Institute by Horowitz *et al.* (1958). Rosen had defined "recovery" as

"...not meaning merely that the patient is able to live comfortably outside an institution, but rather that such a degree of integrity is achieved that the emotional stability of the patient and his personality and character structures are so well organized as to withstand at least as much environmental assault as is expected of a normal person, that is, of a person who never experienced a psychotic episode."

Of the 37 patients treated and pronounced recovered by Rosen, Horowitz and his associates were able to identify and follow nineteen. Of the nineteen, twelve were found to have been diagnosed schizophrenic, six had been psychoneurotics, one a manic-depressive. One of the seven nonschizophrenics had subsequently been twice readmitted to a state hospital, given ECT, and again diagnosed as manic-depressive. All seven nonschizophrenics were out in the community at the time of the follow-up. Of the twelve schizophrenics found, five had been readmitted to hospital before his original paper was published (1947), nine had been readmitted to mental hospitals within the decade, two had undergone psychosurgery, and an additional one had requested this radical treatment. Electroshock, insulin, coma, psychotherapy, tranquilizers had been used on at least half of the schizophrenic group in the years subsequent to discharge. None of the twelve had maintained the recovery criterion that Rosen had set up. The therapeutic outcome does not support Rosen's claims; the proportion making a successful adjustment is not larger than that found in other samples of schizophrenics who have been given little more than custodial care.

Some of the reports of successful psychoanalytic therapy, or of the success of its derivative forms, as well as the rival claims of organicists, have been marred by excessive enthusiasm and by the use of cases with an uncertain diagnosis and still less certain depth to the illness. How many of them should be placed in a "nonprocess" group, we have no way of knowing. Some of the studies are little more than descriptions of an "I once had a schizophrenic patient" type, where whatever was done for the patient resulted in recovery, and where the precise causes of improvement cannot be isolated. Recoveries are seldom evaluated by independent judges nor are they followed through the years subsequent to their discharge, or matched by control cases who are equally ill and who are given other therapies or no therapy at all. In short, we have to conclude: The reports of the results of the therapies that have been used with schizophrenics demonstrate the meanings implicit in a theory; they demonstrate the conviction of the therapist; they may even lead to reformulations of a theory; but they have not, so far, proved the value of any therapy.

EPILOG

Perhaps, in concluding our discussion of schizophrenia we should return to the fact that the disease is of unknown origin. Each of the therapies now in use can be rationalized on the basis of certain assumptions. When we review the evidence, as tests of hypotheses they have not proved adequate. In our present stage of therapy and research, the proofs that have been offered have all violated, in one way or another, what we know about research design. Some are even poor as demonstrations.

As a kind of living projection test, they sometimes reveal the personality of the therapist. Ferenczi, full of the milk of human kindness, wanted to do something for these grown-up infants. Freud, disgusted with Ferenczi's childishness, feared the latter's enthusiasms would bring discredit on the whole psychoanalytic enterprise. To some psychoanalysts Freud seemed unusually cautious, a bit cold, overintellectual, aloof; since they viewed his procedures as austere and mechanical, a few went to the opposite extremes. Ferenczi was ever ready to admit his errors to his patient, inclined to let the latter guide him in his interpretations, but Freud, never! Fromm-Reichmann could not imagine herself as a part of Rosen's boisterous (and at times obscene) game. A gentlewoman, she respected the persons she treated, and she succeeded in her way with her patients (whom Rosen might have destroyed, she feared). Sechehaye, full of maternal feelings, embraced and reassured and fed her schizophrenic girl, like a good mother. The types of therapy range from a cool, impersonal enlightenment to the boisterous interchanges and acting-out designed to shock the patient into a response to his surroundings: they express the therapist; they reveal what he feels toward his patients and what he imputes to them. For all that anyone can say, at present, they are of equal worth and at least no more harmful than mere custodial care.

There are seven possible etiologies of schizophrenia, Jackson (1960, p. 13) concluded, as he tried to place within his outline the main trends in the evidence accumulated over the past hundred years. Seven or seventeen, there are bound to be as many divergent therapies as there are theories. In the genes, in the family constellations, in the pressures rooted in the broader culture, in the repressions which—in infancy—had laid the groundwork of primary-process distortion, in the slow and cumulative compounding of bad habits, in a special physiology which produces an "M" substance that, in turn, leads to pathology in behavior, in the interruption of vital contact with reality, and in any combination of any or all of the foregoing "causes," we have sought for a rational design that would enable therapists to attack this most resistant form of psychopathology. Psychogenic, genogenic, biochemical, and physiological, the seven or seventeen types of causes have served as guides for both therapy and research, but the recovery rates have not demonstrated any final mastery of the problem. Manfred Sakel's words to the reporters, as he debarked at New York harbor, suggested to the readers of the morning newspapers that 90 per cent of our schizophrenics were now curable by the new insulin-shock therapy. Two decades later, Rosen's "direct analysis" promised similar cures and recovery rates, as did the claims of Hoffer, who, after having "discovered" the relations between adrenochrome and schizophrenia, later believed that thirteen out of seventeen schizophrenics could be cured by three grains of niacin daily. Sakel's hopes proved premature; Rosen's patients, followed up, were found either not to have been schizophrenic or to have suffered relapses, save for a few who have remained well and out of hospital, as do other schizophrenics who have not had the benefits of his dramatic therapy. In the recent past we have learned of efforts to replicate Hoffer's therapy that have yielded no gains whatsoever. Tomorrow we may discover that, instead of gains, the massive dosages of niacin have produced unfortunate side-effects.

There are thus two pressing problems that call for an active strategy on the part of all directors of clinics where research and therapy for schizophrenics is carried on. They are inherent in the diagnosis and treatment of a disorder of unknown origin. The question of cause must be kept open, as well as the question of whether there is a single, unitary disease process under the rather expanded conceptual tent now covering this group of illnesses. All possible hypotheses have to be given a fair trial. We shall have to find ways of combining data and of utilizing all information from varied disciplines in the planning of our therapy, so that whatever does make a difference can be forced to reveal its role in bringing about recovery. Difficult as it is to accomplish, we must find some way of evaluating these hypotheses (and therapies) that will be superior to what we have employed to date.

At present we know of no single action which will make all the difference for a schizophrenic patient. We know a great many things about what promotes the health of the body, and we have some (often vague) notions about what makes a good life (for a schizoid personality as well as for others). Although each therapist presses his own particular conception of the one essential thing to be done, in our present and painful state of ignorance we would be wise to keep in the foreground the main problems of bodily well-being and a truly human climate in those institutions where the mentally ill are treated.

False hopes and a stubborn clinging to particular therapies which give us something to do (while overlooking our shortcomings) have already proved less than helpful, and for some of them (such as lobotomies and electroshock) we may have actually paid in worsened health and capacities. An impersonal efficiency in drugging, shocking, surgically treating patients can be not only sterile but therapeutically harmful, increasing the threat of a reality already too difficult to adjust to. Therapists, like patients, can be caught up in what one might call "the determinism of ignorance," and, like their patients, be driven to a kind of autistic-dereistic thinking of which Bleuler wrote.

Chapter 12 • Reflections, Generalizations, and Emphases

As we come to the end of our study of the abnormal personality, there are a few generalizations I might make by way of emphasis. In making them, I risk betraying the prejudices with which I began this study; and because this "science of the abnormal" is constantly changing, I risk dating my own views. When Percival Bailey delivered the annual academic lecture to the American Psychiatric Association in 1956, the question which he voiced—as he summed up his reflections on a long life of distinguished service as a neurosurgeon—expressed his puzzlement and dismay as he witnessed the current trends around him. "Why does it flourish?" he asked, referring to psychoanalysis, for he had emerged from a surfeit of study to say "in psychoanalysis I can find no vision." As he developed his thesis by pointing out some of its peculiarities, here and there disgusted members of the psychoanalytic group arose and left the hall, in protest.

Tempted by his role to evaluate the past and to point the way to the future, while emphasizing the solid ground on which we stand today, a speaker in Bailey's role is virtually invited to become prophet, shaper of the future. Yet as he reviewed the seven or more "revolutions" in psychiatric practice and theory that had been successively hailed as measures which would shortly empty the hospitals and straighten out the mentally ill, he was driven to a quite different position. Although he chose to stand with the biochemists, who would, he thought, be the ones to discover the basic nature of the schizophrenic process, he had to admit that his own view was tentative, hypothetical, and still without the scientific underpinning that alone could convert his hunch into valid theory.

Perhaps this image of an aging practitioner, confessing to his doubts and voicing his hunches about the future, while his colleagues leave the hall in which he has been invited to speak as honored guest, too angry to listen further to what the speaker believed to be the spectacle of modern clinical theory and practice, is a good one to symbolize the present state of affairs, for we are divided. We find it all but impossible to agree on a concept of the *normal personality*, which—one might assume—is the goal toward which all theory should be directed. As for such a complex concept as "the structure and dynamics of the self-system," this, too, promptly becomes a bone of contention. Freud had no sooner published his study of the "Anatomy of the Personality" than the revisionists were at work, and Sullivan (1940), Horney (1950), Fromm (1947), and a dozen others have felt it necessary to redo this central organizing concept (see also Offer and Sabshin 1966, and Rogers 1959).

One point most will agree on: The self is neither immaculately conceived nor genetically fixed for a lifetime. It ebbs and flows, grows stronger and weaker, disintegrates in general paresis, takes a shape in infancy (within a family and a culture), and makes contracts which it is not always able to fulfill. One psychologist, at a recent professional meeting, impressed with the number of marriages that fail, suggested that the marriage contract should be made for a period of five years, and then be reviewed by both parties periodically to see whether the first hasty decision was a valid one. Instead of being of flinty substance and immortal, the self emerges (particularly from a study of abnormal ones) as a chameleon-like, changeable thing, taking on new qualities in every new interpersonal context and fluctuating with the "tides of life" (the endocrines, the metabolic changes that come with aging, the process going on silently down among the cells), to say nothing of the burrowing spirochetes and the passing infections in which invading viruses and bacteria take up residence in a body that the self so poorly manages.

Not only is the constancy of the self a limited thing, but its strength at any one time is limited. It can structure a field about it, make promises, set future goals, act like a free man, *up to a point.* The spectacle of free men paying a fee to enter a clinic where someone will help them break a relatively trivial habit like smoking is enough to remind us of the self's limitations. We have not found ways of measuring this type of "force" save in the making of a life that "works" and that seems satisfying. It was Janet's placement of this force, which he called psychological tension, at the center of his analyses of the psychoneuroses and of his plans for therapy that makes the passing of his popularity a matter to be regretted. When I visited the Salpêtrière, not long ago, to pay my respects to the clinic where Charcot and Janet had taught so brilliantly, a half-century ago, I could find no one on the staff who remembered Janet. A young resident told me he had spent a year of study in America under Percival Bailey, from whom he first learned about Janet. The Freudian tide had swept away even the memory of this one-time dean of French psychiatry. In the lecture hall where all of Paris's intellectuals gathered to see and hear Charcot demonstrate cases of hysteria, there was a plaque to mark the fact that Sigmund Freud once studied here, but none to record the fact that Janet spent years practicing and lecturing. The theories of human personality are ephemeral, swept away when the impressive presence of the lecturer who expounds them has gone.

To the degree that psychoanalysis has become a cult, it has crowded out all critical thinking by those who follow the master. Jules Masserman's "stunt" of giving a solemn and straight-faced exposition of the psychosomatic problems connected with the ingrown toenail (with free-wheeling interpretations couched in the "correct" language of libido, cathexis, regression, and sexual symbolism) brought him to a shocking realization of the state of mind of his analytically trained audience when some of them came up to congratulate him on his profound insights. The need for an advance in the scientific and critical quality of clinical thinking in the place of a certain cultist approach to problems is obvious.

One further reflection seems prompted by such anecdotal material. The stress on "current dynamics," on the present life-situation, on facts that are presently visible and verifiable, rather than on a hypothetical character structure, an imagined early infancy, a hypothetical genetic constitution, seems to be a healthy one. This is a common shift in emphasis among various schools of "revisionists." At the same time, the revisionists must avoid their own cultist oversimplifications. Behaviorists especially, whether neo-Pavlovian or Skinnerian, might heed the conclusion of Jerome Bruner (1962, p. 90):

"When learning leads only to pellets of this or that in the short run rather than to mastery in the long run, the behavior can be readily 'shaped' by extrinsic rewards. But when behavior becomes more extended and competence-oriented, it comes under the control of more complex cognitive structures and operates more from the inside out."

Looking back at my first chapter, where I introduced the problem of freedom, I am moved to reflect that there is a built-in and calculated risk in the clinician's role. Dramatically highlighted by the suicide of Hemingway, who was released from hospital after a bout of depression, only to shoot himself shortly thereafter, we have learned that every recovering depressed case is a "risk." In other mental illnesses, such as alcoholism, neurasthenia, hysteria, we have seen how patients assume an attitude in response to their clinician's basic assumptions. If the latter shows by his acts that he believes the patient to be sick, helpless, and without inner resources of his own, he fosters a dependence and a sense of helplessness. If he goes too far in the opposite direction, he can also intensify this same feeling in patients who are simply "not up to it." Indeed, it is a common belief among those who treat alcoholics that, until their patients admit their helplessness and confess their dependence on direction from outside, there is no hope of helping them. "The 'I can manage this myself' alcoholic never does," they say.

Decisions about the management of a patient are not simple matters, since they involve the personality of the therapist. The "big" clinician can often blow up his role unnecessarily, and create some of the very weaknesses he is forced to treat. Not only do we have very poor measures of the success of therapy, but it is also difficult to parse out the portions of a lingering illness that are themselves clinician-caused.

Another point becomes abundantly clear as we study abnormal personalities. We might call it "the problem of the categories." Mental diseases have been classified and reclassified; the psychiatric associations periodically revise their handbooks, so that the statistics reported in one state may be comparable to those found in others and so that everyone can be brought up to date with the latest clinical findings. Yet the best classifications have not yielded firm diagnoses for symptom clusters, with a clear-cut cause, course, and outcome (as would be the case with an "ideal" physical illness). The categories continue to change; the best clinics study patients as persons in unique settings, and when they have made their best analysis of all the relevant conditions they are able to identify, the last question that comes up in staff meeting is, "And what category should we use in reporting this illness to the state authority?" There was a time when the Kraepelinian conviction of the fatal terminus of demential praecox (simple schizophrenia) was so strong in some clinics that they felt called on to reclassify and rediagnose any dementia-praecox patient who recovered. Today the loose concept of "the schizophrenias," which some believe should be broken into twenty or more categories, is less binding. Even the division into process and nonprocess schizophrenia fails to fit the diversity in clinical facts.

The categories, like most of our concepts, are a source of efficiency and at the same time a possible set of blinders that can shut out the living facts: with abnormal personalities, the risk in adhering to clinical stereotypes is greater than usual. We have learned to mistrust the predicted outcomes, the claims about prepsychotic personalities, and to use our categories lightly, with a proper doubt. Adolf Meyer, the greatest teacher of psychiatrists in America in this century, bore down heavily upon any resident physician that he caught reporting a "stereotype" and not what he had actually observed. The neurophysiologist Lashley gave a similar warning in his 1929 presidential address to the American Psychological Association (in Beach *et al.* 1960, p. 208):

". . . The value of theories in science today depends chiefly upon their adequacy as a classification of unsolved problems, or rather as a grouping of phenomena which present similar problems. Behaviorism has offered one such classification, emphasizing the similarity of psychological and biological problems. Gestalt psychology has stressed a different aspect and reached a different grouping: purposive psychology still another. The facts of cerebral physiology are so varied, so diverse, as to suggest that for some of them each theory is true, for all of them every theory is false."

The question of heredity continues to plague us. Its bearing on mental illness has been clearly established, certainly when we confine ourselves to the statistics of large groups. But it is equally clear that there are enthusiasts who have gone far beyond the facts on both sides of the argument, and some of the oft-quoted data have not borne up under subsequent analysis. In the end, as attention narrows to the individual patient, the question has to be resolved much in the manner we have chosen in speaking of the "freedom" of the patient. He is as free as he is, as capable of assuming responsibility as he is, and there is a residue of "capacity to learn productive adjustments" that is as great as it is; only patience, persistent effort, and a willingness to assume occasional risks can prove how great this margin of modifiability is. When one sees an identical twin settle down to a progressively deteriorating simple schizophrenia, while his brother (with an identical inheritance) proceeds to take one position after another with increasing responsibilities and to weather these stresses successfully, one becomes aware of the weighting that must be given to "the other factors." The identical twin pairs, one member of which commits suicide while the other member returns, after a depression that was also experienced by his brother, to face life, remind us that the development of a human personality is not fated in the sense that some geneticists seem prone to believe. The clinician is required to work with what he has, toward what normality he can achieve, and with whatever means there are to outwit or supplement the genetic capacity.

Within the clinical field where abnormal personalities are studied, there is much to praise and much to criticize. One can see how the future historian of this period, acting as a strict judge of what passed scientific muster or was offered as an imaginative and revealing study of a single case in our time, might find much to condemn, some in "high places." Sigmund Freud's "Case of Little Hans" contains much that, from the point of view of method and scientific caution, a conscientious clinician would condemn. It illustrates much that a weatherwise child psychiatrist should not do. Some of the studies that are shining examples of what should be attempted—such as the Cohen and White study of neurocirculatory asthenia—are too seldom mentioned in the literature. One notable example of a neglected study is Janet's *De l'angoisse à l'extase*, the most extended and meticulous report of a cyclothymic in the literature. Searching through the references in Bertram Lewin (1950), a study of ecstasy (which problem Janet treats at length), one can find not a single footnote or bibliographic reference to indicate that he has ever seen Janet's study. One gets the sad impression from such bibliographic voyages that psychoanalysts read only the works of other members of their cult.

I know that comparisons of this sort are odious and do little to advance the "science." Therefore I think I should state an impression which the extended reading of clinical literature, both that published by psychiatrists and that published by clinical psychologists, tends to create. In both "disciplines" the novices are required to study the natural sciences. Perhaps the physicians have had more scientific training than the average clinical psychologist; hence their offense is greater. The published studies, when examined for rigorous proof and well-controlled data, are rather poor. If the training has been in science, there has been too little transfer of training into practice. For the dozens of studies which can be cited in refutation of such a judgment, there are hundreds in which the stricture fits.

We continue the process of "stereotype manufacturing." One clinician draws for us a picture of the schizophrenogenic mother; another provides us with "typical" prepsychotic personalities (on the basis of a study of ten patients) for the manic-depressives he has studied. The sociologist is capable of stereotyping the slum ghetto from which schizophrenics emerge at higher than normal rates, until we are convinced we grasp an interacting system that is pathogenic, even though the free-wheeling picture is drawn in the armchair. Franz Alexander gave us a "gastric personality," and others have given us accident-prone personalities, cardiac personalities, asthenic and pyknic personalities; each of these stereotypes has circulated widely. It is easier to perceive with a stereotype, even if it falsifies the evidence; we seize on such short-cuts. So the convinced typologist who believes that his "seeing eye" can spot a manic-depressive or a schizophrenic at a hundred paces (as soon as he can size up his physique) has no need of facts: they will only confuse him.

In spite of the slow march of science, the literature of the abnormal is enough to teach us that we are still in the Dark Ages. This is not a bright and shining Age of Enlightenment, yet. Even Arnold Toynbee, without ever having studied this lunatic fringe at close hand, can conclude that our deviants have something important to say for our time, a "judgment" to make upon our civilization. The scientific crust that forms on our half-baked culture is still quite thin. The best of us can fall through. Perhaps the greatest lesson to be learned from the study of abnormal personalities is scientific humility.

BIBLIOGRAPHY

Dates cited in the text for references are those of original publication. However, if more than one edition of the book is listed below, the page numbers in the text refer to the last (or English-language) edition listed. Some exceptions to this rule are indicated for specific books.

Abraham, Karl. *Selected Papers on Psychoanalysis.* Hogarth, 1927.

Abrahams, Joseph, and Edith Varon. *Maternal Dependency and Schizophrenia.* International University Press, 1953.

Abse, D. Willard. "Hysteria," in Arieti 1959, pp. 272-292.

Ackerly, S. Spafford, and Arthur Benton. "Report of a case of bilateral frontal lobe defect," *Proc. Assn. Res. nerv. ment. Dis.,* 28 (1948), 479ff.

Adams, Brooks. *The Degradation of the Democratic Dogma.* Macmillan, 1920.

Adler, Alfred. *Understanding Human Nature.* Greenberg, 1927.

Aichorn, August. *Verwahrloste Jugend.* Wiener Psychanalytischer Verlag, 1925. *Wayward Youth.* Viking, 1935.

Aiken, Lewis R., Jr. *General Psychology: A Survey.* Chandler, 1968.

Ainsworth, Mary D., R. G. Andry, R. G. Harlow, S. Lebovici, M. Mead, D. G. Prug, and B. Wootton. *Deprivation of Maternal Care: A Reassessment of Its Effects.* World Health Organization, 1962.

Alanen, Yrjö O. *The Mothers of Schizophrenic Patients.* Munksgaard, 1958.

Aldrich, C. A., and M. M. Aldrich. *Babies Are Human Beings.* Macmillan, 1938.

Alexander, Franz. "The neurotic character," *Int. J. Psychoanal.,* 2 (1930), 292-311.

———. "Emotional factors in essential hypertension," *J. psychosom. Med.,* 1 (1939a), 175ff.

———. "Psychoanalytic study of a case of essential hypertension," *J. psychosom. Med.,* 1 (1939b), 139-152.

———. *Our Age of Unreason.* Lippincott, 1942.

———. "Fundamental concepts of psychosomatic research," *J. psychosom. Med.,* 5 (1943), 205-210.

———. *Fundamentals of Psychoanalysis.* Norton, 1948.

Alexander, Franz, and T. M. French. *Psychoanalytic Therapy.* Ronald, 1946.

Alexander, Franz, and Sydney Portis. "A psychosomatic study of hypoglycaemic fatigue," *J. psychosom. Med.,* 6 (1944), 191-206.

Alexander, Franz, and Helen Ross, eds. *Dynamic Psychiatry.* University of Chicago Press, 1952.

Alexander, Franz, and Thomas Szasz. "The psychosomatic approach to medicine," in Alexander and Ross 1952.

Allen, C., and C. Berg. *The Problem of Homosexuality*. Citadel, 1958.

Allen, Edgar, ed. *Sex and Internal Secretions*. Williams and Wilkins, 1939.

Allport, Floyd. *Social Psychology*. Houghton Mifflin, 1924.

Allport, Gordon W. *Becoming: Basic Considerations for a Psychology of Personality*. Yale University Press, 1955.

Alström, C. H. "A study of epilepsy in its clinical, social, and genetic aspects," *Acta Psychiat. Neurol.*, suppl. 63 (1950), 1-284.

Altmann, M., E. Knowles, and H. D. Bull. "A psychosomatic study of the sex cycle in women," *J. psychosom. Med.*, 3 (1941), 199-225.

Alvarez, Walter C. "The 'little strokes,'" *New England med. J.*, 246 (1952), 155ff.

_____. *Little Strokes*. Register and Tribune Syndicate, 1960.

American Psychiatric Association. *Diagnostic and Statistical Manual of Mental Disorders*. 2nd ed. Washington, D.C., 1968.

Ames, Frances. "A clinical and metabolic study of acute intoxication with cannabis sativa," *J. ment. Sci.*, 104 (1958), 972-999.

Anderson, O. D., and Richard Parmenter. "A long-term study of the experimental neurosis in the sheep and the dog," *Psychosom. Med. Monogr.*, 2, nos. 3 and 4 (1941), 1-150.

Anderson, O. D., Richard Parmenter, and H. S. Liddell. "Some cardiovascular manifestations of the experimental neurosis in sheep," *J. psychosom. Med.*, 1 (1939), 93-104.

Angyal, Andras. *Foundations for a Science of the Personality*. Commonwealth Fund, 1941.

_____. *Neurosis and Treatment: A Holistic Theory*. Wiley, 1965.

Arieti, Silvano, ed. *American Handbook of Psychiatry*. Basic Books, 1959.

_____. "Manic-depressive psychosis," in Arieti 1959, I, 419-454.

_____. "Schizophrenia," in Arieti 1959, I, 455ff.

_____. "Studies of the thought processes in contemporary psychiatry," *Amer. J. Psychiat.*, 120 (1963), 58-64.

Arlow, Jacob. "Identification mechanisms in coronary occlusion," *J. psychosom. Med.*, 7 (1945), 202-209.

Armitage, Stewart G. "An analysis of certain psychological tests used for the evaluation of brain injury," *Psychol. Monogr.*, 59 (1946), 48ff.

Arnold, Matthew. *Culture and Anarchy*. Macmillan, 1905.

Aron, Raymond. *Dimensions de la conscience historique*. Plon, 1961.

Association for Research in Nervous and Mental Diseases. *Heredity in Nervous and Mental Disease*. Hoeber, 1923.

_____. "The frontal lobes," *Proc. Assn. Res. nerv. ment. Dis.*, vol. 28 (1948).

_____. *Neurology and Psychiatry in Childhood*. Williams and Wilkins, 1956.

Aubry, Jenny. *La Carence de soins maternels*. Presses Universitaires de France, 1955.

Augustine, St. *Confessions*. Everyman's, 1907.

Ayllon, T. "Intensive treatment of psychotic behavior by stimulus satiation and food reinforcement," *Behav. Res. Ther.*, 1 (1963), 53-61.

Azima, Hassan, Raul Vispo, and Fern J. Azima. "Observations on anaclitic therapy during sensory deprivation," in Solomon, Kubansky, and Trumbull 1961, pp. 143-160.

Azima, H., E. D. Wittkower, and J. La Tendresse. "Object relations therapy in schizophrenic states," *Amer. J. Psychiat.*, 115 (1958), 60-62.

Babinski, J., and J. Froment. *Hysteria or Pithiatism and Reflex Nervous Disorders in War*. University of London Press, 1917.

Bachrach, A. J., W. J. Erwin, and J. P. Mohr. "The control of eating behavior in an anorexic by operant conditioning techniques," in Ullmann and Krasner 1965.

Bailey, Percival. "The academic lecture," *Amer. J. Psychiat.*, 113 (1956), 387-406.

Bainton, Roland H. *Here I Stand: A Life of Martin Luther.* Abingdon, 1950.

Baldwin, Alfred L., Joan Klahorn, and Fay Breese Huffman. "Patterns of parent behavior," *Psychol. Monogr.,* vol. 58, no. 3 (1945).

—————. "The appraisal of parent behavior,"*Psychol. Monogr.,* vol. 63, no. 4 (1949).

Baldwin, Monica. *The Called and the Chosen.* Farrar, Strauss, and Cudahy, 1957.

Barbusse, Henri. *L'Enfer.* Albin Michel, 1908.

Barker, Roger C., Jacob S. Kounin, and Herbert F. Wright. *Child Behavior and Development.* McGraw-Hill, 1943.

Barker, Wayne. "Studies on epilepsy: The petit mal attack," *J. psychosom. Med.,* 10 (1948a), 73-94.

—————. "Personality pattern, situational stress, and symptoms of narcolepsy," *J. psychosom. Med.,* 10 (1948b), 193-292.

Barry, Herbert. "Significance of maternal bereavement before eight in psychiatric patients," *Arch. Neurol. Psychiat.,* 62 (1949), 630ff.

Barry, Herbert, and E. Lindemann. "Critical ages for maternal bereavement in psychoneuroses," *J. psychosom. Med.,* 22 (1960), 166ff.

Bartlett, F. C. S. *Remembering.* Macmillan, 1932.

Baruk, Henri. "Early experiments leading to a chemical concept of psychosis," in Rinkel and Denber 1958.

Beach, F. A. "Instinctive behavior," in Stevens 1951.

—————, *et al.,* eds., *The Neuropsychology of Lashley.* McGraw-Hill, 1960.

Beard, George M. "Neurasthenia, or nervous exhaustion," *Boston med. surg. J.,* new series 3 (1869), 217ff.

—————. *American Nervousness, with Its Causes and Consequences.* 1880a.

—————. *A Practical Treatise on Nervous Exhaustion.* 1880b.

Beck, A. T., and Marvin Hurvich. "Psychological correlates of depression," *J. psychosom. Med.,* 21 (1959), 50-55.

Beck, A. T., Clyde H. Ward, and Edward Rascoe. "Typical dreams," *Arch. gen. Psychiat.,* 5 (1961), 606-615.

Beck, A. T., C. H. Ward, M. Mendelson, J. Mock, and J. Erbaugh. "An inventory for measuring depression," *Arch. gen. Psychiat.,* 4 (1961), 561-571.

Beers, Clifford. *A Mind That Found Itself.* Longmans, Green, 1908.

Bellak, Leopold. *Dementia Praecox.* Grune and Stratton, 1948.

—————. *Manic-Depressive Psychoses and Allied Conditions.* Grune and Stratton, 1952.

Benda, C. E. *Mongolism and Cretinism.* Grune and Stratton, 1946.

Bender, Lauretta. "Childhood schizophrenia," *Amer. J. Orthopsychiat.,* 17 (1947), 40-56.

—————. "Anxiety in disturbed children," in Hoch and Zubin 1950, pp. 119-139.

—————. *Aggression, Hostility and Anxiety in Children.* Thomas, 1953.

—————. *A Dynamic Psychopathology of Childhood.* Thomas, 1954.

—————. "Schizophrenia in childhood: Its recognition, description, and treatment," *Amer. J. Orthopsychiat.,* 26 (1956), 499-506.

Bender, Lauretta, and A. M. Freedman. "A study of the first three years in the maturation of schizophrenic children," *Quart. J. Child Behav.,* 4 (1952), 245-271.

Bender, Lauretta, and Alvin Grugett. "A study of certain epidemiological factors in a group of children with childhood schizophrenia," *Amer. J. Orthopsychiat.,* 26 (1956), 131-143.

Bender, Lauretta, and Saul Gurewitz. "Results of psychotherapy with young schizophrenic children," *Amer. J. Orthopsychiat.,* 25 (1955), 162-170.

Bender, Lauretta, and William Helme. "A quantitative test of theory and diagnostic indications of childhood schizophrenia," *Arch. Neurol. Psychiat.,* 70 (1953), 413-445.

Benedek, Therese. *Psychosexual Functions in Women.* Ronald, 1952.

Benedek, Therese, and Boris B. Rubenstein. "The correlations between ovarian activity and psychodynamic processes," *J. psychosom. Med.*, 1, no. 2 (April 1939), 245-271; same title, *J. psychosom. Med.*, 1, no. 4 (October 1939), 461-485.

Benedict, Ruth. *Patterns of Culture.* Pelican, 1934.

Benjamin, John. "Some considerations in biological research in schizophrenia," *J. psychosom. Med.*, 20 (1958), 427-445.

Bennett, A. M. "Sensory deprivation in aviation," in Solomon, Kubansky, and Trumbull 1961, pp. 161-173.

Bercel, Nicholas. "A study of the influence of schizophrenic serum on the behavior of the spider zilla-x-notata," in Jackson 1960.

Berger, Ralph J. "Experimental modification of dream content by meaningful verbal stimuli," *Brit J. Psychiat.*, 109 (1963), 722-740.

Bergler, Edmund. *The Battle of Conscience.* Wash. Inst. of Med., 1946.

Bergman, P., and Sybille K. Escalona. "Unusual sensitivities in very young children," in Eissler *et al.* 1949, III, 333-352.

Bernard, L. L. *Instinct.* Holt, 1924.

Bettelheim, Bruno. *Love is Not Enough.* Free Press, 1950.

————. *Truants from Life.* Free Press, 1955.

————. "Schizophrenia as a reaction to extreme situations," *Amer. J. Orthopsychiat.*, 26 (1956), 507-518.

————. *The Informed Heart.* Free Press, 1960.

Bieber, I., Toby B. Bieber, H. J. Dain, P. R. Dince, M. Drellich, H. Grand, R. Gundlach, Malvina Kremer, A. Rivkin, and Cornelia B. Wilbur, eds. *Homosexuality.* Basic Books, 1962.

Binger, C. A., N. W. Ackerman, A. E. Cohn, H. A. Schroder, and J. M. Steele. "Personality in arterial hypertension," *Psychosom. Med. Monogr.*, vol. 4, no. 8 (1945).

Binzwanger, Ludwig. "Traum und Existenz" (1930); *Le Rêve et l'existence.* Desclée de Brouwer, 1954.

————. *Schizophrénie.* Neske, 1957; *Le Cas Suzanne Urban: Étude sur la schizophrénie.* Desclée de Brouwer, 1957.

Bleuler, Eugen. *Dementia Praecox oder die Gruppe der Schizophrenen*, 1911. *Dementia Praecox: The Group of Schizophrenias*, trans. by Joseph Zinken. International University Press, 1950.

————. *Das Autistisch-Undiziplinierte Denken in der Medizin und Seine Überwindung.* Springer, 1927.

Bleuler, Manfred. "Schizophrenia: Review of the work of Prof. Eugen Bleuler," *Arch. Neurol. Psychiat.*, 26 (1931), 610-627.

Bliss, Eugene, and C. H. Hardin Branch. *Anorexia Nervosa.* Hoeber, 1960.

Block, H., E. Harvey, H. Jennings, and E. Simpson. "Clinicians' conceptions of the asthmatogenic mother," *Arch. gen. Psychiat.*, 15 (1966), 610-619.

Boisen, A. T. *The Exploration of the Inner World.* Willet, Clark, 1936.

Bolles, Mary M., and Kurt Goldstein. "A study of impairment of abstract behavior in schizophrenic patients," *Psychiat. Quart.*, 12 (1938), 42ff.

Bolt, Robert. *A Man for All Seasons.* Random House, 1966.

Bonaparte, Marie. *De la Sexualité de la femme.* Presses Universitaires de France, 1951.

Bonaparte, Marie, Anna Freud, and Ernst Kris, eds. *Sigmund Freud's Letters: The Origins of Psychoanalysis.* Basic Books, 1954.

Bond, Earl D. "Recovery from a long neurosis," *Psychiat.*, 15 (1952), 161-177.

Bone, Edith. *Seven Years Solitary.* Hamish Hamilton, 1957.

Bourget, Paul. *Le Disciple.* 1889.

Boutonier, Juliette. *L'Angoisse.* Presses Universitaires de France, 1949.

————. *Les Défaillances de la volonté.* Presses Universitaires de France, 1951.

Boveri, Margret. *Treason in the Twentieth Century.* Putnam, 1961.

Bowlby, John. *Maternal Care and Mental Health.* World Health Organization, 1952.
———. *Child Care and the Growth of Love.* Heath, 1953a.
———. "Some pathological processes set in train by early mother-child separation," *J. ment. Sci.,* 99 (1953b), 265-272.
———. "Childhood mourning and its implications for psychiatry," *Amer. J. Psychiat.,* 118 (1961a), 481-498.
———. "Separation anxiety: A critical review of the literature," *Psychol. Psychiat.,* 1 (1961b), 251-269.
Bowlby, John, M. D. Ainsworth, M. Boston, and Rosenbluth. "The effects of mother-child separation: A follow-up study," *Brit. J. med. Psychol.,* 29 (1961), 211-240.
Brenman, Margaret, and Merton Gill. *Hypnotherapy.* International University Press, 1947.
Breuer, Joseph, and Sigmund Freud. *Studien über Hysterie,* 1895; *Studies in Hysteria,* trans. by A. A. Brill, *Nerv. ment. Dis. Monogr.,* 1937. Also available in Freud, *Collected Papers,* vol. III.
Brickner, Richard M. *The Intellectual Functions of the Frontal Lobes.* Macmillan, 1936.
———. "A human cortical area producing repetitive phenomena when stimulated," *J. Neurophysiol.,* 3 (1940), 128-130.
———. "Brain of patient A after bilateral frontal lobectomy: Status of the frontal lobe problem," *Arch. Neurol. Psychiat.,* 68 (1952), 293-313.
Brickner, Richard M., Albert A. Rosner, and Ruth Munro. "Physiological aspects of the obsessive state," *J. psychosom. Med.,* 2 (1940), 369-383.
Bridger, Wagner, Beverly Birns, and Marion Blank. "A comparison of behavioral ratings and heart rate measurements in human neonates," *J. psychosom. Med.,* 27 (1965), 123-134.
Briffault, Robert. *Sin and Sex.* Macauley, 1931.
Brill, A. A., ed. *The Basic Writings of Sigmund Freud.* Modern Library, 1938a.
———. *Lectures on Psychoanalytic Psychiatry.* Knopf, 1938b.
Brill, Henry. "Postencephalitic psychiatric conditions," in Arieti 1959.
Brinton, Crane. *Nietzsche.* Harvard University Press, 1941.
———. *Ideas and Men.* Prentice-Hall, 1950.
British Medical Journal. "Disciplinary treatments of shell shock: Abstracts of notes from the German and Austrian journals," *Brit. med. J.,* 2 (1916), 882ff.
———. "Editorial: The ethics of leucotomy," 2 (1952), 909.
Brody, E. B., and F. C. Redlich, eds. *Psychotherapy with Schizophrenics.* International University Press, 1952.
Brody, Sylvia. *Patterns of Mothering.* International University Press, 1956.
Brooks, Van Wyck, and Charles Van Wyck Brooks, trans. *The Private Journal of Henri Frédéric Amiel.* Macmillan, 1935.
Brown, Felix. "The bodily complaint: A study of hypochondriasis," *J. ment. Sci.,* 82 (1936), 1-65.
———. "Heredity in psychoneuroses," *Proc. Royal Soc. Med.,* 35 (1942), 785-790.
———. "Depression and childhood bereavement," *J. ment. Sci.,* 107 (1961), 754ff.
Bruch, Hilde. "Obesity in childhood, III: Physiologic and psychologic aspects of the food intake of obese children," *Amer. J. Dis. Childh.,* 59 (1940), 739-778.
———. "Obesity in childhood and personality development," *Amer. J. Orthopsychiat.,* 11 (1941), 467-474.
———. "Psychological aspects of obesity," *Psychiat.,* 10 (1947), 373-381.
———. "Psychological aspects of reducing," *J. psychosom. Med.,* 14 (1952), 337-347.
———. *The Importance of Overweight.* Norton, 1957.
Bruch, Hilde, and G. Touraine. "The family frame of obese children," *J. psychosom. Med.,* 2 (1940), 181-206.
Bruetsch, Walter. "Neurosyphilitic conditions," in Arieti 1959, II, 1003-1020.

Bruner, Jerome. *On Knowing: Essays for the Left Hand.* Belknap Press of Harvard University Press, 1962.

Bumke, O., ed. *Handbuch der Geisteskranken.* Springer, 1928.

Bunney, W. E., E. L. Hartmann, and J. W. Mason. "Study of a patient with 48-hour manic-depressive cycles, II: Strong positive correlation between endocrine factors and manic defense patterns," *Arch. gen. Psychiat.,* 12, no. 6 (1965), 619-625.

Bunzel, Ruth. "Introduction to Zuñi ceremonialism," Forty-Seventh Annual Report of the Bureau of Ethnology (1929-1930), 467-545.

Cain, Jacques. *Le Problème des névroses expérimentales.* Desclée de Brouwer, 1959.

Cameron, Norman. "Reasoning, regression, and communication in schizophrenics," *Psychol. Rev. Monogr.,* no. 221 (1938).

——————. "Schizophrenic thinking in a problem situation," *J. ment. Sci.,* 85 (1939), 1-24.

——————. "The Functional Psychoses," in Hunt 1944, II, 861-921.

——————. *Personality Development and Psychopathology: A Dynamic Approach.* Houghton Mifflin, 1963.

Cannon, W. B. *Bodily Changes in Pain, Hunger, Fear, and Rage.* Appleton-Century, 1929.

——————. "Voodoo death," *J. psychosom. Med.,* 19 (1957), 182-190.

Cannon, W. B., J. T. Lewis, and S. W. Britton. "The dispensability of the sympathetic division of the autonomic nervous system," *Boston med. surg. J.,* 197 (1927), 514-515.

Caplan, G., ed. *Prevention of Mental Disorders in Childhood.* Basic Books, 1961.

Cattell, J. P. "The dynamics of post-topectomy: Psychotherapy in patients with pseudoneurotic schizophrenia," *Amer. J. Psychiat.,* 109 (1952), 450ff.

Cavan, R. S. *Suicide.* University of Chicago Press, 1932.

Cazeneuve, Jean. *La Psychologie du prisonnier de la guerre.* Presses Universitaires de France, 1945.

Cerletti, U., and L. Bini. "L'Electrochoc," *Arch.-psicol. Neurol. Psichiat.,* 19 (1938), 266ff.

——————. "Old and new information about electroshock," *Amer. J. Psychiat.,* 107 (1950), 87-94.

Chertok, L. *L'Hypnose.* Masson, 1961.

Chertok, L., and M. Cahen. "Facteurs transférentiels en hypnose," *Acta Psychother. psychosom. orthopádag.,* suppl. 3 (1955), 334-342.

Child, C. M. *Physiological Foundations of Behavior.* Holt, 1924.

Chrzanowski, Gerard. "Neurasthenia and hypochondriasis," in Arieti 1959, I, 258-271.

Clark, L. P. "The psychobiologic concept of essential epilepsy," *Proc. Assn. Res. nerv. ment. Dis.,* 7 (1922), 55ff.

——————. "A further contribution to the psychology and psychotherapy of essential epilepsy," *J. nerv. ment. Dis.,* 67 (1926), 63ff.

Cleckley, Hervey. *The Mask of Sanity: An Attempt to Clarify Some Issues about the So-Called Psychopathic Personality.* Mosby, 1950.

——————. "Psychopathic states," in Arieti 1959, I, chap. 28.

Cleveland, Sidney, E. Edward Reitman, and Catherine Bentinck. "Therapeutic effectiveness of sensory deprivation," *Arch. gen. Psychiat.,* 8 (1963), 453-460.

Cobb, Stanley. *Borderlands of Psychiatry.* Harvard University Press, 1943.

——————. "Personalities as affected by lesions of the brain," in Hunt 1944, I, 550-581.

Cohen, Mandel, and Paul White. "Life situations, emotions, and neurocirculatory asthenia," *J. psychosom. Med.,* 13 (1951), 335-357.

Cole, Jonathan O. "The influence of drugs on the individual," in Farber and Wilson 1961, pp. 116ff.

Cole, L. E. "A comparison of the factors of practice and knowledge of experimental procedure in conditioning the eyelid response of human subjects," *J. gen. Psychol.,* 20 (1939a), 349-375.

————. *General Psychology.* McGraw-Hill, 1939b.

————. "Metapsychology and the right to believe," *Amer. J. Orthopsychiat.,* 21 (1951), 461-471.

————. *Human Behavior: Psychology as a Biosocial Science.* World Book, 1953.

Cole, L. E., and William Bruce. *Educational Psychology.* World Book, 1950; rev. ed., 1958.

Committee on Public Health, New York Academy of Sciences. *Homosexuality.* N.Y. Acad. Sci., 1964.

Condee, Ralph. "A case in point: Bedlam at Edinburgh," *The Reporter* (Oct. 11, 1962).

Conrad, K. "Erbanlage und Epilepsie: Untersuchung an einer Serie von 253 Zwillingspaaren," *Z. ges. Neurol. Psychiat.,* 153 (1935), 271-326.

Cook, Stuart. "The production of 'experimental neurosis' in the white rat," *J. psychosom. Med.,* 1 (1939), 293-308.

Courbon, P. "Sur la psychologie de la vieillesse," *J. Psychol.,* 24 (1927), 455-463.

Creak, E. Mildred. "Childhood psychosis," *Brit. J. Psychiat.,* 109 (1963), 84-89.

Crémieux, Albert. *Les Difficultés alimentaires de l'enfant.* Presses Universitaires de France, 1954.

Custance, John. *Wisdom, Madness, and Folly: The Philosophy of a Lunatic.* Pellegrini and Cudahy, 1952.

Dalbiez, Roland. *Psychoanalytical Method and the Doctrine of Freud.* Longmans, Green, 1941.

D'Allonnes, G. Revault. *Psychologie d'une religion.* 1908.

Darmstatter, Herbert J. "The superiority attitude and rigidity of ideas," *Arch. Neurol. Psychiat.,* 61 (1949), 621-643.

Darr, George, and Frederic Worden. "Case report twenty-eight years after an infantile autistic disorder," *Amer. J. Orthopsychiat.,* 21 (1951), 559-568.

Davidson, H. A. "The new war on psychiatry," *Amer. J. Psychiat.,* 121 (1964), 528-534.

Davis, W. Allison. "Child training and social class," in Barker, Kounin, and Wright 1943, 607-620.

————. *Father of the Man.* Houghton Mifflin, 1947.

Davis, W. Allison, and John Dollard. *Children of Bondage.* Amer. Council on Education, 1940.

Davis, W. Allison, and R. J. Havighurst, "Social class and color differences in child-rearing," *Amer. sociol. Rev.,* 11 (1946), 698-710.

Davis, W. L., and R. W. Husband. "A study of hypnotic susceptibility in relation to personality traits," *J. abnorm. soc. Psychol.,* 26 (1931), 175-182.

Dayton, Neil. *New Facts on Mental Disorders.* Thomas, 1940.

De Auriaguerra, J., and G. Bonvalot-Soubiran. "Indications et techniques de rééducation psychomotrice en psychiatrie infantile," in De Auriaguerra, Diatkine, and Lebovici 1959, II, 423-494.

De Auriaguerra, J., R. Diatkine, and S. Lebovici, eds. *La Psychiatrie de l'enfant.* Presses Universitaires de France, 1959, 2 vols.

De Beauvoir, Simone. *Le Deuxième sexe.* Gallimard, 1949, 2 vols; *The Second Sex.* Knopf, 1953.

————. "Faut-il brûler Sade?" *Les Temps modernes* (Dec. 1951 and Jan. 1952); *The Marquis de Sade.* Calder, 1962.

————. *Mémoires d'une jeune fille rangée.* Gallimard, 1956. *Memoirs of a Dutiful Daughter.* World, 1959.

————. *La Force de l'âge.* Gallimard, 1960.

————. *La Force des choses.* Gallimard, 1963.

De Gaultier, Jules. *La Fiction universelle.* 1903.

De Grazia, Sebastian. *Errors of Psychotherapy.* Doubleday, 1952.

————. *Work, Time, and Leisure.* Twentieth-Century Fund, 1962.

Déjerine, J., and E. Gauckler. *Les Manifestations fonctionelles des psychonévroses, leur traitement par la psychothérapie.* Masson, 1911; *The Psychoneuroses and Their Treatment by Psychotherapy.* Lippincott, 1913.

Delay, Jean. *Les Dérèglements de l'humeur.* Presses Universitaires de France, 1946.

————. *Les Dissolutions de la mémoire.* Presses Universitaires de France, 1950.

————. *Aspects de la psychiatrie moderne.* Presses Universitaires de France, 1956a.

————. *La Jeunesse d'André Gide.* Gallimard, vol. I, 1956b; vol. II, 1957.

Demant, V. A. *Christian Sex Ethics.* Hodder and Stoughton, 1963.

Dement, W., and E. Wolpert. "The relation of eye movements, body motility, and external stimuli to dream content," *J. exp. Psychol.,* 55 (1958), 543-553.

Denker, R. "Results of treatment of psychoneuroses by the general practitioner: A follow-up of 500 cases," *N.Y. State J. Med.,* 46 (1946), 2164ff.

De Rougement, Denis. *L'Amour et l'occident.* Plon, 1956.

————. *The Myths of Love.* Faber and Faber, 1963.

Deschamps, Albert. *Les Maladies de l'énergie: Les asthénies générales.* 1908.

————. *Les Maladies de l'esprit et les asthénies.* Alcan, 1919.

Despert, J. L. "Prophylactic aspect of schizophrenia in childhood," *Nerv. Child.,* 1 (1942), 199-231.

Deutsch, A. *The Mentally Ill in America.* Doubleday, 1937.

Deutsch, Helene. *The Psychology of Women.* Grune and Stratton, 1945, 2 vols.

Devereux, George. *Reality and Dream: Psychotherapy of a Plains Indian.* International University Press, 1951.

De Wardener, H. E., and B. Lennox. "Wernicke's encephalopathy," *Lancet,* 252 (1947), 11-17.

Diamond, Edwin. *The Science of Dreams.* Doubleday, 1962.

Diem, O. "Die psycho-neurotische erbliche Balastung der Geistesgesunden und der Geisteskranken," *Arch. Rassen u. Ges. Biol.,* 2 (1905), 215-236; summarized and evaluated in *Assn. Res. nerv. ment. Dis.* 1923.

Diethelm, Oskar. "Epileptic convulsions and the personality setting," *Arch. Neurol. Psychiat.,* 31 (1934), 755-767.

————. "A historical review of psychiatric treatment," *J. psychosom. Med.,* 3 (1941), 286-294.

————. *Treatment in Psychiatry.* Thomas, 1950.

————. *Etiology of Chronic Alcoholism.* Thomas, 1955.

Dollard, J., and N. E. Miller. *Personality and Psychotherapy.* McGraw-Hill, 1950.

Domarus, V. E., "Zur Theorie des schizophrenen Denken," *Z. ges. Neurol. Psychiat.,* 108 (1927), 703-714.

Domhoff, B., and J. Kamiya. "Problems in dream content study with objective indicators," *Arch. gen. Psychiat.,* 11 (1964), 519-533.

Donnelly, John. "Aspects of the psychodynamics of the psychopath," *Amer. J. Psychiat.,* 120 (1964), 1149-1154.

Dostoevsky, Fyodor. *Idiót (The Idiot),* 1868. Modern Library, 1935.

————. *Bésy (The Possessed),* 1872. Modern Library, 1936.

Douvan, E., and J. Adelson. "The psychodynamics of social mobility in adolescent boys," *J. abnorm. soc. Psychol.,* 56 (1958), 31-44.

Dragstedt, L. R. "Peptic ulcer—an abnormality in the mechanism of gastric secretion," *Bull. Alumni Assn. Northwestern Univ. Med. School,* 14 (1958), 2-5.

Drake, St. Clair, and Horace Cayton. *Black Metropolis.* Harcourt, Brace, 1945.

Draper, G. *Disease and the Man.* Kegan Paul, 1930.

Dreyfus, G. L. *Die Melancholie: Ein Zustandbild des Manisch-Depressiven Irreseins,* 1907.

Dublin, Louis. *Suicide*. Ronald, 1963.

Dubos, René. *Medical Utopias*. Daedalus, 1959.

―――――. *The Dreams of Reason*. Columbia University Press, 1961.

Dunbar, Flanders. *Emotions and Bodily Changes*. 2nd ed.; Columbia University Press, 1938.

―――――. *Mind and Body: Psychosomatic Medicine*. Random House, 1947.

Duncan, Charles, Ian P. Stevenson, and Harold G. Wolff. "Life situations, emotions, and exercise tolerance," *J. psychosom. Med.*, 13 (1951), 36-50.

Dunlap, Charles B. "Dementia praecox: Some preliminary observations on brains from carefully selected cases, and a consideration of certain sources of error," *Amer. J. Psychiat.*, 81 (1924), 403-421.

Dunn, William H. "Emotional factors in neurocirculatory asthenia," *J. psychosom. Med.*, 4 (1942), 353ff.

Durant, Will, and Ariel Durant. *The Story of Civilization, IV: The Age of Faith*. Simon and Schuster, 1950.

Duycaerts, F. *La Notion de normal en psychologie clinique*. Vrin, 1954.

Eaton, Joseph, and Robert Weil. *Culture and Mental Disorders*. Free Press, 1955.

Ebin, David, ed. *The Drug Experience*. Orion, 1961.

Edwards, Allen E., and Loren E. Acker. "A demonstration of the long-term retention of a conditioned GSR," *J. psychosom. Med.*, 24 (1962), 459-463.

Eisenberg, Leo. "The fathers of autistic children," *Amer. J. Orthopsychiat.*, 27 (1957), 715-724.

Eisenberg, L., and L. Kanner. "Early infantile autism, 1943-1955," *Amer. J. Orthopsychiat.*, 26 (1956), 556-566.

Eissler, K. R., ed. *Searchlights on Delinquency: New Psychoanalytic Studies*. International University Press, 1949.

Eissler, Ruth S., Anna Freud, Heinz Hartmann, and Ernst Kris, eds. *Psychoanalytic Studies of Children*. International University Press: vol. I, 1945; vol. II, 1946; vols. III and IV, 1949; vol. V, 1950; vol. VI, 1951; vol. VII, 1952; vol. VIII, 1953; vol. IX, 1954; vol. X, 1955.

Eitinger, Leo. "Concentration-camp survivors in the post-war world," *Amer. J. Orthopsychiat.*, 32 (1962), 367-375.

Ekstein, R. "The space child's time machine: On 'reconstruction' in the psychotherapeutic treatment of a schizophrenoid child," *Amer. J. Orthopsychiat.*, 24 (1954), 492-506.

―――――. "Special training problems in psychotherapeutic work with psychotic and borderline children," *Amer. J. Orthopsychiat.*, 32 (1962), 569-581.

Eliade, Mircea. *Le Yoga: Immortalité et liberté*. Payot, 1954.

Elliott, K. A. C., and W. Bremner. "A program for prefrontal lobotomy with report of effect on intractable pain," *Ottawa Dept. of Veterans Affairs Treatment Service Bull.* 3 (1948), 26-35.

Erikson, Erik H. *Childhood and Society*. Norton, 1950.

―――――. "The problem of ego identity," *J. Amer. psychoanal. Assn.*, 4 (1956), 4ff.

―――――. *Young Man Luther*. Norton, 1962.

―――――. *Insight and Responsibility*. Norton, 1964.

Escalona, Sibylle K. "Some considerations regarding psychotherapy with psychotic children," *Bull. Menninger Clin.*, 12 (1948), 126-134.

Escover, Harold, Sidney Malitz, and Barnard Wilkins. "Clinical profiles of paid normal subjects volunteering for hallucinogenic drug studies," *Amer. J. Psychiat.*, 117 (1961), 910-915.

Esquirol, Jean Étienne Dominique. *Oeuvres*, vol. I, 1838; *Mental Maladies: A Treatise on Insanity*, trans. by E. K. Hunt, 1845.

Essen-Möller, E. "Psychiatrische Untersuchungen an einer Serie von Zwillingen," *Acta Psychiat. Neurol.*, supp. 23 (1941).

Estes, Hubert R., Clarice Haylett, and Adelaide M. Johnson. "Separation anxiety," *Amer. J. Psychother.,* 10 (1956), 682-695.

Evans-Pritchard, E. E. *Witchcraft, Oracles, and Magic Among the Azande.* Oxford University Press, 1937.

Ewalt, J. T., G. C. Randall, and Harry Morris. "The phantom limb," *J. psychosom. Med.,* 9 (1947), 118-123.

Ey, Henri. *Études psychiatriques.* Desclée de Brouwer: vol. I, 1948; vol. II, 1950; vol. III, 1954.

———. "Unity and diversity of schizophrenia: Clinical and logical analysis of the concept of schizophrenia," *Amer. J. Psychiat.,* 115 (1959), 706-714.

———. "The reality of mental disease and the disease of reality," *J. comprehensive Psychiat.,* 1 (1960), 2-7.

Ey, Henri, P. Bernard, and C. Brisset. *Manuel de psychiatrie.* Masson, 1963.

Eysenck, H. J. *Dimensions of the Personality.* Kegan Paul, 1947.

———. "The effects of psychotherapy," *J. consult. Psychol.,* 16 (1952), 319-324.

———. *Behavior Therapy and the Neuroses.* Pergamon, 1960.

———. *The Effects of Psychotherapy.* International Science Press, 1966.

Eysenck, H. J., and D. B. Prell. "The inheritance of neuroticism: An experimental study," *J. ment. Sci.,* 97 (1951), 441-465.

Eysenck, H. J., and S. Rachman. *The Causes and Cures of Neurosis.* Routledge and Kegan Paul, 1965.

Farber, Leslie, and Charles Fisher. "An experimental approach to dream psychology through the use of hypnosis," in Tomkins 1943.

Farber, Seymour, and Roger H. Wilson, eds. *Control of the Mind.* McGraw-Hill, 1961.

Farberow, N. L. "Personality patterns of suicidal mental hospital patients," *Genet. Psychol. Monogr.,* 42 (1950), 3-80.

Faris, Robert E. L. "Demography of urban psychotics with special reference to schizophrenics," *Amer. sociol. Rev.,* 3 (1938), 203-209.

———. *The Ecological Study of Insanity in the City.* University of Chicago Press, 1939.

———. "Ecological factors in human behavior," in Hunt 1944, I, 736-760.

Faris, Robert E. L., and W. Dunham. *Mental Disorders in Urban Areas.* University of Chicago Press, 1939.

Farrar, Clarence B. "Suicide," *J. clin. exp. Psychopathol.,* 12 (1951), 83ff.

Faulkner, William B. "Severe esophageal spasm," *J. psychosom. Med.,* 2 (1940), 139-140.

Federn, Paul. "Discussion of Rosen's paper," *Psychiat. Quart.,* 21 (1947), 23ff.

———. *Ego Psychology and the Psychoses.* Basic Books, 1952.

Feldberg, Wilhelm S. "Catatonia, anesthesia, and sleeplike conditions," in Rinkel and Denber 1958, pp. 277-291.

Fenichel, Otto. *The Psychoanalytic Theory of Neurosis.* Norton, 1945.

Ferraro, Armando, "Senile psychoses" 1959a, in Arieti 1959.

———. "Psychoses with cerebral arteriosclerosis" 1959b, in Arieti 1959.

Ferster, C. B. "Positive reinforcement and behavioral deficits of autistic children," *Child Develpm.,* 32 (1961), 437ff.

Ferster, C. B., and M. de Meyer. "A method for the experimental analysis of the behavior of autistic children," *Amer. J. Orthopsychiat.,* 32 (1962), 89-98.

Field, Margaret J. *Religion and Medicine of the Ga People.* Oxford University Press, 1937.

———. "Witchcraft as a primitive interpretation of mental disorder." *J. ment. Sci.,* 101 (1955), 827-833.

———. "Mental disorder in rural Ghana," *J. ment. Sci.,* 104 (1958), 1043-1051.

Finan, John. "Effects of frontal lobe lesions on temporally organized behavior in monkeys," *J. Neurophysiol.,* 2 (1939), 208-226.

————. "Delayed response with pre-delay reinforcement in monkeys after the removal of the frontal lobe," *J. Amer. Psychol.*, 55 (1942) 202-214.

Fink, P. J., M. J. Goldman, and I. Lyons, "Morning glory seed psychosis," *Arch. gen. Psychiat.*, 15 (1966), 209-213.

Fish, Barbara, Theodore Shapiro, Florence Halpern, and Renee Wile. "The prediction of schizophrenia in infancy, III: A ten-year follow-up report of neurological and psychological development," *Amer. J. Psychiat.*, 121 (1965), 765-768.

Fish, F. J. "The classification of schizophrenia: The views of Kleist and his coworkers," *J. ment. Sci.*, 103 (1957), 443-463.

Fisher, C. "Psychoanalytic implications of recent research on sleep and dreaming: I— Empirical findings; II—Implications for psychoanalytic theory," *J. Amer. psychoanal. Assn.*, 13 (1965), 197-203.

Fleck, Stephen, Theodore Lidz, and Alice Cornelison. "Comparison of parent-child relationships of male and female schizophrenic patients," *Arch. gen. Psychiat.*, 8 (1963), 1-7.

Flournoy, Th. *Des Indes à la planète Mars*, 1898; *From India to the Planet Mars*. University Books, 1963.

————. *Esprits et médiums*. Kündig, 1911.

Foss, B. M., ed. *Determinants of Infant Behavior*. Methuen, 1963.

Frankl, Viktor E. *Ärztliche Seelsorge*. Denticke, 1946. *The Doctor and the Soul*. Knopf, 1959.

————. *Die Psychotherapie der Praxis*. Denticke, 1947.

————. *Theorie und Therapie der Neurosen*: *Einfürung in Logotherapie und Existenzanalyse*. Urban und Schwartzenberg, 1956; *Man's Search for Meaning*: *An Introduction to Logotherapy*. Hodder and Stoughton, 1964.

————. *From Death Camp to Existentialism*: *A Psychiatrist's Path to a New Therapy*. Beacon, 1959.

————. "Beyond self-actualization and self-expression," *J. exist. Psychiat.*, 1 (1960), 5-20.

Franz, S. I. *Persons One and Three*. McGraw-Hill, 1933.

Freedman, Paul. "Sexual deviations," in Arieti 1959.

Freeman, Walter. "Symptomatic epilepsy in one of identical twins," *J. Neurol. Psychopath.*, 15 (1935), 210-218.

————. "Psychosurgery," in Arieti 1959, II, 1521-1540.

————. "Review of psychiatric progress in 1963: Psychosurgery," *Amer. J. Psychiat.*, 120 (1964), 648-650.

Freeman, Walter, and James W. Watts. "Some observations on obsessive ruminative tendencies following interruption of the frontal association pathways," *Bull. Los Angeles neurol. Soc.*, 3 (1938), 51-66.

————. "The frontal lobes and consciousness of the self," *J. psychosom. Med.*, 3 (1941), 111ff.

————. *Psychosurgery*. Thomas, 1942.

————. "Prefrontal lobotomy," *Amer. J. Psychiat.*, 99 (1943), 798-806.

French, T. M., and Franz Alexander. "Psychogenic factors in bronchial asthma," *Psychosom. Med. Monogr.*, 1941.

Freud, Anna. *Psychoanalysis for Teachers and Parents*. Emerson, 1947.

Freud, Sigmund. "Die Abwehr Neurosen," 1894; "The defense neuro-psychoses," in *Collected Papers*, I, 59-75.

————. *The Interpretation of Dreams*, 1896. 3rd ed.; Allen and Unwin, 1913.

————. "Fragment of an analysis of a case of hysteria" 1905a, in *Collected Papers*,

————. "Drei Abhandlungen zur Sexualtheorie," 1950b; "Three contributions to the theory of sex," *Nerv. ment. Dis. Monogr.*, 1930.

————. "Analysis of a phobia in a five-year-old boy: The case of little Hans," 1909, in *Collected Papers*, III, 149-295.

————. "Psychoanalytical notes upon an autobiographical account of a case of paranoia," 1911, in *Collected Papers,* III, 390-472.

————. "Über einige Übereinstimmungen im Seelenleben der Wilden und der Neurotiker," 1912; "Totem and taboo," in Brill 1938a, pp. 807-931.

————. "The history of the psychoanalytic movement," 1914, in Brill 1938a, pp. 933-977.

————. "Mourning and melancholia," 1917, in *Collected Papers,* IV, chap. 8.

————. *Jenseits des Lust Prinzips,* 1920; *Beyond the Pleasure Principle,* Liveright, 1950.

————. *Selbstdarstellung,* 1925; *An Autobiographical Study.* Hogarth, 1935.

————. *Hemmung, Symptem, und Angst.* Internationaler Psychanalytischer Verlag, 1926; *The Problem of Anxiety.* Norton, 1936.

————. "Dostoevsky and parricide," 1928a, in *Collected Papers,* V, 222-243.

————. *The Future of an Illusion,* 1928b. Liveright, 1949.

————. *Das Unbehagen in der Kultur,* 1930; *Civilization and Its Discontents,* trans. by Joan Riviere. Hogarth, 1949.

————. *Neue Folge der Vorlesungen für Einführung in die Psychanalyse,* 1933; *New Introductory Lectures.* Norton, 1933.

————. *Der Mann Moses und die Monotheistische Religion,* 1937; *Moses and Monotheism.* Hogarth, 1939.

————. *Abriss der Psycho-analyse,* 1940; *An Outline of Psychoanalysis.* Norton, 1949.

————. *Collected Papers.* Hogarth, 1950.

Freud, Sigmund, and Oskar Pfister. *Psychoanalysis and Faith.* Basic Books, 1963.

Freyhan, Fritz. "Bleuler's concept of the schizophrenias," *Amer. J. Psychiat.,* 114 (1958), 769-779.

Friedan, Betty. *The Feminine Mystique.* Norton, 1963.

Fromm, Erich. *Escape from Freedom.* Farrar and Rinehart, 1941.

————. *Man For Himself.* Rinehart, 1947.

————. *The Forgotten Language.* Rinehart, 1951.

————. *The Sane Society.* Rinehart, 1955.

————. *The Mission of Sigmund Freud: An Analysis of His Personality and Influence.* Harper, 1959.

————. *May Man Prevail?* Doubleday, 1961.

Fromm-Reichmann, Frieda. "Transference problems in schizophrenics," *Psychoanal. Quart.,* 8 (1939), 412-426.

————. "Remarks on the philosophy of mental disorder," *Psychiat.,* 9 (1946), 293-308.

————. *Principles of Intensive Psychotherapy.* University of Chicago Press, 1950.

————. "Some aspects of psychoanalytic psychotherapy with schizophrenics," in Brody and Redlich 1952.

————. "Basic problems in the psychotherapy of schizophrenia," *Psychiat.,* 21 (1958), 1ff.

Fuller, Dorothy S. "A schizophrenic behavior pattern in a child with brain injury," *Bull. Menninger Clin.,* 18 (1954), 52-58.

Fuller, John L., and W. Robert Thompson. *Behavior Genetics.* Wiley, 1960.

Fulton, John F. *Frontal Lobotomy and Affective Behavior.* Norton, 1951.

Fulton, J. F., and C. F. Jacobsen. "The functions of the frontal lobes: A comparative study in monkeys, chimpanzees, and man," *Advances in mod. Biol.* (Moscow), 4 (1935), 113-123.

Gandhi, Mahatma. *Guide de la santé.* Fournier, 1949.

————. *Letters to a Disciple.* Harper, 1950.

Gantt, W. Horseley. "Principles of nervous breakdown—schizokinesis and autokinesis," in Miner 1953, pp. 143-163.

Gantt, W. H., and W. C. Hoffmann. "Conditioned cardiorespiratory changes accompanying conditioned food reflexes," *Amer. J. Physiol.*, 129, no. 2 (1940), 360ff.

Garcia, Blanche, and Mary A. Sarvis. "Evaluation and treatment planning for autistic children," *Arch. gen. Psychiat.*, 10 (1964), 530-541.

Gautier, Théophile. "Hemp," in Ebin 1961.

Gellhorn, Ernst. "Factors modifying conditioned reactions and their relation to the autonomic nervous system," 1953a, in Miner 1953, pp. 200-213.

————. *Physiological Foundations of Neurology and Psychiatry.* University of Minnesota Press, 1953b.

Gellhorn, Ernst, and G. N. Loofburrow. *Emotions and Emotional Disorders.* Hoeber, 1963.

Gerard, D. L., and L. G. Houston. "Family setting and the social ecology of schizophrenia," *Psychiat. Quart.*, 27 (1953), 90-91.

German, G. A. "The effect of serum from schizophrenics on evoked cortical potentials in the rat," *Brit. J. Psychiat.*, 109 (1963), 616-623.

Gesell, Arnold, Catherine Amatruda, Burton Castner, and Helen Thompson. *Biographies of Child Development.* Hoeber, 1939.

Gesell, Arnold, and Frances Ilg. *Infant and Child in the Culture of Today.* Harper, 1943.

Gibby, R. G., H. B. Adams, and R. N. Carrera. "Therapeutic changes in psychiatric patients following partial sensory deprivation," *Arch. gen. Psychiat.*, 3 (1960), 33-42.

Gide, André. *Si le grain le meurt.* Gallimard, 1928.

————. *Journal.* Knopf, 1951, 4 vols.

Gillespie, R. D. "Amnesia," *Arch. Neurol. Psychiat.*, 37 (1937), 748-764.

Gjessing, R. "Beiträge zur Somatologie der periodischen Katatonie," *Arch. Psychiat.*, 191 (1953), 291-326.

Glass, Bentley. "Symposium of genetics: Discussion," *Amer. J. Psychiat.*, 113 (1956), 504ff.

Glueck, S., and E. T. Glueck. *Unraveling Juvenile Delinquency,* Commonwealth Fund, 1950.

————. *Predicting Delinquency and Crime.* Harvard University Press, 1959.

Golden, Mandel, Bernard Glueck, Jr., and Zetta Feder. "A summary description of fifty 'normal' white males," *Amer. J. Psychiat.*, 119 (1962), 48-60.

Goldfarb, W. "The effects of early institutional care on adolescent personality." *J. exp. Educ.* 12 (1943), 106ff.

Goldstein, Kurt. "The modification of behavior consequent to cerebral lesions," *Psychiat. Quart.*, 10 (1936a), 586-610.

————. "The problem of meaning of words based upon observations of aphasic patients," *J. Psychol.*, 2 (1936b), 301-316.

————. "The significance of the frontal lobes for mental performance," *J. Neurol. Psychopathol.*, 17 (1936c), 27-40.

————. *The Organism: A Holistic Approach to Biology Derived from Pathological Data in Man.* American Book, 1939.

————. *Human Nature in the Light of Psychopathology.* Harvard University Press, 1940.

————. *Aftereffects of Brain Injuries in War.* Grune and Stratton, 1942.

————. *Language and Language Disturbances.* Grune and Stratton, 1948.

————. "The effect of brain damage on the personality," *Psychiat.*, 15 (1952) 245-260.

————. "Functional disturbance in brain damage," in Arieti 1959, I, 775ff.

Goldstein, Kurt, and Siegfried Katz. "The psychopathology of Pick's disease," *Arch. Neurol. Psychiat.*, 38 (1937), 473-490.

Goldstein, Kurt, and Martin Scheerer. "Abstract and concrete behavior: An experimental study with special tests," *Psychol. Monogr.,* vol. 53 (1941).

Gottlieb, Anthony A., Goldine Gleser, and Louis Gottschalk. "Verbal and physiological responses to hypnotic suggestions of attitudes," *J. psychosom. Med.,* 29 (1967), 172-183.

Gottlieb, Jacques S., M. Coulson Ashby, and John R. Knott. "Primary behavior disorders and psychopathic personality," *Arch. Neurol. Psychiat.,* 56 (1946), 381-400.

Grace, William J., and David T. Graham. "Relationship of specific attitudes and emotions to certain bodily diseases," *J. psychosom. Med.,* 14 (1952), 243-251.

Graham, David T. "Cutaneous vascular reactions in Raynaud's disease and in states of hostility, anxiety, and depression," *J. psychosom. Med.,* 17 (1955), 200-207.

Graham, David T., R. M. Lundy, Lorna Benjamin, J. D. Kabler, William C. Lewis, Nancy Kunish, and Frances Graham. "Specific attitudes in initial interviews with patients having different psychosomatic diseases," *J. psychosom. Med.,* 24 (1962), 257-273.

Green, Arnold W., ed. *Class, Status, and Power: A Reader in Social Stratification.* Free Press, 1953.

————. "The middle-class male child and neurosis," in Green 1953.

Green, R. G., W. E. Carlson, and C. A. Evans. "Deficiency disease of foxes produced by feeding fish; B_1 avitaminosis analogous to Wernicke's disease." *J. Nutrition,* 21 (1941), 243-256.

Greenacre, Phyllis. *Trauma, Growth, and Personality.* Norton, 1952.

Greenberg, N. H. "Studies in psychosomatic differentiation during infancy," *Arch. gen. Psychiat.,* 7 (1962), 389-406.

Grégoire, Ménie. "Un Dernier mot," *L'Esprit* (Nov. 1960), pp. 1951ff.

Gregory, I. "Factors influencing first admission rates to Canadian mental hospitals," *Canadian psychiat. Assn. J.,* 1 (1956), 115-143.

Grinker, Roy R. *Neurology.* Thomas, 1937.

————. "Hypothalamic functions in psychosomatic interrelations," *J. psychosom. Med.,* 1 (1939), 33ff.

Grinker, R. R., and R. R. Grinker, Jr., "Mentally healthy young males (homoclites)," *Arch. gen. Psychiat.,* 6 (1962), 405-453.

Groddeck, Georg Walther. *The Book of the It,* auth. trans. by V. M. E. Collins. Funk and Wagnalls, 1950.

Groen, J. "Psychogenesis and psychotherapy of ulcerative colitis," *J. psychosom. Med.,* 9 (1947), 151-174.

Grosskurth, Phyllis. *John Addington Symonds.* Longmans, Green, 1964.

Grünthal, E. "Zur Kenntniss der Psychopathologie der K. Syndrom-komplexen," *Mschr. Psychol.,* 53 (1923), 99ff.

————. "Über der Symptom der Einstellungsstörungen bei exogener Psychosen," *Z. ges. Neurol.,* 92 (1924) pp. 266-355.

————. "Zur Kenntnis der Psychopathologie des Korsakowschen Symptomkomplexen," in Bumke 1928, vol. VII, part 3.

Grünthal, E., and G. E. Storring. "Über das Verhalten bei umbeschriebener völliger Merkung fähigkeit," *Mschr. Psychol.,* 74 (1930), 354-368.

Guillain, Georges, *J.-M. Charcot, 1825-1893, His Life, His Work,* ed. and trans. by Pearce Bailey. Hoeber, 1959.

Guiraud, Paul. *Psychiatrie générale.* Librairie le Français, 1950.

Gutheil, Emil, A., ed. *The Autobiography of Wilhelm Stekel: The Life Story of a Pioneer Psychoanalyst.* Liveright, 1950.

Guze, Samuel B., and Michael Perley. "Observations on the natural history of hysteria," *Amer. J. Psychiat.,* 119 (1963), 960-965.

Hall, Calvin S. "Temperament: A survey of animal studies," *Psychol. Bull.,* 38 (1941), 909-943.

————. *The Meaning of Dreams*. Harper, 1953.

Halliday, H. L. *Psychosocial Medicine*. Norton, 1948.

Halstead, Ward. *Brain and Intelligence: A Quantitative Study of the Frontal Lobes*. University of Chicago Press, 1947.

Hamilton, Donald, and Warren Mann. "The hospital treatment of involutional psychoses," in Hoch and Zubin 1954.

Hamilton, G. V. *Objective Psychopathology*. Mosby, 1925.

Hammond, J. L., and Barbara Hammond. *The Town Laborer*. Longmans, 1932a.

————. *The Village Laborer*. Longmans, 1932b.

Hanfmann, Eugenia. "Analysis of the thinking disorder in a case of schizophrenia," *Arch. Neurol. Psychiat.*, 41 (1939), 568-579.

Hanfmann, E., and J. A. Kasanin. "Conceptual thinking in schizophrenia," *Nerv. ment. Dis. Monogr.*, no. 68 (1942).

Hare, E. H. "Family setting and the urban distribution of schizophrenia," *J. ment. Sci.*, 102 (1956), 753-760.

Harlow, H. F. "The nature of love," *Amer. Psychologist*, 13 (1958), 673ff.

————. "Primary affectional patterns in primates," *Amer. J. Orthopsychiat.*, 30 (1960), 676ff.

————. "The development of affectional patterns in infant monkeys," in Foss 1963.

Harrington, Michael. *The Other America*. Macmillan, 1962.

————. *The Accidental Century*. Macmillan, 1965.

Harris, A. "Sensory deprivation and schizophrenia," *J. ment. Sci.*, 105 (1959), 235-236.

Harris, Harold J. "Brucellosis: A case report illustrating a psychosomatic problem," *J. psychosom. Med.*, 6 (1944), 334-335.

Harrower-Erickson, M. K. "Psychological studies of patients with epileptic seizures," in Penfield and Erickson 1941, pp. 546-574.

Hartenberg, Paul. *Les Timides et la timidité*. Alcan, 1921.

————. *Les Psychonévroses anxieuses*. Alcan, 1922.

Havighurst, Robert, and Ruth Albrecht. *Older People*. Longmans, Green, 1953.

Head, Henry. *Aphasia and Kindred Disorders of Speech*. Macmillan, 1926.

Heath, Robert G. "Electrical self-stimulation of the brain in man," *Amer. J. Psychiat.*, 120 (1963), 571-578.

Heath, Robert G., Sten Martens, Byron Leach, Matthew Cohen, and Charles Angel. "Effect on behavior in humans with the administration of taraxein," *Amer. J. Psychiat.*, 114 (1957), 14-24.

Hebb, D. O. "Intelligence in man after large removals of cerebral tissue: Report of four left frontal lobe cases," *J. gen. Psychol.*, 21 (1939), 73-87.

————. "Man's frontal lobes," *Arch. Neurol. Psychiat.*, 54 (1945), 10-24.

————. *The Organization of Behavior*. Wiley, 1949.

Hebb, D. O., and Wilder Penfield. "Human behavior after extensive bilateral removal of the frontal lobes," *Arch. Neurol. Psychiat.*, 44 (1940), 421-438.

Hecht, Jacqueline, and Jean-Claude Chasteland. "Démographie et connaissance de la sexualité," *L'Esprit* (Nov. 1960), pp. 1789-1791.

Heilbroner, Robert. *The Limits of American Capitalism*. Harper and Row, 1966.

Henderson, D. K., and R. D. Gillespie. *A Textbook in Psychiatry*. 4th ed.; Oxford University Press, 1936.

Hendrick, Ives. *Facts and Theories of Psychoanalysis*. Knopf, 1941.

Henry, George W. *Sex Variants: A Study of Homosexual Patterns*. Hoeber, 1941, 2 vols.

Heron, Alastair, ed. *Towards a Quaker View of Sex: An Essay by a Group of Friends*. Friends Home Service Committee, 1963.

Herrick, C. J. *The Brains of Rats and Men*. University of Chicago Press, 1926.

Hesnard, A. *Les Troubles de la personnalité dans les états d'asthénie psychique*. Alcan, 1909.

————. "Le Mechanisme psychanalytique de la psychonévrose hypochondriaque," *Rev. Psychanal.,* 3, no. 1 (1929), 110-121.

————. *L'Univers morbide de la faute.* Presses Universitaires de France, 1949.

Hicklin, George, William Sacks, Hans Wehrheim, George Simpson, John Saunders, and Nathan Kline. "Crosstransfusion in schizophrenia," *Amer. J. Psychiat.,* 116 (1959), 334-336.

Hilgard, E. R. *Hypnotic Suggestibility.* Harcourt, Brace, 1965.

Hilgard, E., and D. Marquis. *Conditioning and Learning.* Appleton-Century-Crofts, 1956.

Hilgard, J. R., and M. F. Newman. "Evidence for functional genesis in mental illness: Schizophrenia, depressive psychoses, and psychoneuroses," *J. nerv. ment. Dis.,* 132 (1961), 3-16.

Hill, D. J., and D. Watterson. "Electroencephalographic studies of psychopathic personalities," *J. Neurol. Psychiat.,* 5 (1942), 47-65.

Hill, Lewis B. *Psychotherapeutic Intervention in Schizophrenia.* University of Chicago Press, 1955.

Hillyer, J. *Reluctantly Told.* Macmillan, 1927.

Hinsie, Leland. *Concepts and Problems of Psychotherapy.* Columbia University Press, 1937.

Hirschberg, J. Cotter, and Keith N. Bryant. "Problems in the differential diagnosis of childhood schizophrenia," in Assn. Res. nerv. ment. Dis., 1956.

Hoaken, P. C. S., Mary Clarke, and Marianne Breslin, "Psychopathology in Klinefelter's syndrome," *J. psychosom. Med.,* 26 (1964), 207-223.

Hoch, A., and J. T. MacCurdy. "The prognosis of involutional melancholia," *Arch. Neurol. Psychiat.,* vol. 7 (1922).

Hoch, Paul, and Joseph Zubin, eds. *Anxiety.* Grune and Stratton, 1950.

————. *Depression.* Grune and Stratton, 1954.

————. *Psychopathology of Childhood.* Grune and Stratton, 1955.

Hoenig, J., E. W. Anderson, J. C. Kenna, and Ruth Blunden. "Clinical and pathological aspects of the amnestic syndrome," *J. ment. Sci.,* 108 (1962), 541-599.

Hoffer, Abram, Humphrey Osmond, and John Smythies. "Schizophrenia, a new approach, II: Result of a year's research," *J. ment. Sci.,* 100 (1954), 29-45.

Hoffman, M. "Psychiatry, nature, and science," *Amer. J. Psychiat.,* 117 (1960), 205-210.

Hollingshead, A. B., and F. C. Redlich, eds. *Proceedings of the Conference on Community Structure and Psychiatric Disorders.* Milbank Fund, 1952.

————. *Social Class and Mental Illness.* Wiley, 1958.

Holt, Robert. "A critical review of Sheldon's *Varieties of Delinquent Youth,*" *J. abnorm. soc. Psychol.,* 45 (1950), 790-795.

Holt, Simma. *Terror in the Name of God.* Crown, 1965.

Holzinger, Rudolf, Ray Mortimer, and Wilson Van Dusen. "Aversion conditioning treatment of alcoholism," *Amer. J. Psychiat.,* 124 (1967), 246ff.

Horney, Karen. *The Neurotic Personality of Our Time.* Norton, 1937.

————. *New Ways in Psychoanalysis.* Norton, 1939.

————. *Neurosis and Human Growth.* Norton, 1950.

Horowitz, W. A., P. Polatin, L. C. Kolb, and P. H. Hoch. "A study of cases of schizophrenia treated by 'direct analysis,'" *Amer. J. Psychiat.,* 114 (1958), 780ff.

Horton, D. "The functions of alcohol in primitive societies: A cross-cultural study," *Quart. J. Stud. Alcohol,* 4 (1943), 199ff.

Hoskins, Roy G. *The Biology of Schizophrenia.* Norton, 1946.

Hotchner, A. E. *Papa Hemingway.* Random House, 1966.

Hull, Clark L. "Quantitative aspects of the evolution of concepts," *Psychol. Monogr.,* 28 (1920), 1-86.

_____. *Hypnosis and Suggestibility: An Experimental Approach.* Appleton-Century, 1933.

Hunt, J. McV., ed. *Personality and the Behavior Disorders.* Ronald, 1944.

Hunt, W. A., and Carney Landis. "The overt behavior pattern in startle," *J. exp. Psychol.,* 19 (1936), 312ff.

Huschka, Mabel. "The incidence and character of masturbation threats in a group of problem children," *Psychoanal. Quart.,* 7 (1938), 338-356.

Huston, P. E., and L. M. Locher. "Manic-depressive psychosis," *Arch. Neurol. Psychiat.,* 60 (1948), 37-48.

Huxley, Aldous. *Brave New World.* Harper, 1932.

_____. *Ends and Means.* Harper, 1937.

_____. *The Devils of Loudon.* Harper, 1953.

_____. *Brave New World Revisited.* Harper, 1958.

_____. *The Doors of Perception: Heaven and Hell.* Chatto and Windus, 1960.

Isaacs, Susan. *Social Development in Young Children.* Routledge, 1948.

_____. *Les Premières années de l'enfant.* Delachaux et Niestle, 1955.

Isberg, Emil. "Sudden death precipitated by anxiety complicating aortic stenosis (constriction)," *Amer. J. Psychiat.,* 112 (1956), 743ff.

Jackson, Don D., ed. *The Etiology of Schizophrenia.* Basic Books, 1960a.

_____. "A critique of the literature on the genetics of schizophrenia," in Jackson 1960b.

Jackson, J. Hughlings. *Selected Writings,* ed. by James Taylor. Hodder and Stoughton: vol. I, 1931; vol. II, 1932.

Jacobsen, C. F. "Studies of cerebral functions in primates," *Comp. Psychol. Monogr.,* 13, no. 63 (1936), 3-60.

Jacobsen, C. F., and G. M. Haselrud. "Studies of cerebral functions in primates, III: The effect of motor and premotor area lesions on the delayed alternation response in monkeys," *Comp. Psychol. Monogr.,* 13, no. 63 (1936), 66-68.

Jacobsen, Edmund. *Progressive Relaxation.* University of Chicago Press, 1929.

James, William. *Principles of Psychology.* Holt, 1890, 2 vols.

_____. *The Will to Believe and Other Essays in Popular Philosophy,* 1896. Longmans, Green, 1919.

_____. *Varieties of Religious Experience,* 1902. Longmans, Green, 1919.

James, William T. "Morphological and constitutional factors in conditioning," in Miner 1953, pp. 171-183.

Janet, Pierre. *L'Automatisme psychologique,* doctoral thesis, 1889. 2nd ed.; Alcan, 1919.

_____. *L'État mental des hystériques.* Alcan, 1893-1894; 2nd rev. ed., 1911; 3rd ed., 1931; *The Major Symptoms of Hysteria.* Macmillan, 1907. All citations in text, unless otherwise noted, are to the 1911 edition.

_____. *Les Névroses et les idées fixes.* Alcan, 1898, 2 vols.

_____. *Les Obsessions et la psychasthénie.* Alcan, 1903; 2nd rev. ed., 1911, 2 vols. All citations in text, unless otherwise noted, are to the 1911 edition.

_____. *Les Névroses.* Flammarion, 1909.

_____. *Les Médications psychologiques.* Alcan, 1919, 3 vols.; *Psychological Healing.* Macmillan, 1925, 2 vols.

_____. *La Médecine psychologique.* Flammarion, 1924; *Principles of Psychotherapy.* Macmillan, 1924.

_____. *De l'Angoisse à l'extase.* Alcan: vol. I, 1926; vol. II, 1928.

_____. *L'Évolution psychologique de la personnalité.* Chahine, 1929.

_____. *La Force et la faiblesse psychologique.* Maloine, 1932.

Jaspers, Karl. *The Future of Mankind.* University of Chicago Press, 1961.

Jelliffe, S. E. "Psychopathology of forced movements in oculogyric crises," *Nerv. ment. Dis. Monogr.,* no. 55 (1932).

Jellinek, E. M., and H. J. Clinebel. *Understanding and Counseling the Alcoholic.* Abingdon, 1956.

Jenkins, Richard. "The nature of the schizophrenic process," *Arch. Neurol. Psychiat.,* 64 (1950), 243ff.

————. "The schizophrenic sequence," *Amer. J. Orthopsychiat.,* 22 (1952), 738-748.

Jesperson, Otto. *Language: Its Nature, Development, and Origins.* Holt, 1922.

Johnson, A. M. "Sanctions for superego lacunae of adolescents," in Eissler 1949.

Johnson, Adelaide M., E. I. Falstein, S. A. Szurek, and Margeret Svendsen. "School phobia," *Amer. J. Orthopsychiat.,* 11 (1941), 702ff.

Johnson, A. M., and S. A. Szurek. "Etiology of antisocial behavior in delinquents and psychopaths," *J. Amer. med. Assn.,* 154 (1954), 814-817.

Jones, Ernest. *Papers on Psychoanalysis.* Balliere, Tindall, and Cox, 1938.

————. *The Life and Work of Sigmund Freud.* Basic Books: vol. I, 1953; vol. II, 1955; vol. III, 1957.

Jones, Maxwell. "Society and the sociopath," *Amer. J. Psychiat.,* 119 (1962), 410-414.

Jost, Hudson, and L. W. Sontag. "The genetic factor in autonomic nervous system function," *J. psychosom. Med.,* 6 (1944), 308-310.

Jouvet, M. "Telencephalic and rhombencephalic sleep in the cat," in Wolstenholme and O'Connor 1961, pp. 188-206.

Jung, Carl G. *Psychologie der Dementia Praecox,* 1907; "The psychology of dementia praecox," trans. by A. A. Brill, *Nerv. ment. Dis. Monogr.,* 1936.

————. *Wandlungen und Symbole der Libido,* 1912; *Psychology of the Unconscious.* Dodd, Mead, 1947.

————. *Modern Man in Search of a Soul.* Harcourt, Brace, 1947.

Kalinowsky, L. B. "Problems of psychotherapy and transference in shock treatment and psychosurgery," *J. psychosom. Med.,* 18 (1956), 399-403.

Kalinowsky, L. B., and Paul H. Hoch. *Shock Treatments, Psychosurgery, and Other Somatic Treatments in Psychiatry.* Grune and Stratton, 1952.

Kallmann, Franz. *The Genetics of Schizophrenia.* Augustin, 1938.

————. "Review of psychiatric progress: Heredity and eugenics," *Amer. J. Psychiat.,* 100 (1944), 551-555.

————. "The concept of induced insanity in family units," *J. nerv. ment. Dis.,* 104 (1946a), 303-315.

————. "The genetic theory of schizophrenia," *Amer. J. Psychiat.,* 103 (1946b), 309-322.

————. "Comparative twin study on genetic aspects of male homosexuality," *J. nerv. ment. Dis.,* 115 (1952), 283-298.

————. *Heredity in Health and Mental Disorder.* Norton, 1953.

————. "Genetic principles in manic-depressive psychosis," in Hoch and Zubin 1954.

Kallmann, Franz J., and M. M. Anastasia. "Twin studies of the psychopathology of suicide," *J. Hered.,* 37 (1946), 171-180.

Kallmann, F., and S. E. Barrera. "The heredo-constitutional mechanisms of predisposition and resistance to schizophrenia," *Amer. J. Psychiat.,* 98 (1942), 544-550.

Kanner, Leo. *Child Psychiatry.* Thomas, 1937.

————. "Autistic disturbances of affective contact," *Nerv. Child,* 2 (1943), 217-250.

————. "Early infantile autism," *J. Pediat.,* 15 (1944), 211-217.

————. "Problems of nosology and psychodynamics of early infantile autism," *Amer. J. Orthopsychiat.*, 19 (1949), 416-426.

————. "The conceptions of wholes and parts of early infantile autism," *Amer. J. Psychiat.*, 108 (1951), 23-26.

————. "Childhood schizophrenia," *Amer. J. Orthopsychiat.*, 24 (1954), 526ff.

————. *In Defense of Mothers.* Thomas, 1958.

————. "Trends in child psychiatry," *J. ment. Sci.*, 105 (1959), 581-593.

————. *Child Psychiatry.* Blackwell, 1960.

Kanner, L., and L. Eisenberg. "Notes on the follow-up studies of autistic children," in Hoch and Zubin 1955.

Kardiner, Abram. *Sex and Morality.* Charter, 1954.

Kardiner, Abram, Ralph Linton, Cora DuBois, and James West. *The Psychological Frontiers of Society.* Columbia University Press, 1945.

Karpman, Benjamin. "Conscience in the psychopath," *Amer. J. Orthopsychiat.*, 18 (1948), 455-491.

————. *The Hangover.* Thomas, 1957.

Kasanin, J. A. "Pavlov's theory of schizophrenia," *Arch. Neurol. Psychiat.*, 28 (1932), 210-218.

————. "A case of schizophrenia in only one of identical twins," *Amer. J. Psychiat.*, 91 (1934), 751-759.

Kasanin, J. A., and E. Hanfmann. "Disturbances in concept formation in schizophrenia," *Arch. Neurol. Psychiat.*, 40 (1938a), 1276-1282.

————. "An experimental study of concept formation in schizophrenia, I: Quantitative analysis of the results," *Amer. J. Psychiat.*, 95 (1938b), 35-48.

Katz, Louis N., 1964, in "Timberline conference," q. v.

Katz, Sandor. *Freud: On War, Sex, and Neurosis.* Arts and Science Press, 1947.

Kaufman, Walter. *Nietzsche: Philosopher, Psychologist, Antichrist.* Princeton University Press, 1950.

Kay, D. W., and Martin Roth. "Environmental and hereditary factors in the schizophrenias of old age ('late paraphenia') and their bearing on the general problem of causation in schizophrenia," *J. ment. Sci.*, 107 (1961), 649-687.

Kazin, Alfred. "The bitter 30's," *Atlantic Monthly*, 209 (1962), 82-98.

Kelley, Sr. M. William. "Depression in the psychoses of members of religious communities of women," *Amer. J. Psychiat.*, 188 (1961), 423-425.

Kempf, Edward J. *Psychopathology.* Mosby, 1921a.

————. "Autonomic functions and the personality," *Nerv. ment. Dis. Monogr.*, no. 28 (1921b).

Kimmelman, George. "Moral maturity and psychology," *Amer. J. Orthopsychiat.*, 18 (1948), 552-554.

Kindwall, Joseph A., and Elaine Kinder. "Postscript on a benign psychosis," *Psychiat.*, 3 (1940), 527-534.

Kinsey, Alfred C., Wardell B. Pomeroy, and Clyde E. Martin. *Sexual Behavior in the Human Male.* Saunders, 1948.

Kinsey, Alfred C., Wardell B. Pomeroy, Clyde E. Martin, and Paul H. Gebhard. *Sexual Behavior in the Human Female.* Saunders, 1953.

Klein, Melanie. *The Psychoanalysis of Children.* Hogarth, 1949.

Klein, Melanie, and Joan Riviere. *Love, Hate, and Reparation.* Norton, 1964.

Kleitman, Nathaniel. *Sleep and Wakefulness.* University of Chicago Press, 1963.

Kline, Nathan S. "LSD: The latch of disinhibition," *Psychiat. soc. Sci. Rev.*, 1, no. 5 (1967), 4ff.

Kluckhohn, Clyde. *Mirror for Man: The Relation of Anthropology to Modern Life.* Whittlesey House, 1949.

Klüver, H., and P. C. Bucy. "Preliminary analysis of functions of the temporal lobes in monkeys," *Arch. Neurol. Psychiat.*, 42 (1939), 979-1000.

Knapp, Peter, Charles Bliss, and Harriet Wells. "Addictive aspects in heavy cigarette smoking," *Amer. J. Psychiat.*, 119 (1963), 966-972.

Knight, Robert. "Psychotherapy of an adolescent catatonic schizophrenic with mutism," *Psychiat.*, 9 (1946), 323-340.

Knowles, J. B., and C. J. Lucas. "Experimental studies of the placebo response," *J. ment. Sci.*, 106 (1960), 231-240.

Knox, R. A. *Enthusiasm: A Chapter in the History of Religion.* Oxford University Press, 1950.

Koch, S., ed. *Psychology: A Study of a Science.* McGraw-Hill, 1959.

Koestler, Arthur. *The Act of Creation.* Hutchinson, 1964.

Koffka, Kurt. *Die Grundlagen der Psychischen Entwicklung.* Osterwieck am Harz: Zickfeldt, 1921. *The Growth of the Mind.* Harcourt, Brace, 1924.

––––––. *Principles of Gestalt Psychology.* Harcourt, Brace, 1935.

Köhler, Wolfgang. *Intelligenzprüfungen an Menschenaffen.* Springer, 1917; *The Mentality of Apes.* Harcourt, Brace, 1925.

Kolb, Lawrence C. *The Painful Phantom.* Thomas, 1954.

Kolb, Philip. *Marcel Proust: Correspondence avec sa mère.* Plon, 1953.

Korsakoff, S. "Erinnerungstäuschungen bei Polyneuritischer Psychosen," in Bumke 1928, vol. VII, part 3.

Kraines, Samuel H. *The Therapy of the Neuroses and Psychoses.* Lea and Febiger, 1941.

––––––. *Mental Depressions and Their Treatment.* Macmillan, 1957.

Krauch, E. *A Mind Restored.* Putnam, 1937.

Kretschmer, E. *Körperbau und Charakter.* Springer, 1925.

Kroeber, Alfred L. *The Nature of Culture.* University of Chicago Press, 1952.

Krutch, Joseph Wood. *The Modern Temper.* Harcourt, Brace, 1929.

––––––. *The Voice of the Desert.* Sloane, 1956.

Laforgue, René. *Psychopathologie de l'échec.* Payot, 1950.

Landis, Carney. "Studies of emotional reactions: General behavior and facial expression," *J. comp. Psychol.*, 4 (1924), 447-501.

Landis, Carney, and Marjorie Bolles. *Personality and Sexuality of the Physically Handicapped Woman.* Hoeber, 1942.

––––––. *Textbook of Abnormal Psychology.* Macmillan, 1950.

Landis, Carney, and James D. Page. *Modern Society and Mental Disease.* Farrar and Rinehart, 1938.

Langfeldt, G. *Prognosis in Schizophrenia.* Levin and Munksgaard, 1937.

––––––. "The significance of a dichotomy in clinical psychiatric classifications," *Amer. J. Psychiat.*, 116 (1959), 537-539.

La Piere, Richard. *The Freudian Ethic.* Duell, Sloane, 1959.

Lashley, K. S. *Brain Mechanisms and Intelligence: A Quantitative Study of the Effects of Brain Injury.* University of Chicago Press, 1929.

Lazarus, A. "The results of behavior therapy in 126 cases of severe neurosis," *Behav. Res. Ther.*, 1 (1963), 65-78.

Leighton, Alexander H., T. A. Lambo, C. C. Hughes, Dorothea Leighton, Jane Murphy, and David B. Macklin. *Psychiatric Disorders Among the Yoruba.* Cornell University Press, 1963.

Leighton, Dorothea. "The distribution of psychiatric symptoms in a small town," *Amer. J. Psychiat.*, 112 (1956), 716-723.

Leighton, Dorothea, and Clyde Kluckhohn. *Children of the People.* Harvard University Press, 1947.

Leighton, Dorothea, A. H. Leighton, J. S. Hardin, David B. Macklin, and A. M. Macmillan. *The Character of Danger: Psychiatric Symptoms in Selected Communities.* Basic Books, 1963.

Lennox, W. G. *Science and Seizures.* Harper, 1941.

————. "Seizure states," in Hunt 1944, vol. II, chap. 31.

Lennox, W. G., and S. Cobb. "Varieties of aura in epilepsy," *Arch. Neurol. Psychiat.,* 30 (1933), 374ff.

Lennox, W. G., E. L. Gibbs, and F. A. Gibbs. "Inheritance of cerebral dysrhythmia and epilepsy," *Arch. Neurol. Psychiat.,* 44 (1940), 1155-1183. Summarized in Fuller and Thompson 1960.

Leonard, K. J. *Aufteilung der Endogenen Psychosen.* Akademie Verlag, 1957.

————. "Cycloid psychoses and endogenous psychoses which are neither schizophrenic nor manic-depressive," *J. ment. Sci.,* 107 (1961), 633-648.

Leonard, William Ellery. *The Locomotive God.* Century, 1927.

Leroy, Bernard-Eugene. *Les Visions du demi-sommeil.* Alcan, 1926.

Leuba, James H. *Psychologie du mysticisme religieux.* Alcan, 1925.

Levey, H. B. "Oral trends and oral conflicts in a case of duodenal ulcer," *Psychoanal. Quart.,* 3 (1934), 515ff.

Levitt, Eugene, John P. Brady, Donald R. Ottinger, and Roger Kinesley. "The effect of sensory restriction on hypnotizability," *Arch. gen. Psychiat.,* 7 (1962), 343-344.

Levy, David M. *Maternal Overprotection.* Columbia University Press, 1943.

————. "Animal psychology in its relation to psychiatry," in Alexander and Ross 1952.

————. *Behavioral Analysis: Analysis of Clinical Observations of Behavior, as Applied to Mother-Newborn Relationships.* Thomas, 1958.

Lévy-Bruhl, Claude. *La Mentalité primitive.* Alcan, 1925.

Lewin, Bertram. *The Psychoanalysis of Elation.* Norton, 1950.

Lewis, Aubrey. "Between guesswork and certainty in psychiatry," *Lancet,* 1 (1958), 170-227.

Lewis, Julian, and T. R. Sarbin. "Studies in psychosomatics, I: The influence of hypnotic stimulation on gastric hunger contractions," *J. psychosom. Med.,* 5 (1943), 125-131.

Lewis, Nolan D. C., and Zygmunt Piotrowski. "Clinical diagnoses of manic-depressive psychosis," in Hoch and Zubin 1954.

Lewis, Oscar. *La Vida: A Puerto Rican Family in the Culture of Poverty—San Juan and New York.* Random House, 1965.

Lhermitte, Jean. *Les Hallucinations.* Doin, 1951.

Liddell, H. S. "Instinctual processes and conditioned reflexes," *J. psychosom. Med.,* 4 (1942), 390-395.

————. "Animal origins of anxiety," in Reymert 1950.

————. *Emotional Hazards in Animals and Man.* Thomas, 1956.

Liddell, H. S., and T. L. Bayne. "The development of 'experimental neurasthenia' in the sheep during the formation of difficult conditioned reflexes," *Amer. J. Physiol.,* 81 (1927), 494-512.

Liddell, H. S., W. T. James, and O. D. Anderson. "The comparative physiology of the conditioned motor reflex (based on experiments with the pig, dog, sheep, goat, and rabbit)," *Comp. Psychol. Monogr.,* vol. II, 1934.

Lidz, R. W., and T. Lidz. "The family environment of schizophrenic patients," *Amer. J. Psychiat.,* 106 (1949), 332ff.

Lidz, Theodore. "The amnestic syndrome," *Arch. Neurol. Psychiat.,* 47 (1942), 588-605.

————. "Analysis of a prefrontal lobe syndrome and its theoretic implications," *Arch. Neurol. Psychiat.,* 62 (1949), 1-62.

Lidz, Theodore, and Stephen Fleck. "Schizophrenia, human integration, and the role of the family," in Jackson 1960a.

Lidz, T., S. Fleck, Alice Cornelison, and Dorothy Terry. "The intrafamilial environment of the schizophrenic patient, VI: The transmission of irrationality," *Arch. Neurol. Scand.,* suppl. 112 (1957).

Lief, Alfred, ed. *The commonsense Psychiatry of Adolf Meyer.* McGraw-Hill, 1948.

Lindner, Robert. *Must You Conform?* Rinehart, 1956.

Linton, Ralph. *Culture and Personality: Three Lectures to Educators.* Amer. Council on Education, 1941.

Lipset, S. M., and R. Bendix. *Social Mobility in Industrial Society.* University of California Press, 1959.

Lipton, E. L., A. Steinschneider, and J. Richmond. "Autonomic function of the neonate, IV: Individual differences in cardiac reactivity," *J. psychosom. Med.,* 23 (1961), 427ff.

Ljungberg, L. "Hysteria: A clinical, prognostic, and genetic study," *Acta Psychiat. Neurol. Scand.,* suppl. 112 (1957).

London, Perry. *The Modes and Morals of Psychotherapy.* Holt, Rinehart and Winston, 1964.

Lorenz, Konrad Z. *King Solomon's Ring.* Crowell, 1952.

_____. *On Aggression.* Harcourt, Brace, 1963.

Lorenz, M., and Stanley Cobb. "Language behavior in manic patients," *Arch. Neurol. Psychiat.,* 67 (1952), 763-670.

Losse, H., M. Kretschmer, G. Kuban, and K. Bottger. "Die vegetative Struktur des Individiuums," *Acta Neuroveg.,* 13 (1956), 374-399.

Lowie, Robert H. *Primitive Religion.* Bone and Liveright, 1924.

Lu Li-chuang. "Contradictory parental expectations in schizophrenia," *Arch. gen. Psychiat.,* 6 (1962), 219-234.

Ludwig, A. M., and F. Farrelly. "The code of chronicity," *Arch. gen. Psychiat.,* 15 (1966), 562-568.

Lundberg, Ferdinand, and Maryna F. Farnham. *Modern Woman: The Lost Sex.* Harper, 1947.

Luxenburger, H. "Vorläufigen Bericht über psychiatrische Serienuntersuchungen an Zwillingen," *Z. ges. Neurol. Psychiat.* 116 (1928), 297-326.

_____. "Psychiatrische-neurologische Zwillingspathologie," *Zbl. ges. Neurol. Psychiat.,* 14 (1930), 145-180.

_____. *Handbuch der Erbkrankheiten.* Vol. IV; Leipzig: Thieme, 1942.

McCarthy, Dorothea. "Language development in the preschool child," in Barker, Kounin, and Wright, 1943.

McClelland, David C. *Studies in Motivation.* Appleton-Century-Crofts, 1955.

MacDermott, Neil, and Stanley Cobb. "A psychiatric survey of bronchial asthma," *J. psychosom. Med.,* 1 (1939), 203-244.

McFarland, R. A. *The Psychological Effects of Oxygen Deprivation on Human Behavior. Arch. Psychol.,* no. 145 (1932).

McGeer, Edith, and Patrick McGeer. "Physiologic effects of schizophrenic body fluids," *J. ment. Sci.,* 105 (1959), 1-18.

MacKenzie, Norman. *Dreams and Dreaming.* Vanguard, 1965.

MacLean, Paul D. "Psychosomatic disease and the 'visceral brain,'" *J. psychosom. Med.,* 11 (1949), 338-353.

MacLeish, Archibald. *Poetry and Experience.* Houghton Mifflin, 1961.

McLoughlin, Emmett. *People's Padre.* Beacon, 1954.

MacRobert, Russell G. "Hallucinations of the sane," *J. Insurance Med.,* 5 (1950), 1-12.

Magnan, J. J. V. *Maladies mentales* (1893-1897).

Mahl, George. "Effect of chronic fear on the gastric secretion of HCl in dogs," *J. psychosom. Med.,* 11 (1949), 30-44.

_____. "Anxiety, HCl secretion, and peptic ulcer etiology," *J. psychosom. Med.* 12 (1950), 158-169.

_____. "Physiological changes during chronic fear," in Miner 1953.

Mahl, George, and Richard Karpe. "Emotions and hydrochloric acid secretion during the psychoanalytic hour," *J. psychosom. Med.,* 15 (1953), 312-327.

Mahler, M. S. "On child psychosis and schizophrenia: Autistic and symbiotic infantile psychoses," in Eissler *et al.* 1952, pp. 286-305.

Mahler, M. S., J. R. Ross, and Z. DeFries. "Clinical studies in benign and malignant cases of childhood psychosis (schizophrenia-like)," *Amer. J. Orthopsychiat.,* 19 (1949), 295-305.

Mahoney, J. F., R. C. Arnold, and A. Harris. "Penicillin treatment of early syphilis," *Venereal Dis. Information,* 24 (1943), 355ff.

Maier, N. R. F. "Studies of abnormal behavior in the rat, XIV: Strain differences in the inheritance of susceptibility to convulsions," *J. comp. Psychol.,* 35 (1943), 327-335.

_____. *Frustration: The Study of Behavior Without a Goal.* McGraw-Hill, 1949.

Maine de Biran, François-Pierre. *Journal,* 1845. Baconnière, 1954.

Malamud, William, S. L. Sands, and I. Malamud. "The involutional psychoses: A socio-psychiatric study," *J. psychosom. Med.,* 3 (1941), 410-426.

Malebranche, Nicolas. *Traité de l'amour de dieu.* Bossard, 1922.

Malmo, R. B., J. F. Davis, and S. Barza. "Total hysterical deafness: An experimental case study," in Eysenck 1960.

Malzberg, Benjamin. "Important statistical data about mental illness," in Arieti 1959.

Mandell, Arnold J., and Mary P. Mandell. "Biochemical aspects of rapid eye movement sleep," *Amer. J. Psychiat.,* 122 (1965), pp. 391-401.

Mannheim, Karl. *Man and Society in an Age of Reconstruction,* Harcourt, 1935.

Maslow, Abraham H. *Motivation and Personality.* Harper, 1954.

_____. *Toward a Psychology of Being.* Van Nostrand, 1962.

Masserman, Jules. "Is the hypothalamus a center of emotion?" *J. psychosom. Med.,* 3 (1941), 3-20.

_____. *Behavior and Neurosis.* University of Chicago Press, 1943.

_____. "Experimental neurosis and group aggression," *Amer. J. Orthopsychiat.,* 14 (1944), 636ff.

_____. *Principles of Dynamic Psychiatry.* Saunders, 1946.

_____. "A biodynamic and psychoanalytic approach to the problems of feeling and emotion," in Reymert 1950, pp. 65ff.

_____. *The Practice of Dynamic Psychiatry.* Saunders, 1955.

Masserman, Jules, and Curtis Pechten. "Neuroses in monkeys: A preliminary report on experimental observations," in Miner 1953.

Masserman, Jules, and Paul W. Siever. "Dominance, neurosis, and aggression," *J. psychosom. Med.,* 6 (1944), 7-16.

Masserman, Jules, and K. S. Yum. "An analysis of the influence of alcohol on experimental neuroses in cats," *J. psychosom. Med.,* 8 (1946), 36-52.

Matthiessen, F. O. *The James Family.* Knopf, 1947.

Maugham, Robin. *Somerset and All the Maughams.* Longmans, Heinemann, 1966.

Mauriac, François. *Thérèse.* Grasset, 1927.

Maurois, André. *À la Recherche de Marcel Proust.* Hachette, 1949; *Proust: Portrait of a Genius.* Harper, 1950.

_____. *Prometheus: The Life of Balzac.* Harper and Row, 1965.

Mauz, F. *Die Prognostik der Endogenen Psychosen.* Leipzig: Thieme, 1930.

May, Rollo. "The origins and significance of the existential movement in psychology," in May, Angel, and Ellenberger 1959, pp. 3-36.

_____, ed. *Existential Psychology.* Random House, 1961.

May, Rollo, Ernest Angel, and Henri F. Ellenberger, eds. *Existence: A New Dimension in Psychiatry and Psychology.* Basic Books, 1959.

Mead, Margaret. *Competition and Cooperation Among Primitive Peoples.* McGraw-Hill, 1937.

Memmi, Albert. *Portrait of a Jew.* Orion, 1962.

Menninger, Karl. *Man Against Himself.* Harcourt, Brace, 1938.

————. *Love and Hate.* Harcourt, Brace, 1942.

Menzies, R. "Conditioned vasomotor responses in human subjects," *J. Psychol.,* 4 (1937), 75-120.

————. "Further studies of conditioned vasomotor responses in human subjects," *J. exp. Psychol.,* 29 (1941), 457-482.

Mettler, Fred, ed. *Selective Partial Ablation of the Frontal Cortex.* Hoeber, 1949.

Meyer, Adolf. "Fundamental conceptions of dementia praecox," *J. nerv. ment. Dis.,* 34 (1907), 331-336. Also in Lief 1948 and in Winters 1951.

————. "The dynamic interpretation of dementia praecox," *Amer. J. Psychol.,* 21 (1910), 385-403. Also in Lief 1948 and in Winters 1951.

————. "The nature and conception of dementia praecox," *J. abnorm. Psychol.,* 5 (1910-1911), 274-285. Also in Winters 1951, II, 459.

Millar, W. M. "Hysteria—A reevaluation," *J. ment. Sci.,* 104 (1958), 813-821.

Miller, James. "The Individual Response to Drugs," in Farber and Wilson 1961.

Miller, Perry. *The New England Mind.* Macmillan, 1939.

Minc, Salek, Gavin Sinclair, and Ronald Taft. "Some psychological factors in coronary heart disease," *J. psychosom. Med.,* 25 (1963), 132-139.

Miner, Roy, ed. *Comparative Conditioned Neuroses.* N.Y. Acad. Sci., 1953.

Minkowski, E. *La Schizophrénie: Psychopathie des schizoides et des schizophrènes.* Payot, 1927; Desclée de Brouwer, 1953.

————. *Le Temps vécu: Études phénoménologiques et psychopathologiques.* Collection de L'Évolution Psychiatrique, 1933.

Mitchell, Silas Weir. *Fat and Blood.* 1877.

Mittelmann, Bela, and Harold G. Wolff (with M. Scharf). "Experimental studies on patients with gastritis, duodenitis, and peptic ulcer," *J. psychosom. Med.,* 4 (1942), 5-61.

Money, John. "Components of eroticism in man, I: The hormones in relation to sexual morphology and sexual desire," *J. nerv. ment. Dis.,* 132 (1961), 239-248.

————. "Cytogenetic and psychosexual incongruities with a note on space-form blindness," *Amer. J. Psychiat.,* 119 (1963), 820ff.

Money, John, Joan Hampson, and J. L. Hampson. "Imprinting and the establishment of gender roles," *Arch. Neurol. Psychiat.,* 77 (1957), 333-336.

Montaigne, Michel. *Essays.* Stanford University Press, 1957.

Montherlant, Henri. *Selected Essays.* Macmillan, 1961.

Moore, Gerald. *Seven African Writers.* Oxford University Press, 1962.

More, Sir Thomas. *Utopia,* 1516, in Negley and Patrick 1952.

Morris, J. V., and M. B. MacGillvray. "Mongolism in one of twins," *J. ment. Sci.,* 99 (1953), 557-559.

Moscovici, Serge. *La Psychanalyse: Son image et son public.* Presses Universitaires de France, 1960.

Mosse, Hilde. "The misuse of the diagnosis of childhood schizophrenia," *Amer. J. Psychiat.,* 114 (1958), 791-794.

Mowrer, O. H. "Learning theory and the neurotic paradox," *Amer. J. Orthopsychiat.,* 18 (1948), 571-610.

————. *Psychotherapy: Theory and Research.* Ronald, 1953a.

————. "Neurosis: A disorder of conditioning or problem solving," 1953b, in Miner 1953.

————. *The Crisis in Psychiatry and Religion.* Van Nostrand, 1961.

Mowrer, O. H., and Clyde Kluckhohn. "A dynamic theory of the personality," in Hunt 1944, I, 69-131.

Muller, H. J. "Genetic principles in human populations," *Amer. J. Psychiat.,* 113 (1956), 481-491.

Muncie, Wendell. *Psychobiology and Psychiatry.* Mosby, 1939; 2nd ed., 1948.

————. "Chronic fatigue," *J. psychosom. Med.,* 3 (1941), 277-285.

Munthe, Axel. *The Story of San Michele.* Dutton, 1937.

Myerson, Abraham. "The relationship of hereditary factors to mental processes," *Proc. Assn. Res. nerv. ment. Dis.,* 19 (1939a), 16-49.

————. "Theory and principles of the 'total push' method in the treatment of chronic schizophrenia," *Amer. J. Psychiat.,* 95 (1939b), 1197-1208.

Myrdal, Gunnar. *An American Dilemma.* Harper, 1944.

Nadel, Aaron B. "A qualitative analysis of behavior following cerebral lesions," *Arch. Psychol.,* no. 224 (1938).

Natenberg, Maurice. *The Case History of Sigmund Freud: A Psychobiography.* Regent House, 1955.

Naville, Ernest. *Maine de Biran: Sa Vie et ses pensées,* 1857.

Neel, J. V., and W. J. Schull. *Human Heredity.* University of Chicago Press, 1954.

Negley, Glenn, and J. Max Patrick. *The Quest for Utopia: An Anthology of Imaginary Societies.* Schuman, 1952.

Nehru, Jawaharlal. *Toward Freedom: The Autobiography of Jawaharlal Nehru.* John Day, 1941.

Newman, John Henry, Cardinal. *Sermons and Discourses.* Longmans, Green, 1949.

Nichols, Ira C., and J. McVickers Hunt. "A case of partial bilateral frontal lobectomy," *Amer. J. Psychiat.,* 96 (1940), 1063-1083.

Nietzsche, Friedrich. *Also Sprach Zarathustra,* 1885. Modern Library, 1917.

Noyes, Arthur P., and Lawrence C. Kolb. *Modern Clinical Psychiatry.* Saunders, 1963.

Nunberg, H. "Practice and theory of psychoanalysis," *Nerv. ment. Dis. Monogr.* (1948).

O'Connor, John F., George Daniels, Aaron Karush, Leon Moses, Charles Flood, and Lenore Stern. "The effects of psychotherapy on the course of ulcerative colitis— a preliminary report," *Amer. J. Psychiat.,* 120 (1964), 738-742.

Offer, D., and M. Sabshin. *Normality: Theoretical and Clinical Concepts of Mental Health.* Basic Books, 1966.

Oken, D., R. Grinker, H. A. Heath, M. Herz, S. Korchin, M. Sabshin, and N. Schwartz. "Relation of physiological response to affect expression," *Arch. gen. Psychiat.,* 6 (1962).

Olsen, Willard. "Growth of the child as a whole," in Barker, Kounin, and Wright 1943, pp. 199-208.

O'Neal, Patricia, and Lee N. Robins. "Childhood patterns predictive of adult schizophrenia: A 30-year follow-up study," *Amer. J. Psychiat.,* 115 (1958), 385-391.

O'Neal, Patricia, Lee N. Robins, Lucy J. King, and Jeanette Schaefer. "Parental deviance and the genesis of sociopathic personality," *Amer. J. Psychiat.,* 118 (1962), 1114-1124.

Opler, Marvin. *Culture, Psychiatry, and Human Values.* Thomas, 1956.

Orlansky, Harold. "Infant care and personality," *Psychol. Bull.,* 46 (1949), 1-48.

Ort, Robert. "A study of role-conflict as related to class level," *J. abnorm. soc. Psychol.,* 47 (1952), 425-432.

Øster, J. *Mongolism.* Munksgaard, 1953.

Owen, Robert. *A New View of Society,* 1813. Everyman's, 1963.

Pacella, B. L., N. Kopeloff, S. E. Barrera, and L. M. Kopeloff. "Experimental production of focal epilepsy," *Arch. Neurol. Psychiat.,* 52 (1944), 189-196.

Palmer, H. D. "Involutional melancholia," *Public Health Reports,* suppl. 168 (1942), 118-124.

————. "Mental disorders of old age," *Geriat.,* 1 (1946), 60-69.

Palmer, H. D., and F. J. Jardon. "Hereditary patterns in involutional melancholia," *Arch. Neurol. Psychiat.,* 46 (1941), 740ff.

Palmer, H. D., and S. H. Sherman. "The involutional melancholia process," *Arch. Neurol. Psychiat.,* 40 (1938), 762-768.

Parfitt, D. N. "The neurology of schizophrenia," *J. ment. Sci.,* 102 (1956), 671-718.

Parran, Thomas. *Shadow on the Land: Syphilis.* Reynal and Hitchcock, 1937.

Parrinder, Geoffrey. *Witchcraft: European and African.* Barnes and Noble, 1963.

Pasamanick, Benjamin. "Prevalence and distribution of psychosomatic conditions in an urban population according to social class," *J. psychosom. Med.,* 24 (1962), 352-356.

Pasamanick, B., and Hilda Knobloch. "Epidemiologic studies on the complications of pregnancy and the birth process," in Caplan 1961, pp. 74-95.

Pasqualine, R. Q., G. Vidal, and G. E. Bur. "Psychopathology of Klinefelter's syndrome," *Lancet,* 2 (1957), 164-172.

Pastore, Nicholas. "The genetics of schizophrenia," *Psychol. Bull.,* 46 (1949a), 285-302.

_____. *The Nature-Nurture Controversy.* King's Crown Press, 1949b.

Pauling, Linus. "The molecular basis of genetics," *Amer. J. Psychiat.,* 113 (1956), 492-495.

Pavlov, Ivan. *Lectures on Conditioned Reflexes.* Liveright, 1928.

_____. *Conditioned Reflexes and Psychiatry,* trans. by W. H. Gantt. International University Press, 1941.

Peckham, G. W., and E. G. Peckham. "Some observations on the mental powers of spiders," *J. Morphol.,* 1 (1887), 383ff.

Penfield, Wilder. *The Excitable Cortex in Conscious Man.* Thomas, 1958.

Penfield, Wilder, and T. Erickson, eds. *Epilepsy and Cerebral Localization.* Thomas, 1941.

Penfield, Wilder, and J. Evans. "The frontal lobe in man: A clinical study of maximum removals," *Brain,* 58 (1935), 115-133.

Penfield, Wilder, and Herbert Jasper. *Epilepsy and the Functional Anatomy of the Human Brain.* Little, Brown, 1954.

Penfield, Wilder, and Theodore Rasmussen. *The Cerebral Cortex in Man.* Macmillan, 1950.

Perry, John Weir. *The Self in Psychotic Process.* University of California Press, 1953.

Petrie, Asenath. *Personality and the Frontal Lobes.* Routledge and Kegan Paul, 1952.

Pfeffer, Arnold Z. *Alcoholism.* Grune and Stratton, 1958.

Pfeiffer, C. C., and E. H. Jenney. "The inhibition of the conditioned response and the counteraction of schizophrenia by muscarinic stimulation of the brain," *Ann. N.Y. Acad. Sci.,* 66 (1957), 753ff.

Pieper, Josef. *Leisure: The Basis of Culture.* Pantheon, 1952.

Pieron, Henri. *Thought and the Brain.* Harcourt, Brace, 1927.

Piotrowski, Z. J. "The Rorschach inkblot method in organic disturbances of the central nervous system," *J. nerv. ment. Dis.,* 86 (1937), 525-537.

Pitres, A., and E. Régis. *Les Obsessions et les impulsions.* 1902.

Pollard, J. C., L. Uhr, and C. W. Jackson. "Studies in sensory deprivation," *Arch. gen. Psychiat.,* 8 (1963), 435-454.

Pollin, William, and Seymour Perlin. "Psychiatric evaluation of 'normal control' volunteers," *Amer. J. Psychiat.,* 115 (1958), 129-133.

Porter, R. W., J. V. Brady, D. Conrad, J. W. Mason, R. Galambos, and D. M. Rioch. "Some experimental observations on gastrointestinal lesions in behaviorally conditioned monkeys," *J. psychosom. Med.,* 20 (1958), 379-394.

Prince, Morton. *The Dissociation of a Personality.* Longmans, Green, 1905.

_____. *Clinical and Experimental Studies in Personality.* Sci-Art, 1939.

Prince, Raymond. "The 'brain fag' syndrome in Nigerian students," *J. ment. Sci.,* 106 (1960), 559-570.

Pritchard, Michael. "Homosexuality and genetic sex," *J. ment. Sci.,* 108 (1962), 616-623.

Proust, Marcel. *Swann's Way.* Thomas Seltzer, 1924; Modern Library, 1956.

Puner, Helen W. *Freud: His Life and His Mind.* Grosset and Dunlap, 1947.

Purtell, J. J., E. Robins, and M. Cohen. "Observations on clinical aspects of hysteria," *J. Amer. med. Assn.,* 146 (1953), pp. 902-909.

Quercy, Pierre. *L'Hallucination.* Alcan, 1930, 2 vols.

Rado, Sandor. "Obsessive behavior: So-called obsessive-compulsive neurosis," in Arieti 1959, I, 324ff.

Rainer, John D., Alvin M. Mesnikoff, Lawrence C. Kolb, and Arthur C. Carr. "Homosexuality and heterosexuality in identical twins," *J. psychosom. Med.,* 22 (1960), 251-259.

Rand, Ayn. *For the New Intellectual.* Random House, 1961.

Redfield, Robert, and Alfonso Villa Rojas. *Chan Kom: A Maya Village.* Carnegie Institute, 1934.

Redlich, Frederick C. "The concept of schizophrenia," 1952a, in Brody and Redlich 1952.

————. *Psychotherapy with Schizophrenic Patients.* International University Press, 1952b.

Rees, Linford. "Psychosomatic aspects of vagotomy," *J. ment. Sci.,* 99 (1953), 505-512.

Régis, E., and A. Hesnard. *La Psychanalyse des névroses et des psychoses.* Alcan, 1914; 2nd ed., 1922; 3rd ed., 1929.

Reich, Wilhelm. "Über den Epileptischen Anfall," *Int. Z. Psychanal.,* 17 (1931), 263ff.

Reichard, S. A. "A re-examination of 'Studies on Hysteria,'" *Psychoanal. Quart.,* 25 (1956), 156ff.

Reichard, S., and C. Tillman. "Patterns of parent-child relationships in schizophrenia," *Psychiat.,* 13 (1950), 247-257.

Reik, Theodore. *Geständniszwang und Strafbedürfnis.* Internationaler Psychanalytischer Verlag, 1925. *Masochism and Modern Man.* Farrar and Rinehart, 1941.

————. *Listening with the Third Ear.* Farrar, Strauss, 1948.

Reiser, Morton F., and Hyman Bakst. "Psychology of cardiovascular disorders," in Arieti 1959.

Rennie, T. A. C. "Prognosis in manic-depressive psychosis," *Amer. J. Psychiat.,* 98 (1942), 801ff.

————. "Present status of shock therapy," *Psychiat.,* 6 (1943), 127-137.

Rennie, T. A. C., and J. E. Howard. "Hypoglycaemia and tension-depression," *J. psychosom. Med.,* 4 (1942), 273-282.

Reymert, Martin, ed. *The Mooseheart Symposium on Feelings and Emotions.* McGraw-Hill, 1950.

Ribble, Margaret A. "Infantile Experience in Relation to Personality Development," in Hunt 1944, II, 621-651.

Ribot, Th. *Les Maladies de la volonté.* Alcan, 1914.

Richards, Esther Loring. "Study of the invalid reaction," *Arch. Neurol. Psychiat.,* 1919.

————. "Practical features in the study and treatment of anxiety cases," *New England J. Med.,* 210 (1934), 633-637.

Richter, Curt. "On the phenomenon of sudden death in animals and men," *J. psychosom. Med.,* 19 (1957), 191-198.

Rimland, Bernard. *Infantile Autism.* Appleton-Century-Crofts, 1964.

Rinkel, Max, and H. C. B. Denber, eds. *Chemical Concepts of Psychosis.* McDowell-Obolensky, 1958.

Rioch, David M., J. V. Brady, and J. McV. Hunt. "Experimental aspects of anxiety," *Amer. J. Psychiat.,* 113 (1956), 435-442.

Rivers, W. H. R. *Instinct and the Unconscious.* Cambridge University Press, 1922.

Robinson, John A. T. *Honest to God.* Westminster, 1963.

Roe, Anne. "Children of alcoholic parents raised in foster homes," *Quart. J. Stud. Alcohol,* memoir no. 3 (1945).

Rogers, Carl. *Client-Centered Therapy.* Houghton Mifflin, 1951.

————. "A theory of therapy, personality, and interpersonal relationships as developed in a clinical framework," in Koch 1959.

Rogow, Arnold. *James Forrestal: A Study of Personality, Politics, and Policy.* Macmillan, 1963.

Rokeach, Milton. *The Three Christs of Ypsilanti: A Psychological Study.* Knopf, 1964.

Rosanoff, A. J., and L. M. Handy. "Huntington's chorea in twins," *Arch. Neurol. Psychiat.,* 33 (1935), 839ff.

Rosanoff, A. J., L. M. Handy, I. R. Plesset, and S. Brush. "The etiology of the so-called schizophrenic psychoses, with special reference to their occurrence in twins," *Amer. J. Psychiat.,* 91 (1934), 247-286.

————. "The etiology of manic-depressive syndromes with special reference to their occurrence in twins," *Amer. J. Psychiat.,* 91 (1935), 725-762.

Rosanoff, A. J., L. M. Handy, and I. A. Rosanoff. "Etiology of epilepsy with special reference to its occurrence in twins," *Arch. Neurol. Psychiat.,* 31 (1934), 1165ff. Summarized in Fuller and Thompson 1960.

Rose, J. A. "Eating inhibitions in children in relation to anorexia nervosa," *J. psychosom. Med.,* 5 (1943), 117-124.

Rosen, John N. "The treatment of schizophrenic psychosis by direct analytic therapy," *Psychiat. Quart.,* 21 (1947), 117-119.

————. *Direct Analysis.* Grune and Stratton, 1953.

Ross, I. S. "An autistic child," *Pediat. Conf.,* 2, no. 2 (1959) 1-13.

Ross, T. A. *The Common Neuroses.* Wood, 1938.

Roussel, Raymond. *La Doublure.* Pauvert, 1963.

Rovetta, P. "Effect of mescaline and LSD on evoked responses, especially of the optic system of the cat," *Electroenceph. clin. Neurophysiol.* 8 (1956), 15-24.

Sandison, R. A. "Psychological aspects of the LSD treatment of the neuroses," *J. ment. Sci.,* 100 (1954), 508-515.

Sandison, R. A., and A. M. Spencer. "The therapeutic value of lysergic acid diethylamide in mental illness," *J. ment. Sci.,* 100 (1954), 491-507.

Santayana, George. *Skepticism and Animal Faith.* Scribner's, 1923.

Sarbin, T. R. "Role theory," in G. Lindzey, ed. *Handbook of Social Psychology.* vol. 1, Addison-Wesley, 1954.

Sartre, Jean-Paul. *La Nausée.* Gallimard, 1938.

Sarvis, Mary A., and Blanche Garcia. "Etiological variables in autism," *Psychiat.,* 24 (1961), 307-317.

Schiele, Burtrum C., and Josef Brozek. " 'Experimental neurosis' resulting from semi-starvation in man," *J. psychosom. Med.,* 10 (1948), 31-50.

Schilder, Paul. *Über das Wesen der Hypnosis.* Springer, 1921. *The Nature of Hypnosis.* International University Press, 1956, part I.

————. "The organic background of obsessions and compulsions," *Amer. J. Psychiat.,* 94 (1938), 1397ff.

Schilder, Paul, and Otto Kauders. *Lehrbuch der Hypnosis.* Springer, 1926. *The Nature of Hypnosis.* International University Press, 1956, part II.

Schwartz-Bart, André. *The Last of the Just.* Atheneum, 1961.

Sclare, A. Balfour. "The psychiatric patient in America," *J. ment. Sci.,* 99 (1953), pp. 572-579.

Scott, John Paul. *Aggression.* University of Chicago Press, 1958.

Seabrook, W. *Asylum.* Harcourt, Brace, 1935.

Sears, R. R., and L. H. Cohen. "Hysterical anesthesia, analgesia, and astereognosis" 1933, in Eysenck 1960.

Sechahaye, M. A. *Autobiography of a Schizophrenic Girl.* Grune and Stratton, 1951a.

_____. *Symbolic Realization.* International University Press, 1951b.

Seitz, P. F. D. "Infantile experience and adult behavior in animal subjects, II: Age of separation from the mother and adult behavior in the cat," *J. psychosom. Med.,* 21 (1959), 353ff.

Shapiro, Arthur. "The placebo effect in the history of medical treatment: Implications for psychiatry," *Amer. J. Psychiat.,* 116 (1959), 298-303.

Shaw, E. B., R. V. Dermott, R. Lee, and T. N. Burbridge. "Phenothiazine tranquilizers as a cause of severe seizures," *Pediat.,* 23 (1959), 485-492.

Sheen, Fulton J. *Peace of Soul.* McGraw-Hill, 1949.

Sheldon, W. H., S. S. Stevens, and W. B. Tucker. *The Varieties of Human Physique.* Harper, 1940.

Sherrington, C. S. *Integrative Action of the Nervous System.* Yale University Press, 1906.

_____. *Man on His Nature.* Cambridge University Press, 1940; 2nd rev. ed., 1951.

Siegel, Malcolm, Donald Niswander, Ernest Sachs, Jr., and Dino Stavros. "Taraxein, fact or artifact?" *Amer. J. Psychiat.,* 115 (1959), 819-820.

Simmons, Leo. *Sun Chief: The Autobiography of a Hopi Indian.* Yale University Press, 1942.

Simmons, Leo, and Harold G. Wolff. *Social Science in Medicine.* Russell Sage, 1954.

Skinner, B. F. *Walden Two.* Macmillan, 1948.

Slater, Eliot. "Genetic investigations in twins," *J. ment. Sci.,* 99 (1953), 44-52.

_____. "Hysteria 311," *J. ment. Sci.,* 107 (1961), 359-381.

Slocum, Jonathan, C. L. Bennet, and J. Lawrence Pool. "The role of prefrontal lobe surgery as a means of eradicating intractable anxiety," *Amer. J. Psychiat.,* 116 (1959), 222-230.

Smith, Huston. "Do drugs have religious import?" in Solomon and Leary 1964.

Smith, L. H. "Progress in psychiatry," *J. Amer. med. Assn.,* 158 (1955), 46-48.

Smuts, J. C. *Holism and Evolution.* 2nd ed.; Macmillan, 1927.

Snow, C. P. *The Two Cultures.* Cambridge University Press, 1959.

Snyder, F. "The new biology of dreaming," *Arch. gen. Psychiat.,* 8 (1963), 381-392.

_____. "Progress in the new biology of dreaming," *Amer. J. Psychiat.,* 122 (1965), 377-390.

Solomon, David, and Timothy Leary, eds. *LSD: The Consciousness-Expanding Drug.* Putnam, 1964.

Solomon, Philip. "Sensory deprivation: Its meaning and significance," *State of Mind,* vol. 2, no. 9 (1958).

Solomon, Philip, Philip Kubansky, and Richard Trumbull, eds. *Sensory Deprivation: A Symposium.* Harvard University Press, 1961.

Solomon, Philip, P. Leiderman, Jack H. Mendelsohn, and Donald Wexler. "Sensory deprivation: A review," *Amer. J. Psychiat.,* 114 (1957), 357-365.

Sontag, L. W. "Differences in modifiability of fetal behavior and physiology," *J. psychosom. Med.,* 6 (1944), 151-154.

Sontag, L. W., and G. Comstock. "Striae in the bones of a set of monozygotic triplets," *Amer. J. Dis. Childh.,* 56 (1938), 301-308.

Sontag, L. W., and V. L. Nelson. "Comparison of the physical and mental traits of a set of monozygotic triplets," *J. Hered.,* 24 (1933a), 473-480.

_____. "Behavior of a set of identical triplets," *Pediat. Sem. and J. genet. Psychol.,* 42 (1933b), 406-422.

Sorokin, Pitirim. *The American Sex Revolution.* Porter Sargent, 1956.

Sperber, Manès. *The Achilles Heel.* Doubleday, 1960.

Sperry, Warren M. "The biochemistry of depressions," in Hoch and Zubin 1954.

Spiegel, Herbert. "Is symptom removal dangerous?" *Amer. J. Psychiat.*, 123 (1967), 1279-1283.

Spielmayer, Walther. "The problem of the anatomy of schizophrenia," *Proc. Assn. Res. nerv. ment. Dis.*, 10 (1931), 105-110.

Srole, Leo, Thomas S. Langner, Stanley T. Michael, Marvin K. Opler, and T. A. C. Rennie. *Mental Health in the Metropolis.* McGraw-Hill, 1962.

Stearns, A. W. "Suicide in Massachusetts," *Ment. Hygiene,* 5 (1924), 752-777.

Stein, C. "Hereditary factors in epilepsy: A comparative study of 1,000 institutionalized epileptics and 1,115 non-epileptic controls," *Amer. J. Psychiat.*, 89 (1933), 989-1037.

Stendhal (Henri Beyle). *Vie de Henri Brulard,* 1890. *The Life of Henry Brulard.* Noonday, 1958.

Stephen, Karin. *The Wish to Fall Ill.* Cambridge University Press, 1960. Preface by Ernest Jones.

Stephens, Joseph H., and Christian Astrup. "Prognosis in 'process' and 'non-process' schizophrenia," *Amer. J. Psychiat.*, 119 (1963), 945-959.

Stetson, R. H., and H. D. Bouman. "The coordination of simple skilled movements," *Arch. Néerlandaises de physiol. de l'homme et des animaux,* 20 (1935), 177-254.

Stevens, S. S., ed. *Handbook of Experimental Psychology.* Wiley, 1951.

Stevenson, Robert Louis. "Familiar studies of men and books," *Cornhill,* 1876; *Memories and Portraits,* Chatto and Windus, 1887; Scribner's, 1911.

Stockings, G. T. "Clinical study of the mescaline psychosis with special reference to the mechanisms of the genesis of schizophrenia and other psychotic states," *J. ment. Sci.,* 86 (1940), 29-47.

Stoyva, J. M. "Posthypnotically suggested dreams and the sleep cycle," *Arch. gen. Psychiat.,* 12 (1965), 287-294.

Strauss, Hans. "Epileptic disorders," in Arieti 1959.

Strindberg, August. *Inferno,* 1897. Hutchinson, 1962.

Sullivan, Harry Stack. "The relation of onset to outcome in schizophrenia," *Proc. Assn. Res. nerv. ment. Dis.,* 10 (1931), 111-118.

————. *Conceptions of Modern Psychiatry,* 1940, in *Collected Works,* vol. I.

————. *The Interpersonal Theory of Psychiatry.* Norton, 1953.

————. *Clinical Studies in Psychiatry.* Norton, 1956.

————. *Collected Works.* Norton, 1964.

Syz, Hans. "Psycho-galvanic studies on sixty-four medical students," *Brit. J. Psychol.,* 17 (1926), 54-69.

————. "Recovery from loss of mnemic retention after head trauma," *J. gen. Psychol.,* 17 (1937), 355-387.

Szasz, Thomas S. "Factors in the psychogenesis of peptic ulcer," *J. psychosom. Med.,* 11 (1949), 300ff.

————. "Psychiatric aspects of vagotomy, III: The problem of diarrhea after vagotomy," *J. nerv. ment. Dis.,* 115 (1952), 394-402.

————. "The myth of mental illness," *Amer. Psychologist,* 15 (1960), 115ff.

————. *The Myth of Mental Illness.* Hoeber-Harper, 1961.

————. *Law, Liberty, and Psychiatry.* Macmillan, 1963.

————. "The moral dilemma of psychiatry: Autonomy or homonomy?" *Amer. J. Psychiat.,* 121 (1964), 521-528.

————. *Psychiatric Justice.* Macmillan, 1965.

Szasz, Thomas, E. Levin, J. B. Kirsner, and W. L. Palmer. "The role of hostility in pathogenesis of peptic ulcer: Theoretical considerations with the report of a case," *J. psychosom. Med.,* 9 (1947), 331-336.

Szurek, Stanislaus. "Notes on the genesis of psychopathic personality trends," *Psychiat.,* 5 (1942), 1-6.

————. "Experiences with delinquents," in Eissler 1949.

Taggart, S. R., S. B. Russell, and E. B. Price. "Report of syphilis follow-up program among veterans after World War II," *J. chronic Dis.,* 4 (1956), 579ff.

Tarsis, Valeriy. *Ward 7.* Dutton, 1965.

Terhune, William. "The phobic syndrome," *Arch. Neurol. Psychiat.,* 62 (1949), 162-172.

Terman, Lewis M. *Genetic Study of Genius, Vol. I: Mental and Physical Traits of a Thousand Gifted Children.* Stanford University Press, 1925.

————. *Psychological Factors in Marital Happiness.* McGraw-Hill, 1938.

Terry, Gladys, and T. A. C. Rennie. "Analysis of parergasia," *Nerv. ment. Dis. Monogr.* (1938).

Theresa, St. *The History of Her Foundations,* trans. by Sr. Agnes Mason. Cambridge University Press, 1909.

Thigpen, Corbett H., and Hervey M. Cleckley. *The Three Faces of Eve.* McGraw-Hill, 1957.

Thompson, Clara. "Ferenczi's contribution to psychoanalysis," *Psychiat.,* 7 (1944), 245-252.

Thompson, Clara, Milton Mazer, and Earl Witenberg, eds. *An Outline of Psychoanalysis.* Rev. ed.; Random House, 1955.

Thompson, Clara, and Patrick Mullahy. *Psychoanalysis: Evolution and Development.* Hermitage, 1950.

Thompson, George N. *The Psychopathic Delinquent and Criminal.* Thomas, 1953.

————. "Acute and chronic alcoholic conditions," in Arieti 1959, II, 1203-1221.

Thompson, Laura. *Culture in Crisis.* Harper, 1950.

Tietze, Trude. "A study of mothers of schizophrenic patients," *Psychiat.,* 12 (1949), 55-65.

"Timblerline conference of psychophysiological aspects of cardiovascular disease," *J. psychosom. Med.,* 26 (1964), 413-541.

Tinkelpaugh, O. L. "The self-mutilation of a male macacus rhesus monkey," *J. Mammals,* 9 (1928), 293-300.

Titley, W. B. "Prepsychotic personality of patients with agitated depression," *Arch. Neurol. Psychiat.,* 39 (1938), 333-342.

Tomkins, Silvan, ed. *Contemporary Psychopathology.* Harvard University Press, 1943.

Toynbee, Arnold J. *A Study of History.* Oxford University Press: vols. I-III, 1934; vols. IV-VI, 1939; vols. VII-X, 1954; vol. XI, 1959; vol. XII, 1961.

————. *Change and Habit.* Oxford University Press, 1966.

Travis, J. H. "Precipitating factors in manic-depressive psychoses," *Psychiat. Quart.,* 7 (1933), 411-418.

Ullmann, L. P., and L. Krasner, eds. *Case Studies in Behavior Modification.* Holt, 1965.

Unger, Sanford. "Mescaline, LSD, psilocybin, and personality change," in Solomon and Leary 1964, pp. 200ff.

United States Department of Health, Education, and Welfare, Public Health Service, National Institute of Mental Health, Research Grants Branch. *Current Research on Sleep and Dreams.* Public Health Service, publ. no. 1389 (1966).

Unwin, J. D. *Sex and Culture.* Oxford University Press, 1934.

Van Amburg, Robert. "A study of women psychopathic personalities requiring hospitalization," *Psychiat. Quart.,* 18 (1944), 61-77.

Van Paassen, Pierre. *A Crown of Fire.* Scribner's, 1960.

Veith, Ilsa. *Hysteria: The History of a Disease.* University of Chicago Press, 1965.

Vernon, Jack. *Inside the Black Room: Studies of Sensory Deprivation.* Souvenir, 1963.

Vessie, P. R. "On the transmission of Huntington's chorea for 300 years: The Bures family group," *J. nerv. ment. Dis.,* 76 (1932), 553-573.

Vigotsky, L. S. "Thought in schizophrenia," *Arch. Neurol. Psychiat.,* 31 (1934), 1063-1077.

_____. "Thought and speech," *Psychiat.,* 2 (1939), 29-54.

Vogt, C., and O. Vogt. "Über anatomische Substrate-Bemerkungen zum pathol-anatomische Befunden bei Schizophrenen," *Ärztliche Forschung,* 2 (1948), 101ff.

_____. "Importance of neuroanatomy in the field of neuropathology," *Neurol.,* 1 (1951), 205ff.

Wagner, Philip S. "Psychiatric activities during the Normandy offensive," *Psychiat.,* 9 (1946), 341-364.

Wall, J. H., and E. B. Allen. "Results of hospital treatment of alcoholism," *Amer. J. Psychiat.,* 100 (1944), 474-479.

Waller, J., M. Ralph Kaufman, and Felix Deutsch. "Anorexia nervosa: A psychosomatic entity," *J. psychosom. Med.,* 2 (1940), 1-16.

Walsh, Chad. *From Utopia to Nightmare.* Bles, 1962.

Walton, D., and D. A. Black. "The application of learning theory to the treatment of chronic hysterical aphonia," in Eysenck 1960.

Wang, G. H. "Relation between 'spontaneous' activity and oestrus cycle in the white rat," *Comp. Psychol. Monogr.,* vol. 2, no. 6 (1923).

Wardman, H. W. *Ernest Renan.* Athlone, 1964.

Warner, W. Lloyd. *A Black Civilization: A Study of an Australian Tribe.* Harper, 1941.

Warner, W. Lloyd, Buford H. Junker, and Walter A. Adams. *Color and Human Nature.* Amer. Council on Education, 1941.

Warner, W. Lloyd, and Paul S. Lunt. *The Social Life of a Modern Community.* Yale University Press, 1941.

Warner, W. Lloyd, and Leo Srole. *The Social Systems of American Ethnic Groups.* Yale University Press, 1945.

Wasserman, Jacob. *Wedlock.* Boni and Liveright, 1926.

Watkins, John G. *Hypnotherapy of War Neuroses.* Ronald, 1949.

Watson, John B. *Behavior.* Holt, 1914.

Wechsler, Henry, George Grosser, and Bernard Busfield. "The depression rating scale," *Arch. gen. Psychiat.,* 9 (1963), 334-344.

Weisenberg, Theodore. "A study of aphasia," *Arch. Neurol. Psychiat.,* 31 (1934) 1-33.

Weisenberg, Theodore, and Katherine McBride. *Aphasia: A Clinical and Psychological Study.* Oxford University Press, 1935.

Weiss, Edward. "Recent advances in pathogenesis and treatment of hypertension," *J. psychosom. Med.,* 1 (1939), 193ff.

_____. "Neurocirculatory asthenia," *J. psychosom. Med.,* 14 (1952), 150-153.

Weiss, E., and O. S. English. *Psychosomatic Medicine.* Saunders, 1943.

Wenger, M. A., and M. Ellington. "The measurement of autonomic balance in children," *J. psychosom. Med.,* 5 (1943), 241-253.

Werner, Heinz. "Abnormal and subnormal rigidity," *J. abnorm. soc. Psychol.,* 41 (1946), 15-24.

West, Rebecca. *The New Meaning of Treason.* Viking, 1964.

Wheeler, E. O., P. D. White, E. W. Reed, and M. E. Cohen. "Familial incidence of neurocirculatory asthenia," *J. clin. Invest.,* 27 (1948), 562ff.

_____. "Neurocirculatory asthenia: A 24-year follow-up study of 173 patients," *J. Amer. med. Assn.,* 142 (1950), pp. 878-889.

Wheeler, W. M. *Social Life Among the Insects.* Harcourt, Brace, 1923.

White, James C. "Autonomic discharge from stimulation of the hypothalamus in man," *Proc. Assn. Res. nerv. ment. Dis.,* 20 (1940), 854-863.

White, Paul D., Howard Rusk, Philip Lee, and Bryan Williams. *Rehabilitation of the Cardiovascular Patient.* McGraw-Hill, 1958.

White, R. W. "A preface to the theory of hypnotism," *J. abnorm. soc. Psychol.,* 36 (1941), 477-505.

Whitehorn, John. "Stress and emotional health," *Amer. J. Psychiat.,* 112 (1956), 773-781.

Whiting, John W. M., and Irvin L. Child. *Child Training and Personality: A Cross-Cultural Study.* Yale University Press, 1953.

Whiting, P. W., and E. J. Winstrup. "Fertile gynandromorphs in Habsobracon," *J. Hered.,* 23 (1932), 31-38.

Whitman, Charles O. *The Behavior of Pigeons.* Carnegie Institute, 1919.

Whitman, R. M., M. Kramer, and B. Baldridge. "Which dreams does the patient tell?" *Arch. gen. Psychiat.,* 8 (1963), 277-282.

Williams, H. W., and Charles Rupp. "Observations on confabulations," *Amer. J. Psychiat.,* 95 (1938), 395-405.

Wilson, Angus. *Émile Zola: An Introductory Study of His Novels.* Morrow, 1952.

Winters, Eunice, ed. *The Collected Papers of Adolf Meyer.* Johns Hopkins Press, 1951.

Wittkower, E., E. F. Rodger, and I. T. Wilson. "Macbeth effort syndrome," *Lancet,* 1 (1941), 531ff.

Wittson, C. L. "Involutional melancholia," *Psychiat. Quart.,* 14 (1940), 167-184.

Wolberg, Lewis R. *Hypnoanalysis.* Grune and Stratton, 1945.

————. "Hypnotic experiments in psychosomatic medicine," *J. psychosom. Med.,* 9 (1947), 337-342.

Wolf, Stewart, Phillippe Cardon, Edward M. Shepard, and Harold G. Wolff. *Life Stress and Essential Hypertension.* Williams and Wilkins, 1955.

Wolf, Stewart, and Harold G. Wolff. *Human Gastric Functions.* Oxford University Press, 1943.

Wolfenden Report. *Report of the Committee on Homosexual Offenses and Prostitution Prepared for the British Parliament.* H.M.S.O., 1957; Stein and Day, 1963; Lancet, 1964. Also included in Allen and Berg, 1958.

Wolff, Harold G. *Stress and Disease.* Thomas, 1953.

Wolpe, J. "The systematic desensitization treatment of neuroses," *J. nerv. ment. Dis.,* 132 (1961), 189-203.

Wolpert, E. A., and H. Trosman. "Studies in psychophysiology of dreams," *Arch. Neurol. Psychiat.,* 79 (1958), 603-606.

Wolstenholme, G. E., and M. O'Connor, eds. *The Nature of Sleep.* Little, Brown, 1961.

Woolf, Virginia. *A Writer's Diary.* Harcourt, Brace, 1954.

Wortis, Joseph. *Soviet Psychiatry.* Williams and Wilkins, 1950.

————. "Physiological treatment," *Amer. J. Psychiat.,* 116 (1960), 595-600.

————. "A psychiatric study tour of the USSR," *J. ment. Sci.,* 107 (1961), 119-156.

————. "Physiological treatment," *Amer. J. Psychiat.,* 118 (1962), 595-597.

————. "Psychopharmacology and physiological treatment," *Amer. J. Psychiat.,* 120 (1963), 621-626.

————. "Psychopharmacology and physiological treatment," *Amer. J. Psychiat.,* 120 (1964), 643-648.

Wortis, Joseph, and David Frendlich. "Psychiatric work therapy in the Soviet Union," *Amer. J. Psychiat.,* 121 (1964), 123-128.

Wulf, F. "Über die Veränderung von Vorstellungen," *Psychol. Forsch.,* 1 (1922) 337ff.

Yahraes, Herbert. *Epilepsy: The Ghost Is Out of the Closet.* Public Affairs Committee, pamphlet no. 98 (1944).

Yerkes, R. M. "Social behavior of chimpanzees: Dominance between mates, in relation to sexual status," *J. comp. Psychol.,* 30 (1940), 147-186.

Yudkin, Simon, and Anthea Holme. *Working Mothers and Their Children.* Joseph, 1963.

Zabriskie, Edwin G., and A. Louise Brush. "Psychoneuroses in wartime," *J. psychosom. Med.*, 3 (1941), 295-329.

Ziegler, Frederick J., John B. Imboden, and Eugene Meyer. "Contemporary conversion symptomology," *Amer. J. Psychiat.*, 116 (1960), 901-910.

Zilboorg, Gregory. *History of Medical Psychology.* Norton, 1941.

————. *Mind, Medicine, and Man.* Harcourt, Brace, 1943.

Zipf, G. K. *Human Behavior and the Principle of Least Effort.* Addison-Wesley, 1949.

Zola, Émile. *Thérèse Raquin,* 1867, trans. by. Willard Trask. Bantam, 1960.

Zublin, W. "Zur Psychologie des Klinefelter-Syndrome," *Acta Endocrinol.,* 14 (1953), 137ff.

Zwerling, Israel, and Milton Rosenbaum. "Alcoholic addiction and personality," in Arieti 1959, II, 623-646.

INDEX
OF NAMES

INDEX

OF TOPICS